**Cancer Immune Therapy**

*Edited by*
*G. Stuhler and P. Walden*

# Cancer Immune Therapy

Current and
Future Strategies

*Edited by*
*G. Stuhler and P. Walden*

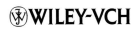

**Editors:**

*Dr. Gernot Stuhler*
University of Tübingen
Medical Clinic
Department of Hematology, Oncology
and Immunology
Otfried-Müller-Strasse 10
72076 Tübingen
Germany

*Prof. Dr. Peter Walden*
Humboldt University Berlin
Charité
Department of Dermatology
Schumann Strasse 20/21
10117 Berlin
Germany

**Cover Illustration**
Human tumor cell and MHC molecule.
With permission adapted from electron
micrograph by E. Kaiserling, University of
Tübingen, Medical School and molecule
structure by C. Ciatto, A. C. Tissot,
M. Tschopp, G. Capitani, F. Pecorari,
A. Plückthun & M.G. Grütter: Crystal
structure of the LCMV peptidic epitope
NP396 in complex with the murine class I
MHC molecule H2 - MMDB: 17707 - PDB:
1JPG.

**Library of Congress Card No.: applied for**

**British Library Cataloguing-in-Publication
Data:** A catalogue record for this book is
available from the British Library

**Die Deutsche Bibliothek –
CIP Cataloguing-in-Publication-Data**
A catalogue record for this publication is
available from Die Deutsche Bibliothek

Printed in the Federal Republic of Germany.
Printed on acid-free paper.

**Composition**   ProSatz Unger, Weinheim
**Printing**   betz-druck gmbh, Darmstadt
**Bookbinding**   J. Schäffer GmbH & Co. KG,
Grünstadt

**ISBN**   3-527-30441-X

# Preface

Although there may be elements of heritable predisposition, cancers are genetic diseases, and are essentially determined by somatic genetics and, often on-going, somatic evolution. As for the evolution of species, diversification, isolation or compartmentalization and selection are expected, and found, to be guiding principles in the ontology and the development of malignant diseases; tumors may become extinct when their propagation is not in balance with the resources of their environment, when the environmental conditions change to become less permissive or when they are eliminated by selection. On the other hand, tumor cells in manifest cancer are expected, and have been shown, to be selected for survival and adapted to escape the various surveillance systems of the body.

Our knowledge of the molecular and cell biology of the ontology and evolution of cancer has grown considerably over recent years. Despite recurring themes of oncogene functions and tumor suppressor gene defects, we are faced with a picture of considerable heterogeneity of the factors, events and paths that lead to malignant transformation and that control malignant development. Such heterogeneity is expected in the context of evolutionary biological concepts of cancer which emphasize the adaptability and developmental capacity of tumor cells as well as the impact of selection processes on these adaptations and developments – be they inborn, such as the action of tumor suppressor gene products and the immune system, or the result of therapeutic interventions, such as chemotherapy or immune therapy.

Heterogeneity of tumor cells in cancer has been reported in terms of the morphology, histology, cytogenetics, molecular genetics, phenotypes, gene expression profiles and cell biology of the tumors. A one-to-one relation of a particular genetic aberration with a particular cancer type, as in the case of the *bcr–abl* translocation in chronic myelocytic leukemia and some acute leukemias, is the exception rather than the rule. It is this heterogeneity, acquired in successive selection processes as a necessary result of the ontogenesis of cancer by evolutionary processes, that is the basis for new evasion mechanisms that make it so very difficult to develop effective therapies. The immune system, of all the surveillance systems of the body, appears to be the best suited to handle such heterogeneity. Its specificity and capacity to quickly adapt to new antigens and to expand in order to mount effective cytolytic responses are instrumental in this context. However, manifest cancer testifies to the failure of the immune system and all the other tumor suppressor mechanisms.

Recent years have seen a great increase of our knowledge about tumor antigenicity and the mechanisms of antitumor immune responses, and much of this new knowledge has been translated into new cancer immune therapies and clinical trials. While some of the trials yielded promising results that were hailed to herald future breakthroughs, others have disappointed. With all the progress made, and the many interesting and important clinical results, there is still no effective cancer immune therapy with a predictable therapeutic outcome, and there are still many questions to be answered in the development of such therapies. How should effective immune therapies of cancer be designed? What are the conditions and what are the best tools for successful therapeutic intervention? Which strategy best suits a particular cancer and the state of the disease in a particular patient? Are there parameters that would allow for early evaluation of the therapeutic effects to direct disease management and therapeutic intervention? Are preventive vaccinations possible? These are only some of the strategic questions addressed in the field.

This volume reviews our current understanding of tumor immunology with special emphasis on the inter-relationship of the tumor and immune system, and cancer immune therapy. The different chapters dissect the antigenicity of tumors, the instruments utilized by the immune system to battle these diseases and the reasons for their failure, such as T cell anergy and immune evasion mechanisms from the tumor's side. With this background, current therapeutic strategies are reviewed and critically evaluated to identify novel approaches and future directions in the development of new cancer immune therapies.

*Peter Walden*
*Department of Dermatology*
*Charité, Humboldt University Medical School*
*Berlin*
*Germany*

*Gernot Stuhler*
*Department of Hematology and Oncology*
*Eberhard-Karls University Tübingen*
*Tübingen*
*Germany*

# Contents

List of Contributors   *XVII*

Color Plates   *XIX*

Part 1     Tumor Antigenicity

1          **Search for Universal Tumor-Associated T Cell Epitopes**   *3*
           ROBERT H. VONDERHEIDE and JOACHIM L. SCHULTZE
1.1        Introduction   *3*
1.2        T Cell Epitopes as the Basis for Anti-Cancer Therapy   *4*
1.3        Identification of Tumor-Associated Antigens   *5*
1.4        Search for Universal Tumor Antigens   *6*
1.5        Epitope Deduction   *6*
1.6        Identification of the Telomerase Reverse Transcriptase (hTERT) as a
           Widely Expressed Tumor-Associated Antigen   *8*
1.7        Linking Cancer Genomics to Cancer Immunotherapy   *10*
1.8        Prospects for Additional Universal Tumor Antigens   *11*
1.9        Prospect of Universal Tumor Antigens as a Clinical Target for
           Immunotherapy   *11*
1.10       Conclusions   *12*
           References   *13*

2          **Serological Determinants On Tumor Cells**   *17*
           CARSTEN ZWICK, KLAUS-DIETER PREUSS, CLAUDIA BORMANN,
           FRANK NEUMANN and MICHAEL PFREUNDSCHUH
2.1        Introduction   *17*
2.2        SEREX: The Approach   *18*
2.3        Searching for Human Antigens by SEREX   *19*
2.4        Molecular Characterization of SEREX Antigens   *19*
2.5        Specificity of SEREX Antigens   *20*
2.5.1      Shared Tumor Antigens   *20*
2.5.2      Differentiation Antigens   *21*

2.5.3 Antigens Encoded by Mutated Genes  *21*
2.5.4 Viral Genes  *22*
2.5.5 Antigens Encoded by Over-expressed Genes  *22*
2.5.6 Amplified Genes  *22*
2.5.7 Splice Variants of Known Genes  *22*
2.5.8 Cancer-Related Autoantigens  *22*
2.5.9 Non-Cancer-Related Autoantigens  *23*
2.5.10 Products of Underexpressed Genes  *23*
2.6 Incidence of Antibodies to SEREX Antigens and Clinical Significance  *23*
2.7 Functional Significance of SEREX Antigens  *24*
2.8 Reverse T Cell Immunology  *24*
2.9 Towards a Definition of the Human Cancer Immunome  *24*
2.10 Consequences for Cancer Vaccine Development  *25*
2.11 Conclusions and Perspectives  *26*
References  *27*

**3 Processing and Presentation of Tumor-associated Antigens**  *30*
Peter-M. Kloetzel and Alice Sijts
3.1 The Major Histocompatibility Complex (MHC) Class I Antigen-Processing Pathway  *30*
3.2 Immuno-Proteasomes  *31*
3.2.1 The Function of Immuno-Proteasomes  *31*
3.2.2 The Role of the Proteasome Activator PA28 in Antigen Processing  *33*
3.3 The Proteasome System and Tumor Antigen Presentation  *34*
3.3.1 Impaired Epitope Generation by Immuno-Proteasomes  *35*
3.4 PA28 and Tumor Epitope Processing  *35*
3.5 Exploiting Proteasome Knowledge  *36*
References  *37*

**4 T Cells In Tumor Immunity**  *40*
Pedro Romero, Mikael J. Pittet, Alfred Zippelius, Danielle Liénard, Ferdy J. Lejeune, Danila Valmori, Daniel E. Speiser and Jean-Charles Cerottini
4.1 Introduction  *40*
4.2 Morphological Evidence of T Cell Immunity in Human Tumors  *41*
4.3 Approaches to the Molecular Identification of Cytolytic T Lymphocyte (CTL)-defined Tumor Antigens  *41*
4.4 Monitoring the Spontaneous CTL Responses to Tumor Antigens  *44*
4.4.1 Monitoring Specific CTL in the PBMC Compartment  *44*
4.4.2 Evidence of Tumor Antigen-specific T Cell Responses at the Tumor Sites  *46*
4.5 CD4 T Cells in Tumor Immunity  *49*
4.6 Concluding Remarks  *51*
References  *52*

**Part 2    Immune Evasion and Suppression**    *57*

**5**        **Major Histocompatibility Complex Modulation and Loss**    *59*
            BARBARA SELIGER and ULRIKE RITZ
5.1         The Major Histocompatibility Complex (MHC) Antigen-Processing
            and -Presentation Pathways    *59*
5.1.1       The MHC Class I Antigen-Processing Machinery (APM)    *60*
5.1.2       The MHC Class II APM    *61*
5.2         The Physiology of the Non-classical HLA-G Molecule    *63*
5.3         Determination of the Expression of Classical and Non-classical
            MHC Antigens    *63*
5.4         Interaction between Tumor and the Immune System    *65*
5.5         The Different MHC Class I Phenotypes and their Underlying Molecular
            Mechanisms    *66*
5.5.1       MHC Class I Loss    *67*
5.5.2       MHC Class I Down-regulation    *69*
5.5.3       Selective Loss or Down-regulation    *72*
5.6         MHC Class I Alterations: Impact on Immune Responses
            and Clinical Relevance    *76*
5.7         The Role of MHC Class II Processing and Presentation in Tumors    *79*
5.7.1       Frequency and Clinical Impact of MHC Class II Expression
            on Tumors    *79*
5.7.2       Molecular Mechanisms of Deficiencies in the MHC class II APM    *81*
5.7.3       Modulation of Immune Response by Altered MHC Class II
            Expression    *81*
5.7.4       MHC Class II Expression in Antitumor Response    *82*
5.8         Role of IFN-γ in Immunosurveillance    *83*
5.8.1       IFN-γ-dependent Immunosurveillance of Tumor Growth    *84*
5.8.2       Deficiencies in the IFN Signal Transduction Pathway    *85*
5.9         HLA-G Expression: an Immune Privilege for Malignant Cells?    *85*
5.9.1       HLA-G Expression in Tumor Cells of Distinct Origin    *86*
5.9.2       Clinical Impact of HLA-G Expression    *88*
5.9.3       Induction of Tolerance by HLA-G Expression    *88*
5.10        Conclusions    *88*
            Acknowledgments    *89*
            References    *89*

**6**        **Immune Cells in the Tumor Microenvironment**    *95*
            THERESA L. WHITESIDE
6.1         Introduction    *95*
6.2         The Immune System and Tumor Progression    *95*
6.3         Immune Cells in the Tumor Microenvironment    *97*
6.4         Phenotypic and Functional Characteristics of Immune Cells Present
            at the Tumor Site    *99*
6.4.1       T Cells    *99*

6.4.2      Natural Killer (NK) Cells   *101*
6.4.3.     DCs   *105*
6.4.4      Macrophages   *107*
6.4.5      B Cells   *108*
6.5        Mechanisms Linked to Dysfunction of Immune Cells in Cancer   *108*
6.5.1      The CD95–CD95 Ligand (CD95L) Pathway   *110*
6.5.2      T Lymphocyte Apoptosis in Patients with Cancer   *111*
6.5.3      Tumor Sensitivity to FasL-Mediated Signals   *111*
6.5.4      A Dual Biologic Role of FasL   *112*
6.5.5      Contributions of other Pathways to Lymphocyte Demise in Cancer   *112*
6.6        Conclusions   *113*
           References   *115*

**7**        **Immunosuppressive Factors in Cancer**   *119*
           RICHARD BUCALA and CHRISTINE N. METZ
7.1       *Introduction*   *119*
7.1       *Transforming Growth Factor (TGF)-β*   *119*
7.1.1      Sources of TGF-β   *121*
7.1.2      Effects of TGF-β   *121*
7.1.2.1    Effects of TGF-β on monocytes/macrophages   *121*
7.1.2.2    Effects of TGF-β on T lymphocytes   *122*
7.1.2.3    Effects of TGF-β on NK and lymphokine-activated killer (LAK) activity   *123*
7.1.2.4    Effects of TGF-1;b on dendritic cells (DCs)   *123*
7.1.3      Inhibition of TGF-β: Implications for Therapy   *124*
7.2        IL-10   *125*
7.2.1      Sources of IL-10   *125*
7.2.2      Effects of IL-10   *126*
7.2.2.1    Effects of IL-10 on monocytes/macrophages   *126*
7.2.2.2    Effects of IL-10 on T lymphocytes   *126*
7.2.2.3    Effects of IL-10 on NK cells   *128*
7.2.2.4    Effects of IL-10 on DCs   *128*
7.2.3      Inhibition of IL-10: Implications for Therapy   *128*
7.2.3.1    Antibodies   *129*
7.2.3.2    Drugs   *129*
7.2.3.3    Removal of the source of IL-10   *129*
7.3        Macrophage Migration Inhibitory Factor (MIF)   *130*
7.4        Prostaglandin (PG) $E_2$   *131*
7.4.1      Sources of $PGE_2$   *131*
7.4.2      Effects of $PGE_2$   *131*
7.4.2.1    Effects of $PGE_2$ on monocytes/macrophages   *131*
7.4.2.2    Effects of $PGE_2$ on T lymphocytes   *131*
7.4.2.3    Effects of $PGE_2$ on NK cells and LAK activity   *132*
7.4.3      Inhibition of $PGE_2$: Implications for Therapy   *132*
7.5        Polyamines   *132*

7.5.1        Sources of Polyamines   *133*
7.5.2        Effects of Polyamines   *133*
7.5.2.1      Effects of polyamines on monocytes/macrophages   *133*
7.5.2.2      Effects of polyamines on T lymphocytes   *134*
7.5.2.3      Effects of polyamines on NK cells   *134*
7.5.3        Inhibition of Polyamine Biosynthesis: Implications for Therapy   *134*
7.6          Tumor-Shed Immunosuppressive Molecules   *134*
7.7          Conclusion   *135*
             References   *136*

**8**          **Interleukin-10 in Cancer Immunity**   *155*
             ROBERT SABAT and KHUSRU ASADULLAH
8.1          Introduction   *155*
8.2          IL-10 Protein and IL-10 Receptor (IL-10R)   *155*
8.2.1        IL-10 Structure and Expression   *155*
8.2.2        IL-10R   *156*
8.2.3        IL-10 Homologs   *157*
8.3          Biological Activities of IL-10   *157*
8.3.1        Effects on Myeloid Antigen-Presenting Cells (APC)   *158*
8.3.2        Effects on T Cells   *159*
8.3.3        Effects on Natural Killer (NK) Cells   *160*
8.3.4        Effects on other Immune Cells   *160*
8.3.5        IL-10's Role in the Immune System   *160*
8.4          IL-10 Expression in Cancer Patients   *161*
8.4.1        Cellular Sources of IL-10 in Cancer Patients   *161*
8.4.2        Selectivity of IL-10 Production   *162*
8.4.3        IL-10 Presence: Local or Systemic?   *163*
8.4.4        Prognostic Value of Enhanced IL-10 Expression   *163*
8.5          Effects of IL-10 in Cancer Models   *164*
8.5.1        Tumor-Promoting Effects of IL-10   *164*
8.5.2        Tumor-Inhibiting Effects of IL-10   *165*
8.6          Conclusions   *166*
             Acknowledgements   *167*
             References   *168*

**Part 3**     **Strategies for Cancer Immunology**   *177*

**9**          **Dendritic Cells and Cancer: Prospects for Cancer Vaccination**   *179*
             DEREK N. J. HART, DAVID JACKSON and FRANK NESTLE
9.1          Introduction   *179*
9.2          DC Properties   *179*
9.3          DC in Human Cancer   *182*
9.4          Blood DC Counts and DC Mobilization   *183*
9.5          DC Preparations for Immunotherapy   *184*

9.6      Loading DC with Antigens   *186*
9.7      Dose Delivery and Vaccination Schedule   *187*
9.8      Phase I/II Clinical Trials   *188*
9.9      Phase III Clinical Trials   *193*
9.10     Side Effects   *194*
9.11     Monitoring Immune Responses   *194*
9.12     Tumor Escape   *195*
9.13     New Developments in DC Immunotherapy   *196*
9.14     Conclusion   *197*
         References   *197*

**10       The Immune System in Cancer: If It Isn't Broken, Can We Fix It?**   *204*
         RICHARD G. VILE
10.1     Commitment and the Modern Immune System   *204*
10.2     Evolutionary Tuning   *206*
10.3     Tumor Antigens and Responses to Them   *209*
10.4     Antigen Presentation – A Resume   *209*
10.5     Playing to Strengths   *211*
10.6     Exploiting Weaknesses: Autoimmunity   *214*
10.7     Combining the Best of Both Worlds   *218*
10.8     The Way Forward   *221*
         Acknowledgments   *223*
         Appendix: Glossary   *223*
         References   *225*

**11       Hybrid Cell Vaccination for Cancer Immune Therapy**   *230*
         PETER WALDEN, GERNOT STUHLER and UWE TREFZER
11.1     Introduction   *230*
11.2     Immunological Basis of the HCV Approach to Cancer Immune
         Therapy   *231*
11.2.1   Tumor Antigenicity   *231*
11.2.2   T–T Cell Collaboration in the Induction of Cellular Cytotoxic Immune
         Responses   *233*
11.3     Vaccination Strategies for Cancer Immune Therapy   *235*
11.4     HCV   *236*
11.4.1   Conceptual Basis   *236*
11.4.2   HCV in Preclinical Studies   *237*
11.4.3   Clinical Experience with HCV   *238*
11.5     Conclusion and Prospects   *240*
         References   *241*

**12       Principles and Strategies Employing Heat Shock Proteins
         for Immunotherapy of Cancers**   *253*
         ZIHAI LI
12.1     The Thesis   *253*

12.1.1    HSPs *per se are rarely Tumor Antigens*   254
12.1.2    HSPs are Molecular Chaperones for Antigenic Peptides   254
12.1.3    HSPs are Adjuvants   255
12.1.4    HSPs are Involved in Cross-Priming   255
12.1.5    Other Roles   256
12.2      Cancer Immunotherapy Strategies with HSPs   256
12.2.1    Strategy 1: Autologous HSPs as Tumor-Specific Vaccines   256
12.2.2    Strategy 2: HSPs as Adjuvant   258
12.2.2.1  *Non-covalent complex between HSP and antigenic peptides*   259
12.2.2.2  *Covalent complex between HSP and antigenic peptides*   259
12.2.3    Strategy 3: Whole Cell Vaccine based on the Modulation
          of the Expression of HSPs   260
12.2.3.1  Modulation of the level of HSPs for cancer immunotherapy   261
12.2.3.2  Modulation of the site of HSP expression for cancer
          immunotherapy   262
12.3      Conclusion and Perspectives   263
          References   264

13        **Applications of CpG Motifs from Bacterial DNA in Cancer
          Immunotherapy**   268
          ARTHUR M. KRIEG
13.1      History of Cancer Immunotherapy with Bacterial Extracts and Nucleic
          Acids   268
13.2      CpG Motifs in bDNA Explain its Immune Stimulatory Activity   270
13.3      Identification of a Specific Receptor for CpG motifs, Toll-like Receptor
          (TLR)-9   271
13.4      Backbone-dependent Immune Effects of CpG Motifs and Delineation of
          CpG-A versus CpG-B Classes of ODN   272
13.5      Applications of CpG DNA in Immunotherapy of Cancer   274
13.5.1    CpG-A or CpG-B DNA as a Monotherapy   274
13.5.2    CpG DNA as an Adjuvant for Cancer Vaccines   276
13.5.3    Application of CpG DNA to Enhance ADCC for Treating Cancer   277
13.6      Conclusion   278
          Acknowledgments   278
          References   279

14        **The T-Body Approach: Towards Cancer Immuno-Gene Therapy**   287
          JEHONATHAN H. PINTHUS and ZELIG ESHHAR
14.1      Background   287
14.2      CRs with Antitumor Specificity   288
14.2.1    Optimizing the CR Design   288
14.2.1.1  The single-chain CR   288
14.2.1.2  Direct recruitment of intracellular triggering molecules   288
14.2.1.3  Combining stimulatory and co-stimulatory signals   289
14.2.2    Anticancer Specificities of CRs   290

14.2.2.1   Cancer-specific antibodies   *290*
14.2.2.2   Ligands and receptors recognition units   *290*
14.2.3.   Pre-Clinical Experimental Models   *292*
14.2.4.   Clinical Trials   *293*
14.3   Conclusions and Perspectives   *294*
Acknowledgments   *295*
References   *295*

**15**   **Bone Marrow Transplantation for Immune Therapy**   *299*
Fabio Ciceri and Claudio Bordignon
15.1   Introduction   *299*
15.2   Graft-versus-Host (GvH) Reactions   *299*
15.3   Graft-versus-Tumor (GvT) Effect   *301*
15.4   Donor Lymphocyte Infusions (DLIs)   *301*
15.5   Complications of DLI: GvHD and Marrow Aplasia   *303*
15.6   Strategies to reduce GvHD while preserving GvT   *303*
15.7   The Suicide Gene Strategy   *304*
15.8   HSV-*tk Lymphocyte Add-backs after Haploidentical Transplantation*   *306*
15.9   Reduced Intensity versus Conventional Conditioning Regimens   *307*
References   *307*

**16**   **Immunocytokines: Versatile Molecules for Biotherapy of Malignant Disease**   *311*
Holger N. Lode, Rong Xiang, Jürgen C. Becker, Andreas G. Niethammer, F. James Primus, Stephen D. Gillies and Ralph A. Reisfeld
16.1   Introduction   *311*
16.1.1   Immunocytokines   *311*
16.1.2   Construction of Immunocytokines   *312*
16.1.3   Binding and Cytokine Activity of IL-2 Immunocytokines   *313*
16.2   Treatment of Tumor Metastases with Immunocytokines   *313*
16.2.1   Colorectal Carcinoma   *313*
16.2.2   Long-lived Tumor-Protective Immunity is Boosted by Non-curative Doses of huKS1/4–IL-2 Immunocytokine   *316*
16.2.3   Carcinoembryonic Antigen (CEA)-based DNA Vaccines for Colon Carcinoma Boosted by IL-2 Immunocytokine   *319*
16.2.4   T Cell-mediated Protective Immunity against Colon Carcinoma Induced by a DNA Vaccine encoding CEA and CD40 Ligand Trimer (CD40LT)   *322*
16.3   Non-small Cell Lung Carcinoma   *324*
16.3.1   Boost of a CEA-based DNA Vaccine by the huKS1/4–IL-2 Immunocytokine   *324*
16.4   Prostate Carcinoma   *327*
16.4.1   Suppression of Human Prostate Cancer Metastases by an IL-2 Immunocytokine   *327*
16.5   Melanoma   *330*

16.5.1     Treatment of Tumor Metastases with Immunocytokines   *330*
16.5.2     Tumor Targeting of LT-α Induces a Peripheral Lymphoid-like Tissue
           Leading to an Efficient Immune Response against Melanoma   *333*
16.5.3     ch14.18–IL-2 Immunocytokine Boosts Protective Immunity Induced
           by an Autologous Oral DNA Vaccine against Murine Melanoma   *334*
16.6       Neuroblastoma   *337*
16.6.1     Treatment with ch14.18–IL-2 Immunocytokine   *337*
16.6.2     Immunocytokine Treatment of Bone Marrow and Liver Metastases   *337*
16.6.3     Mechanism of Immunocytokine-mediated Immune Responses   *338*
16.6.4     Amplification of Suboptimal CD8$^+$ T Memory Cells by a Cellular
           Vaccine   *340*
16.6.5     Synergy between Targeted IL-2 and Antiangiogensis   *341*
16.7       Conclusions and Perspectives   *342*
           Acknowledgments   *342*
           References   *343*

**17**     **Immunotoxins and Recombinant Immunotoxins in Cancer Therapy**   *347*
           YORAM REITER and AVITAL LEV
17.1       Introduction   *347*
17.2       First- and Second-Generation Immunotoxins   *350*
17.3       The Development of Recombinant DNA-based Immunotoxins: Design of
           Recombinant Immunotoxins   *351*
17.3.1     The Toxin Moiety   *351*
17.3.1.1   Plant toxins   *351*
17.3.1.2   Bacterial toxins: DT and DT derivatives   *352*
17.3.1.3   Bacterial toxins: PE and PE derivatives   *353*
17.3.2     The Targeting Moiety – Recombinant Antibody Fragments   *354*
17.4       Construction and Production of Recombinant Immunotoxins   *357*
17.5       Preclinical Development of Recombinant Immunotoxins   *358*
17.6       Application of Recombinant Immunotoxins   *360*
17.6.1     Recombinant Immunotoxins against Solid Tumors   *360*
17.6.2     Recombinant Immunotoxins against Leukemias and Lymphomas   *361*
17.7       Isolation of New and Improved Antibody Fragments as Targeting
           Moieties: Display Technologies for the Improvement of Immunotoxin
           Activity   *363*
17.8       Improving the Therapeutic Window of Recombinant Immunotoxins:
           The Balance of Toxicity, Immunogenicity and Efficacy   *366*
17.8.1     Immune Responses and Dose-limiting Toxicity   *367*
17.8.2     Specificity Dictated by the Targeting Moiety   *368*
17.9       Conclusions and Perspectives   *369*
           References   *369*

           **Glossary**   *380*

           **Index**   *395*

# List of Contributors

Richard Bucala
Section of Rheumatology
Department of Internal Medicine
School of Medicine
Yale University
New Haven, 06520-8031
USA

Fabio Ciceri and Claudio Bordignon
Fondazione Centro S. Raffaele/
Monte Tabor
Istituto Di Ricovero E Cuva A Carattere
Scientifico
Via Olgettina 60
20132 Milano
Italy

Prof. Zelig Eshhar
Department of Chemical Immunology
The Weizmann Institute of Science
P.O. Box 26
Rehovot 76100
Israel

Prof. Derek Hart
Mater Medical Research Institute
Aubigny Place
Raymond Terrace
South Brisbane QLD 4101
Australia

Peter-M. Kloetzel and Alice Sijts
Charité-Humboldt Universität zu Berlin
Institut für Biochemie
Monbijoustrasse 2
10117 Berlin
Germany

Arthur M. Krieg, MD
Coley Pharmaceutical Group
93 Worcester St.
Suite 101
Wellesley, MA 02481
USA

Zihai Li, M.D., PhD.
Center for Immunotherapy of Cancer
and Infectious Diseases, MC 1601
University of Connecticut School of
Medicine
263 Farmington Avenue
Farmington, CT 06030-1601
USA

Christine Metz, PhD
Assistant Investigator
NS-LIJ Research Institute
350 Community Drive
Manhasset, NY 11030
USA

Prof. Dr. med. M. Pfreundschuh
Med. Klinik und Poliklinik,
Innere Medizin I
Universitätsklinikum Saarland
66421 Homburg
Germany

Ralph A. Reisfeld
The Scripps Research Institute
10550 North Torrey Pines Road, IMM-13
La Jolla, CA 92037
USA

Dr. Yoram Reiter
Faculty of Biology
Technion-Israel Institute of Technology
Room 333, Technion City
Haifa 32000
Israel

Dr. Pedro Romero
Division of Clinical OncoImmunology
Ludwig Institute for Cancer Research
Hôpital Orthopédique, Niveau 5
Aile Est, Avenue Pierre Decker, 4
1005 Lausanne
Switzerland

Robert Sabat and Khusru Asadullah
Research Business Area Dermatology
Schering AG
Müllerstr. 178
13342 Berlin
Germany

Barbara Seliger and Ulrike Ritz
Johannes Gutenberg University
III. Department of Internal Medicine
Langenbeckstr. 1
55101 Mainz
Germany

Richard G. Vile
Molecular Medicine Program
Guggenheim 18, Mayo Foundation
200 First Street SW
Rochester, MI 55902
USA

Dr. Robert H. Vonderheide, MD., D.Phil.
Abramson Family Cancer Research
Institute
University of Pennsylvania
Cancer Center
Philadelphia, PA 19104
USA

Prof. Dr. Peter Walden
Universitätsklinikum Humboldt
Universität Berlin
Campus Charité Mitte,
Klinik für Dermatologie
Schumannstr. 20/21
10117 Berlin
Germany

Theresa L. Whiteside, Ph.D.
W1041 Biomedical Science Tower
200 Lothrop Street
Pittsburgh, PA 15213-2582
USA

## Color Plates

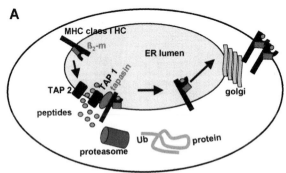

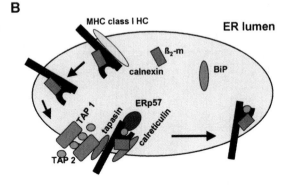

**Fig. 5.2** The MHC class I APM. Ubiquitinylated proteins are cleaved into peptides by the multicatalytic proteasome subunits which are then transported via the TAP heterocomplex into the ER. In the ER, peptides assemble with the MHC class I HC and $\beta_2$-m to form the trimeric MHC class I complex, which is then transported through the Golgi complex to the cell surface for presentation to CD8$^+$ cytotoxic T cells (A). The MHC class I/peptide assembly is assisted by various chaperones, such as calnexin, calreticulin, ERp57 and tapasin, which partially form the multimeric TAP complex (B).

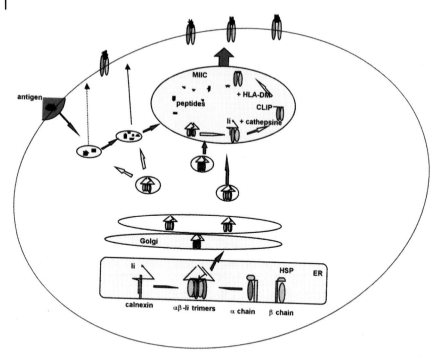

**Fig. 5.3** The MHC class II APM. MHC class II molecules present peptides derived from exogenous antigens internalized into the endocytic pathway. Briefly, HLA class II heterodimers assemble in the ER with the Ii to form nonameric α/β/Ii complexes. These are targeted to the MHC class II endocytic compartment where the MHC class II-associated Ii is degraded, leaving the CLIP peptide within the MHC class II binding groove. CLIP can be exchanged for antigenic peptides catalyzed by HLA-DM molecules. The HLA-DM-dependent peptide loading is controlled by HLA-DO. The peptide-loaded MHC class II molecules are then transported to the cell surface for presentation to CD4[+] T lymphocytes.

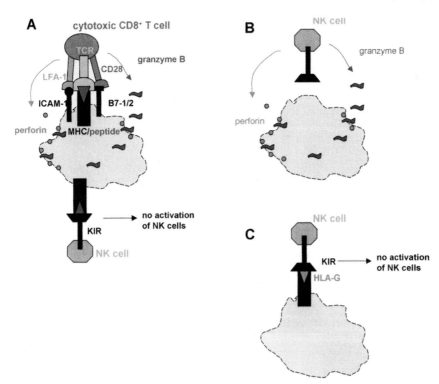

**Fig. 5.5** Different immune effector mechanisms. (A) MHC class I molecules are crucial structures for antigen presentation to T lymphocytes and the physiological ligands for NK receptors. Two distinct signals are required for the initiation and maintenance of an effective immune response. The first is provided by the interaction of MHC class I/peptide complex with the TCR, the second is mediated by a number of co-stimulatory molecules, e.g. B7/CD28. MHC class I molecules often disappear from the tumor cell surface to escape T cell recognition. Therefore patients must be monitored for the expression of these molecules prior to T cell-based immunotherapy. (B) Tumor cells lacking MHC class I molecules could be efficiently recognized by NK cells. (C) HLA-G expression of tumor cells can inhibit NK cell-mediated lysis suggesting that HLA-G expression is a novel immune escape mechanism.

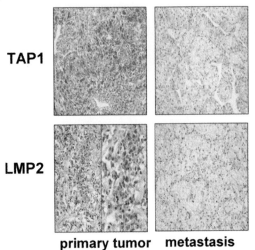

**TAP1**

**LMP2**

**primary tumor    metastasis**

**Fig. 5.11** Association of deficient TAP expression with the metastatic phenotype. A representative example of immunohistochemical staining of a primary and metastatic RCC lesion with an anti-TAP1 mAb is shown. TAP1 expression is strongly down-regulated in the metastasis when compared to the primary tumor lesion.

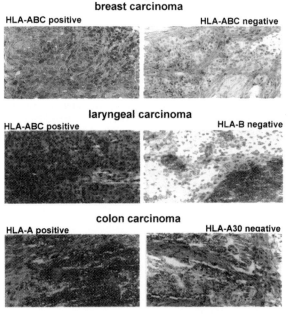

**breast carcinoma**

HLA-ABC positive                    HLA-ABC negative

**laryngeal carcinoma**

HLA-ABC positive                    HLA-B negative

**colon carcinoma**

HLA-A positive                    HLA-A30 negative

**Fig. 5.13** Representative examples of defects in HLA class I antigen expression in surgically removed carcinoma lesions of distinct origin. Frozen tissue sections were stained in the immunoperoxidase reaction with respective anti-HLA class I mAbs. (Top panels) The lack of staining of the breast carcinoma lesions in the right top panel by the anti-HLA-A, -B and -C mAbs indicates a total HLA class I antigen loss in this lesion. (Middle panels) The lack of staining of the lesion with an anti-HLA-B mAb indicates a selective loss of the gene products of HLA-B loci. (Bottom panels) The lack of staining of the lesion with the anti-HLA-A30 mAb indicates selective loss of the HLA class I allospecificity.

**Fig. 5.17** Possible pathway for the generation of an antitumor response dependent on the MHC class II expression of tumor cells (according to Blanck [95]). (I) The pathway which is directly affected by a tumor cell mutation leading to the generation of an antigenic, tumor-associated peptide. (II) The pathway which is directly affected by a tumor cell mutation due to inhibition of the $T_h1$ response or secretion of immunosuppressive cytokines. These mutations include defects in the retinoblastoma gene preventing MHC class II activation in response to IFN-$\gamma$. (III) The non-inducible expression could be caused by deficiencies in the IFN-$\gamma$ signed transduction pathway.

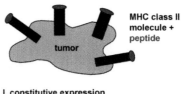

MHC class II molecule + peptide

**I. constitutive expression**

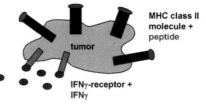

MHC class II molecule + peptide

IFN$\gamma$-receptor + IFN$\gamma$

**II. inducible expression**

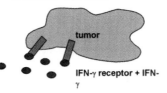

IFN-$\gamma$ receptor + IFN-$\gamma$

**III. non-inducible expression**

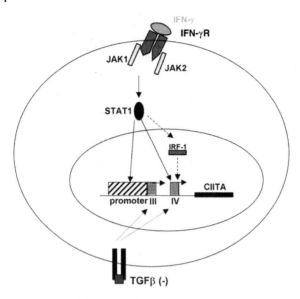

**Fig. 5.19**  Model of the regulation of MHC class II genes by IFN-·
The constitutive expression of CIITA is mediated by a proximal 5′
flanking sequence of the CIITA promoter III. In contrast, the induction of this promoter by IFN-γ is mediated by distal upstream
sequences. Binding of IFN-γ to its receptor activates the JAK kinases which subsequently results in the phosphorylation of
STAT1. STAT1 activation is accompanied by the activation of the
CIITA promoter directly via STAT1 binding to sequences in this region. In addition, STAT1 activation induces the transcription of
the CIITA promoter IV both by binding directly to sequences in
this promoter or by inducing the transcription of IRF1 which is
also required for the promoter activation. CIITA then activates the
transcription of MHC class II antigens, the Ii and HLA-DM genes
through common sequences located in the promoter regions of
these genes.

**Fig. 6.2** T lymphocytes in the tumor microenvironment. In (A), a mass of HLA-DR$^+$ T cells surrounds the tumor. Immunoperoxidase staining of the biopsy obtained from a patient with head and neck cancer. Original magnification: × 400. In (B), a cluster of CD8$^+$ T cells (red) infiltrating a human head and neck cancer. Apoptotic T cells (TUNEL$^+$ whitish) are evident among the CD8$^+$ T cells. A TUNEL reagent was used in combination with immunoperoxidase staining. Original magnification: × 400. Dr T. E. Reichert, U. Mainz, Germany contributed Fig. 2(B).

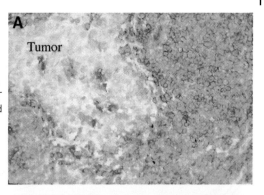

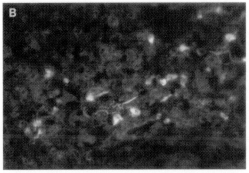

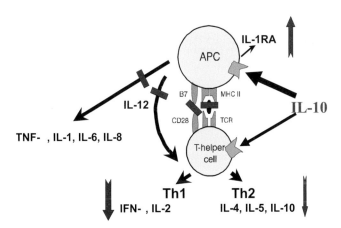

**Fig. 8.1** Effects of IL-10 on APC–T cell interaction. IL-10 suppresses the expression of pro-inflammatory cytokines and enhances the formation of anti-inflammatory mediators. Moreover, IL-10 inhibits the capacity of monocytes and macrophages to present antigen to T cells.

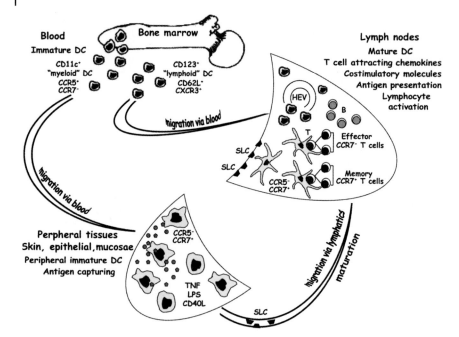

**Fig. 9.1** The DC Life Cycle. Hematopoietic stem cells in bone marrow produce DCs into the blood stream. Blood myeloid DCs and lymphoid DCs use adhesion molecules and chemokine receptors (CD62L, CXCR3 and CCR5) to traffic to peripheral tissues (CD11c$^+$ myeloid) or directly to lymph nodes (DC123$^+$ lymphoid) via HEVs. In peripheral tissues immature myeloid DCs which encounter antigens and accompany microbial products (TNF and lipopolysaccharide) and signals from activated T cells (CD40L) start to differentiate. These DCs move toward lymphatics using chemokine receptors (CCR7), whose ligand SLC, is found both in lymphatic endothelium and in secondary lymphoid tissue. In the lymph node mature DCs produce chemokines, which attract naive and activated T cells. Complex interactions with the local microenvironment (perhaps including lymphoid DCs) increase co-stimulatory molecules, optimize antigen presentation, and induce further lymphocyte activation and the production of effector and memory T lymphocytes. DCs also contribute to B lymphocyte activation and antibody production.

**Part 1**
**Tumor Antigenicity**

# 1
# Search for Universal Tumor-Associated T Cell Epitopes

Robert H. Vonderheide and Joachim L. Schultze

## 1.1
## Introduction

Definitive proof over the last 10 years that human cancers express antigens which can be specifically targeted by cellular immunity has accelerated efforts to design strategies for T lymphocyte-based anti-cancer immunotherapy. To date, the promise of such strategies has outweighed clinical results, but knowledge gained from early trials coupled with the impressive development of novel adjuvants and delivery modalities justifies continued enthusiasm. Clinical immunologists and oncologists involved in T cell immunotherapy make note of the long road required for monoclonal serotherapy to emerge as a powerful new therapeutic tool after years of frustrating results. For the development of both humoral and cellular immunotherapy, the identification of tumor-associated targets is the keystone of the approach. Since 1990, a growing array of tumor-associated T cell epitopes have been identified for particular malignant histologies, driving clinical trials particularly in melanoma that test these targets either alone or in combination. Despite the fact that most tumor antigens described thus far are restricted to a few tumor types – and to a subset of patients who have these tumors – the demonstration that tumor-associated antigens do exist in human cancer also provides part of the rationale behind tumor cell-based therapies in which the targeted antigens are not expressly defined. In this chapter, we explore the hypothesis that recent developments in T cell biology and tumor immunology make it possible to extend the search for appropriate targets to universal, or near-universal, tumor-associated antigens. Furthermore, the results of the Human Genome Project, improved bioinformatics tools and optimized immunological analytical tools enable any given protein to be screened for immunogenic eptitopes that might be incorporated into new therapies. The bench-to-bedside transition from cancer genomics to cancer immunology to clinical oncology is now underway.

## 1.2
## T Cell Epitopes as the Basis for Anti-Cancer Therapy

The potential clinical power of mobilizing T lymphocytes against human cancer has been extensively reviewed elsewhere [1, 2]. T cell-directed cytokine therapy, for example, has achieved remarkable clinical responses in certain patients. Results of donor lymphocyte infusions for chronic myelogenous leukemia in relapse after stem cell transplantation have been even more impressive, reliable and durable [3]. These clinical experiments and other work in both animal and human models support the hypothesis that T cells can under certain circumstances be triggered to induce meaningful anti-tumor responses. Antigen-specific T cell responses are vital in each case, and include the hallmark features of (i) peptide specificity and (ii) restriction to the major histocompatibility complex (MHC). As protein antigens expressed by tumors are degraded in the cytosol, peptides derived from these proteins are incorporated into a peptide-binding groove of MHC molecules before these molecules become expressed on the cell surface. Based on recognition by a clonally unique T cell receptor, specific T cells – if they exist in the repertoire – recognize peptide in the context of the peptide–MHC complex. In the case of CD8$^+$ cytotoxic T lymphocytes (CTL), peptide is generally recognized in the context of MHC class I. Tumor cells expressing peptide–MHC complexes can trigger an effector T cell response, which for CD8$^+$ CTL may involve lysis of the target tumor cell. These peptide epitopes derive following cytolplasmic proteosomal digestion of proteins which may or may not be cell surface antigens. Indeed, most tumor antigens discovered to date are intracytoplasmic self-antigens that are selectively expressed by tumor cells. The hypothesis that these immunogenic peptide epitopes expressed by tumor cells can drive robust effector T cell responses has become a major focus of clinical tumor immunology.

With tumor antigens in hand, how can they be used therapeutically? Two main approaches – adoptive T immunotherapy and therapeutic vaccination – have been envisioned to exploit these findings for novel anti-cancer immunotherapy. In the first strategy, tumor-specific T cells are expanded *ex vivo* and subsequently reinfused into cancer patients. Antigen-specific adoptive T cell therapy for cytomegalovirus disease and Epstein–Barr virus-related lymphoproliferative disorders that complicate allogeneic bone marrow transplantation is safe and highly effective [4, 5]. Efforts are underway to provide autologous antigen-specific T cell therapy for non-transplant cancer patients [6, 7], although these strategies have been more difficult and hindered by the need to generate sufficient numbers of patient-derived, tumor-specific T cells that retain cytotoxic activity. In a second approach, patients are vaccinated against tumor-specific or tumor-associated antigens in order to activate specific cellular and/or humoral immunity against cancer. Most vaccination approaches have been shown to be highly feasible and numerous trials – which are not reviewed here – are currently underway. Many vaccine formulations have been tested, ranging from the use of single antigens or parts of single antigens in peptide or nucleic acid form to the use of tumor cells themselves as the substrate for tumor antigen inoculation. Early reports in melanoma and hematologic malignancies suggest that antigen-specific vaccination is safe and feasible [8–10]. Despite the enthusiasm generated by these early clinical trials, however, it is clear that most vaccination trials have achieved immunological responses without significant clinical responses. To be sure, these are largely phase I trials designed to test safety not efficacy. The issues involved in the design of cancer vaccine trials are complicated and particular to the field [11]. Successful approaches in antigen-specific T cell immunotherapy will need to repair host immune deficits in antigen presentation and T cell function, circumvent immunosuppressive factors of the tumor, and possibly most importantly, optimize target antigens with regard to clinical applicability and risk of immune escape.

## 1.3
## Identification of Tumor-Associated Antigens

Given the scarcity of clinically significant tumor-specific immune responses in cancer patients, there had been reasonable doubt through the 1970s and 1980s that tumor-associated antigens existed in human cancer outside of oncogenic viral proteins or the immunoglobulin idiotype in B cell tumors. However, in landmark studies in the early 1990s, Boon and colleagues and Rosenberg and colleagues molecularly dissected the specificity of measurable T cell responses in melanoma patients [12, 13]. Tumor-associated antigens were rapidly characterized in several other malignancies [12–14] and this initiated the hypothesis that most, if not all, tumors express antigens that T cells can potentially attack [2].

The classical methods to identify tumor antigens have been extensively reviewed elsewhere [1, 15, 16]. Tumor antigens have been identified by analyzing patients T cell responses or by antibody-based techniques analyzing the humoral anti-tumor immune response. Importantly, the phrase "tumor-associated antigen" cannot be used interchangeably with "tumor rejection antigen" or "tumor regression antigen" [17]. Clearly, not all tumor antigens identified so far induce immune responses that lead to tumor rejection. Of course, minimal clinical responses may relate as much to an inferior mode of delivery or to a phase I design with limited power to detect efficacy as it does to the antigen itself. There is no consensus as to whether cellular or non-cellular modalities, active or passive immunization, or antigen-specific or tumor-specific strategies are to be favored. Unfortunately, this area of research is still primarily empirical, and the judgment of whether a particular antigen is useful or not is a complex function of immunology, oncology, pharmacology and biostatistics. As described by Gilboa, "tumor rejection antigen is an operational term describing how well an immune response elicited against a tumor antigen will impact on the tumor growth" [17]. This depends not only on the nature of the tumor antigen but also on the nature of the immune response to the tumor antigen. Variables such as T cell avidity, tolerance and frequency play a major role for a tumor antigen to qualify as a tumor rejection antigen. Potent tumor rejection antigens would elicit high avidity T cell responses and recruit a high frequency of T cells with a high diversity in T cell receptor usage. The establishment of immunological memory in the wake of therapy is vital.

## 1.4
## Search for Universal Tumor Antigens

The biggest practical problem of currently described tumor-associated antigens is the lack of wide expression. Clinical studies have been limited as strategies have been tested one malignancy at a time and, in some cases (such as the immunoglobulin idiotypic antigen in B cell malignancies), patient by patient [10]. To circumvent these obstacles, we proposed a method of identifying tumor antigens with universal or near universal expression in cancer, such that CTL responses against a broad range of tumor types could be triggered [18]. Rather than analyzing patient-derived T cells or antibody responses to tumor, an alternative strategy can be used in which tumor antigens and their CTL epitopes are deduced from genes known to be selectively expressed in tumors [18]. This method, often called "epitope deduction" or "reverse immunology", does not rely on the presence of an innate anti-tumor T cell response, which is then dissected by molecular immunology. This is important because the T cell response against the most common types of cancers is felt to be weak or absent.

Given the hallmark features of T cell recognition outlined above, we began a search for antigens that met the following criteria:

- Expression by the vast majority of human cancers.
- Expression of peptide sequences that bind to MHC molecules.
- Adequate processing by tumor cells such that antigen-derived peptides are available for binding to MHC molecules.
- Recognition by the T cell repertoire in an MHC-restricted fashion, permitting the expansion of naive CTL precursors bearing specific T cell receptors.

## 1.5
## Epitope Deduction

The method of epitope deduction postulates that candidate T cell peptide epitopes can be chosen based on predicted binding affinities of peptide to MHC and then scrutinized for immunogenicity based on the capacity of experimentally generated peptide-specific T lymphocytes to kill tumors *in vitro* or *in vivo*. Table 1.1 outlines several algorithms publicly available for predicting the MHC class I-binding affinities of peptides. Candidate peptides are screened systematically against the criteria described above. Any gene product can be subjected to this analysis without the need to dissect anti-tumor immune responses from cancer patients. Such dissection is the cornerstone of the classical discovery approach, but becomes limited as efforts move beyond melanoma to the majority of common cancers in which patient immunoreactivity is weak. To be sure, the method is not restricted to the field of tumor antigens and has been richly exploited elsewhere, particularly in the search for immunogenic targets of infectious agents.

Epitope deduction has been used to characterize numerous epitopes from candidate tumor-associated antigens (Tab. 1.2) [19]. Most commonly, MHC class I-restricted

**Tab. 1.1.** Publicly available alogorithms for epitope deduction

| Algorithm | Internet site |
|---|---|
| BioInformatics & Molecular Analysis Section | http://bimas.dcrt.nih.gov/molbio/hla_bind/ |
| SYFPEITHI | http://www.uni-tuebingen.de/uni/kxi/ |
| SEREX | http://www-ludwig.unil.ch/SEREX/mhc_pep.html |

**Tab. 1.2** Tumor-associated antigens with peptide epitopes identified by the method of deduction

| Antigen | Reference |
|---|---|
| Ig idiotype | 26 |
| Telomerase hTERT | 28 |
| Survivin | 47 |
| Mage-3 | 48 |
| P53 | 49 |
| Ras | 50 |
| Bcr-abl | 51 |
| Proteinase-3 | 52 |
| Wilm's tumor antigen-1 | 53 |
| CEA | 54 |
| PSA | 55 |
| Her2-neu | 56 |
| MUC-1 | 57 |
| Folate-binding protein | 58 |
| Ep-CAM | 59 |

candidate epitopes are used to generate specific CTLs that are then evaluated for cytotoxicity against tumor cells expressing the antigen and the appropriate MHC allele. A similar approach shows promise for the identification of MHC class II-restricted epitopes [20].

In some cases, due to mutation, protein fusion or recombination, the deduced peptide epitopes are truly tumor-specific. Typically, the antigen from which the epitope is deduced is a self-protein, for which the existence of T cell tolerance may be formidable [21, 22]. Tolerance is less probable against epitopes derived from oncogenic viral proteins, but the clinical applicability of such deduced epitopes is restricted to a few tumor types. For epitopes identified by deduction, we speculate that most – but certainly not all [23, 24] – are probably ignored by the immune system, even in the setting of measurable cancer, raising the hypothesis that targeting such epitopes might draw upon a naïve T cell repertoire that has been spared functional inactivation [18].

It is controversial how well HLA/peptide affinity is predicted by available algorithms and whether or not this truly indicates immunogenicity. For some antigens, such as human papillomavirus [25] or the human immunoglobulin idiotype [26], there is a good correlation between peptide prediction and MHC affinity. For other classically discovered antigens, such as MART-1/Melan A or gp100, not all well-characterized peptide epitopes receive high predictive binding scores, either because the peptides are of low affinity or because the algorithms fail to pick out high-affinity peptides with unusual motifs. The ability to alter certain peptide sequences to increase peptide affinity for MHC without affect T cell specificity has been used both for enhanced immune assessment [24, 27] and formulation of vaccines [8].

## 1.6
### Identification of the Telomerase Reverse Transcriptase (hTERT) as a Widely Expressed Tumor-Associated Antigen

For a prototype of a universal tumor-associated antigens, we recently evaluated the immunogenic profile of hTERT by epitope deduction [28]. hTERT is expressed in more than 85% of all tumors, but rarely in normal cells [29, 30]. In tumors that express telomerase activity, hTERT appears to be found in nearly all tumor cells within a given lesion. Based on *in situ* hybridization studies, hTERT expression appears to increase as tumors progress from carcinoma *in situ* to primary tumors to metastatic tumors [31]. hTERT is the most widely expressed tumor antigen yet described.

Evidence that hTERT can function as a tumor-associated antigen comes from epitope deduction: peptides derived from hTERT were shown to be naturally processed by tumor cells, presented in an MHC class I-restricted fashion and function as a target for antigen-specific CTL [28, 32]. The first such peptide described, I540 (ILAKFLHWL), is found within the middle of the deduced amino acid sequence of hTERT, roughly 70 amino acids to the N-terminus of the first reverse transcriptase motif. The I540 peptide is restricted to the MHC class I allele HLA-A2, the most frequently expressed HLA allele found among nearly 50% of Caucasian, Asians and Hispanics, and 33% of African-Americans. This peptide was initially deduced from the sequence of hTERT based on computer-assisted analysis of MHC-binding motifs, and was subsequently shown experimentally to bind strongly to HLA-A2 [28]. CTL generated using the hTERT peptide in an *ex vivo* expansion system were specific for the I540 hTERT peptide in more than 70% of normal donors tested. *In vitro*, these CTL lines killed a wide range of hTERT$^+$ tumor cell lines and primary tumors in a peptide-specific, MHC-restricted fashion. Importantly, CTL were shown to lyse U2OS cells retrovirally infected with full-length hTERT but not U2OS cells infected with vector alone. The HLA-A2$^+$ sarcoma cell line U2OS is one of the rare human cancer cell lines that does not express hTERT. Monoclonal antibodies against HLA-A2 blocked CTL lysis of hTERT-infected U2OS cells. These observations strongly suggested that the I540 peptide from hTERT is naturally processed by tumor cells and is presented in the context of MHC class I on the cell surface where it can be recognized by specific T cells [28]. Parallel work in murine systems [33] and other human *in vitro* systems [32, 34, 35] has corroborated these findings. Additional hTERT-derived epitopes have been identified that are restricted to other common HLA alleles, including HLA-A3 [36] and HLA-A24 [37]. Table 1.3 describes currently described hTERT CTL epitopes.

**Tab. 1.3**  hTERT-derived CTL epitopes

| Epitope [Reference] | Sequence | Restriction element |
|---|---|---|
| I540 [28] | ILAKFLHWL | HLA-A2 |
| R865 [32] | RLVDDFLLV | HLA-A2 |
| K973 [36] | KLFGVLRLK | HLA-A3 |
| V324 [37] | VYAETKHFL | HLA-A24 |
| V461 [37] | VYGFVRACL | HLA-A24 |

Unlike most other tumor antigens, the expression of hTERT in tumor cells has been linked to tumor growth and development. The expression of hTERT was shown to contribute essentially to oncogenic transformation by permitting unlimited replicative potential [38, 39]. In a landmark paper by Hahn, Counter, Weinberg and colleagues, ectopic expression of hTERT in combination with two oncogenes (the simian virus 40 large-T oncoprotein and an oncogenic allele of H-*ras*) resulted in direct tumorigenic conversion of normal human epithelial and fibroblast cells, demonstrating that disruption of the intracellular pathways regulated by large-T, oncogenic *ras* and telomerase suffices to create a human tumor cell [38]. Moreover, inhibition of telomerase activity in hTERT$^+$ tumor cells leads to telomere shortening and cell death by apoptosis [40, 41]. This latter observation is critical in considering telomerase as a tumor-associated antigen because it is already well-established that therapeutic strategies targeting antigens not involved in tumor growth can result in the selection of antigen-loss tumor mutants that are clinically progressive [6, 42].

hTERT-specific CTL have been generated *ex vivo* from cancer patients in multiple experimental systems, suggesting that T cells specific to hTERT are neither fully deleted nor irreversibly tolerized even in the setting of active neoplasia. In our series, CTL from HLA-A2 patients with a variety of diseases, stages and treatment histories were generated *ex vivo* and demonstrated hTERT-specific cytotoxicity in standard cytotoxicity assays. In another experimental approach, hTERT-specific CTL were generated *ex vivo* from cancer patients using autologous dendritic cells transduced with hTERT mRNA [33]. These CTL were shown to kill primary human tumors in an antigen-specific fashion. Finally, polyclonal anti-tumor cell T cells generated *ex vivo* from patients following stimulation with autologous dendritic cells transduced with *whole tumor* mRNA [34, 35] killed tumors but with multiple antigen specificities. For prostate and renal cell carcinoma, a significant portion of the specific response of these polyclonal T cell lines was against hTERT [34, 35].

A major concern in considering hTERT as a tumor antigen is the potential cytolysis of rare normal cell types that express telomerase activity. Telomerase activity is absent in nearly every major organ including heart, lung, liver, kidney and brain; however, hematopoietic stem cells, activated lymphocytes, basal keratinocytes, gonadal cells and certain epithelial cells have been reported to be telomerase-positive [31, 43–45]. In our experiments, neither HLA-A2-restricted nor HLA-A3-restricted hTERT CTL lyse telomerase-positive peripheral blood CD34$^+$ cells, despite adequate target expression of MHC class I [28]. Similar observations were made if CD34$^+$ peripheral cells were first activated with a combination of cytokines [36]. Anti-hTERT CTL also fail to lyse activated T cells, including phytohemagglutinin-activated $CD8^+$ or $CD4^+$ T cells or $hTERT^+$ CTL themselves. As with stem cells, this finding may reflect relatively low levels of hTERT or, alternatively, may indicate that hTERT is not properly processed and presented in certain normal cells. In contrast, activated B cells, in either the HLA-A2 or HLA-A3 system, were susceptible to hTERT-specific lysis. Activated B cells function well as antigen presenting cells and notably represent the only cell other than tumor cells that to date have been demonstrated to undergo hTERT-specific lysis.

Mouse model systems have confirmed these *in vitro* observations. In mice vaccinated with dendritic cells transduced with murine TERT RNA [33], anti-murine TERT prophylactic immunity can be demonstrated in three individual tumor models. These results are particularly interesting because of the much broader expression of TERT in mice compared with humans. Vaccinated mice in this study were reported to remain healthy and without injury to hematopoietic cells or other murine tissues that express mTERT such as the liver [33].

It is not yet known whether hTERT is a tumor rejection antigen. However, if efficient immunity can be successfully induced without the induction of autoimmunity, hTERT clearly becomes a prime candidate for a widely applicable anti-cancer vaccine. In the US, at least two clinical trials targeting hTERT peptide in HLA-A2 advanced cancer patients are underway and similar trials have been initiated in Europe. A feasibility vaccination study of hTERT peptide-pulsed dendritic cells was initiated at the Dana-Farber Cancer Institute and a peptide/adjuvant/cytokine trial was initiated at the National Cancer Institute. Results have not yet been reported.

## 1.7
### Linking Cancer Genomics to Cancer Immunotherapy

hTERT represents only one example of a nearly universal tumor-associated antigen identified by epitope deduction. Now, after the unveiling of the human genome [46], it becomes possible to explore systematically gene products critical to the cancer process as potential targets for immunotherapy, following the analysis of hTERT as a guide. From advances in genomics and cancer biology, discoveries regarding genetic regulation and dysregulation in cancer will be advanced. Facilitated by genomic and proteomic technology, there will be sufficient data about these genes so that a direct link can be made between genomic information and the discovery of antigens [18].

Gene expression profiling in cancer can be used to reveal overexpressed gene products including oncogenes, mutations, fusion products, and viral genes, which are expressed in tumor cells but not in normal tissue. Differential gene expression analysis on the transcriptome level can be performed by a variety of techniques including serial analysis of gene expression (SAGE), reverse transcription-polymerase chain reaction-based differential display techniques and subtractive hybridization. Ideal candidate genes would be restricted to the malignant phenotype, expressed in the great majority of all human cancers and present at the earliest stages of malignant transformation. Moreover, gene expression profiling need not be restricted to tumor cells themselves for the discovery of antigens. The comparison of normal versus malignant stroma or endothelium, for example, may uncover non-tumor derived T cell epitopes against which cellular immunotherapy can be developed.

## 1.8
### Prospects for Additional Universal Tumor Antigens

At least two antigens other than hTERT are already being evaluated as candidate universal tumor antigens. Our group has preliminary data demonstrating that a carcinogen metabolizing enzyme, a member of the cytochrome P450 gene family, is not only widely expressed in human cancer but also a target for immune intervention (J. L. Schultze, unpublished). Analyzing publicly available SAGE databases revealed a marked overexpression of this gene in breast cancer cells. Analysis of more than 120 tumor samples revealed that more than 95% of tumors overexpress this protein, whereas it is absent in nearly all normal tissues. In preliminary experiments, peptides identified from this gene by epitope deduction have been shown to be presented by tumor cell MHC and that the peptide-specific T cell repertoire in healthy individuals and in cancer patients is intact (J. L. Schultze, unpublished). Similarly, the newly identified apoptosis inhibitor protein survivin has been recognized as a widely occurring tumor-associated antigen capable of inducing cytolytic specific CD8$^+$ T cells *in vitro* [24, 47]. At least one peptide predicted by epitope deduction was shown to result from natural intracellular processing of survivin.

## 1.9
### Prospect of Universal Tumor Antigens as a Clinical Target for Immunotherapy

There are several reasons to consider that universal tumor-associated antigens, characterized by epitope deduction might offer a useful advance in the development of cellular immunotherapy. Most directly, a wide expression across all types of tumors would enable novel strategies for antigen-specific immunotherapy to extend to more patients with common cancers. In the case of telomerase, HLA-A2, -A3 or -A24 is expressed by more than 75% of cancer patients, such that nearly three quarters of all cancer patients could already be considered for hTERT-specific therapies based on the hTERT CTL epitopes currently described.

Second, targeting gene products vital to the oncogenic process may help to circumvent the difficulties of immune escape. Molecules like hTERT, if restricted to tumor cells and naturally processed for presentation by MHC, might be able to function as effective immune targets for which mutation or loss as a means of immune escape is incompatible with sustained tumor growth [18]. Small mutations, particularly within targeted epitopes, as well as down-regulation or functional loss of the presenting HLA allele, would remain problematic, of course, but these issues might be addressed by polyepitope and polyallelic vaccines.

Third, host T cell responses to antigens characterized by epitope deduction may be naïve and therefore less likely to be limited by anergy or tolerance. Our data suggests, for example, that hTERT-specific T cells in cancer patients are spared functional inactivation *in vivo* owing to immunological ignorance. Of course, a naïve precursor T cell frequency to hTERT or other similar antigens would impose upon any therapeutic strategy the need to *prime* specific response in patients, which may be far more difficult than *boosting* ongoing anti-tumor responses against "recall" tumor antigens.

Finally, and probably most importantly, the characterization of universal tumor-associated antigens opens the door to consideration of preventative immunotherapy [18]. Although new candidate antigens are necessarily tested for safety in a *therapeutic* clinical setting, it is an important reminder that post-exposure vaccination is rarely, if ever, clinically effective. In cancer patients, tumor burden negatively impacts attempts at therapeutic vaccination and, accordingly, there is considerable effort to test strategies that pass phase I safety testing in patients with minimal residual tumor [11]. Cancer risk assessment based on genetic factors and medical history is a fast-growing and rapidly expanding part of clinical oncology, and therefore, it makes sense that the first preventative cancer vaccines may be tested in individuals at high-risk for cancer. Any preventative cancer vaccine would require a very narrow toxicity profile and it remains to be seen if this is truly possible when targeting antigens expressed even at low levels in normal tissue. Nevertheless, immunoprevention should be a major goal and one that necessarily requires knowledge of the targeted antigen up front. Any vaccine or immunotherapeutic strategy that requires autologous tumor cells as part of the formulation – whether for gene transfer, cell fusion, DNA extraction or otherwise – obviously mandates that patients already have a diagnosis of cancer, for which a truly preventative approach is essentially impossible to envisage.

## 1.10
## Conclusions

Clinically successful specific cancer immunotherapy depends on the identification of tumor regression antigens. Historically, tumor antigens have been identified by either analyzing cancer patients' own T cell or antibody responses. The unveiling of the human genome, improved bioinformatics tools and optimized immunological analytical tools have made it possible to screen any given protein for immunogenic epitopes. These advancements enable the characterization of universal or nearly universal tumor-associated gene products that mediate critical functions for tumor growth and development. The extent to which the telomerase reverse transcriptase hTERT represents a prototype for this new class of tumor antigens remains to be seen; however, immunological profiling of hTERT and other candidate antigens justifies efforts to begin testing this hypothesis in the clinic. Universal tumor antigens represent one hope for immunoprevention of cancer.

# References

1 ROSENBERG, S. A. A new era for cancer immunotherapy based on the genes that encode cancer antigens, *Immunity* 10: 281–7, 1999.

2 ROSENBERG, S. A. Progress in human tumour immunology and immunotherapy, *Nature* 411: 380–4, 2001.

3 ALYEA, E. Adoptive immunotherapy: insights from donor lymphocyte infusions, *Transfusion* 40: 393–5, 2000.

4 HESLOP, H. E. and ROONEY, C. M. Adoptive cellular immunotherapy for EBV lymphoproliferative disease, *Immunol Rev* 157: 217–22, 1997.

5 WALTER, E. A., GREENBERG, P. D., GILBERT, M. J., FINCH, R. J., WATANABE, K. S., THOMAS, E. D. and RIDDELL, S. R. Reconstitution of cellular immunity against cytomegalovirus in recipients of allogeneic bone marrow by transfer of T-cell clones from the donor, *N Engl J Med* 333: 1038–44, 1995.

6 YEE, C., THOMPSON, J. A., ROCHE, P., BYRD, D. R., LEE, P. P., PIEPKORN, M., KENYON, K., DAVIS, M. M., RIDDELL, S. R. and GREENBERG, P. D. Melanocyte destruction after antigen-specific immunotherapy of melanoma: direct evidence of T cell-mediated vitiligo, *J Exp Med* 192: 1637–44, 2000.

7 SCHULTZE, J. L., ANDERSON, K. C., GILLEECE, M. H., GRIBBEN, J. G. and NADLER, L. M. A pilot study of combined immunotherapy with autologous adoptive tumour-specific T-cell transfer, vaccination with CD40-activated malignant B cells and interleukin 2, *Br J Haematol* 113: 455–60, 2001.

8 ROSENBERG, S. A., YANG, J. C., SCHWARTZENTRUBER, D. J., HWU, P., MARINCOLA, F. M., TOPALIAN, S. L., RESTIFO, N. P., DUDLEY, M. E., SCHWARZ, S. L., SPIESS, P. J., WUNDERLICH, J. R., PARKHURST, M. R., KAWAKAMI, Y., SEIPP, C. A., EINHORN, J. H. and WHITE, D. E. Immunologic and therapeutic evaluation of a synthetic peptide vaccine for the treatment of patients with metastatic melanoma, *Nat Med* 4: 321–7, 1998.

9 NESTLE, F. O., ALIJAGIC, S., GILLIET, M., SUN, Y., GRABBE, S., DUMMER, R., BURG, G. and SCHADENDORF, D. Vaccination of melanoma patients with peptide- or tumor lysate-pulsed dendritic cells, *Nat Med* 4: 328–32, 1998.

10 HSU, F. J., BENIKE, C., FAGNONI, F., LILES, T. M., CZERWINSKI, D., TAIDI, B., ENGLEMAN, E. G. and LEVY, R. Vaccination of patients with B-cell lymphoma using autologous antigen-pulsed dendritic cells, *Nat Med* 2: 52–8, 1996.

11 SIMON, R. M., STEINBERG, S. M., HAMILTON, M., HILDESHEIM, A., KHLEIF, S., KWAK, L. W., MACKALL, C. L., SCHLOM, J., TOPALIAN, S. L. and BERZOFSKY, J. A. Clinical trial designs for the early clinical development of therapeutic cancer vaccines, *J Clin Oncol* 19: 1848–54, 2001.

12 VAN PEL, A., VAN DER BRUGGEN, P., COULIE, P. G., BRICHARD, V. G., LETHE, B., VAN DEN EYNDE, B., UYTTENHOVE, C., RENAULD, J. C. and BOON, T. Genes coding for tumor antigens recognized by cytolytic T lymphocytes, *Immunol Rev* 145: 229–50, 1995.

13 ROSENBERG, S. A. Cancer vaccines based on the identification of genes encoding cancer regression antigens, *Immunol Today* 18: 175–82, 1997.

14 VAN DEN EYNDE, B. J. and VAN DER BRUGGEN, P. T cell defined tumor antigens, *Curr Opin Immunol* 9: 684–93, 1997.

15 BOON, T., CEROTTINI, J. C., VAN DEN EYNDE, B., VAN DER BRUGGEN, P. and VAN PEL, A. Tumor antigens recognized by T lymphocytes, *Annu Rev Immunol* 12: 337–65, 1994.

16 SAHIN, U., TURECI, O. and PFREUNDSCHUH, M. Serological identification of human tumor antigens, *Curr Opin Immunol* 9: 709–16, 1997.

17 GILBOA, E. The makings of a tumor rejection antigen, *Immunity* 11: 263–70, 1999.

18 SCHULTZE, J. L. and VONDERHEIDE, R. H. From cancer genomics to cancer immunotherapy: toward second-generation tumor antigens, *Trends Immunol* 22: 516–23, 2001.

**19** RENKVIST, N., CASTELLI, C., ROBBINS, P. F. and PARMIANI, G. A listing of human tumor antigens recognized by T cells, *Cancer Immunol Immunother* **50**: 3–15, 2001.

**20** STURNIOLO, T., BONO, E., DING, J., RADDRIZZANI, L., TUERECI, O., SAHIN, U., BRAXENTHALER, M., GALLAZZI, F., PROTTI, M. P., SINIGAGLIA, F. and HAMMER, J. Generation of tissue-specific and promiscuous HLA ligand databases using DNA microarrays and virtual HLA class II, *Nat Biotechnol* **17**: 555–561, 1999.

**21** THEOBALD, M., BIGGS, J., HERNANDEZ, J., LUSTGARTEN, J., LABADIE, C. and SHERMAN, L. A. Tolerance to p53 by A2.1-restricted cytotoxic T lymphocytes, *J Exp Med* **185**: 833–41, 1997.

**22** SHERMAN, L. A., MORGAN, D. J., NUGENT, C. T., HERNANDEZ, F. J., KREUWEL, H. T., MURTAZA, A., KO, A. and BIGGS, J. Self-tolerance and the composition of T cell repertoire, *Immunol Res* **21**: 305–13, 2000.

**23** MOLLDREM, J. J., LEE, P. P., WANG, C., FELIO, K., KANTARJIAN, H. M., CHAMPLIN, R. E. and DAVIS, M. M. Evidence that specific T lymphocytes may participate in the elimination of chronic myelogenous leukemia, *Nat Med* **6**: 1018–23, 2000.

**24** ANDERSEN, M. H., PEDERSEN, L. O., BECKER, J. C. and STRATEN, P. T. Identification of a cytotoxic T lymphocyte response to the apoptosis inhibitor protein survivin in cancer patients, *Cancer Res* **61**: 869–72, 2001.

**25** RESSING, M. E., SETTE, A., BRANDT, R. M., RUPPERT, J., WENTWORTH, P. A., HARTMAN, M., OSEROFF, C., GREY, H. M., MELIEF, C. J. and KAST, W. M. Human CTL epitopes encoded by human papillomavirus type 16 E6 and E7 identified through *in vivo* and *in vitro* immunogenicity studies of HLA-A*0201-binding peptides, *J Immunol* **154**: 5934–43, 1995.

**26** TROJAN, A., SCHULTZE, J. L., WITZENS, M., VONDERHEIDE, R. H., LADETTO, M., DONOVAN, J. and GRIBBEN, J. G. Immunoglobulin framework-derived peptides function as cytotoxic T cell epitopes commonly expressed in B cell malignancies, Nat. Med. **6**: 667–672, 2000.

**27** ROMERO, P., DUNBAR, P. R., VALMORI, D., PITTET, M., OGG, G. S., RIMOLDI, D., CHEN, J. L., LIENARD, D., CEROTTINI, J. C. and CERUNDOLO, V. *Ex vivo* staining of metastatic lymph nodes by class I major histocompatibility complex tetramers reveals high numbers of antigen-experienced tumor-specific cytolytic T lymphocytes, *J Exp Med* **188**: 1641–50, 1998.

**28** VONDERHEIDE, R. H., HAHN, W. C., SCHULTZE, J. L. and NADLER, L. M. The telomerase catalytic subunit is a widely expressed tumor-associated antigen recognized by cytotoxic T lymphocytes, *Immunity* **10**: 673–9, 1999.

**29** KIM, N. W., PIATYSZEK, M. A., PROWSE, K. R., HARLEY, C. B., WEST, M. D., HO, P. L., COVIELLO, G. M., WRIGHT, W. E., WEINRICH, S. L. and SHAY, J. W. Specific association of human telomerase activity with immortal cells and cancer, *Science* **266**: 2011–5, 1994.

**30** SHAY, J. W. and BACCHETTI, S. A survey of telomerase activity in human cancer, *Eur J Cancer* **33**: 787–91, 1997.

**31** KOLQUIST, K. A., ELLISEN, L. W., COUNTER, C. M., MEYERSON, M., TAN, L. K., WEINBERG, R. A., HABER, D. A. and GERALD, W. L. Expression of TERT in early premalignant lesions and a subset of cells in normal tissues, *Nat Genet* **19**: 182–6, 1998.

**32** MINEV, B., HIPP, J., FIRAT, H., SCHMIDT, J. D., LANGLADE-DEMOYEN, P. and ZANETTI, M. Cytotoxic T cell immunity against telomerase reverse transcriptase in humans, *Proc Natl Acad Sci USA* **97**: 4796–801, 2000.

**33** NAIR, S. K., HEISER, A., BOCZKOWSKI, D., MAJUMDAR, A., NAOE, M., LEBKOWSKI, J. S., VIEWEG, J. and GILBOA, E. Induction of cytotoxic T lymphocyte responses and tumor immunity against unrelated tumors using telomerase reverse transcriptase RNA transfected dendritic cells, *Nat Med* **6**: 1011–7, 2000.

**34** HEISER, A., MAURICE, M. A., YANCEY, D. R., WU, N. Z., DAHM, P., PRUITT, S. K., BOCZKOWSKI, D., NAIR, S. K., BALLO, M. S., GILBOA, E. and VIEWEG, J. Induction of polyclonal prostate cancer-specific CTL using dendritic cells transfected with amplified tumor RNA, *J Immunol* **166**: 2953–60, 2001.

**35** HEISER, A., MAURICE, M. A., YANCEY, D. R., COLEMAN, D. M., DAHM, P. and VIEWEG, J. Human dendritic cells transfected with renal tumor RNA stimulate polyclonal T-cell responses against antigens expressed by primary and metastatic tumors, *Cancer Res* **61**: 3388–93, 2001.

**36** VONDERHEIDE, R., ANDERSON, K., HAHN, W., BUTLER, M., SCHULTZE, J. and NADLER, L. Characterization of HLA-A3-restricted cytotoxic T lymphocytes reactive against the widely expressed tumor antigen telomerase, *Clin Cancer Res* **61**: 8366–8370, 2001.

**37** ARAI, J., YASUKAWA, M., OHMINAMI, H., KAKIMOTO, M., HASEGAWA, A. and FUJITA, S. Identification of human telomerase reverse transcriptase-derived peptides that induce HLA-A24-restricted antileukemia cytotoxic T lymphocytes, *Blood* **97**: 2903–7, 2001.

**38** HAHN, W. C., COUNTER, C. M., LUNDBERG, A. S., BEIJERSBERGEN, R. L., BROOKS, M. W. and WEINBERG, R. A. Creation of human tumour cells with defined genetic elements, *Nature* **400**: 464–8, 1999.

**39** GREENBERG, R. A., CHIN, L., FEMINO, A., LEE, K. H., GOTTLIEB, G. J., SINGER, R. H., GREIDER, C. W. and DEPINHO, R. A. Short dysfunctional telomeres impair tumorigenesis in the INK4a(delta2/3) cancer-prone mouse, *Cell* **97**: 515–25, 1999.

**40** HAHN, W. C., STEWART, S. A., BROOKS, M. W., YORK, S. G., EATON, E., KURACHI, A., BEIJERSBERGEN, R. L., KNOLL, J. H., MEYERSON, M. and WEINBERG, R. A. Inhibition of telomerase limits the growth of human cancer cells, *Nat Med* **5**: 1164–70, 1999.

**41** HERBERT, B., PITTS, A. E., BAKER, S. I., HAMILTON, S. E., WRIGHT, W. E., SHAY, J. W. and COREY, D. R. Inhibition of human telomerase in immortal human cells leads to progressive telomere shortening and cell death, *Proc Natl Acad Sci USA.* **96**: 14276–81, 1999.

**42** JAGER, E., RINGHOFFER, M., KARBACH, J., ARAND, M., OESCH, F. and KNUTH, A. Inverse relationship of melanocyte differentiation antigen expression in melanoma tissues and CD8+ cytotoxic-T-cell responses: evidence for immunoselection of antigen-loss variants *in vivo, Int J Cancer* **66**: 470–6, 1996.

**43** HARLE-BACHOR, C. and BOUKAMP, P. Telomerase activity in the regenerative basal layer of the epidermis inhuman skin and in immortal and carcinoma-derived skin keratinocytes, *Proc Natl Acad Sci USA* **93**: 6476–81, 1996.

**44** YASUMOTO, S., KUNIMURA, C., KIKUCHI, K., TAHARA, H., OHJI, H., YAMAMOTO, H., IDE, T. and UTAKOJI, T. Telomerase activity in normal human epithelial cells, *Oncogene* **13**: 433–9, 1996.

**45** NORRBACK, K. F. and ROOS, G. Telomeres and telomerase in normal and malignant haematopoietic cells, *Eur J Cancer* **33**: 774–80, 1997.

**46** BALTIMORE, D. Our genome unveiled, *Nature* **409**: 814–6, 2001.

**47** SCHMITZ, M., DIESTELKOETTER, P., WEIGLE, B., SCHMACHTENBERG, F., STEVANOVIC, S., OCKERT, D., RAMMENSEE, H. G. and RIEBER, E. P. Generation of survivin-specific CD8+ T effector cells by dendritic cells pulsed with protein or selected peptides, *Cancer Res* **60**: 4845–9, 2000.

**48** VAN DER BRUGGEN, P., BASTIN, J., GAJEWSKI, T., COULIE, P. G., BOEL, P., DE SMET, C., TRAVERSARI, C., TOWNSEND, A. and BOON, T. A peptide encoded by human gene MAGE-3 and presented by HLA-A2 induces cytolytic T lymphocytes that recognize tumor cells expressing MAGE-3, *Eur J Immunol* **24**: 3038–43, 1994.

**49** MELIEF, C. J. and KAST, W. M. T-cell immunotherapy of cancer, *Res Immunol* **142**: 425–9, 1991.

**50** GEDDE-DAHL, T., III, FOSSUM, B., ERIKSEN, J. A., THORSBY, E. and GAUDERNACK, G. T cell clones specific for p21$^{ras}$-derived peptides: characterization of their fine specificity and HLA restriction, *Eur J Immunol* **23**: 754–60, 1993.

**51** CHEN, W., PEACE, D. J., ROVIRA, D. K., YOU, S. G. and CHEEVER, M. A. T-cell immunity to the joining region of p210$^{BCR–ABL}$ protein, *Proc Natl Acad Sci USA* **89**: 1468–72, 1992.

**52** Molldrem, J., Dermime, S., Parker, K., Jiang, Y. Z., Mavroudis, D., Hensel, N., Fukushima, P. and Barrett, A. J. Targeted T-cell therapy for human leukemia: cytotoxic T lymphocytes specific for a peptide derived from proteinase 3 preferentially lyse human myeloid leukemia cells, *Blood* **88**: 2450–7, 1996.

**53** Gaiger, A., Reese, V., Disis, M. L. and Cheever, M. A. Immunity to WT1 in the animal model and in patients with acute myeloid leukemia, *Blood* **96**: 1480–9, 2000.

**54** Tsang, K. Y., Zaremba, S., Nieroda, C. A., Zhu, M. Z., Hamilton, J. M. and Schlom, J. Generation of human cytotoxic T cells specific for human carcinoembryonic antigen epitopes from patients immunized with recombinant vaccinia-CEA vaccine, *J Natl Cancer Inst* **87**: 982–90, 1995.

**55** Correale, P., Walmsley, K., Zaremba, S., Zhu, M., Schlom, J. and Tsang, K. Y. Generation of human cytolytic T lymphocyte lines directed against prostate-specific antigen (PSA) employing a PSA oligoepitope peptide, *J Immunol* **161**: 3186–94, 1998.

**56** Ioannides, C. G., Fisk, B., Jerome, K. R., Irimura, T., Wharton, J. T. and Finn, O. J. Cytotoxic T cells from ovarian malignant tumors can recognize polymorphic epithelial mucin core peptides, *J Immunol* **151**: 3693–703, 1993.

**57** Brossart, P., Heinrich, K. S., Stuhler, G., Behnke, L., Reichardt, V. L., Stevanovic, S., Muhm, A., Rammensee, H. G., Kanz, L. and Brugger, W. Identification of HLA-A2-restricted T-cell epitopes derived from the MUC1 tumor antigen for broadly applicable vaccine therapies, *Blood* **93**: 4309–17, 1999.

**58** Peoples, G. E., Anderson, B. W., Lee, T. V., Murray, J. L., Kudelka, A. P., Wharton, J. T. and Ioannides, C. G. Vaccine implications of folate binding protein, a novel cytotoxic T lymphocyte-recognized antigen system in epithelial cancers, *Clin Cancer Res* **5**: 4214–23, 1999.

**59** Trojan, A., Witzens, M., Schultze, J. L., Vonderheide, R. H., Harig, S., Krackhardt, A. M., Stahel, R. A. and Gribben, J. G. Generation of cytotoxic T lymphocytes against native and altered peptides of human leukocyte antigen-A*0201 restricted epitopes from the human epithelial cell adhesion molecule, *Cancer Res* **61**: 4761–5, 2001.

# 2
# Serological Determinants On Tumor Cells

CARSTEN ZWICK, KLAUS-DIETER PREUSS, CLAUDIA WAGNER, FRANK NEUMANN and MICHAEL PFREUNDSCHUH

## 2.1
## Introduction

The identification and molecular characterization of tumor antigens that elicit specific immune responses in the tumor-bearing host is a major task in tumor immunology. In the 1970s and 1980s monoclonal antibody technology was exploited for the identification of molecules on tumor cells that could be used as diagnostic markers or as target structures for immunotherapeutic approaches with monoclonal antibodies. While some of these efforts have yielded new therapeutic tools, such as the anti-CD20 antibody rituximab that shows considerable activity and has been licensed for the treatment of B cell lymphomas [1], approaches of *active* immunotherapy require the identification of target structures which are immunogenic in the autologous tumor-bearing host.

The analysis of humoral and cellular immune responses against such antigens in cancer patients had indicated for a long time that cancer-specific antigens do indeed exist which are recognized by the patient's immune system [2]. To define the molecular nature of these antigens, cloning techniques were developed that used established cytotoxic T lymphocyte (CTL) clones [3] or circulating antibodies [4] as probes for screening tumor-derived expression libraries. While the molecular characterization of the first human tumor antigens was accomplished with cloning techniques that used established CTL clones [3], it is now commonly accepted that immune recognition of tumors is a concerted action. Thus, high-titered circulating tumor-associated antibodies of the IgG class may reflect a significant host–tumor interaction and may identify such gene products to which at least cognate T cell help, but also specific cytotoxic T cells, should exist. This rationale prompted us to design a novel strategy using the antibody repertoire of cancer patients for the molecular definition of antigens. Serologically defined antigens could then be subjected to procedures of "reverse" T cell immunology for the definition of epitopes which are presented by MHC class I or II molecules, respectively, and are recognized by T lymphocytes.

## 2.2
### SEREX: The Approach

To identify tumor antigens recognized by the antibody repertoire of cancer patients we developed a serological cloning approach, termed SEREX (serological analysis of tumor antigens by recombinant cDNA expression cloning). It allows a systematic and unbiased search for antibody responses against proteins and the direct molecular definition of the respective tumor antigens based on their reactivity with autologous patient serum. For SEREX, cDNA expression libraries are constructed from fresh tumor specimens, cloned into λ phage expression vectors and phages are used to transfect *Escherichia coli*. Recombinant proteins expressed during the lytic infection of the bacteria are transferred onto nitrocellulose membranes, which are then incubated with diluted (1:500–1:1000) and, most important, extensively pre-absorbed serum from the autologous patient. Clones reactive with high-titered antibodies are identified using an enzyme-conjugated second antibody specific for human IgG. Positive clones are subcloned to monoclonality thus allowing the direct molecular characterization by DNA sequencing.

The SEREX approach is technically characterized by several features [5, 6]:

1. There is no need for established tumor cell lines and pre-characterized CTL clones.
2. The use of fresh tumor specimens restricts the analysis to genes that are expressed by the tumor cells *in vivo* and circumvents *in vitro* artifacts associated with short- and long-term tumor cell culture.
3. The use of the polyclonal (polyspecific) patient's serum allows for the identification of multiple antigens with one screening course.
4. The screening is restricted to clones against which the patient's immune system has raised high-titered IgG or/and IgA antibody responses indicating the presence of a concomitant T helper lymphocyte response *in vivo*.
5. As both the expressed antigenic protein and the coding cDNA are present in the same plaque of the phage immunoscreening assay, identified antigens can be sequenced immediately. Sequence information of excised cDNA inserts can be directly used to determine the expression spectrum of identified transcripts by Northern blot and reverse transcription polymerase chain reaction (RT-PCR).
6. The release of periplasmatic proteins involved in protein folding during phage-induced bacterial lysis allows at least partial folding of recombinant proteins and provides the basis for the identification of linear as well as non-linear epitopes. This has been confirmed by the expression of transcripts that code for enzymatically active proteins [7]. In contrast, epitopes derived from eukaryotic post-translational modification (e.g. glycosylation) are not detected by the phage immunoscreening assay.

Meanwhile, a number of modifications of the original method have been implemented. Immunoglobulins, which are also recombinantly expressed due to the presence of B lymphocytes and plasma cells in the tumor specimens used for the cDNA library, may represent more than 90% of all "positive" clones in libraries derived from certain tissues. They can be identified by a modified initial screening procedure whereby the nitrocellulose membrane is incubated with enzyme-conjugated anti-human IgG followed by visualization with the appropriate enzymatic color reaction prior to the incubation of the autologous patient's serum [8]. Screening of tumor cell lines rather than fresh tumor specimen circumvents this problem and additionally provides a pure RNA source which is not contaminated with normal stroma [9]. Subtractive approaches allow enriching the cDNA library for tumor-specific transcripts [10]. cDNA libraries may also be prepared from sources of specific interest, such as amplified chromosomal regions obtained by microdissection [11].

## 2.3
### Searching for Human Antigens by SEREX

Expression libraries were constructed and analyzed by SEREX from a variety of different neoplasms, including three different renal cell carcinomas of the clear cell type, two melanomas, one ovarian carcinoma, one hepatocarcinoma, 10 gliomas, two colorectal cancers, one pancreatic cancer, two breast cancers, two Hodgkin's lymphomas, two acute T cell leukemias and two acute myelogenous leukemias. Primary libraries with at least $1 \times 10^6$ independent clones were established. The screening of at least $1 \times 10^6$ clones per library revealed multiple reactive clones in each library. Some transcripts were detected repeatedly, indicating that they were multiply represented in the library. In order to bias for the detection of antigens of the cancer testis class, libraries were constructed from normal testis tissue and screened with allogeneic tumor patients' sera.

## 2.4
### Molecular Characterization of SEREX Antigens

Clones were selected for more in-depth analysis on the basis of:

1. Their sequence data and comparison with databases to reveal identity or homologies with known genes and to identify domains or motifs informative for a putative function or cellular localization.
2. The analysis of the expression pattern of the respective antigen in normal tissues and tumors by RT-PCR, by Northern blot hybridization with specific probes and by analysis in expressed sequence tag-containing databases.
3. An initial survey for antibodies in the sera from healthy controls and allogeneic tumor patients to evaluate the incidence of serum antibodies to the respective antigen.

Four different groups of genes coding for antigens were identified. The first group codes for known tumor antigens such as the melanoma antigens MAGE-1, MAGE-4a and tyrosinase. A second group encodes known classical autoantigens for which immunogenicity is associated with autoimmune diseases, e. g. anti-mitochondrial antibodies or antibodies to U1-snRNP. When patients known to have autoimmune or rheumatic disorders are excluded from SEREX analysis, the incidence of such antigens is not higher than 1%. A third group codes for transcripts that are either identical or highly homologous to known genes, but have not been known to elicit immune responses in humans. Examples are restin, which had originally been identified by a murine monoclonal antibody specific for Hodgkin and Reed-Sternberg cells, and lactate dehydrogenase, an enzyme overexpressed in many human tumors. The fourth group of serologically defined antigens represents products of previously unknown genes.

## 2.5
## Specificity of SEREX Antigens

According to their expression pattern in normal and malignant tissues, several classes of tumor antigens can be distinguished (Tab. 2.1): (1) shared tumor antigens, (2) differentiation antigens, products of (3) mutated, (4) viral, (5) overexpressed and (6) amplified genes, as well as (7) splice variants, (8) widely expressed, but cancer-associated autoantigens, the immunogenicity of which is restricted to cancer patients, (9) common autoantigens to which antibodies are found in sera from patients with other than malignant diseases, and, finally, (10) products of genes which are *underexpressed* in the autologous tumor compared to normal tissues.

**Tab. 2.1**  Specificity of tumor antigens detected by SEREX

| Specificity | Example | Source |
|---|---|---|
| (1) Shared tumor antigens | HOM-MEL-40 | melanoma |
| (2) Differentiation antigens | HOM-MEL-55 (tyrosinase) | melanoma |
| (3) Mutated genes | NY-COL-2 (p53) | colorectal carcinoma |
| (4) Splice variants | HOM-HD-397 (restin) | Hodgkin's disease |
| (5) Viral antigens | HOM-RCC-1.14 (HERV-K10) | renal cell cancer |
| (6) Overexpression | HOM-HD-21 (galectin-9) | Hodgkin's disease |
| (7) Gene amplifications | HOM-NSCLC-11 (eIF-4γ) | lung cancer |
| (8) Cancer-related autoantigens | HOM-MEL-2.4 (CEBP) | melanoma |
| (9) Cancer-independent autoantigens | NY-ESO-2 (U1-snRNP) | esophageal carcinoma |
| (10) Underexpressed genes | HOM-HCC-8 | hepatocellular carcinoma |

### 2.5.1
### Shared Tumor Antigens

Shared tumor antigens are expressed in a variable proportion of human tumors (10–70%, depending on the type of tumor). Interestingly, all human shared tumor antigens identified to date are expressed in a variety of human cancers, but not in normal tissues, except for testis; therefore, the term *cancer testis antigens* has been coined for them [9]. Since it is not the whole testis organ, but only the spermatocytes that express these antigens, the term *cancer germline antigens* might be more appropriate. Many of the genes coding for these antigens exist as multi-member gene families. The prototypes of this category, MAGE [3], BAGE [12] and GAGE [13], were initially identified as targets for cytotoxic T cells. The HOM-MEL-40 antigen, which was detected in a melanoma library, is the first cancer/testis antigen identified by SEREX. It is encoded by the SSX-2 gene [8]. Members of the SSX gene family, SSX1 and SSX2, have been shown to be involved in the t(X;18)(p11.2; q11.2) translocation which is found in the majority of human synovial sarcomas [14] and fuses the respective SSX gene with the SYT gene from chromosome 18. Using homology cloning, additional members of the SSX-family were identified [15] revealing at least five genes, of which four (SSX-1, -2, -4 and -5) demonstrate a CT antigen-like expression [16]. Using SEREX, Chen *et al.* [9] identified NY-ESO-1 as a new CT antigen. NY-ESO-1 mRNA expression is detectable in a wide array of human cancers, including melanomas, breast cancer, bladder cancer and prostate cancer. A homologous gene, named LAGE-1, was subsequently isolated by a subtractive cloning approach [17] demonstrating that NY-ESO-1 belongs to a gene family with at least two members. NY-ESO-1 as well as its homolog LAGE-1 were discovered by independent groups using tumor specific CTL or tumor-infiltrating lymphocytes (TIL) derived from melanoma patients as probes, thus disclosing several HLA-A0201- and HLA-A31-restricted epitopes [18], and demonstrating that NY-ESO-1 is a target for both antibody and CTL responses in the same patient [18, 19]. IgG antibody responses, sometimes at very high titers (up to 1:100 000), directed against NY-ESO-1 are present in up to 50% of antigen-expressing patients, demonstrating the extraordinary immunogenicity of NY-ESO-1 and proving this antigen as a frequent target for $CD4^+$ T lymphocytes [20]. Another new CT antigen is HOM-TES-14 [10], which is encoded by the gene coding for the synaptonemal complex protein SCP-1.

## 2.5.2
### Differentiation Antigens

Differentiation antigens are expressed in tumors in a lineage-associated expression, but are also found in normal cells of the same origin; examples are tyrosinase and glial fibrillary acidic protein (GFAP), which are antigenic in malignant melanoma and glioma [21], but are also expressed in melanocytes or brain cells, respectively.

## 2.5.3
### Antigens Encoded by Mutated Genes

Antigens encoded by mutated genes have been demonstrated only rarely by the serological approach, with mutated p53 being one example [22]. However, it is very difficult to rule out that an antibody response detected by SEREX is not initiated by a mutated antigen, since such antibody responses may be directed to epitopes shared between the wild-type and mutated form of the antigen. Thus, wild-type alleles may be picked up during the immunoscreening and sequencing of several independent clones from the same library as well as exclusion of polymorphisms is mandatory.

### 2.5.4
### Viral Genes

A virus-encoded antigen that elicits an autologous antibody response is the env protein of the human endogenous retrovirus HERV-K10, which was found in a renal cell cancer and in a seminoma.

### 2.5.5
### Antigens Encoded by Over-expressed Genes

Over-expressed genes code for many tumor antigens identified by SEREX, which has an inherent methodological bias for the detection of abundant transcripts. The members of this antigen class are expressed at low levels in normal tissues (usually detectable by RT-PCR, but often missed by Northern blot analysis), but are up to 100-fold overexpressed in tumors. Examples are HOM-RCC-3.1.3, a new carbonic anhydrase CA), which is overexpressed in a fraction of renal cell cancers [7], and the Bax inhibitor protein 1, which is overexpressed in gliomas [21].

### 2.5.6
### Amplified Genes

Amplified genes may also code for tumor antigens. The overexpression of a transcript resulting from a gene amplification has been demonstrated for the translation initiation factor eIF-4$\gamma$ in a squamous cell lung cancer [11].

### 2.5.7
### Splice Variants of Known Genes

Splice variants of known genes were also found to be immunogenic in cancer patients. Examples are NY-COL-38 and restin, which represents a splice variant of the formerly described cytoplasmic linker protein CLIP-170 [23].

### 2.5.8
### Cancer-Related Autoantigens

Cancer-related autoantigens are expressed ubiquitously and at a similar level in healthy as well as malignant tissues. The encoding genes are not altered in tumor samples. However, they elicit antibody responses only in cancer patients, but not in healthy individuals. This might result from tumor-associated post-translational modifications or changes in the antigen processing and/or presentation in tumor cells. An example is HOM-MEL-2.4, which represents the CCAAT enhancer binding protein.

## 2.5.9
### Non-Cancer-Related Autoantigens

Non-cancer-related autoantigens are expressed in most human tissues; in contrast to cancer-related autoantigens, antibodies against these antigens are found in non-tumor bearing controls at a similar frequency as in tumor patients. An example is HOM-RCC-10 which represents mitochondrial DNA and HOM-TES-11 which is identical to pericentriol material (PCM-1).

## 2.5.10
### Products of Underexpressed Genes

An antigen was detected during the SEREX analysis of a hepatocellular carcinoma, which was underexpressed in the malignant tissue when compared to normal liver [24].

## 2.6
### Incidence of Antibodies to SEREX Antigens and Clinical Significance

The analysis of sera from patients with various malignant diseases and from healthy controls showed that different patterns of serological responses against SEREX antigens exist. Clinically most interesting is the group of antibodies that occurs exclusively in patients with cancer. Such strictly tumor-associated antibody responses are detected with varying frequencies only in the sera of patients with tumors that express the respective antigen. Examples are antibodies against HOM-TES-14/SCP-1 [10], NY-ESO-I [9] and against several antigens cloned from colon cancer [22]. The incidence of tumor-associated antibodies in unselected tumor patients ranges between 5 and 50% depending on the tumor type and the respective antigen. The antibodies against many SEREX antigens are only detected in the patient whose serum was used for the SEREX assay. A third group of antibodies occurs in cancer patients and healthy controls at a similar rate. While most of these antibodies are directed against non-cancer-associated, widely expressed autoantigens, e.g. poly-adenosyl-ribosyl transferase, antibodies of this category are also found to be directed against antigens with a very restricted expression pattern, e.g. restin. Restin represents a differentiation antigen, since its expression is limited to Hodgkin and Reed-Sternberg cells and immature dendritic cells.

There is little information on the clinical significance of antibody responses and their correlation with the clinical course of the malignant disease. Well-designed prospective studies are necessary to answer the question, whether and which antibodies are (alone or in combination with others) valuable for the diagnosis and/or the evaluation of the response to therapy of malignant diseases. Why only a minority of the patients with an antigen-positive tumor develop antibodies to the respective antigen, remains enigmatic. From anecdotal observations we have the impression that antibodies are only found in a patient's serum, if the tumor expresses the respective antigen. Antibody titers drop and often disappear when the tumor is removed or the patient is in remission.

## 2.7
### Functional Significance of SEREX Antigens

Antigens with a known function identified by SEREX include HOM-RCC-3.1.3 [7], which was shown to be a novel member of the CA family, designated as CA XII. Overexpression of this transcript was observed in 10% of renal cell cancers (RCC), suggesting a potential significance in this tumor type. In fact, the same transcript was cloned shortly thereafter by another group based on its downregulation by the wild-type von-Hippel-Lindau tumor suppressor gene, the loss of function of which is known to be associated with an increased incidence of RCC [25]. Since the invasiveness of RCC cell lines expressing CA XII has been shown to be inhibited by acetazolamide [26], CA XII might be exploited therapeutically. Bax inhibitor protein 1, which was found to be overexpressed in gliomas, is an anti-apoptotic molecule [21].

The first cancer testis antigen to which a physiological function could be ascribed is HOM-TES-14, which is encoded by the SCP-1 gene [10]. SCP-1 is known to be selectively expressed during the meiotic prophase of spermatocytes and is involved in the pairing of homologous chromosomes, an essential step for the generation of haploid cells in meiosis I. Transfection of diploid cell lines with SCP-1 induces polyploidy, suggesting that the aberrant expression of this meiosis-specific gene product in the somatic cells of human tumors is involved in the induction of chromosomal instabilities in cancer cells (unpublished data).

## 2.8
### Reverse T Cell Immunology

SEREX may also be useful for the analysis of the CD4$^+$ and CD8$^+$ T cell repertoire against tumor antigens, in a strategy which is also known as "reverse T cell immunology". Serologically defined antigens are valuable tools for the identification and determination of peptide epitopes reacting in the context of MHC molecules with the antigen-specific receptor of T cells, since the isotope switching and the development of high-titered IgG *in vivo* requires cognate CD4$^+$ T cell help. Several CD4$^+$ binding epitopes of the NY-ESO-1 antigen have been identified [27]. With regard to CD8$^+$ T-lymphocytes that recognize SEREX antigens, CTL responses have been demonstrated for NY-ESO-1 and HOM-MEL-40 [27, 28].

## 2.9
### Towards a Definition of the Human Cancer Immunome

SEREX allows for the identification of an entire profile of antigens using the antibody repertoire of a single cancer patient. The analysis of a variety of neoplasms demonstrated that all hitherto investigated neoplasms are immunogenic in the tumor-bearing host and that immunogenicity is conferred by multiple antigens. For the systematic documentation and archivation of sequence data and immunological characteristics of identified antigens an electronical SEREX database was initiated by the Ludwig Cancer Research Institutes, which is accessible to the public (www.licr.org/ SEREX.html). By December 2001, more than 2000 entries had been made into the SEREX database, the majority of them representing independent antigens. The SEREX database is not only meant as a computational interface for discovery information management, but also as a tool for mapping the entire panel of gene products which elicit spontaneous immune responses in the tumor bearing autologous host, for which the name "cancer immunome" has been coined by L. J. Old (LICR, New York Branch). The cancer immunome which is defined by using spontaneously occurring immune effectors from cancer patients as probes gains increasing interest, since it has been shown that many antigens may be valuable as new molecular markers of malignant disease. The value of each of these markers or a combination of them for diagnostic or prognostic evaluation of cancer patients has to be determined by studies which correlate the presence or absence of these markers with clinical data.

The multitude of tumor-specific antigens identified by the SEREX approach demonstrates that there is ample immune recognition of human tumors by the autologous host's immune system. Together with the identification of T lymphocyte epitopes a picture of the immunological profile of cancer is emerging. Knowledge of the cancer immunome provides a new basis for understanding tumor biology, and for the development of new diagnostic and therapeutic strategies for cancer. The specificities of the antigens expressed by human tumors and detected by SEREX vary widely, ranging from tumor-specific antigens to common autoantigens. This surprising finding together with the observation that some ubiquitously expressed antigens elicit immune responses only in cancer patients suggest that the context in which a protein is presented to the immune system (e.g. the context of "danger) is more decisive for its immunogenicity (and breaking of tolerance) than its more or less tumor-restricted expression. Our results obtained with the SEREX analysis of many human tumors also show that, besides the rare tumor-specific antigens, there is a great majority of widely expressed autoantigens which are presented by the tumor and recognized by the immune system. The presentation of common autoantigens by a given tumor (presumably in the context of "danger") induces a broad range of autoimmunity, and it is only if the tumor happens to express and present tumor-specific molecules that tumor-specific autoimmunity can occur: specific tumor immunity is just a small part of broad autoimmunity that is commonly induced by malignant growth.

## 2.10
## Consequences for Cancer Vaccine Development

The fact that tumors present a majority of molecules that are also expressed in normal tissue and only a minority of tumor-specific molecules in the context of their MHC molecules also implies that vaccines using whole tumor cell preparations are rather unlikely to be successful, because the induction of tumor-specific immunity by such vaccines would be a negligible quantity compared to the majority of immune responses (or tolerance) induced to normal autoantigens by such a vaccine.

The main goal of cancer vaccination is the induction of an effective specific catalytic response against tumor cells which spares the cells of normal tissues. With respect to specificity several classes of antigens may be suitable targets; in addition to the CT antigens, these include differentiation antigens, tumor-associated overexpressed gene products, mutated gene products and tumor-specific splice variants. Clinically the most interesting class of antigens is that of the shared tumor antigens or cancer-testis antigens. To cope with the rapidly growing number of CT antigens, a new nomenclature has been suggested for them [29]. According to the order of their initial identification the individual genes are designated by enumeration. Since individual CT antigens are expressed only in a variable proportion of tumors, only the availability of several CTA could significantly enlarge the proportion of patients eligible for vaccination studies. In this regard it is interesting that members of a given gene family tend to be expressed in a co-regulated fashion whereas different gene families are preferentially expressed in other sets of tumors. It is therefore reasonable to choose antigens from different CT families to cover as many tumors as possible. Despite the fact that SEREX enlarged the pool of available tumor antigens, the proportion of tumors for which no tumor antigen is known is still high, particularly in frequent neoplasms such as colon and prostate cancer. Moreover, immunohistological investigations for MAGE antigens have demonstrated a heterogeneity of antigen expression even in the same tumor specimen [30, 31]. Thus, the use of a mixture of several antigens to vaccinate in a patient would have the potential of reducing or even preventing the *in vivo* selection of antigen-negative clones and would also address the problem of a heterogeneous expression of a given antigen in an individual tumor specimen.

For the development of molecular vaccine strategies, the knowledge of antigen-derived peptide epitopes which are capable of priming or activating specific CTL or T helper cells is an indispensable prerequisite. Because of the diversity of peptides presented by the highly polymorphic HLA alleles, the definition of these epitopes by "reverse T cell immunology" represents an enormous challenge. However, we and others have demonstrated that by using straight-forward strategies, the identification of epitopes from SEREX-defined antigens which bind and activate either $CD8^+$ or $CD4^+$ is feasible and has been successful for each SEREX antigen for which the definition of such epitopes has been pursued.

## 2.11
### Conclusions and Perspectives

The knowledge and availability of a large number of human tumor antigens and their MHC-binding epitopes has opened the perspective for the development of polyvalent vaccines for a wide spectrum of human cancers using pure preparations of antigenic proteins or peptide fragments. Moreover, the study and long-term follow-up of large numbers of patients will help to determine the diagnostic and prognostic relevance of tumor-related/specific autoantibodies in patients' sera and of antigen expression in tumors, as well as the correlation with CTL responses and specific T helper cells. Well-designed clinical trials will answer the question whether our increased knowledge about these antigens can be translated into immuno- and gene therapeutic strategies with an improved prognosis for patients with malignant disease not curable by current standard therapy. Finally, the knowledge of the functional role of cancer-associated antigens provides us with a more profound insight into genetic and molecular alterations that play a role in the pathogenesis and growth of cancer.

## References

1 MALONEY, D. G., GRILLO, L. A., WHITE, C. A., BODKIN, D., SCHILDER, R. J., NEIDHART, J. A., *et al.* (1997) IDEC-C2B8 (Rituximab) anti-CD20 monoclonal antibody therapy in patients with relapsed low-grade non-Hodgkin's lymphoma. *Blood*, **90**, 2188–2195.

2 OLD, L. J. (1981) Cancer immunology: the search for specificity. G. H. A. Clowes Memorial lecture. *Cancer Res.*, **41**, 361–375.

3 VAN DER BRUGGEN, P., TRAVERSARI, C., CHOMEZ, P., LURQUIN, C., DE PLAEN, E., VAN DEN EYNDE, B., KNUTH, A. and BOON, T. (1991) A gene encoding an antigen recognized by cytolytic T lymphocytes on a human melanoma. *Science*, **254**, 1643–1647.

4 SAHIN, U., TÜRECI, Ö., SCHMITT, H., COCHLOVIUS, B., JOHANNES, T., SCHMITS, R., STENNER, F., LUO, G., SCHOBERT, I. and PFREUNDSCHUH, M. (1995) Human neoplasms elicit multiple immune responses in the autologous host. *Proc. Natl Acad. Sci. USA*, **92**, 1180–11813.

5 SAHIN, U., TÜRECI, Ö. and PFREUNDSCHUH, M. (1997) Serological identification of human tumor antigens. *Curr. Opin. Immunol.*, **9**, 709–716.

6 TÜRECI, Ö., SAHIN, U. and PFREUNDSCHUH, M. (1997) Serological analysis of human tumor antigens: molecular definition and implications. *Mol. Med. Today*, **3**, 342–349.

7 TÜRECI, Ö., SAHIN, U., VOLLMAR, E., SIEMER, S., GÖTTERT, E., SEITZ, G., PARKKILA, A. K., SHAH, G., GRUBB, J. H., PFREUNDSCHUH, M. and SLY, W. S. (1998) Carbonic anhydrase XII: cDNA cloning, expression, and chromosomal localization of a novel carbonic anhydrase gene that is overexpressed in some renal cell cancers. *Proc. Natl Acad. Sci. USA*, **95**, 7603–7613

8 TÜRECI, Ö., SAHIN, U., SCHOBERT, I., KOSLOWSKI, M., SCHMITT, H., SCHILD, H. J., STENNER, F., SEITZ, G., RAMMENSEE, H. G. and PFREUNDSCHUH, M. (1996) The SSX2 gene, which is involved in the t(X,18) translocation of synovial sarcomas, codes for the human tumor antigen HOM-MEL-40. *Cancer Res.*, **56**, 4766–4772.

9 CHEN, Y. T., SCANLAN, J., SAHIN, U., TÜRECI, Ö., GÜRE, A. O., TSANG, S., WILLIAMSON, S., STOCKERT, E., PFREUNDSCHUH, M. and OLD, L. J. (1997) A testicular antigen aberrantly expressed in human cancers detected by autologous antibody screening. *Proc. Natl Acad. Sci. USA*, **94**, 1914–1918.

10 TÜRECI, Ö., SAHIN, U., ZWICK, C., KOSLOWSKI, M., SEITZ, G. and PFREUNDSCHUH, M. (1998) Identification of a meiosis-specific protein as new member of the cancer/testis antigen superfamily. *Proc. Natl Acad. Sci. USA*, **95**, 5211–5216.

11 BRASS, N., HECKEL, D., SAHIN, U., PFREUNDSCHUH, M., SYBRECHT, G. W. and MEESE, E. (1997) Translation initiation factor eIF-4 gamma is encoded by an amplified gene and induces an immune response in squamous cell lung carcinoma. *Hum. Mol. Genet.*, **6**, 33–39.

**12** BOEL, P., WILDMANN, C., SENSEI, M. L., BRASSEUR, R., RENAULD, M., COULIE, P., BOON, T. and VAN DER BRUGGEN, P. (1995) BAGE: a new gene encoding an antigen recognized on human melanomas by cytolytic T lymphocytes. *Immunity*, **2**, 167–175.

**13** VAN DEN EYNDE, B., PEETERS, O., DE BACKER, O., GAUGLER, B., LUCAS, S. and BOON, T. (1995) A new family of genes coding for an antigen recognized by autologous cytolytic T lymphocytes on a human melanoma. *J. Exp. Med.*, **182**, 689–698.

**14** CLARK, J., ROQUES, J. P., CREW, J., GILL, S., SHIPLEY, J., CHAND, A., GUSTERSON, B. and COOPER, C. S. (1994) Identification of novel genes SYT and SSX involved in the t(X,18)(p11.2,q11.2) translocation found in human synovial sarcoma. *Nat. Genet.*, **7**, 502–508.

**15** GÜRE, A. O., TÜRECI, Ö., SAHIN, U., TSANG, S., SCANLAN, M., JÄGER, E., KNUTH, A., PREUNDSCHUH, M., OLD, L. J. and CHEN, Y. T. (1997). SSX, a multigene family with several members transcribed in normal testis and human cancer. *Int. J. Cancer*, **72**, 965–971.

**16** TÜRECI, Ö., CHEN, Y. T., SAHIN, U., GÜRE, A. O., ZWICK, C., VILLENA, C., TSANG, S., SEITZ, G., OLD, L. J. and PFREUNDSCHUH, M. (1998) Expression of SSX genes in human tumors. *Int. J. Cancer*, **77**, 19–23.

**17** LETHE, B., LUCAS, S., MICHAUX, L., DE SMET, C., GODELAINE, D., SERRANO, A., DE PLAEN, E. and BOON, T. (1998) LAGE-1, a new gene with tumor specificity. *Int. J. Cancer*, **76**, 903–908.

**18** JÄGER, E., CHEN, Y. T., DRIJFHOUT, J. W., KARBACH, J., RINGHOFFER, M., JÄGER, D., ARAND, M., WADA, H., NOGUCHI, Y., STOCKERT, E., OLD. L. J. and KNUTH A. (1998) Simultaneous humoral and cellular immune response against cancer-testis antigen NY-ESO-1: definition of human histocompatibility leukocyte antigen (HLA)-A2-binding peptide epitopes. *J. Exp. Med.*, **187**, 265–270.

**19** JÄGER, E., STOCKERT, E., ZIDIANAKIS, Z., CHEN, Y. T., KARBACH, J., JAGER, D., ARAND, M., RITTER, G., OLD, L. J. and KNUTH, A. (1999) Humoral immune responses of cancer patients against "Cancer-Testis" antigen NY-ESO-1: correlation with clinical events. *Int. J. Cancer*, **84**, 506–10.

**20** STOCKERT, E., JÄGER, E., CHEN, Y. T., SCANLAN, M. J., GOUT, I., KARBACH, J., ARAND, M., KNUTH, A. and OLD, L. J. (1998) A survey of the humoral immune response of cancer patients to a panel of human tumor antigens. *J. Exp. Med.*, **187**, 1349–1354.

**21** SCHMITS, R., COCHLOVIUS, B., TREITZ, G., KETTER, R., PREUSS, K.-D., ROMEIKE, B. F. M. and PFREUNDSCHUH, M. (2001) Analysis of the antibody repertoire of astrocytoma patients against antigens expressed by gliomas. *Int. J. Cancer*, in press. vUpdate?v

**22** SCANLAN, M. J., CHEN, Y. T., WILLIAMSON, B., GÜRE, A. O., STOCKERT, E., GORDAN, J. D., TÜRECI, Ö., SAHIN, U., PFREUNDSCHUH, M. and OLD, L. J. (1997) Characterization of human colon cancer antigens recognized by autologous antibodies. *Int. J. Cancer*, **76**, 652–658.

**23** PIERRE, P., SCHEEL, J., RICKARD, J. E. and KREIS, T. (1992) CLIP-170 links endocytic vesicles to microtubules. *Cell*, **70**, 887–892.

**24** STENNER-LIEWEN, F., LUO, G., SAHIN, U., TÜRECI Ö., KOSLOWSKI, M, KAUTZ, I., LIEWEN, H. and PFREUNDSCHUH, M. (2000) Definition of tumor-associated antigens in hepatocellular carcinoma. *Cancer Epidemiol. Biomarkers Prevention*, **9**, 285–290.

**25** IVANOV, S. V., KUZMIN, I., WEI, M. H., PACK, S., GEIL, L., JOHNSON, B. E., STANBRIDGE, E. J. and LERMAN, M. I. (1998) Down-regulation of transmembrane carbonic anhydrases in renal cell carcinoma cell lines by wild-type von Hippel-Lindau transgenes. *Proc. Natl Acad. Sci. USA*, **95**, 12596–601.

**26** PARKKILA, S., RAJANIEMI, H., PARKKILA, A. K., KIVELA, J., WAHEED, A., PASTOREKOVA, S., PASTOREK, J. and SLY, W. S. (2000) Carbonic anhydrase inhibitor suppresses invasion of renal cancer cells *in vitro*. *Proc. Natl Acad. Sci. USA*, **97**, 2220–2224.

**27** JÄGER, E., JÄGER, D., KARGACH, J., CHEN, Y.-T., RITTER, G., NAGAT, Y., GNJATIC, S., STOCKERT, E., ARAND, M., OLD,

L. J. and KNUTH, A. (2000) Identification of NY-ESO-1 epitopes presented by human histocompatibility antigen (HAL)-DRB4*0101–0103 and recognized by CD4$^+$ T lymphomcates of patients with NY-ESO-1-expressing melanoma. *J. Exp. Med.*, **191**, 625–630.

28  AYYOUB, M., STEFANOVIC, S., SERVIS, C., SAHIN, U., GUILLAUME, P., RIMOLDI, D., RUBIO-GODY, V., VALMORI, D., ROMERO, P., CEROTTINI, J.-C., RAMMENSEE, H.-G., PFREUNDSCHUH, M., LEVY, F. and SPEISER, D. (2002) Protesasome-assisted identification of a SSX-2 derived epitope recognized by tumor reactive cytllytic T lymphocytes infiltrating metastatic melanoma. *J. Immunol.*, in press.

29  OLD, L. J. and CHEN, Y. T. (1998) New paths in human cancer serology. *J. Exp. Med.*, **187**, 1163–1167.

30  HOFBAUER, G. F., SCHAEFER, C., NOPPEN, C., BONI, R., KAMARASHEV, J., NESTLE, F. O., SPAGNOLI, G. C. and DUMMER, R. (1997) MAGE-3 immunoreactivity in formalin-fixed, paraffin-embedded primary and metastatic melanoma: frequency and distribution. *Am. J. Pathol.*, **151**, 1549–53.

31  JUNGBLUTH, A. A., CHEN, Y. T., STOCKERT, E., BUSAM, K. J., KOLB, D., IVERSEN, K., WILLIAMSON, B., ALTKORI, N. and OLD, L. J. (2001): Immunohistochemical analysis of NY-ESO-1 antigen expressed in normal and malignant tissues. *Int. J. Cancer*, **92**, 856–860.

# 3

# Processing and Presentation of Tumor-associated Antigens

Peter-M. Kloetzel and Alice Sijts

## 3.1

## The Major Histocompatibility Complex (MHC) Class I Antigen-Processing Pathway

As part of the vertebrate immune surveillance system cytotoxic T cells recognize antigens which are bound by MHC class I proteins. To allow binding to MHC class I molecules a protein has to be proteolytically processed to peptides. The recognition of the MHC–peptide complex on the plasma membrane by a T cell receptor (TCR) which is specific for a given antigenic peptide bound to a specific MHC class I molecule eventually leads to T cell activation [1].

Considering the complexity of the MHC class I sequence motifs, any proteolytic system involved in the generation of immuno-dominant MHC class I epitopes has to be able to produce peptides of the appropriate size (8–10 residues) and amino acid sequence diversity, and it has to be able to generate peptides with defined C-terminal anchor residues in sufficient efficiency from a large variety of different proteins in the cytosol and nucleus. Today it is widely accepted that the proteasome system is responsible for the generation of the majority MHC class I ligands [2–4].

The proteasome is the major cytosolic protease complex in eukaryotic cells. It is composed of a proteolytically active core, i.e. the 20S proteasome and two 19S regulator complexes which attach to both sides of the barrel-shaped 20S proteasome. The complex formed by the cylinder-shaped 20S proteasome and the two regulators is called the 26S proteasome. The 20S proteasome consists of 14 non-identical subunits ranging in molecular weight from 31 to 21 kDa and is composed of four stacked rings of seven subunits each. The seven different $\alpha$ subunits form the two outer rings, while the two inner rings are formed by the seven different $\beta$ subunits [3]. The proteolytically active sites are restricted to the lumen of the cylinder and are formed by three of the seven $\beta$ subunits, i.e. subunits $\delta$ ($\beta$1), Z ($\beta$2) and MB1 ($\beta$5). In total, the 20S proteasome therefore possesses six active sites within the two inner $\beta$ rings [5, 6].

Proteasome function can be modulated through the interaction with several regulatory proteins and in order to enter the catalytic chamber protein substrates have to be in an unfolded or extended conformation [7, 8]. Unfolding of substrates is thought to be performed by the six ATPases of the 19S regulator complex which directly attach to the 20S proteasome and form the so-called base structure of the 19S regulator.

## 3.2
## Immuno-Proteasomes

One characteristic feature of the MHC class I antigen presentation pathway is that several of its components are induced by the cytokine interferon (IFN)-γ. This includes the MHC class I heavy chain, the transporter associated with antigen processing (TAP) proteins, several of the 20S proteasome subunits and the proteasome activator PA28 – a protein complex that can influence proteasome behavior by substituting for one of the two 19S regulator complexes [9–11].

Three of the 20S proteasome's β subunits, all of which exhibit proteolytic activity, are IFN-γ inducible: β1i (LMP2), β5i (LMP7) and β2i (MECL-1). These are referred to as the immuno-subunits and their incorporation into the 20S core requires its *de novo* assembly. In consequence, new 20S complexes are formed in which the constitutive subunits, β1 (delta), β2 (z) and β5 (MB1), are replaced by the three immuno-subunits [12, 13].

Incorporation of the immuno-subunits seems to be a cooperative event implying that the immuno-subunits are incorporated together guaranteeing that a defined population of proteasome complexes with altered cleavage properties are formed [14]. The situation is, however, probably more complex than this since IFN-γ not only induces the formation of pure immuno-proteasomes, but also that of 20S complexes in which immuno-subunits and constitutive subunits coexist [15].

### 3.2.1
### The Function of Immuno-Proteasomes

Two different approaches were employed to further elucidate the role of the IFN-γ-inducible subunits in the production of antigenic peptides. Proteasomes containing the constitutive or facultative active-site subunits were purified from cells and tested for reactivity against the three different categories of fluorogenic substrates that cover the hydrolyzing specificity of the different active-site subunits [16–21]. Although these studies showed a clear reduction of the caspase-like activity (cleavage after acidic residues) upon incorporation of immuno-subunits, only inconsistent changes in the activities displayed by the two other active site were observed. More importantly, a further analysis of cleavage products generated from larger polypeptides and protein substrates demonstrated that the activities of the three different catalytic centers towards longer substrates are less well defined [22]. Thus cleavages after basic residues in fluorogenic tripeptides are solely mediated by the β2/β2i pair of catalytic subunits [23]. Cleavage after the same residues within polypeptides substrates appears to be performed by different active-site subunits. Overall, these studies failed to reveal the essence of immuno-subunits.

The analysis of mutant cell lines with defective LMP2 and LMP7 expression did not reveal any major consequences of the absence of these subunits for antigen presentation [24–26]. The restoration of TAP expression in the T2 and 712.174 lymphoblastoid cell lines which lack the genomic region encoding TAP, LMP2 and LMP7 re-established MHC class I surface expression and antigenic peptide presentation. Thus β1i and β5i expression did not appear to be essential. On the other hand, it was found that LMP7 expression was essential for the processing of an influenza-derived cytotoxic T lymphocyte (CTL) epitope [27]. These experiments suggested that immuno-subunits, while not being essential of antigen presentation, may be of importance for the generation of specific CTL epitopes.

More detailed investigations over the recent years have changed this initial skeptical view concerning the hypothetical function of immuno-subunits in antigen processing.

The analysis of by now almost 20 different MHC class I epitopes (mostly viral) shows that the liberation of some epitopes is greatly improved by, or absolutely dependent on, the function of immuno-proteasomes, but the generation of others is not affected at all [28–31] (Tab. 3.1).

*In vitro* digestion experiments with purified 20S proteasomes and synthetic polypeptides encompassing the antigenic peptide and their natural flanking sequences as substrates confirmed the observations made in intact cellular systems. Quantitative analysis of *in vitro* produced peptide fragments by mass spectrometry showed that that immuno-subunit incorporation changed the cleavage site preference of proteasomes [28–30].

Interestingly, in none of the above analysis was a negative effect of immuno-subunit expression on viral CTL epitope production observed. Remarkably, recent studies have indicated that that this may be different in the case of self-antigen-derived CTL epitopes (Tab. 3.1) [32]. Morel *et al.* reported that the incorporation of immuno-subunits into the proteasome abrogated the production of two antigenic peptides, one derived from the self protein RU1 and one derived from the melanoma differentiation antigen Melan-A. On the other hand, we recently observed that such a down-regulation of tumor epitope generation upon exposure to IFN-γ can also occur in the absence of induction of immuno-subunits expression [33].

**Tab. 3.1**  Effects of immuno-proteasomes and PA28 on MHC class I antigen processing

| Antigen | Epitope | Effect of immuno-subunits | Effect of PA28 |
| --- | --- | --- | --- |
| Ovalbumin | 257–264 | no effect | ND |
| HY antigen | ND | + | ND |
| Influenza A nucleoprotein | 366–374 | + | ND |
| Murine cytomegalovirus pp89 | 168–176 | ND | + |
| JAK1 tyrosine kinase | 355–363 | ND | + |
| Influenza A/PR/8 nucleoprotein | 146–154 | ND | + |
| Hepatitis B virus core antigen | 141–151 | + | ND |
| Adenovirus E1A | 234–243 | no effect | no effect |
| Adenovirus E1B | 192–200 | + | ND |
| LCMV nucleoprotein | 118–126 | + | no effect |
| Moloney murine leukemia virus *gag* pr75 | 75–83 | + | + |
| Moloney murine leukemia virus *env* gp70 | 189–196 | no effect | no effect |
| RU1 tumor antigen | 34–42 | – | ND |
| Melan-A tumor antigen | 26–35 | – | ND |

Although it is still not entirely clear how immuno-subunits influence the antigen-processing capacity of the proteasome, one emerging concept is that incorporation of immuno-subunits may result in subtle structural changes of the whole 20S complex and thus, in turn, influence its processing properties [28]. For example, although the concerted presence of all three immuno-subunits was essential for the generation of an epitope from the HBV core antigen, an inactive β5i subunit also supported epitope generation. This result indicates that incorporation of β5i influences the structural architecture of the 20S proteasomes, and consequently affects the cleavage-site preferences of the β1i and β2i active sites.

## 3.2.2
### The Role of the Proteasome Activator PA28 in Antigen Processing

Biochemical screens performed by the groups of DeMartino and Rechsteiner have identified several additional regulatory molecules [9, 10]. The best characterized is the proteasome activator PA28/11S regulator, a heptameric 180–200 kDa complex composed of α and β subunits [11, 34]. PA28 attaches in an ATP-independent way to the outer α rings of the 20S proteasome and replaces the 19S regulator on at least one side of the 20S core, resulting in the formation of so-called hybrid proteasomes [35]. PA28 is expressed in all cells types of higher eukaryotes, suggesting that it displays a basal cellular function [36]. On the other hand, PA28 gene-deficient mice are viable, which may argue in favor of a more specialized function [37]. In support, the expression of both of its subunits is controlled by IFN-γ and professional antigen-presenting cells generally express PA28 at high levels, which is in agreement with the described function of this complex in MHC class I antigen processing [38].

The same biochemical screens that allowed the identification of PA28 also resulted in the characterization of a molecule that inhibits proteasome function, PI31 [39]. PI31 is a protein of approximately 31 kDa that presumably functions as homodimer. *In vitro* PI31 inhibits 20S mediated cleavage of short fluorogenic substrates and of polypeptides and competes the binding of PA28 to 20S proteasomes. This suggests that PI31 binds the α rings of the 20S proteasome and thereby obstructs the access to the catalytic cavity [40, 41]. Nevertheless, transfection of PI31 into intact cells does not interfere with cell cycle progression or protein degradation, indication that the *in vivo* function of PI31 may differ from the proposed function as a general inhibitor of proteasome activity (own unpublished observation).

Cell systems that express PA28 independently of IFN-γ showed that PA28 enhances the presentation of several viral antigens without increasing overall protein turnover or turnover of viral protein substrates [31]. Furthermore, this enhanced peptide presentation is independent of the presence of immuno-subunits in the 20S proteasome [30, 31], excluding the possibility that PA28 might exert its function by increasing immuno-proteasome formation as proposed recently [37].

Similar to the immuno-proteasomes, PA28 does not affect presentation of all MHC class I epitopes equally (Table 3.1). Kinetic studies imply that binding of PA28 to the 20S core increases substrate affinity without changing the maximal activity of the enzyme complex and that PA28 activates the proteasome by enhancing either the uptake of substrates or the release of peptide products [42]. A structural explanation was given by Whitby *et al.* [43]. In their studies it was shown that PA26, the trypanosome homolog of PA28, induces conformational changes in the α subunits of the 20S proteasome core complex. Based on this and the observation that PA28 facilitates product exit, it was proposed that that such an open conformation may allow the release of slightly longer peptides. Thus these peptides would be rescued from further degradation, which may support the generation of certain CTL epitope precursor peptides in particular of epitopes that are produced as N-terminally extended epitope precursor peptides. Nevertheless, since not only PA28 but also the 19S regulator can induce the opening of the central gate, it remains unclear whether the above observations indeed fully explain the effects of PA28 on substrate cleavage.

Detailed analysis of the effects of PA28 on proteasomal cleavage usage have shown that PA28 does not confer new cleavage specificities nor has it a major impact on the rate of substrate degradation. Instead, PA28 markedly enhances the frequency of usage of specific, already preferred or minor cleavage sites resulting in an immediate liberation of the intervening peptide fragments [44 and unpublished observation]. These data and also a recent mutational analysis of PA28 [45] suggest that PA28 binding may induce conformational changes within the 20S complex which changes the accessibility of the active sites. Thus the dramatic effects of PA28 on antigenic peptide liberation are unlikely to be explained by the opening of the 20S catalytic channel alone.

## 3.3
## The Proteasome System and Tumor Antigen Presentation

Despite its central role in the generation of tumor epitopes which bind to HLA class I molecules, and therefore its potential role in tumor surveillance and control of tumor growth, the analysis of proteasome function in tumor cells is still at its beginning. So far the experimental analysis of proteasomes in tumors has mainly concentrated on the constitutive expression of IFN-γ induced proteasome subunits LMP2 (iβ1) and LMP7 (iβ7), which both are encoded within the HLA region in the direct neighborhood to the TAPs [46, 47]. More recent studies also included the analysis of MECL-1 (iβ2) and the PA28 subunits, both of which are encoded on different chromosomes. Reverse transcription-polymerase chain reaction (RT-PCR) analysis of a large number of different tumors shows that in many instances LMP2 and LMP7 expression is down-regulated, where the extent of their down-regulation is variable and does not appear to be specific for a given type of tumor nor follow a specific pattern [48]. In these studies the expression of the MECL-1 subunit and PA28 appeared not be affected. Concomitant with the down-regulation of LMP expression, one often also observes an impaired expression of TAP mRNAs, suggesting that these neighboring genes possess common regulators whose activity is affected in tumor cells. With regard to LMP subunit expression, a similar observation was also made in Adeno type 5-induced tumors [49]. However, it is important to mention that expression of LMP2 and LMP7 (and TAPs) in all these cases was restored upon treatment with IFN-γ. Thus, while the reversible down-regulation of components of the proteasomal antigen-processing machinery seems to be a widespread phenomenon, so far there exists no experimental evidence that this has any significant functional consequences for the processing of tumor antigens, since the vast majority of epitopes will also be generated by constitutive proteasomes.

### 3.3.1
### Impaired Epitope Generation by Immuno-Proteasomes

Morel *et al.* [32] recently reported that immuno-proteasomes are unable to produce several self-antigen-derived CTL epitopes, including an important CTL epitope derived from the melanoma differentiation antigen, Melan-A. These data represent the first example of CTL epitopes that are generated by constitutive but not by immuno-proteasomes and may have a large impact on our understanding of tumor immunology. Since it is likely that thymic dendritic cells involved in T cell selection predominantly contain immuno-proteasomes, it was suggested that this observations could explain how CTLs against self-antigens escape destruction in the thymus. These T cells could be recruited for tumor therapy using vaccination strategies. Although this seems to be an interesting hypothesis, further studies involving more tumor-derived CTL epitopes will be required to elucidate the underlying molecular mechanism and how CTLs specific for self-antigens can survive negative selection in the thymus.

Biochemical analysis of stimulated dendritic cells (DC) shows that during maturation of DCs the synthesis of immuno-proteasomes increases and that at day 6 most of the newly synthesized proteasomes are immuno-proteasomes [38]. Nevertheless, considering the long half-live of proteasomes, DCs still ought to contain a considerable amount of constitutive proteasomes even at day 6 after stimulation. Thus upregulation of immuno-proteasomes may not be the only explanation for impaired tumor epitope processing. In fact, in our own studies of melanoma cells we identified a tyrosinase-related protein 2 (TRP2)-derived epitope whose presentation diminishes upon treatment of melanoma cells with IFN-$\gamma$. However, this reduction of antigenic peptide presentation was found on all IFN-$\gamma$-treated melanoma cells, including one cell line which lacks constitutive expression of immuno-proteasomes and PA28, and in which immuno-subunit and PA28 expression are not up-regulated following IFN-$\gamma$ treatment. These data indicate that there must exist other IFN-$\gamma$ inducible factors which can negatively influence tumor epitope presentation and which are distinct from immuno-proteasomes or even the proteasome system.

### 3.4
### PA28 and Tumor Epitope Processing

Under non-inflammatory conditions many cell types lack immuno-subunit expression and express PA28$\alpha\beta$ only at low levels. One plausible explanation for the apparent necessity to regulate immuno-subunit and PA28 expression may lie in their possible role in the development of the CD8 T cell repertoire. In particular, the observation that immuno-subunits may influence antigen processing of foreign and self-antigen differentially seems indicative of this assumption. Since the DC lineage also expresses PA28 at high levels, the role of PA28 in the processing of self-protein-derived epitopes may be a great interest. We recently analyzed the processing and presentation of two CTL epitopes derived from a melanoma differentiation antigen, i. e. TRP2. In these studies we found that several of our melanoma cell lines failed to present one of the two antigenic peptides. This deficiency of epitope presentation correlated with the absence of PA28 in these cells. In support of this we found that restoration of PA28αβ expression rescued the presentation of this CTL epitope. These data could be further supported by *in vitro* experiments demonstrating that only in the presence of PA28 was the proteasome able to liberate detectable amounts of the TRP2 epitope. Therefore the effects of PA28 on tumor epitope processing are not fundamentally different from those on viral epitope processing and that, apparently, the CD8 T cell repertoire available for tumor antigen recognition is not biased towards epitopes that are processed in a PA28-independent manner.

## 3.5
## Exploiting Proteasome Knowledge

With regard to the development of epitope-based vaccines, a detailed knowledge of proteasomal cleavage properties is of great practical relevance as it would allow the identification of CTL epitope candidates within protein stretches. Kessler *et al.* first exploited such a "reverse immunology" method to characterize HLA-A2-presented CTL epitopes in PRAME, a tumor-associated antigen that is expressed in a wide variety of tumors [50]. The PRAME protein sequence was first screened for the presence of nonamer and decamer peptides with the HLA-A*0201-binding motif. Identified peptides were synthesized and tested for actual HLA binding. Putative epitope candidates found to bind with high affinity were synthesized as part of larger polypeptides, encompassing the potential antigenic sequences and their natural flanking residues, and offered as substrates to purified 20S immuno-proteasomes. The analysis of the digestion products led to the identification of four epitope candidates that were generated by the proteasome. Each of the PRAME-derived peptides induced specific CTL responses *in vitro* and CTL clones established by this method specifically lysed PRAME-expressing HLA*0201$^{+}$ tumor cells.

To simplify CTL epitope identification strategies, computer prediction programs that predict cleavage site usage within proteins have been established [51–53]. So far two prediction programs based on different parameters have been published. One program was trained using 20S cleavage data of the enolase-1 protein; the other program is based on polypeptide cleavage data generated in a large number of studies. Both programs predict proteasomal cleavages with high fidelity, whereby the latter program not only identifies proteasome cleavage sites but also predicts the probability with which specific fragments are generated. Indeed, the application of this program in combination with a program that predicts MHC class I binding affinity led to the identification of eight CTL epitopes derived from the entire deduced proteome of *Chlamydia trachomatis* that are presented by HLA-B27 molecules [54].

In summary, these computer-assisted approaches enable a rapid and easy identification of CTL epitopes that can be included in the proposed CTL-inducing vaccine and will help the selection of epitope flanking spacers that improve proteasome-mediated epitope processing. The existing proteasome cleavage programs are currently being tested for general applicability, whereby the availability of new cleavage data obtained through *in vitro* digestion of designed constructs with purified proteasomes in turn will allow the designers to improve their programs.

## References

1 KLOETZEL, P.-M. (2001) *Nat Rev Mol Cell Biol* **2**: 179–187.

2 PAMER, E. and CRESSWELL, P. (1998) *Annu Rev Immunol* **16**: 323–358.

3 COUX, O., TANAKA, K. and GOLDBERG, A. L. (1996) *Annu Rev Biochem* **65**: 801–847.

4 COFFINO, P. (2001) *Nat Rev Mol Cell Biol* **2**: 188–194.

5 GROLL, M., DITZEL, L., LÖWE, J., *et al.* (1997) *Nature* **386**: 463–471.

6 BOCHTLER, M. DITZEL, L., GROLL, M., HARTMANN, C. and HUBER, R (1999) *Annu Rev Biophys Biomol Struct* **28**: 295–317.

7 BRAUN, B. C., GLICKMAN, M., KRAFT, R., DAHLMANN, B., KLOETZEL, P.-M., FINLEY, D. and SCHMIDT, M. (1999) *Nat Cell Biol* **1**: 221–226.

8 STRICKLAND, E., HAKALA, K., THOMAS, P. J. and DEMARTINO, G. N. (2000) *J Biol Chem.* **275**: 5565–5572.

9 DUBIEL, W., PRATT, G., FERRELL, K. and RECHSTEINER, M. (1992) *J Biol Chem* **267**: 22369–22377.

10 MA, C. P., SLAUGHTER, C. A. and DEMARTINO, G. N. (1992) *J Biol Chem* **267**: 10515–23.

11 KNOWLTON, J. R., JOHNSTON, S. C., WHITBY, F. G., REALINI, C., ZHANG, Z., RECHSTEINER, M. and HILL, C. P. (1997) *Nature* **390**: 639–643.

12 GRIFFIN, T. A., NANDI, D., CRUZ, M., FEHLING, H. J., VAN KAER, L., MONACO, J. J. and COLBERT, R. A. (1998) *J Exp Med* **187**: 97–104.

13 GROETTRUP, M., STANDERA, S., STOHWASSER, R. and KLOETZEL, P.-M. (1997) *Proc Natl Acad Sci USA* **94**: 8970–8975.

14 SCHMIDT, M. and KLOETZEL, P.-M. (1997) *FASEB J* **11**: 1235–1243.

15 NANDI, D., WOODWARD, E., GINSBURG, D. B. and MONACO J. J. (1997) *EMBO J* **16**: 5363–5375.

16 ELEUTERI, A. M., KOHANSKI, R. A., CARDOZO, C. and ORLOWSKI, M. (1997) *J Biol Chem* **272**: 11824–11831.

17 BOES, B., HENGEL, H., RUPPERT, T., MULTHAUP, G., KOSZINOWSKI, U. H. and KLOETZEL, P.-M. (1994) *J Exp Med* **179**: 901–909.

18 DRISCOLL, J., BROWN, M. G., FINLEY, D. and MONACO, J. J. (1993) *Nature* **365**: 262–264.

19 GACZYNSKA, M., ROCK, K. L. and GOLDBERG, A. L. (1993) *Nature* **365**: 264–267.

20 USTRELL, V., PRATT, G. and RECHSTEINER, M. (1995) *Proc Natl Acad Sci USA* **92**: 584–588.

21 GROETTRUP, M., RUPPERT, T., KUEHN, L., SEEGER, M., STANDERA, S., KOSZINOWSKI, U. and KLOETZEL, P.-M. (1995) *J Biol Chem* **270**: 23808–23815.

22 NUSSBAUM, A. K., DICK, T. P., KEILHOLZ, W., SCHIRLE, M., STEVANOVIC, S., DIETZ, K., HEINEMEYER, W., GROLL, M., WOLF, D. H., HUBER, R., RAMMENSEE, H. G. and SCHILD, H. (1998) *Proc Natl Acad Sci USA* **95**: 12504–12509.

23 SALZMANN, U., KRAL, S., BRAUN, B., STANDERA, S., SCHMIDT, M., KLOETZEL, P. M. and SIJTS, A. (1999) *FEBS Lett* **454**: 11–15.

24 ARNOLD, D., DRISCOLL, J., ANDROLEWICZ, M., HUGHES, E., CRESSWELL, P. and SPIES, T. (1993) *Nature* **360**: 171–174.

25 MOMBURG, F., ORTIZ-NAVARRETE, V., NEEFJES, J., GOULMY, E., VAN-DE-WAL, Y.,

Spits, H., Powis, S. J., Butcher, G. W., Howard, J. C., Walden, P. and Haemmerling, G. (1993) *Nature* **360**: 174–177.

26 Yewdell, J., Lapham, C., Bacik, I., Spies, T. and Bennink, J. (1994) *J Immunol* **152**: 1163–1170.

27 Cerundolo, V., Kelly, A., Elliot, T., Trowsdale, J. and Townsend, A. (1995) *Eur J Immunol* **25**: 554–562.

28 Sijts, A. J., Ruppert, T., Rehermann, B., Schmidt, M., Koszinowski, U. and Kloetzel, P.-M. (2000) *J Exp Med* **191**: 503–514.

29 Sijts, A. J., Standera, S., Toes, R. E., Ruppert, T., Beekman, N. J., van Veelen, P. A., Ossendorp, F. A., Melief, C. J. and Kloetzel, P.-M. (2000) *J Immunol* **164**: 4500–4506.

30 Schwarz, K., Van Den Broek, M., Kostka, S., Kraft, R., Soza, A., Schmidtke, G., Kloetzel, P.-M. and Groettrup, M. (2000) *J Immunol* **165**: 768–778.

31 van Hall, T., Sijts, A., Camps, M., Offringa, R., Melief, C., Kloetzel, P.-M. and Ossendorp, F. (2000) *J Exp Med* **192**: 483–494.

32 Morel, S., Levy, F., Burlet-Schiltz, O., Brasseur, F., Probst-Kepper, M., Peitrequin, A. L., Monsarrat, B., Van Velthoven, R., Cerottini, J. C., Boon, T., Gairin, J. E. and Van den Eynde, B. J. (2000) *Immunity* **12**: 107–117.

33 Sun, Y., Sijts, A. et al. (2002) *Cancer Res.* **62**, 2875–2882.

34 Zhang, Z., Krutchinsky, A., Endicott, S., Realini, C., Rechsteiner, M. and Standing, K. G. (1999) *Biochemistry* **38**: 5651–5658.

35 Hendil, K. B., Khan, S. and Tanaka, K. (1998) *Biochem J* **332**: 749–754.

36 Jiang, H. and Monaco, J. J. (1997) *Immunogenetics* **46**: 93–98.

37 Preckel, T., Fung-Leung, W. P., Cai, Z., Vitiello, A., Salter-Cid, L., Winqvist, O., Wolfe, T. G., Von Herrath, M., Angulo, A., Ghazal, P., Lee, J. D., Fourie, A. M., Wu, Y., Pang, J., Ngo, K., Peterson, P. A., Fruh, K. and Yang, Y. (1999) *Science* **286**: 2162–2165.

38 Macagno, A., Gilliet, M., Sallusto, F., Lanzavecchia, A., Nestle, F. O. and Groettrup, M. (1999) *Eur J Immunol* **29**: 4037–4042.

39 Chu-Ping, M., Slaughter, C. A. and DeMartino, G. N. (1992) *Biochim Biophys Acta* **1119**: 303–311.

40 McCutchen-Maloney, S. L., Matsuda, K., Shimbara, N., Binns, D. D., Tanaka, K., Slaughter, C. A. and DeMartino, G. N. (2000) *J Biol Chem* **275**: 18557–18565.

41 Zaiss, D. M., Standera, S., Holzhutter, H., Kloetzel, P. and Sijts, A. J. (1999) *FEBS Lett* **457**: 333–338.

42 Groettrup, M., Soza, A., Eggers, M., Kuehn, L., Dick, T. P., Schild, H., Rammensee, H. G., Koszinowski, U. H. and Kloetzel, P.-M. (1996) *Nature* **381**: 166–168.

43 Whitby, F. G., Masters, E. I., Kramer, L., Knowlton, J. R., Yao, Y., Wang, C. C. and Hill, C. P. (2000) *Nature* **408**: 115–120.

44 Dick, T. P., Ruppert, T., Groettrup, M., Kloetzel, P. M., Kuehn, L., Koszinowski, U. H., Stevanovic, S., Schild, H. and Rammensee, H. G. (1996) *Cell* **86**: 253–262.

45 Li, J., Gao, X., Ortega, J., Nazif, T., Joss, L., Bogyo, M., Steven, A. C. and Rechsteiner, M. (2001) *EMBO J* **20**: 3359–3369.

46 Seliger, B., Hohne, A., Knuth, A., Bernhard, H., Meyer, T., Tampe, R., Momburg, F. and Huber, C. (1996) *Cancer Res* **56**: 1756–1760.

47 Kageshita, T., Hirai, S., Ono, T., Hicklin, D. J. and Ferrone, S. (1999) *Am J Pathol* **154**: 745–754.

48 Seliger, B., Wollscheid, U., Momburg, F., Blankenstein, T. and Huber, C. (2001) *Cancer Res* **61**: 1095–1099.

49 Rotem-Yehudar, R., Groettrup, M., Soza, A., Kloetzel, P.-M. and Ehrlich, R. (1996) *J Exp Med* **183**: 499–514.

50 Kessler, J. H., Beekman, N. J., Bres-Vloemans, S. A., Verdijk, P., van Veelen, P. A., Kloosterman-Joosten, A. M., Vissers, D. C., ten Bosch, G. J., Kester, M. G., Sijts, A., Drijfhout, J. W., Ossendorp, F., Offringa, R. and Melief, C. J. (2001) *J Exp Med* **193**: 73–88.

**51** KUTTLER, C., NUSSBAUM, A. K., DICK, T. P., RAMMENSEE, H. G., SCHILD, H. and HADELER, K. P. (2000) *J Mol Biol* **298**: 417–429.

**52** HOLZHUTTER, H. G., FROMMEL, C. and KLOETZEL, P.-M. (1999) *J Mol Biol*, **286**: 1251–1265.

**53** HOLZHUTTER, H. G. and KLOETZEL, P.-M. (2000) *Biophys J* **79**: 1196–1205.

**54** KUON, W., HOLZHUTTER, H. G., APEL, H., GROLMS, M., KNOLLNBERGER, S., TRAEDER, A., HENKLEIN, P., WEISS, E., THIEL, A., LAUSETR, R., BOWNESS, P., RADBRUCH, A., KLOETZEL, P.-M. and SIEPER, J. (2001) *J Immunol* **167**, 4738–4746.

# 4
# T Cells In Tumor Immunity

Pedro Romero, Mikael J. Pittet, Alfred Zippelius, Danielle Liénard, Ferdy J. Lejeune, Danila Valmori, Daniel E. Speiser and Jean-Charles Cerottini

## 4.1
## Introduction

Experimental work during the last decades of last century firmly established the concept that T cell immunity may limit tumor progression and even mediate tumor rejection. However, this conclusion was achieved through a twisted road. For instance, the role of T cells in tumor immunity was seriously challenged in the 1970s. Rigorous experimentation in the last 30 years has clearly demonstrated the important role of immunity in protecting against cancer. Moreover, recent results in well-defined animal models have rekindled the immunosurveillance hypothesis. Both interferon (IFN)-$\gamma$ and T lymphocytes were found to contribute to reducing the incidence of chemically induced tumors as well as to shaping the antigenic make-up of emerging tumors [1]. The measurement of incidence of malignancies in pharmacologically immunosuppressed patients has also provided clues for the role of immunesurveillance in tumor control. Indeed, a long-term study of kidney transplant patients clearly indicates an increased risk of neoplasia [2].

As suggested by Burnett, thymus-dependent lymphocytes, i.e. T cells, are the most important effectors of immunosurveillance [3]. Decisive evidence of the involvement of T cells in antitumor immunity has finally emerged during the past 10 years with the cloning of genes encoding tumor antigens and the subsequent molecular identification of tumor-associated T cell epitopes. In turn, the detailed knowledge of T cell-defined tumor antigens has opened the possibility to dissect the interplay between tumors and lymphocytes, to monitor the natural immune response against tumors, to design therapeutic-specific cancer vaccines, and to assess their impact in immunized patients. In this chapter, we will focus on the work concerning T cell-mediated immunity in human cancer.

## 4.2
## Morphological Evidence of T Cell Immunity in Human Tumors

It has been shown in animal models that infiltration of tumors by tumor-reactive T lymphocytes is required for efficient tumor regression [4, 5]. In humans, histopathology analysis of various types of cancers has shown that they can be infiltrated by lymphocytes, which are routinely referred to as tumor-infiltrating lymphocytes (TILs) [6, 7]. Immunohistochemical studies in colorectal carcinomas indicated that the presence of CD8$^+$ T lymphocytes correlated with improved overall survival [8, 9]. Similarly, the presence of TILs in primary melanoma lesions has also been associated with improved prognosis [10]. In particular, it was shown that when categories of TILs are defined as brisk (when the infiltrating lymphocytes gain access to the tumor mass), non-brisk (peritumoral accumulations of T lymphocytes) and absent, they in fact have strong prognostic value for primary cutaneous melanomas in the vertical growth phase. Similar studies have also been performed in tumors from the upper gastrointestinal tract. Analysis of infiltrating CD8$^+$ T cells in Epstein–Barr virus (EBV)-associated gastric cancer showed increased rates of proliferative activity and perforin granules [11]. In three independent studies, the presence of inflammatory cells infiltrating esophageal squamous cell carcinoma correlated positively with prognosis [12–14]. Immunostaining of esophageal carcinomas revealing decreasing levels of MHC class I antigen expression as compared to normal tissues was correlated to reduced survival selectively in the squamous, but not in the adeno, cell carcinomas [15]. In a recent report, it was shown that intratumoral CD8$^+$ T cell infiltration more than peritumoral infiltration was associated with a favorable clinical outcome in both squamous cell and adenocarcinomas of the esophagus [16].

An important advance was the possibility to efficiently expand *in vitro* TIL populations, recovered from enzymatically dissociated tumor masses, by culture in the presence of high doses of IL-2. These were shown to have a more potent antitumor activity than lymphokine-activated killer (LAK) cells in animal models of adoptive transfer therapy [17]. Importantly, autologous TILs transferred to cancer patients persisted in the peripheral blood for periods ranging between 6 and 60 days [18], and were able to home to the tumor site [19]. Significant antitumor activity was observed in clinical trials of adoptive transfer of expanded autologous TILs mainly in melanoma, but also in other tumors such as renal cell carcinoma. These observations, coupled to the difficulties associated with isolation, *in vitro* expansion and adoptive transfer of TILs, provided the impetus at the end of the 1980s to undertake the isolation of individual tumor-reactive T cell clones from TILs and to identify their targets on the tumor cells.

## 4.3
## Approaches to the Molecular Identification of Cytolytic T Lymphocyte (CTL)-defined Tumor Antigens

The initial experimental system which allowed to unequivocally reveal the presence of tumor-reactive T cells in humans was the so called "mixed lymphocyte tumor cell culture" (MLTC). This consisted of the repeated periodical *in vitro* stimulation of peripheral blood lymphocytes with the autologous tumor cell line in medium supplemented with interleukin (IL)-2. Under these conditions, tumor-reactive T lymphocytes were observed in 50% of melanoma patients [20]. Thus, since this *in vitro* procedure presupposes the availability of autologous tumor cell lines, the majority of tumor-reactive T cells were initially isolated from melanoma. Because this is the tumor type among human tumors allowing a relatively high efficiency isolation of *in vitro* adapted, continuously growing, tumor cell lines. Indeed, the proportion of tumors from which it is possible to establish a cell line varies from 30 to 40% in different laboratories. The only other human tumor type from which cell lines can be isolated with a relatively high rate of success is the renal cell carcinoma. This rate ranges from 10%, [21] to even 60% of attempts [22], and may attain 80% for short-term tumor cell lines [23]. As mentioned above, another rich and reliable source of tumor-reactive T cells were the TILs mainly from melanoma lesions but also from other tumors such as colon or renal cell carcinomas readily expandable in *in vitro* culture with high-dose IL-2 [24].

The advent of techniques for both cloning antigen-specific T cells and measuring their cytolytic activity facilitated the isolation of tumor-reactive T cell clones from both MLTC and TIL cultures. Stable *in vitro* growing CTL clones were the critical tools which allowed the molecular identification of the first tumor antigens. Several strategies were successfully used to achieve this goal. The first involved the cloning of the genes encoding the tumor antigens from genomic or cDNA libraries created from the corresponding autologous melanoma tumor cells [25, 26]. The second strategy was the direct isolation and sequencing of the active antigenic peptide species bound to MHC class I molecules on the surface of the tumor cells [27]. In both cases, tumor-reactive CTL clones are used to monitor each of the multiple steps leading to cloning of the gene or to biochemically identifying the antigenic peptide. It was later realized that expression cloning in *Escherichia coli* of B cell-defined tumor antigens was also feasible using autologous sera from cancer patients [28]. This technology has been given the name of SEREX, for Serological Identification of Antigens by Recombinant Expression cloning. More than 1200 genes cloned to date have been listed [29]. Interestingly, several genes were independently cloned by both approaches indicating the existence of both T and B cell responses directed against the same target gene product naturally induced in the course of tumor progression. Examples of these genes are the MAGE-1, tyrosinase and NY-ESO-1. Other variants of molecular cloning of tumor antigens have been successfully used such as for instance representational difference analysis [30]. Thus, relatively large numbers of CTL-defined tumor antigens have been identified in the last 10 years. Several recent reviews contain complete listings of the tumor antigens [31, 32].

As expected from the understanding of molecular events involved in antigen recognition by CTL [33], tumor antigens are non-covalently associated tri-molecular complexes. The three molecular components are a polymorphic heavy chain encoded by sets of three pairs of alleles inherited co-dominantly in the class I MHC, a non-polymorphic $\beta_2$-microglobulin and a small antigenic peptide. The latter is generated by a dedicated antigen-processing machinery that involves proteolytic degradation of proteins in the cytosolic compartment and transport of peptides across the membrane of the endoplasmic reticulum. Virtually any protein that is synthesized in the cell may be the source of peptides for association with MHC class I and $\beta_2$-microglobulin in the lumen of the endoplasmic reticulum. The rules governing the interaction between antigenic peptides and MHC class I molecules are now well understood and supported by abundant structural data, including relatively numerous crystal structures. Recently, two MHC class I molecule/tumor antigenic peptide complexes have been crystallized [34, 35]. Simple peptide-binding motifs have now been defined for numerous MHC class I alleles. They contain three major components: a defined length and two preferred amino acid residues at fixed positions within the short peptide. The latter are referred to as anchor residues. Additional refinements can be introduced such as secondary residues that influence binding either positively or negatively. Thus, it became obvious that one could predict the set of peptides with the ability to bind to a given MHC class I allele by scanning the gene product sequence of interest with appropriate algorithms. This procedure had the advantage to be independent of the availability of pairs of specific CTL clones and autologous tumor cell lines and became known as "reverse immunology" [36, 37].

Although straightforward, two important limitations in the reverse immunology approach have been identified. First, it turned out that only one in four predicted peptides do actually bind efficiently to the MHC class I molecule of interest. Additional refinements to the prediction algorithms allow to improve the accuracy of MHC binding scores and to reduce the number of peptides to be tested in binding assays. Some of these good binder peptides can efficiently induce peptide-specific CTL upon *in vitro* stimulation of peripheral blood mononuclear cells (PBMC). However, the second limitation relates to the generation of the predicted peptide by the antigen-processing machinery of the cell. Indeed, some predicted good binder peptides have been shown to be either poorly generated by the proteasome or destroyed upon proteolytic degradation by the proteasome [38, 39]. In addition, the proteasome and immunoproteasome may significantly differ in their ability to modulate the generation of antigenic peptides [40]. These results impose the need to incorporate the new dimension of the "processability" of candidate peptides in the prediction algorithms. This is not an easy task as the factors involved are only partially understood at present. It seems that the main parameter in this regard is the proteasome itself. Efficient prediction of CTL epitopes from the PRAME tumor-associated protein was demonstrated using a combination of peptide-binding motifs and experimental digestion of long peptides by purified proteasome preparations [41]. Attempts are underway to define algorithms incorporating these new elements in the prediction process ([42, 43] and http://www.syfpeithi.de). Clearly, this type of approaches hold great promise to mine new tumor antigens from the human genome which can be expected to be completed in the foreseeable future [44].

New technologies are constantly applied to the task of tumor antigen identification. For instance, in an effort to obviate both the need for large numbers of tumor cells (biochemical identification of the antigenic peptide) and of cloning the gene encoding the tumor-associated antigen (genetic approaches), randomized and combinatorial peptide libraries have been used to probe the specificity of human tumor-reactive T cells [45, 46]. In one case, several mimotopes efficiently recognized by a CTL clone directed against a cutaneous T cell lymphoma (CTCL) in an HLA-B8-restricted fashion were identified. Moreover, close to 80% of a panel of HLA-B8 CTCL patients appeared to have detectable frequencies of mimotope-reactive CD8 T cells in the circulating lymphocyte compartment. However, the native tumor antigenic peptide could not be identified in the current gene databases [45]. In the other case, a validation of the combinatorial peptide library approach was conducted using tumor-reactive CTL clones of well-defined specificity and restricted by the commonly expressed HLA-A2 molecule [46]. To better guide the identification of the stimulating peptides present in the highly complex peptide mixtures of the libraries, a biometric matrix was designed [47]. This is used to search protein databases. Millions of peptides are retrieved with a score that reflects the relative T cell-stimulating weight. Clearly, the antigenic peptide is consistently placed among the first thirty peptides in the list of peptides ranked according to their score. Although encouraging, these results indicate the need to further refine this promising approach to T cell ligand(s) identification.

## 4.4
### Monitoring the Spontaneous CTL Responses to Tumor Antigens

Knowledge of the molecular identity of CTL-defined tumor antigens opened the possibility to track well-defined antigen-specific CTL responses in cancer patients. Again, technological advances in the detection of antigen-specific T lymphocytes have greatly facilitated monitoring CTL responses directly *ex vivo* without the need for repeated *in vitro* stimulation to obtain expansion of the specific T cells. Indeed, a direct approach for the visual identification of antigen-specific CD8 T cells was introduced for the first time in 1996 [48]. It is based on the use of soluble and fluorescently labeled tetramers of MHC class I molecules complexed with the antigenic peptide of interest [49, 50]. The question we have tried to address is whether the specific CTL clones isolated from a limited number of cancer patients, for tumor antigen identification, reflect frequent responses arising in all the patients with the appropriate expression of both antigen and MHC presenting allele or whether, in contrast, they represent only rare responses in isolated cases.

### 4.4.1
### Monitoring Specific CTL in the PBMC Compartment

The initial screening was obviously performed using the first tumor antigenic peptides that became available after the identification of the genes encoding tumor antigens, i.e. MAGE-A1 161–169 presented by HLA-A1 [51], MAGE-A3 168–176 also presented by HLA-A1 [52] and several melanoma differentiation antigens presented by the HLA-A2 molecule [53–55]. The most widely used screening procedure was applied to the latter antigens using PBMCs. It consisted of three or more rounds of weekly *in vitro* stimulations with peptide and cytokines followed by an assay to assess functionally active antigen-specific T cells expanded in this culture system. The assays most often used were chromium release to measure cytolytic activity and an ELISA-based detection of specific release of IFN-$\gamma$. It became obvious that melanoma patients frequently responded to stimulation with melanoma differentiation antigens such as Melan-A/MART-1 or gp100 [56, 57]. In contrast, there was an apparent paucity of responses to the two MAGE-derived peptides [58]. An in-depth search for the CTL precursors specific for the MAGE-A3 peptide indicated that they occur at very low frequencies in HLA-A1 individuals [59].

The next wave of screening for tumor antigen-specific T cells was performed with fluorescently labeled class I MHC/peptide complexes commonly referred to as tetramers [48, 49]. *Ex vivo*, a high frequency of A2/Melan-A/MART-1 tetramer$^+$ CD8$^+$ T lymphocytes is readily detectable in two-thirds of HLA-A2$^+$ melanoma patients [60]. Interestingly, a comparable proportion of healthy HLA-A2$^+$ individuals also contain a high frequency of these Melan-A/MART-1-specific T cells in their circulating CD8 compartment. The mean frequency is around 0.07%, which implies the presence of one specific cell in 1400 CD8$^+$ lymphocytes. Extensive characterization of the surface phenotype of these cells directly *ex vivo* indicates that in healthy donors they display a functionally naive phenotype. This is characterized mainly by the expression of the high molecular weight of the common lymphocyte antigen, CD45RA and the CCR7 chemokine receptor. In addition, these cells are also CD45RO$^-$, CD28$^+$, CD27$^+$, CD57$^-$, CD62L$^{high}$. In contrast, in about 30% of melanoma patients with circulating Melan-A/MART-1 tetramer$^+$ T cells, these express a mixed surface phenotype. Indeed variable proportions of these T cells display characteristics of an activated/memory phenotype (CD45RA$^{low}$, CCR7$^-$) [60, 61]. The majority of these cells are also CD45RO$^{high}$, CD28$^+$, CD27$^+$.

Apart from the Melan-A/MART-1 specific T cell repertoire, few other tumor antigen specificities are directly detectable *ex vivo* in the circulation with tetramers. In one report, a high frequency of tyrosinase-specific T cells were found to make up to 2% of the circulating CD8$^+$ T lymphocyte pool. These cells displayed the characteristics of activated cells but were found to be profoundly anergic in *in vitro* functional assays of antigen recognition [62]. However, the latter seems to be a special case because other studies, while confirming the existence of high levels of HLA tumor antigen peptide-specific T cells, fail to detect major functional defects [63–65].

The apparent paucity of directly detectable HLA-tumor antigen peptide tetramer$^+$ lymphocytes, other than Melan-A/MART-1, in the blood of the majority of cancer patients may reflect either a specific lack of responsiveness to CTL-defined tumor antigens or low frequencies of specific T cells below the detection limit of tetramers. In this regard, the detection limit for tetramers is imposed largely by background in the flow cytometers and it may be around one in 5000 lymphocytes. Purification of CD8$^+$ from PBMC to close to 100% purity brings the possibility to establish a power of detection down to a frequency of 0.02% within this subpopulation. This limit may vary for different tetramers and may depend on the relative quality of the commercially available fluorescent streptavidin conjugates. Introduction of a single round of *in vitro* stimulation with peptide allows us to expand the tumor-specific T cells to a level that is easily detectable by tetramers. This turned out to be clearly the case for a number of tumor antigens starting by the tyrosinase peptide 368–376 and presented to T cells by the HLA-A2 molecule. About 60% of HLA-A2$^+$ melanoma patients have a vigorous response that becomes detectable with tetramers in 1-week peptide-stimulated cultures of PBMCs [66]. Responses to several other antigens also become detectable in this short-term assay, including gp100, NY-ESO-1 157–165 [67] and MAGE-A10 [68]. However, as mentioned above, other responses occur at much lower frequencies such as the MAGE-A3.A1-specific T cells. In this case, a frequency below one in 1 000 000 was estimated based on polymerase chain reaction with clonotypic-specific primers [69].

### 4.4.2
### Evidence of Tumor Antigen-specific T Cell Responses at the Tumor Sites

The successful use of TILs as a rich source of tumor-reactive CTL lines and clones was an early indication of selective accumulation of tumor antigen-specific T cells at the tumor sites, particularly in melanoma, renal cell carcinoma or ovarian carcinoma. Several TIL lines obtained by continuous culture of melanoma TILs in high-dose IL-2 were used to clone several melanoma associated tumor antigens including gp100, tyrosinase and Melan-A/MART-1 [70]. When it became possible to directly address the presence of antigen-specific T cells in melanoma using fluorescent tetramers, it was clear that Melan-A/MART-1 tetramer$^+$ CD8$^+$ lymphocytes were readily detectable at relatively high frequencies in both TILs and tumor-infiltrated lymph nodes (TILNs) [71]. As illustrated in Fig. 4.1, these frequencies can be very high. In a series of HLA-A2$^+$ TILNs analyzed *ex vivo*, most lesions had detectable high frequencies of Melan-A$^+$ CD8$^+$ lymphocytes with frequencies directly *ex vivo* ranging around 1–15% of the CD8$^+$ subpopulation.

High as the frequencies of Melan-A/MART-1-specific T lymphocytes may appear, they still constitute a numerically small contingent of specific T cells in the metastasis cell suspension analyzed directly *ex vivo*. As illustrated in Fig. 4.2 in cartoon fashion, the majority of the cells recovered from reducing the metastatic lymph nodes to single-cell suspensions are melanoma tumor cells. Only 10% or less of the cells may be lymphocytes. Most of these cells are CD3$^+$ T cells when analyzed by flow cytometry and, in the majority of cases analyzed in our laboratory, over 80% of these are sin-

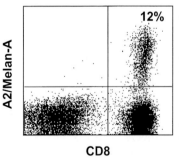

**Fig. 4.1** Melan-A/MART-1 tetramer$^+$ lymphocytes accumulate at tumor sites. Using tetramers, we have observed that Melan-A/MART-1-specific T cells are frequently accumulated at metastatic melanoma lesions. Here, TILs from a metastasis in the back from a HLA-A2$^+$ melanoma patient were stained with A2/Melan-A tetramers and anti-CD8 antibody *ex vivo*. Among the CD8 T cells in the lesion, 12% were specific for the Melan-A peptide directly *ex vivo*, i.e. in a cell suspension freshly prepared by dissociation of the tumor mass. These data confirm previous findings that patients with metastatic melanoma develop substantial CD8 T cell responses against their tumor [71]. Reprinted with permission from [50]

gle CD4$^+$ T cells. Short-term culture of these cell suspensions in medium supplemented with human serum, and recombinant IL-2 and IL-7 leads to dramatic changes of the cellular composition. In about two-thirds of the cultured tumor cell suspensions there is marked lymphocyte proliferation that peaks between days 14 and 21. Tumor cells rapidly decline because of both dilution and death in the culture dish. Proliferation of T lymphocytes does not preserve the original CD4/CD8 ratio. In fact, the dominant expanding population is CD3$^+$CD8$^+$. Monitoring of the expansion at the antigen-specific level is possible using tetramers. For Melan-A/MART-1 tetramers, a 2000-fold expansion has been measured in the period of 21 days. Since the size of the initial population could be determined with tetramers, it was possible to make a minimal estimate of 10–11 cell divisions during the culture period [71]. Thus, two conclusions can be drawn from these observations. On one hand, the sheer numerical inferiority of Melan-A-reactive T cells accumulated in metastases may in itself account for the apparent lack of efficient antitumor activity. No additional defects may be invoked. Rapid tumor growth rates together with the lack of appropriate lymphocyte growth support signals in the tumor environment may suffice to explain the failure of T cells to expand at the same or a faster pace than that of tumor cells. Eventually, the tumor would escape CTL control. On the other hand, Melan-A-specific T cells do not seem to bear major functional defects. They can proliferate vigorously in the presence of cytokines and residual tumor cells. The expanded population exhibits potent lytic activity against tumors and can release IFN-γ specifically upon challenge with antigen-bearing tumors.

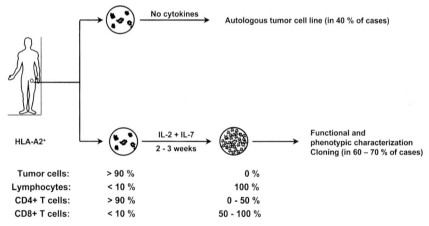

| | | | |
|---|---|---|---|
| Tumor cells: | > 90 % | 0 % | |
| Lymphocytes: | < 10 % | 100 % | |
| CD4+ T cells: | > 90 % | 0 - 50 % | |
| CD8+ T cells: | < 10 % | 50 - 100 % | |

**Fig. 4.2**  Dramatic changes in cellular composition of TILNs upon culture in the presence of cytokines. This cartoon summarizes the outcomes after *in vitro* culture of metastatic lymph node cell suspensions from melanoma patients in our laboratory. Culture in medium supplemented with fetal calf serum but devoid of cytokines favors the outgrowth of melanoma cell lines in close to 40% of cases. In contrast, culture in medium supplemented with human serum, rIL-2 and rIL-7 leads to dramatic expansions of T lymphocytes in about 60–70% of cases. The CD4/CD8 composition of these expanding cells also changes during expansion often resulting in large proportions of CD8$^+$ T lymphocytes. Similar findings can be observed with TILs from dissociated metastatic melanoma tumors [105]. Further details are explained in the text.

Although T cells directed against tumor antigens other than Melan-A are only rarely found in the *ex vivo* TILs or TILNs preparations from melanoma lesions, a much wider spectrum of antigen specificities is found in 2–3 weeks TIL and TILNs cultured in cytokines as described above. As shown in Tab. 4.1, we identified T cells specific for at least four different HLA-A2 tumor-associated antigens other than Melan-A in the same TILN preparation from a melanoma patient. Interestingly, this patient has had an unusually favorable clinical course and remains tumor-free 6 years after removal of this metastatic lymph node. Similar analyses with HLA-A2/peptide tetramers of 2- to 3-week expanded TILs and TILNs reveal a similar trend. The existence of other tumor antigen-specific T cells including melanocyte/melanoma differentiation antigens and the so-called cancer/testis antigens. The latter include MAGE-A10, NY-ESO-1 and CAMEL. These observations suggest that perhaps an important proportion of the CD8$^+$ T lymphocytes present in the TIL/TILN populations may in fact be tumor-specific.

Future studies with panels of tetramers representing a large group of tumor antigens might allow us to catalogue the diversity of antigen-specific T cells in the same individual, at individual tumor sites. Important steps in this direction have recently been reported using panels of cDNAs and transfection approaches. In one study, the reactivity of melanoma TIL populations was analyzed using COS cells co-transfected with individual cDNAs coding for defined melanoma associated antigens and cDNAs encoding HLA class I molecules. Five melanosomal proteins and five HLA-A alleles were included in this analysis [70]. In the other study, this approach was extended to the analysis of 28 cDNAs encoding already defined tumor antigens and 31 HLA class I alleles [72]. It was observed that indeed the spectrum of tumor antigens recognized by a given TIL population can be large. For instance, 10 TIL populations

**Tab. 4.1** The antitumor CTL response can target multiple antigens in the same individual at the same tumor site

| Tumor antigen | Antigenic peptide sequence | Percent lymphocytes tetramer$^+$ CD8$^{+a}$ | Reference |
|---|---|---|---|
| Melan-A/MART-1[b] | ELAGIGILTV[c] | 1.8 | 71 |
| Tyrosinase[b] | YMDGTMSQV | 0.02 | |
| NY-ESO-[d] | SLLMWITQC | 1.1 | 67 |
| MAGE-A10[d] | GLYDGMEHL | 2.1 | 68 |
| CAMEL[d] | MLMAQEALAFL | 0.22 | 96 |
| SSX-2[d] | KASEKIFYV | 0.64 | 97 |

[a] Fluorescently labeled tetramers of HLA-A2 and the corresponding antigenic peptides listed on the first column to the left were used together with anti-CD8–FITC to label a TILN cell suspension from a cutaneous melanoma patient, LAU 50. Labeled cells were analyzed by flow cytometry and the results are reported as percentage of tetramer$^+$ CD8$^+$ among the total CD8$^+$ lymphocytes.

[b] Tetramer measurement was performed in the freshly prepared lymph node cell suspension.

The levels of tyrosinase tetramer$^+$ T cells are below the detection limit and their characterization was not pursued further.

[c] This is a peptide analogue of the Melan-A/MART-1 immunodominant HLA-A2 restricted peptide that has increased antigenicity and immunogenicity as described elsewhere [98].

[d] Tetramer measurement was performed on the TILN populations after two to three weeks in culture in medium supplemented with human serum, rIL-2 and rIL-7, as described [71].

reacted against 10 tumor-specific antigens, in association with eight different HLA molecules. They also revealed the existence of many unknown epitopes derived from 12 different melanoma associated antigens. In conclusion, these studies attest to the selective accumulation of tumor antigen-specific CD8$^+$ T cells at the tumor site. The dynamics of their interactions with tumor cells and the tumor stroma remain to be studied in detail.

## 4.5
## CD4 T Cells in Tumor Immunity

Despite the central role that CD8$^+$ T cell responses have in tumor immunity, there is growing evidence supporting an important role for CD4$^+$ T cells. Murine studies have clearly shown that CD4$^+$ T cells mediate antitumor activity through various mechanisms. First, through the induction phase of antigen-specific CD8$^+$ T cells and of B cells. They also exert direct and indirect effects on tumor cells, even in those that are deficient in MHC class II expression [73]. Initial evidence of CD4$^+$ T cell involvement in antitumor immunity in humans came from studies at the tumor site [74, 75]. An indirect indication of the involvement of CD4$^+$ T cells in immunity against tumor is the detection of tumor-specific IgGs antibodies in cancer patients [28].

As with CD8$^+$ T cells, direct proof of the existence of tumor antigen-specific CD4$^+$ T cell immunity came finally with the identification of several targets of these cells in human tumors. The first epitope identified corresponded to non-mutated peptide of the tyrosinase protein and presented by HLA-DR [76, 77]. Since then the list of MHC class II-restricted T cell epitopes has been growing steadily. In particular, CD4$^+$ T cells recognizing tumor epitopes derived from tyrosinase [77], gp100 [78, 79], triose-phosphate isomerase, CDC27, LDLR-FUT [80], MAGE-A3 [81–83], NY-ESO-1 [84–86] and Melan-A/MART-1 [87] gene products have been identified (Tab. 4.2).

There are several interesting aspects in the knowledge accumulated so far on the CD4 T cell responses to tumor-associated antigens. For instance, tumors need not express MHC class II molecules on their surface. Thus, the priming of the response is likely to have taken place via cross-presentation involving endogenous antigen-presenting cells. The second observation is that several of the CD4 T cell clones or lines have the ability to recognize directly the tumor cells that do express the MHC class II molecule presenting the antigenic peptide. Such is the case for MAGE-3-specific T cells directed against a peptide presented in association with HLA-DP4. Interestingly, however, another peptide derived from the same protein and presented by HLA-DR molecules does not appear to be presented at the surface of tumor cells as the corresponding specific CD4 T cells fail to recognize the tumor. The third point that deserves consideration is the evidence that DP molecules are functional in antigen presentation, an issue that was controversial until recently. This unexpected outcome may have important practical implications for immunotherapy. Indeed, while most of the HLA-DRB alleles occur at low frequency in the population, the HLA-DPB genes have limited polymorphism and the two major alleles, HLA-DPB1*0401 and *0402, are expressed in about 60–70% of the Caucasian population as well as in

**Tab. 4.2** MHC class II-restricted T cell epitopes expressed by human tumors

| Gene | HLA allele | Antigenic peptide sequence | Category | Reference |
|------|-----------|---------------------------|----------|-----------|
| MAGE-A3 | DRB1*1101 | TSYVKVLHHMVKISG | shared tumor specific | 82 |
| MAGE-A1, -A2, -A3, -A6 | DRB1*1301, *1302 | LLKYRAREPVTKAE | | 99 |
| MAGE-A3 | DRB1*1301, *1302 | AELVHFLLLKYRAR | | 81 |
| MAGE-A3 | DPB1*0401, *0402 | TQHFVQENYLEY | | 83 |
| NY-ESO-1 | DRB4*0101 | VLLKEFTVSG | | 84 |
| NY-ESO-1 | DRB4*0101–0103 | PLPVPGVLLKEFTVSGNI VLLKEFTVSGNILTIRLT AADHRQLQLSISSCLQQL | | 85 |
| NY-ESO-1 | DPB1*0401 | SLLMWITQCFLPVF | | 86 |
| Tyrosinase | DRB1*0401 | QNILLSNAPLGPQFP | differentiation | 76 |
| Tyrosinase | DRB1*0401 | SYLQDSDPDSFQD | | 77 |
| Tyrosinase | DRB1*1501 | RHRPLQEVYPEANAPIGHNRE | | 100 |
| Melan-A/ MART-1 | DRB1*0401 | RNGYRALMDKSLHVGTQCALTRR | | 87 |
| Gp100 | DRB1*0401 | WNRQLYPEWTEAQRLD | | 78, 79 |
| PSA | DR4 | ILLGRMSLFMPEDTG SLFHPEDTGQVFQ QVFQVSHSFPHPLYD NDLMLLRLSEPAELT KKLQCVQLHVISM GVLQGITSMGSEPCA | | 101 |
| CDC27 | DRB1*0401 | FSWAMDLDPKGA | mutated/unique | 80 |
| TPI | DRB1*0101 | GELIGILNAAKVPAD | | 102 |
| HPV59-E7 | DRB1*0401 | LFMDTLSFVCPLC | viral | 103 |
| HPV68-E7 | DRB1*0407 | LFMDSLNFVCPWC | | |
| MUC-1 | DR3 | PGSTAPPAHGVT | over-expressed | 104 |

other ethnic groups. Thus, the MAGE-A3 and NY-ESO-1 HLA-DP4-restricted T cell epitopes constitute attractive targets for vaccination. It is going to be interesting in the future to identify additional DP4-restricted epitopes from tumor-associated proteins that have a wide expression in many tumor types. Such targets would indeed cover large segments of the population and help reduce the highly individualized nature of many tumor antigen-based vaccines.

Finally, direct monitoring of tumor antigen-specific CD4[+] T cell responses is its infancy. There are no MHC class II tetramers with tumor antigenic peptides reported yet. Efforts in several laboratories in this direction are underway. Tetramers with a few class II molecules have been successfully generated. For instance, mouse I-A[d] [88], I-E[k] [89], human HLA-DR1 [90], HLA-DR4 [91, 92] and HLA-DQ [93]. Future analyses of the natural or induced class II-restricted antitumor immune responses should greatly benefit from the ability to use fluorescent class II MHC/peptide tetramers.

**4.6**
**Concluding Remarks**

Important progress in the systematic analysis of T cell-mediated immunity against human tumors has finally led to the identification of the targets involved. To date, well over 50 different tumor antigens have been defined at the molecular level. These include both MHC class I- and II-restricted epitopes that can be effectively mimicked by well-defined synthetic peptides. Although some of the antigenic peptides identified thus far represent mutated sequences that uniquely occur in individual tumors, the majority of antigenic peptides are in fact non-mutated self-antigens. Thus tumor immunity can be regarded more as a special case of autoimmune reaction. This fact has important implications. On one hand, interesting observations in some paraneoplastic syndromes would suggest that damage of normal tissue is mediated, at least in part, by T cells directed against antigens whose expression is shared by certain normal cell types and the target tumor cells [94]. It is also possible that the observed increased incidence of vitiligo in melanoma patients treated with high-dose IL-2 [95] reflects the destruction of melanocytes mediated by immunity triggered by the transformed melanocytes. On the other hand, effective antitumor immunity may be limited to variable extents by the processes of central and peripheral tolerance that are essential to avoid the potentially devastating effects of autoimmunity.

The search for new tumor antigens continues. The initial studies which focused on CD8 T cell responses to melanoma have now been extended to many other types of tumors, and to the analysis of specific antibody and CD4 T cells responses. New technologies are constantly applied to this endeavor. Improved reverse immunology approaches for the accurate forecast of new T cell epitopes will be of special value to mine the human genome, soon to be completed and freely available in public databases. The main objective of these efforts is to identify good candidates for the design of cancer vaccines. The ideal candidates should be expressed in a wide variety of tumors and yet absent in normal tissues. They should be efficiently processed by both tumor and professional antigen presenting cells. They should also be strong immunogens, a quality that may critically depend on both their ability to stably bind to MHC molecules and the existence of minimal specific immune tolerance. It is likely that only few in a large palette of tumor antigens may meet these qualities.

The molecular identification of T cell-defined tumor antigens has ushered a new era in tumor immunology. It has provided targets for the design of specific cancer vaccines. Numerous phase I clinical trials of immunization have been completed recently with encouraging results and many more are underway. New adjuvants and antigen delivery systems are being developed. One of the most important advances is the ability to monitor antigen-specific T cells in cancer patients. Direct flow cytometry based assays such as tetramers and cytokine release assays allow the enumeration and functional characterization of single antigen-specific T cells directly *ex vivo*. Results from analyses based on these new tools provide convincing evidence for the existence of frequent natural immune responses against tumors in cancer patients. It is now clear that patients often mount immune responses against their tumors. These can be mediated by both CD8 and CD4 T cells, and target multiple antigens, restricted by several MHC alleles. In spite of these responses tumors progress and multiple mechanisms of escape from immune pressure have been identified. These are explained in another chapter of this book. Thus, the major challenge ahead for specific immunotherapy to achieve clinical benefit is to design intervention procedures allowing us to induce potent as well as sustained immune responses directed against multiple targets on the tumor. The hope is that these types of responses should cope with tumors and minimize the possibilities of escape. To accomplish these colossal tasks, a better understanding of the interplay of tumors and effector lymphocytes in the tumor environment is urgently needed.

## References

1 V. SHANKARAN, H. IKEDA, A. T. BRUCE, J. M. WHITE, P. E. SWANSON, L. J. OLD, R. D. SCHREIBER, *Nature* 2001; **410**: 1107.

2 N. J. LONDON, S. M. FARMERY, E. J. WILL, A. M. DAVISON, J. P. LODGE, *Lancet* 1995; **346**: 403.

3 M. BURNET, *Prog Exp. Tumor Res* 1970; **13**: 1.

4 S. MUKAI, J. KJAERGAARD, S. SHU, G. E. PLAUTZ, *Cancer Res* 1999; **59**: 5245.

5 G. WILLIMSKY, T. BLANKENSTEIN, *Cancer Res* 2000; **60**: 685.

6 A. K. HOUSE, A. G. WATT, *Gut* 1979; **20**: 868.

7 C. M. BALCH, L. B. RILEY, Y. J. BAE, M. A. SALMERON, C. D. PLATSOUCAS, A. VON ESCHENBACH, K. ITOH, *Arch Surg* 1990; **125**: 200.

8 K. M. ROPPONEN, M. J. ESKELINEN, P. K. LIPPONEN, E. ALHAVA, V. M. KOSMA, *J Pathol* 1997; **182**: 318.

9 Y. NAITO, K. SAITO, K. SHIIBA, A. OHUCHI, K. SAIGENJI, H. NAGURA, H. OHTANI, *Cancer Res* 1998; **58**: 3491.

10 C. G. CLEMENTE, M. C. MIHM, JR., R. BUFALINO, S. ZURRIDA, P. COLLINI, N. CASCINELLI, *Cancer* 1996; **77**: 1303.

11 Y. SAIKI, H. OHTANI, Y. NAITO, M. MIYAZAWA, H. NAGURA, *Lab Invest* 1996; **75**: 67.

12 M. IKEGUCHI, H. SAITO, K. KATANO, S. TSUJITANI, M. MAETA, N. KAIBARA, *Oncology* 1997; **54**: 311.

13 Y. MA, M. XIAN, J. LI, T. KAWABATA, S. OKADA, *Apmis* 1999; **107**: 514.

14 Y. OHASHI, S. ISHIBASHI, T. SUZUKI, R. SHINEHA, T. MORIYA, S. SATOMI, H. SASANO, *Anticancer Res* 2000; **20**: 3025.

15 S. B. HOSCH, J. R. IZBICKI, U. PICHLMEIER, N. STOECKLEIN, A. NIENDORF, W. T. KNOEFEL, C. E. BROELSCH, K. PANTEL, *Int J Cancer* 1997; **74**: 582.

16 K. SCHUMACHER, W. HAENSCH, C. ROEFZAAD, P. M. SCHLAG, *Cancer Res* 2001; **61**: 3932.

17 P. J. SPIESS, J. C. YANG, S. A. ROSENBERG, *J Natl Cancer Inst* 1987; **79**: 1067.

18 S. A. ROSENBERG, P. AEBERSOLD, K. CORNETTA, A. KASID, R. A. MORGAN, R. MOEN, E. M. KARSON, M. T. LOTZE, J. C. YANG, S. L. TOPALIAN, *et al.*, *N Engl J Med* 1990; **323**: 570.

19 B. FISHER, B. S. PACKARD, E. J. READ, J. A. CARRASQUILLO, C. S. CARTER, S. L. TOPALIAN, J. C. YANG, P. YOLLES, S. M. LARSON, S. A. ROSENBERG, *J Clin Oncol* 1989; **7**: 250.

20 A. KNUTH, B. DANOWSKI, H. F. OETTGEN, L. J. OLD, *Proc Natl Acad Sci USA* 1984; **81**: 3511.

21 R. UEDA, H. SHIKU, M. PFREUNDSCHUH, T. TAKAHASHI, L. T. LI, W. F. WHITMORE, H. F. OETTGEN, L. J. OLD, *J Exp Med* 1979; **150**: 564.

22 F. BOUET-TOUSSAINT, N. GENETEL, N. RIOUX-LECLERCQ, J. Y. BANSARD, J. LEVEQUE, F. GUILLE, J. J. PATARD, T. LESIMPLE, V. CATROS-QUEMENER, *Eur Cytokine Netw* 2000; **11**: 217.

23 R. O. DILLMAN, L. D. BEUTEL, A. N. CORNFORTH, S. K. NAYAK, *Cancer Biother Radiopharm* 2000; **15**: 161.

24 J. R. YANNELLI, C. HYATT, S. McCONNELL, K. HINES, L. JACKNIN, L. PARKER, M. SANDERS, S. A. ROSENBERG, *Int J Cancer* 1996; **65**: 413.

25 P. van der Bruggen, C. Traversari, P. Chomez, C. Lurquin, E. De Plaen, B. Van den Eynde, A. Knuth, T. Boon, *Science* 1991; **254**: 1643.

26 V. Brichard, A. Van Pel, T. Wolfel, C. Wolfel, E. De Plaen, B. Lethe, P. Coulie, T. Boon, *J Exp Med* 1993; **178**: 489.

27 A. L. Cox, J. Skipper, Y. Chen, R. A. Henderson, T. L. Darrow, J. Shabanowitz, V. H. Engelhard, D. F. Hunt, C. L. Slingluff, Jr, *Science* 1994; **264**: 716.

28 U. Sahin, O. Tureci, H. Schmitt, B. Cochlovius, T. Johannes, R. Schmits, F. Stenner, G. Luo, I. Schobert, M. Pfreundschuh, *Proc Natl Acad Sci USA* 1995; **92**: 11810.

29 V. Jongeneel, *Cancer Immun* 2001; **1**: 3.

30 B. Lethe, S. Lucas, L. Michaux, C. De Smet, D. Godelaine, A. Serrano, E. De Plaen, T. Boon, *Int J Cancer* 1998; **76**: 903.

31 R. F. Wang, *J Mol Med* 1999; **77**: 640.

32 N. Renkvist, C. Castelli, P. F. Robbins, G. Parmiani, *Cancer Immunol Immunother* 2001; **50**: 3.

33 A. Townsend, H. Bodmer, *Annu Rev Immunol* 1989; **7**: 601.

34 P. Sliz, O. Michielin, J. C. Cerottini, I. Luescher, P. Romero, M. Karplus, D. C. Wiley, *J Immunol* 2001; **167**: 3276.

35 J. J. Kuhns, M. A. Batalia, S. Yan, E. J. Collins, *J Biol Chem* 1999; **274**: 36422.

36 E. Celis, V. Tsai, C. Crimi, R. DeMars, P. A. Wentworth, R. W. Chesnut, H. M. Grey, A. Sette, H. M. Serra, *Proc Natl Acad Sci USA* 1994; **91**: 2105.

37 F. Kern, I. P. Surel, C. Brock, B. Freistedt, H. Radtke, A. Scheffold, R. Blasczyk, P. Reinke, J. Schneider-Mergener, A. Radbruch, P. Walden, H. D. Volk, *Nat Med* 1998; **4**: 975.

38 D. Valmori, U. Gileadi, C. Servis, P. R. Dunbar, J. C. Cerottini, P. Romero, V. Cerundolo, F. Levy, *J Exp Med* 1999; **189**: 895.

39 M. Ayyoub, M. Migliaccio, P. Guillaume, D. Lienard, J. C. Cerottini, P. Romero, F. Levy, D. E. Speiser, D. Valmori, *Eur J Immunol* 2001; **31**: 2642.

40 S. Morel, F. Levy, O. Burlet-Schiltz, F. Brasseur, M. Probst-Kepper, A. L. Peitrequin, B. Monsarrat, R. Van Velthoven, J. C. Cerottini, T. Boon, J. E. Gairin, B. J. Van den Eynde, *Immunity* 2000; **12**: 107.

41 J. H. Kessler, N. J. Beekman, S. A. Bres-Vloemans, P. Verdijk, P. A. van Veelen, A. M. Kloosterman-Joosten, D. C. Vissers, G. J. ten Bosch, M. G. Kester, A. Sijts, J. Wouter Drijfhout, F. Ossendorp, R. Offringa, C. J. Melief, *J Exp Med* 2001; **193**: 73.

42 I. Miconnet, C. Servis, J. C. Cerottini, P. Romero, F. Levy, *J Biol Chem* 2000; **275**: 26892.

43 L. Stoltze, A. K. Nussbaum, A. Sijts, N. P. Emmerich, P. M. Kloetzel, H. Schild, *Immunol Today* 2000; **21**: 317.

44 J. L. Schultze, R. H. Vonderheide, *Trends Immunol* 2001; **22**: 516.

45 T. Linnemann, S. Tumenjargal, S. Gellrich, K. Wiesmuller, K. Kaltoft, W. Sterry, P. Walden, *Eur J Immunol* 2001; **31**: 156.

46 C. Pinilla, V. Rubio-Godoy, V. Dutoit, P. Guillaume, R. Simon, Y. Zhao, R. A. Houghten, J. C. Cerottini, P. Romero, D. Valmori, *Cancer Res* 2001; **61**: 5153.

47 Y. Zhao, B. Gran, C. Pinilla, S. Markovic-Plese, B. Hemmer, A. Tzou, L. W. Whitney, W. E. Biddison, R. Martin, R. Simon, *J Immunol* 2001; **167**: 2130.

48 J. D. Altman, P. A. Moss, P. J. Goulder, D. H. Barouch, M. G. McHeyzer-Williams, J. I. Bell, A. J. McMichael, M. M. Davis, *Science* 1996; **274**: 94.

49 A. J. McMichael, C. A. O'Callaghan, *J Exp Med* 1998; **187**: 1367.

50 M. J. Pittet, D. E. Speiser, D. Valmori, D. Rimoldi, D. Lienard, F. Lejeune, J. C. Cerottini, P. Romero, *Int Immunopharmacol* 2001; **1**: 1235.

51 C. Traversari, P. van der Bruggen, I. F. Luescher, C. Lurquin, P. Chomez, A. Van Pel, E. De Plaen, A. Amar-Costesec, T. Boon, *J Exp Med* 1992; **176**: 1453.

52 B. Gaugler, B. Van den Eynde, P. van der Bruggen, P. Romero, J. J. Gaforio, E. De Plaen, B. Lethe, F. Brasseur, T. Boon, *J Exp Med* 1994; **179**: 921.

**53** T. WOLFEL, A. VAN PEL, V. BRICHARD, J. SCHNEIDER, B. SELIGER, K. H. MEYER ZUM BUSCHENFELDE, T. BOON, *Eur J Immunol* 1994; **24**: 759.

**54** Y. KAWAKAMI, S. ELIYAHU, K. SAKAGUCHI, P. F. ROBBINS, L. RIVOLTINI, J. R. YANNELLI, E. APPELLA, S. A. ROSENBERG, *J Exp Med* 1994; **180**: 347.

**55** P. G. COULIE, V. BRICHARD, A. VAN PEL, T. WOLFEL, J. SCHNEIDER, C. TRAVERSARI, S. MATTEI, E. DE PLAEN, C. LURQUIN, J. P. SZIKORA, *et al.*, *J Exp Med* 1994; **180**: 35.

**56** L. RIVOLTINI, Y. KAWAKAMI, K. SAKAGUCHI, S. SOUTHWOOD, A. SETTE, P. F. ROBBINS, F. M. MARINCOLA, M. L. SALGALLER, J. R. YANNELLI, E. APPELLA, *et al.*, *J Immunol* 1995; **154**: 2257.

**57** M. L. SALGALLER, A. AFSHAR, F. M. MARINCOLA, L. RIVOLTINI, Y. KAWAKAMI, S. A. ROSENBERG, *Cancer Res* 1995; **55**: 4972.

**58** P. ROMERO, J. C. CEROTTINI, G. A. WAANDERS, *Mol Med Today* 1998; **4**: 305.

**59** P. CHAUX, V. VANTOMME, P. COULIE, T. BOON, P. VAN DER BRUGGEN, *Int J Cancer* 1998; **77**: 538.

**60** M. J. PITTET, D. VALMORI, P. R. DUNBAR, D. E. SPEISER, D. LIENARD, F. LEJEUNE, K. FLEISCHHAUER, V. CERUNDOLO, J. C. CEROTTINI, P. ROMERO, *J Exp Med* 1999; **190**: 705.

**61** P. R. DUNBAR, C. L. SMITH, D. CHAO, M. SALIO, D. SHEPHERD, F. MIRZA, M. LIPP, A. LANZAVECCHIA, F. SALLUSTO, A. EVANS, R. RUSSELL-JONES, A. L. HARRIS, V. CERUNDOLO, *J Immunol* 2000; **165**: 6644.

**62** P. P. LEE, C. YEE, P. A. SAVAGE, L. FONG, D. BROCKSTEDT, J. S. WEBER, D. JOHNSON, S. SWETTER, J. THOMPSON, P. D. GREENBERG, M. ROEDERER, M. M. DAVIS, *Nat Med* 1999; **5**: 677.

**63** J. F. BAURAIN, D. COLAU, N. VAN BAREN, C. LANDRY, V. MARTELANGE, M. VIKKULA, T. BOON, P. G. COULIE, *J Immunol* 2000; **164**: 6057.

**64** J. J. MOLLDREM, P. P. LEE, C. WANG, K. FELIO, H. M. KANTARJIAN, R. E. CHAMPLIN, M. M. DAVIS, *Nat Med* 2000; **6**: 1018.

**65** V. KARANIKAS, D. COLAU, J. F. BAURAIN, R. CHIARI, J. THONNARD, I. GUTIERREZ-ROELENS, C. GOFFINET, E. V. VAN

SCHAFTINGEN, P. WEYNANTS, T. BOON, P. G. COULIE, *Cancer Res* 2001; **61**: 3718.

**66** D. VALMORI, M. J. PITTET, D. RIMOLDI, D. LIENARD, R. DUNBAR, V. CERUNDOLO, F. LEJEUNE, J. C. CEROTTINI, P. ROMERO, *Cancer Res* 1999; **59**: 2167.

**67** D. VALMORI, V. DUTOIT, D. LIENARD, D. RIMOLDI, M. J. PITTET, P. CHAMPAGNE, K. ELLEFSEN, U. SAHIN, D. SPEISER, F. LEJEUNE, J. C. CEROTTINI, P. ROMERO, *Cancer Res* 2000; **60**: 4499.

**68** D. VALMORI, V. DUTOIT, V. RUBIO-GODOY, C. CHAMBAZ, D. LIENARD, P. GUILLAUME, P. ROMERO, J. C. CEROTTINI, D. RIMOLDI, *Cancer Res* 2001; **61**: 509.

**69** P. G. COULIE, V. KARANIKAS, D. COLAU, C. LURQUIN, C. LANDRY, M. MARCHAND, T. DORVAL, V. BRICHARD, T. BOON, *Proc Natl Acad Sci USA* 2001; **98**: 10290.

**70** Y. KAWAKAMI, N. DANG, X. WANG, J. TUPESIS, P. F. ROBBINS, R. F. WANG, J. R. WUNDERLICH, J. R. YANNELLI, S. A. ROSENBERG, *J Immunother* 2000; **23**: 17.

**71** P. ROMERO, P. R. DUNBAR, D. VALMORI, M. PITTET, G. S. OGG, D. RIMOLDI, J. L. CHEN, D. LIENARD, J. C. CEROTTINI, V. CERUNDOLO, *J Exp Med* 1998; **188**: 1641.

**72** H. BENLALAM, N. LABARRIERE, B. LINARD, L. DERRE, E. DIEZ, M. C. PANDOLFINO, M. BONNEVILLE, F. JOTEREAU, *Eur J Immunol* 2001; **31**: 2007.

**73** D. MUMBERG, P. A. MONACH, S. WANDERLING, M. PHILIP, A. Y. TOLEDANO, R. D. SCHREIBER, H. SCHREIBER, *Proc Natl Acad Sci USA* 1999; **96**: 8633.

**74** P. S. GOEDEGEBUURE, T. J. EBERLEIN, *Immunol Res* 1995; **14**: 119.

**75** C. MACCALLI, R. MORTARINI, G. PARMIANI, A. ANICHINI, *Int J Cancer* 1994; **57**: 56.

**76** S. L. TOPALIAN, L. RIVOLTINI, M. MANCINI, N. R. MARKUS, P. F. ROBBINS, Y. KAWAKAMI, S. A. ROSENBERG, *Proc Natl Acad Sci USA* 1994; **91**: 9461.

**77** S. L. TOPALIAN, M. I. GONZALES, M. PARKHURST, Y. F. LI, S. SOUTHWOOD, A. SETTE, S. A. ROSENBERG, P. F. ROBBINS, *J Exp Med* 1996; **183**: 1965.

**78** K. LI, M. ADIBZADEH, T. HALDER, H. KALBACHER, S. HEINZEL, C. MULLER, J. ZEUTHEN, G. PAWELEC, *Cancer Immunol Immunother* 1998; **47**: 32.

79 C. E. Touloukian, W. W. Leitner, S. L. Topalian, Y. F. Li, P. F. Robbins, S. A. Rosenberg, N. P. Restifo, *J Immunol* 2000; **164**: 3535.

80 R. F. Wang, X. Wang, A. C. Atwood, S. L. Topalian, S. A. Rosenberg, *Science* 1999; **284**: 1351.

81 P. Chaux, V. Vantomme, V. Stroobant, K. Thielemans, J. Corthals, R. Luiten, A. M. Eggermont, T. Boon, P. van der Bruggen, *J Exp Med* 1999; **189**: 767.

82 S. Manici, T. Sturniolo, M. A. Imro, J. Hammer, F. Sinigaglia, C. Noppen, G. Spagnoli, B. Mazzi, M. Bellone, P. Dellabona, M. P. Protti, *J Exp Med* 1999; **189**: 871.

83 E. S. Schultz, B. Lethe, C. L. Cambiaso, J. Van Snick, P. Chaux, J. Corthals, C. Heirman, K. Thielemans, T. Boon, P. van der Bruggen, *Cancer Res* 2000; **60**: 6272.

84 G. Zeng, C. E. Touloukian, X. Wang, N. P. Restifo, S. A. Rosenberg, R. F. Wang, *J Immunol* 2000; **165**: 1153.

85 E. Jager, D. Jager, J. Karbach, Y. T. Chen, G. Ritter, Y. Nagata, S. Gnjatic, E. Stockert, M. Arand, L. J. Old, A. Knuth, *J Exp Med* 2000; **191**: 625.

86 G. Zeng, X. Wang, P. F. Robbins, S. A. Rosenberg, R. F. Wang, *Proc Natl Acad Sci USA* 2001; **98**: 3964.

87 H. M. Zarour, J. M. Kirkwood, L. S. Kierstead, W. Herr, V. Brusic, C. L. Slingluff, Jr, J. Sidney, A. Sette, W. J. Storkus, *Proc Natl Acad Sci USA* 2000; **97**: 400.

88 F. Crawford, H. Kozono, J. White, P. Marrack, J. Kappler, *Immunity* 1998; **8**: 675.

89 I. Gutgemann, A. M. Fahrer, J. D. Altman, M. M. Davis, Y. H. Chien, *Immunity* 1998; **8**: 667.

90 T. O. Cameron, J. R. Cochran, B. Yassine-Diab, R. P. Sekaly, L. J. Stern, *J Immunol* 2001; **166**: 741.

91 B. L. Kotzin, M. T. Falta, F. Crawford, E. F. Rosloniec, J. Bill, P. Marrack, J. Kappler, *Proc Natl Acad Sci USA* 2000; **97**: 291.

92 E. J. Novak, A. W. Liu, G. T. Nepom, W. W. Kwok, *J Clin Invest* 1999; **104**: R63.

93 W. W. Kwok, A. W. Liu, E. J. Novak, J. A. Gebe, R. A. Ettinger, G. T. Nepom, S. N. Reymond, D. M. Koelle, *J Immunol* 2000; **164**: 4244.

94 M. L. Albert, J. C. Darnell, A. Bender, L. M. Francisco, N. Bhardwaj, R. B. Darnell, *Nat Med* 1998; **4**: 1321.

95 S. A. Rosenberg, D. E. White, *J Immunother Emphasis Tumor Immunol* 1996; **19**: 81.

96 D. Rimoldi, V. Rubio-Godoy, V. Dutoit, D. Lienard, S. Salvi, P. Guillaume, D. Speiser, E. Stockert, G. Spagnoli, C. Servis, J. C. Cerottini, F. Lejeune, P. Romero, D. Valmori, *J Immunol* 2000; **165**: 7253.

97 M. Ayyoub, S. Stevanovic, U. Sahin, P. Guillaume, C. Servis, D. Rimoldi, D. Valmori, P. Romero, J. C. Cerottini, M. Rammensee, M. Pfreundschuh, D. Speiser, F. Levy, *J Immunol* 2002; **168**: 1717.

98 D. Valmori, J. F. Fonteneau, C. M. Lizana, N. Gervois, D. Lienard, D. Rimoldi, V. Jongeneel, F. Jotereau, J. C. Cerottini, P. Romero, *J Immunol* 1998; **160**: 1750.

99 P. Chaux, R. Luiten, N. Demotte, V. Vantomme, V. Stroobant, C. Traversari, V. Russo, E. Schultz, G. R. Cornelis, T. Boon, P. van der Bruggen, *J Immunol* 1999; **163**: 2928.

100 H. Kobayashi, T. Kokubo, K. Sato, S. Kimura, K. Asano, H. Takahashi, H. Iizuka, N. Miyokawa, M. Katagiri, *Cancer Res* 1998; **58**: 296.

101 J. M. Corman, E. E. Sercarz, N. K. Nanda, *Clin Exp Immunol* 1998; **114**: 166.

102 R. Pieper, R. E. Christian, M. I. Gonzales, M. I. Nishimura, G. Gupta, R. E. Settlage, J. Shabanowitz, S. A. Rosenberg, D. F. Hunt, S. L. Topalian, *J Exp Med* 1999; **189**: 757.

103 H. Hohn, H. Pilch, S. Gunzel, C. Neukirch, C. Hilmes, A. Kaufmann, B. Seliger, M. J. Maeurer, *J Immunol* 1999; **163**: 5715.

104 E. M. Hiltbold, P. Ciborowski, O. J. Finn, *Cancer Res* 1998; **58**: 5066.

105 D. Valmori, V. Dutoit, D. Lienard, F. Lejeune, D. Speiser, D. Rimoldi, V. Cerundolo, P. Y. Dietrich, J. C. Cerottini, P. Romero, *J Immunol* 2000; **165**: 533.

**Part 2**
**Immune Evasion and Suppression**

# 5
# Major Histocompatibility Complex Modulation and Loss
Barbara Seliger and Ulrike Ritz

## 5.1
### The Major Histocompatibility Complex (MHC) Antigen-Processing
### and -Presentation Pathways

The MHC encodes a number of molecules of immunological significance, in particular in the development of immune responses [1], including the MHC class I and II antigens, and different components of the antigen-processing pathway such as the peptide transporter, some proteasomal subunits and the chaperone tapasin. All these genes are localized in the MHC locus on chromosome 6 (Fig. 5.1). The classical

## MHC class II

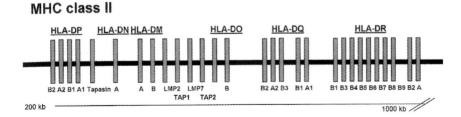

## MHC class I

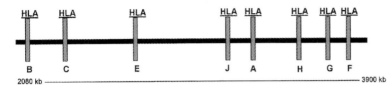

**Fig. 5.1** The MHC locus. The human MHC comprises of the class II region, the class III region and a class I region. The MHC class I and II regions are shown approximately to scale. The MHC class II region is extremely well characterized, and contains components of the MHC class I APM, including TAP1, TAP2, LMP2 and LMP7 as well as tapasin [142, 143]. In contrast, the precise position of many genes in the MHC class I region is as yet unknown.

MHC class I antigens, also termed class Ia, are the human leukocyte antigens (HLA)-A, -B and -C, which play an important role in the antiviral and antitumoral immunity, and are mostly expressed on nucleus-containing cell types. They consist of a highly polymorphic heavy chain (HC) which non-covalently associates with the antigenic peptide and a non-polymorphic light chain, $\beta_2$-microglobulin ($\beta_2$-m), and are characterized by their widespread expression on most tissues, except sperm and brain.

The MHC also encodes a second set of MHC class I molecules, the non-classical or MHC class Ib molecules, which share no homology with the classical MHC class I antigens. These consist of HLA-E, -F and -G, exhibit a limited polymorphism, and demonstrate low levels of tissue expression [2].

In addition to the MHC class Ia and Ib antigens, there exist highly polymorphic MHC class II molecules which are $\alpha/\beta$ heterodimers encoded by three MHC class II isotypes, HLA-DR, -DP and -DQ [3]. The normal expression pattern of MHC class II molecules is restricted to professional antigen-presenting cells (APC), thymic epithelium and B cells.

## 5.1.1
### The MHC Class I Antigen-Processing Machinery (APM)

The molecular steps of the classical MHC class I APM have been well characterized during the last decade and appear to be more complex than initially expected (Fig. 5.2) [4]. *De novo* synthesized MHC class I molecules assemble in the endoplasmic reticulum (ER) with peptides which have been yielded from mainly cytosolic proteins by the multicatalytic proteasome complex or/and other cytosolic proteases [5]. In normal untransformed cells the production of MHC class I peptide ligands by the proteasome is an extremely inefficient process. The delivery of substrates to the proteasome by the molecular chaperone HSC70 might trigger a modification in proteasomes that favors the generation of MHC class I ligands [6]. The constitutive proteasome subunits X, Y and Z are exchanged upon cytokine treatment by the proteasome subunits low molecular weight protein (LMP) 2, LMP7 and LMP10. Their expression, as well as the expression of the proteasome activators PA28$\alpha$ and $\beta$, can be modulated by interferon (IFN)-$\gamma$, tumor necrosis factor (TNF)-$\alpha$, IFN-$\alpha$ as well as interleukin (IL)-10. These inducible subunits are involved in the formation of the immunoproteasome. Changes in the subunit composition sharpen the quantitative and qualitative ability of the proteasome to generate antigenic peptides which limit the production of self peptides. The antigenic peptides are then transported into the ER by the ATP-dependent peptide transporter associated with antigen processing (TAP). TAP, a member of the ABC transporter family, consists of the subunits TAP1 and TAP2, and selects peptides of certain length and specific sequence. Peptides with a preferential length of 8–16 amino acids are efficiently translocated into the ER [7]. TAP is a component of a large macromolecular peptide loading complex incorporating TAP1, TAP2, tapasin as well as the MHC class I HC/$\beta_2$-m dimer in stoichiometrically defined ratios. Tapasin represents a linker between TAP and the MHC class I heterodimer, ensuring high peptide-loading efficiency, optimal ligand

**Fig. 5.2** The MHC class I
APM. Ubiquitinylated proteins
are cleaved into peptides by the
multicatalytic proteasome subunits which are then transported via the TAP heterocomplex into the ER. In the ER, peptides assemble with the MHC
class I HC and $\beta_2$-m to form the
trimeric MHC class I complex,
which is then transported
through the Golgi complex to
the cell surface for presentation
to $CD8^+$ cytotoxic T cells (A).
The MHC class I/peptide assembly is assisted by various
chaperones, such as calnexin,
calreticulin, ERp57 and tapasin,
which partially form the multimeric TAP complex (B).
(see color plates page XIX)

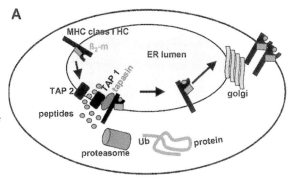

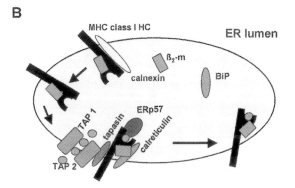

selection and stabilization of the MHC class I-loading complex [8]. In addition, other
ER-resident cofactors, such as the chaperones calnexin and calreticulin, and the thiol
oxidoreductase ERp57, stabilize the MHC class I molecules during their folding
and/or assembly. Moreover, they are also partially involved at different stages in the
formation of the multisubunit loading complex [9–11]. Peptide binding induces the
dissociation of the peptide/MHC class I HC/$\beta_2$-m trimer which is then transported
via the *trans*-Golgi apparatus to the cell surface for presentation to $CD8^+$ cytotoxic T
lymphocytes (CTLs).

### 5.1.2
### The MHC Class II APM

The MHC class II antigen-processing pathway is even more complex than the MHC
class I APM. It allows the formation and delivery of peptide/MHC class II complexes
to the cell surface, where they are presented to $CD4^+$ T cells (Fig. 5.3) [12, 13]. In contrast to MHC class I molecules, MHC class II molecules present peptides that are
mainly derived from exogenous antigens internalized into the endocytic pathway.

The newly synthesized heterodimeric MHC class II molecules consisting of the $\alpha$
and $\beta$ chains associate in the ER with the invariant chains (Ii) that inhibit peptide
binding to MHC class II molecules while they are in the ER. They form a nonameric
complex which is then targeted to specialized MHC class II compartments of the en-

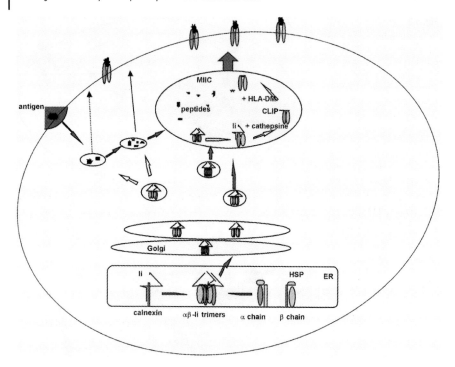

**Fig. 5.3** The MHC class II APM. MHC class II molecules present peptides derived from exogenous antigens internalized into the endocytic pathway. Briefly, HLA class II heterodimers assemble in the ER with the Ii to form nonameric α/β/Ii complexes. These are targeted to the MHC class II endocytic compartment where the MHC class II-associated Ii is degraded, leaving the CLIP peptide within the MHC class II binding groove. CLIP can be exchanged for antigenic peptides catalyzed by HLA-DM molecules. The HLA-DM-dependent peptide loading is controlled by HLA-DO. The peptide-loaded MHC class II molecules are then transported to the cell surface for presentation to CD4$^+$ T lymphocytes. (see color plates page XX)

docytic pathway, termed MIIC [14]. The MHC class II-associated Ii is proteolytically degraded in different steps, leaving only a small fragment, the MHC class II-associated Ii peptide (CLIP), in the MHC class II binding groove. CLIP is then subsequently exchanged by antigenic peptides. This process is catalyzed by the HLA-DM molecule, another HLA-like molecule, that facilitates CLIP removal and stabilizes the peptide-free status of the MHC class II molecules [15]. Thus, HLA-DM acts as a peptide editor that favors presentation of stably bound peptides, thereby critically affecting the peptide repertoire presented to the T cells. The MHC class II-encoded heterodimer HLA-DO consisting of HLA-DOA and -DOB inhibits the HLA-DM-dependent catalysis of peptide loading, suggesting that HLA-DO also affects the antigenic peptide repertoire presented by MHC class II molecules to CD4$^+$ T cells [16, 17], in particular by inhibiting presentation of large-sized peptides [18].

## 5.2
## The Physiology of the Non-classical HLA-G Molecule

The non-classical HLA class I antigens, e.g. HLA-G, are characterized by a limited polymorphism, unique structural features and a tissue-restricted distribution. Under physiological conditions, HLA-G is selectively expressed on trophoblasts of the human placenta, in fetal eye, liver and thymus, and in adult eye, skin, keratinocytes and myelomonocytic cells. A major feature of HLA-G is the alternative splicing of mRNA, thereby encoding four different potentially membrane-bound proteins, HLA-G1, -G2, -G3 and -G4, and three soluble isoforms, HLA-G5, -G6 and -G7 [19, 20]. The HLA-G1 isoform has the classical MHC class I structure consisting of the $\alpha 1$, $\alpha 2$ and $\alpha 3$ extracellular domains non-covalently associated with $\beta_2$-m. Like the full-length HLA-G1 molecule, each truncated HLA-G isoform can also be expressed on the cell surface [21].

The functions of HLA-G are now emerging. HLA-G binds to nonameric peptides and is capable of presenting them to CD8$^+$ T cells [22, 23]. In addition, HLA-G is the ligand of some killer cell immunoglobulin-like receptors presented on lymphocytes, macrophages, dendritic cells (DCs) and natural killer (NK) cells, such as p49, ILT2 and ILT4, and can modulate the expression of HLA-E. Studies on the immunological function have identified HLA-G as a key mediator of immune tolerance, in particular in the interaction between fetus and mother, possibly by inhibiting alloreactivity of maternal NK cells against the fetal tissues [2]. Furthermore, it has been suggested that HLA-G molecules may provide tumor cells with an effective escape mechanism by inhibiting both the lytic activity of *in situ* antigen-specific CD8$^+$ CTLs [24] and the NK cell-mediated cytotoxicity through interaction with killer inhibitory receptors (KIRs) [25].

## 5.3
## Determination of the Expression of Classical and Non-classical MHC Antigens

The pattern of MHC class I and II antigens as well as HLA-G expression has been studied in many tumors of distinct origin using different experimental approaches. In general, immunohistochemical staining of paraffin-embedded, formalin-fixed or frozen tumor sections has been employed [26–28]. However, the lack of standardized protocols that can be applied consistently by different investigators rendered it difficult to compare results obtained in various studies [29]. In addition, such analyses are significantly hampered by both the availability and reliability of reagents. So far, only a limited number of well-characterized anti-MHC class I, class II and non-classical MHC class I pan-reactive antibodies as well as allele- and locus-specific reagents are available and can be successfully employed for staining formalin-fixed tissue sections [30, 31].

Another hurdle is the evaluation and interpretation of the immunohistochemical staining in terms of its classification and scoring, thereby differentiating between a highly significant loss or decrease in expression. This is even more difficult since a heterogeneic MHC expression pattern is often found within the tumor analyzed.

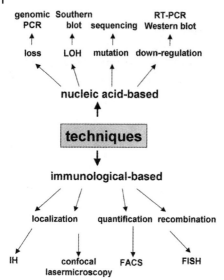

**Fig. 5.4** Different methods for determination of the expression of MHC antigens. The schematic diagram summarizes the different techniques currently employed for the analysis of MHC expression. They can be divided into nucleic acid-based and immunological-based techniques.

Thus, the quality control of experimental approaches and reagents utilized for tumor cell staining as well as the standardization of the interpretation of immunohistochemical results are urgently needed. An alternative method is fluorescence-activated cell sorting (FACS), which is more accurate, sensitive and reliable (Fig. 5.4). For example, tumors considered to be MHC class I⁻ by immunofluorescence have been shown to express low levels of MHC class I antigens as determined by FACS analysis [31–33]. This method can be routinely performed utilizing well-standardized protocols. A further advantage is the simultaneous expression analysis of several markers within a cell population and the concomitant determination of the expression of different antigens on normal versus tumor cells using tumor-specific markers.

In addition, Western blot analysis and nucleic acid-based assays exhibiting a higher sensitivity than immunohistochemistry and flow cytometry are also available, but still utilized less frequently. This includes the mRNA expression profiling by Northern blot analysis or reverse transcriptase polymerase chain reaction (RT-PCR), as well as the gel electrophoresis of specific HLA products using Southern blotting or genomic PCR. The PCR-based methods also allow the identification of structural alterations by direct sequencing of the respective amplification products (Fig. 5.4). However, a major disadvantage of these techniques is the cellular contamination of the tumor samples by stroma cells or by tumor-infiltrating lymphocytes (TILs), which could be minimized or even circumvented by the use of a laser dissection microscope.

## 5.4
## Interaction between Tumor and the Immune System

During the course of disease, the tumor accumulates a series of alterations that lead to dysfunctional regulation of cell growth and differentiation as well as to the escape of immune surveillance. These dynamic and complex changes exhibit a significant intra- and inter-cancer heterogeneity, and are further pronounced during tumor progression. They ultimately affect the efficacy of treatment modalities, such as chemotherapy, radiation and immunotherapy. The latter is reflected by significant heterogeneous responses in patients treated with passive antibody or T cell-based immunotherapy.

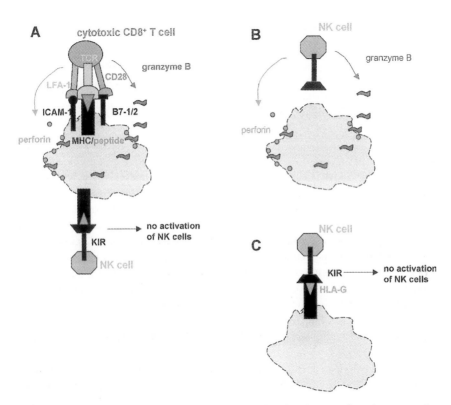

**Fig. 5.5** Different immune effector mechanisms. (A) MHC class I molecules are crucial structures for antigen presentation to T lymphocytes and the physiological ligands for NK receptors. Two distinct signals are required for the initiation and maintenance of an effective immune response. The first is provided by the interaction of MHC class I/peptide complex with the TCR, the second is mediated by a number of co-stimulatory molecules, e.g. B7/CD28. MHC class I molecules often disappear from the tumor cell surface to escape T cell recognition. Therefore patients must be monitored for the expression of these molecules prior to T cell-based immunotherapy. (B) Tumor cells lacking MHC class I molecules could be efficiently recognized by NK cells. (C) HLA-G expression of tumor cells can inhibit NK cell-mediated lysis suggesting that HLA-G expression is a novel immune escape mechanism. (see color plates page XXI)

The interactions between the host and tumor are controlled by the immune system (Fig. 5.5), in particular by CTLs and NK cells. There are several indications that immune responses severely affect the tumor growth:

1. Experimental models have demonstrated that low- or intermediate-affinity CTLs directed against tumor-associated antigens (TAAs) can prevent or treat tumors. This effect is further elicited by CD4$^+$ T helper cells [34–37].
2. During the last decade, T cell-based immunotherapy approaches were successfully implemented and some responders were obtained [38].
3. The course of the natural disease has correlated the type and composition of the T cell infiltrate within tumors with positive clinical outcomes [39].
4. During disease progression and/or immunotherapy based on monospecific CTLs, immune selection can occur resulting in antigen loss or deficiencies in the MHC class I antigen-processing and -presentation pathway. Impaired MHC class I antigen expression causes escape of tumor cells from CTL-mediated elimination, but renders the HLA$^-$ cells sensitive to lysis by NK cells [40–42].
5. The complementary interplay between loss of HLA expression and gain of NK sensitivity can be disrupted by the expression of the non-classical HLA-G antigen on tumors which inhibits NK cell activity by binding to KIRs [43].

## 5.5
### The Different MHC Class I Phenotypes and their Underlying Molecular Mechanisms

Most professional and non-professional APC exhibit normal MHC class I surface expression (Fig. 5.6). However, the immunohistochemical staining of surgically removed lesions with monoclonal antibodies (mAb) and characterization of cell lines originated from these lesions have often demonstrated abnormalities of MHC class I surface expression. So far, different types of defects in the expression of classical MHC class I antigens have been identified. These include (1) HLA class I antigen loss, (2) HLA class I antigen down-regulation and (3) selective loss or down-regulation of HLA class I allospecificities [26, 27, 42]. The frequency of MHC class I alterations has been determined in a large series of studies and occurs at a very high frequency [29, 43, 44]. Tumor sam-

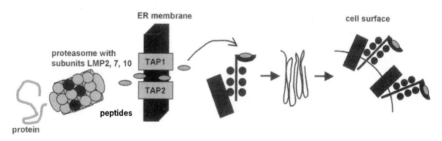

**Fig. 5.6** "Normal" MHC class I surface expression. Normal MHC class I surface expression re- quires proper MHC class I antigen processing and presentation.

ples were derived from either primary cancers or metastases from more than 30 different tumor types. MHC class I alterations appear to occur at a particular step in progression from benign to most aggressive tumors, demonstrating a gradient of expression between normal cells, primary tumors and tumor metastases. Depending on the tumor type analyzed, a loss of MHC class I antigens of 9–52%, an antigen down-regulation of 3–20%, and a selective allele-specific loss or down-regulation varying between 15 and 50% was found. In the following section, the underlying molecular mechanisms of the distinct HLA class I phenotypes are discussed.

### 5.5.1
### MHC Class I Loss

Loss of MHC class I antigens is found in 15% of melanomas, 9% of head and neck carcinomas, and 21% of colorectal tumors [44]. In prostate and breast carcinomas, MHC class I loss varies between 34 and 52%, respectively. Although a variety of molecular mechanisms contribute to this phenotype, it is mainly caused by structural defects in one copy of the $\beta_2$-m gene. This is associated with the loss of the wild-type $\beta_2$-m allele (Fig. 5.7 and Tab. 5.1). The latter is either attributable to a mitotic recombination event or to the loss of chromosome 15, on which the $\beta_2$-m gene is located [45]. This phenotype is consistent with the loss of heterozygosity (LOH) frequently detected in tumor cells due to their genetic instability [46]. Lack of HLA class I antigen expression can be corrected by transfection of cells with the wild-type $\beta_2$-m gene or cDNA [47–49]. This reflects the inability of $\beta_2$-m free HLA class I HC to travel through the *trans*-Golgi apparatus to the cell surface.

The mutations in the $\beta_2$-m gene described in the literature include base pair (bp) substitutions and deletions which range from loss of 1 bp to loss of extensive segments of the gene (Tab. 5.1 and Fig. 5.8). The mutations are randomly distributed through the leader sequences, exon 1, intron 1 and exon 2. In contrast, a dinucleotide CT deletion in an 8-bp CT repeat region in exon 1 appears to represent a mutation "hot spot" within the $\beta_2$-m gene, since the dinucleotide CT deletion has been

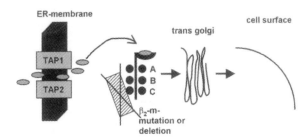

**Fig. 5.7** Loss of MHC class I surface expression due to structural alterations of the $\beta_2$-m gene. Structural alterations in the $\beta_2$-m associated with the loss of one copy of the $\beta_2$-m gene causes lack of MHC class I surface expression. Such defects occur at a high frequency in some tumor entities due to deficient HC/$\beta_2$-m dimer formation.

**Tab. 5.1**  HLA class I loss attributable to alterations in the $\beta_2$-m gene

| Tumor cell line | Tumor type | Molecular alteration | References |
|---|---|---|---|
| GR34 | melanoma | TTCT deletion in leader sequence | 50 |
| BB74-MEL | melanoma | C → G in exon 2 | 144 |
| LB1622-MEL | melanoma | T → A in exon 1 | 144 |
| Me1386 | melanoma | CT deletion in exon 1 | 49 |
| Me18105 | melanoma | A → G in splice acceptor site of intron1 | 49 |
| Me9922 | melanoma | 14-bp deletion in exon 2 | 49 |
| FO-1 | melanoma | deletion of first exon of the 5′ flanking region and of a segment of the first intron | 47 |
| LoVo | colorectal carcinoma | CT deletion in leader sequence | 145 |
| HCT15/DLD1 | colorectal carcinoma | C → A in exon 2/G ← T in intron 1 | 145 |
| SW48 | colorectal carcinoma | CTCT deletion in leader sequence deletion in exon 2 | 145 |
| HRA19 | colorectal carcinoma | TCTT deletion in exon 2 | 146 |
| C84 | colorectal carcinoma | G → A in exon 2 | 146 |
| Daudi | Burkitt's lymphoma | G → C at initiation codon | 147 |
| H2009 | lung adenocarcinoma | A → G in initiation codon | 148 |
| H630 | colorectal carcinoma | CT deletion in exon 1 | 148 |
| SK-MEL | melanoma | G deletion at position 323 in codon 76 | 48 |

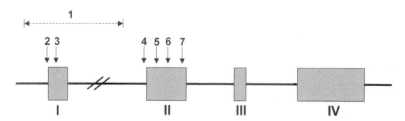

| Cell line | Mutation | Location | Effect | Position |
|---|---|---|---|---|
| FO-1 | large deletion | promoter-intron 1 | inhibits transcription | 1 |
| mel 1074 | T→C transition | initiation codon | inhibits translation | 2 |
| Me 1386, 1106 mel, 1180 mel, 1259 mel | CT deletion | exon 1 | frameshift and early stop codon | 3 |
| Me 18105 | A→G transition | intron 1 splice acceptor site | frameshift and early stop codon | 4 |
| SK-MEL-33 | single base deletion | exon 2 | frameshift and early stop codon | 5 |
| mel 1180 | C→G transversion | exon 2 | early stop codon | 6 |
| Me 9923 | 14 bp deletion | exon 2 | frameshift and early stop codon | 7 |

**Fig. 5.8**  Localization of $\beta_2$-m mutations. The localization of the major $\beta_2$-m mutations are marked demonstrating a "hot spot" region in exon 2.

identified in approximately 30% of cell lines analyzed with HLA class I antigen loss (Tab. 5.1) [50]. This possibility is supported by the higher susceptibility of such nucleotide elements to defective DNA repair mechanisms, and by the association found between the lack of a functional $\beta_2$-m and the presence of a mutator phenotype in a panel of 37 colon carcinoma cell lines [51].

Most of the $\beta_2$-m mutations inhibit their translation rather than their transcription. This mechanism explains the lack of functional $\beta_2$-m protein in spite of the apparently normal $\beta_2$-m mRNA levels in the majority of the cell lines analyzed which do not express HLA class I antigens. Deficient $\beta_2$-m protein expression results in a failure to express trimeric peptide/HC/$\beta_2$-m complexes at the cell surface. Thus, screening of surgically removed tumor lesions and tumor cell lines for functional $\beta_2$-m expression should be performed by Western blot, flow cytometry and/or immunohistochemical staining using anti-$\beta_2$-m antibodies.

The frequency of $\beta_2$-m mutations markedly differs among various types of malignancies. These mutations have been found frequently in colon carcinoma and melanoma, but rarely in other types of malignancies, such as head and neck squamous cell carcinoma (HNSCC), renal cell carcinoma (RCC), and cervical carcinoma [42, 44]. The reason(s) for these differences remain(s) to be determined.

## 5.5.2
### MHC Class I Down-regulation

The molecular mechanisms causing down-regulation of MHC class I antigens have been demonstrated to be quite heterogeneous. Many of them can be corrected by IFN-$\gamma$ treatment. Altered binding of regulatory factors to the MHC class I HC gene enhancer element by methylation or changes in the chromatin structure results in MHC class I HC mRNA down-regulation and consequently in a reduced expression of these molecules on the cell surface (Fig. 5.9) [52, 53].

An alternative mechanism is represented by defects in the peptide loading of HLA class I antigens, resulting in impaired assembly and stability of MHC class I molecules. This is caused by abnormalities in the expression and/or function of different component(s) of the MHC class I antigen-processing and -presentation pathway, such as the proteasomal subunits LMP2, LMP7 and LMP10, the peptide transporter TAP, and the chaperone tapasin [54] (Fig. 5.10 and Tab. 5.2).

So far, the expression of the proteasome subunits has only been determined in a limited number of surgically removed tumor lesions and tumor cell lines of dis-

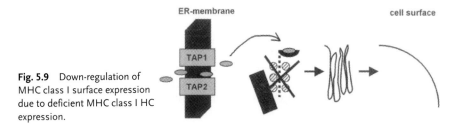

**Fig. 5.9** Down-regulation of MHC class I surface expression due to deficient MHC class I HC expression.

A

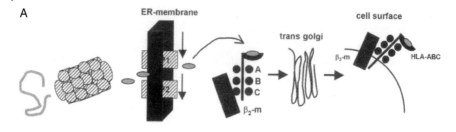

B

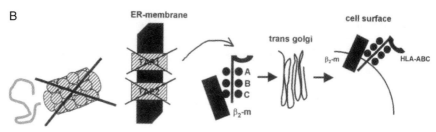

**Fig. 5.10** Association of defects in components of the APM with HLA class I antigen down-regulation. The deficient MHC class I surface expression can be caused by (A) dysregulation of different APM components or (B) structural defects in APM components, in particular of TAP.

**Tab. 5.2** Loss or down-regulation of MHC class I antigens due to deficiencies in the MHC class I APM

| Tumor cell line | Tumor type | Molecular alterations | References |
|---|---|---|---|
| Buf1280 | melanoma | bp deletion in TAP1 | 162., in preparation |
| H1436 | small cell lung carcinoma | CGG → CAG in exon 10 of TAP1 | 148 |
| FM55, FM37, NW16, 453A, 136-2, 823, 634, 603 | melanoma | regulatory defect | 149, 150, 151, 161 |
| PCC-1 | prostate | regulatory defect | 151 |
| H1092, H82 | small cell lung carcinoma | regulatory defect | 152 |
| MZ1257RC, MZ1851RC, MZ1940RC | RCC | regulatory defect | 160 |
| HS C5, HSC 7 | HNSCC | regulatory defect | 60 |

tinct histology (Tab. 5.2). There exists a heterogeneity in terms of quantity and quality of stained cells. In comparison to normal corresponding cells, LMP2 and LMP7 expression is reduced in Burkitt lymphoma lesions, in some breast carcinomas and in melanoma as well as in RCC, although the LMP subunits appear not always to be coordinately down-regulated in these tumor specimens [54]. Similar to the surgically removed lesions, tumor cell lines of distinct histology also exhibit a heterogeneous LMP2 and LMP7 expression pattern. Whether the changes of the LMP subunit expression obtained in tumor lesions or tumor cell lines reflect a transformation-dependent or tissue-specific regulation has not yet been determined. In addition, expression of LMP10 as well as proteasome activator subunits PA28α and β has been investigated in some tumor cell lines, but not in tumor lesions. LMP10 is not constitutively expressed in most tumor cell lines analyzed. This deficiency is frequently associated with the down-regulation of other APM components. In contrast, PA28α and β appear to be comparably expressed in tumor and corresponding normal cells.

Until now, little information has been available on the exact modalities of proteasomal degradation and the specificity as well as the activity of cytosolic proteases in tumor specimen. However, it appears to differ from that of professional APCs, thereby resulting in the generation of a distinct set of antigenic peptides presented to CTLs [55]. The abrogation of CTL epitope processing could also be attributable to single amino acid substitutions in transforming genes [56, 57]. Thus, the expression pattern of proteasome subunits in tumors might tune the generation of antigenic peptides as well as the sensitivity to CTL-mediated lysis which could be further enhanced by accelerated degradation of TAAs [56, 58]. These alterations may have important implications on the success of T cell-based immunotherapies.

Although tapasin has been shown to play an important role in peptide loading of MHC class I molecules, thereby affecting both MHC class I surface expression and immune response, its involvement in immune escape has not been determined. Seliger *et al.* [59] demonstrated deficient mRNA and protein expression of tapasin in colon carcinoma and HNSCC which could be corrected by cytokine treatment. These data were recently extended by Matsui *et al.* [60], providing evidence that the reduced tapasin transcription and CTL-mediated lysis of hepatoma cells can be restored by tapasin gene transfer.

A concomitant HLA class I antigen and TAP down-regulation has been reported in many tumors resulting in the generation of peptide-free, instable MHC class I HC/β$_2$-m heterodimers [59] (Fig. 5.10A). The frequency of TAP down-regulation or loss varies from 10 to 84%, and is particularly high in primary and metastatic cervical carcinomas. The altered frequencies of TAP deficiencies among different tumor types may reflect differences in the characteristics of the patient populations investigated, the immunobiology of various tumor types, the sensitivity of the immunohistochemical methods used as well as changes in the proliferative status of the tumor cells. Indeed, TAP1 expression might be regulated during the cell cycle. Only a few lesions, in particular melanoma and breast carcinoma, have been analyzed for TAP2 protein expression. This is attributable to the lack of TAP2 mAbs which can be routinely used on paraffin-embedded tissues. The frequency of TAP2 down-regulation varied between the tumor types and tumor cell lines analyzed.

The extent of TAP1 and/or TAP2 down-regulation seems to be more pronounced in metastatic than in primary lesions This has been shown in lesions obtained from cervical carcinoma, RCC, HNSCC, colorectal carcinoma, breast carcinoma and uveal or cutaneous melanoma [59, 61, 62] (Fig. 5.11). The impaired TAP expression in mela-

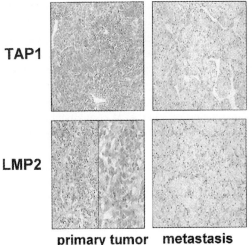

**TAP1**

**LMP2**

**primary tumor  metastasis**

**Fig. 5.11** Association of deficient TAP expression with the metastatic phenotype. A representative example of immunohistochemical staining of a primary and metastatic RCC lesion with an anti-TAP1 mAb is shown. TAP1 expression is strongly down-regulated in the metastasis when compared to the primary tumor lesion. (see color plates page XXII)

noma directly correlates with reduced recognition of metastatic tumor cells by autologous TAA-specific CTLs [63]. The clinical relevance of this observation has only been evaluated in melanoma, demonstrating that TAP down-regulation is associated with reduced patient survival [61, 62, 64] (Fig. 5.12). Thus, down-regulation or loss of TAP1 and TAP2 appear to represent an independent prognostic marker for melanoma [64].

TAP down-regulation can frequently be corrected by IFN-$\gamma$, whereas TAP deficiencies are mainly caused by dysregulation. However, loss of its IFN-$\gamma$ inducibility can also be caused by structural alterations in the peptide transporter subunits or by defects in the early steps of the IFN-$\gamma$ signaling pathway. The latter has recently been shown to occur in RCC cell lines [65]. To the best of our knowledge, structural defects in the TAP genes are a rare event. Until now, mutations in TAP have been identified in two human tumor cell lines, which are associated with the loss of constitutive and IFN-$\gamma$-inducible HLA class I antigen expression due to instability of the empty HLA class I/$\beta_2$-m complex on the cell surface. In a lung carcinoma cell line a point mutation in exon 10 of TAP1 introduces a premature stop codon, thereby resulting in a dysfunctional TAP1 protein [66] (Fig. 5.10B). Recently, Seliger *et al.* [162] have identified a base pair deletion at position 1489 in the TAP1 subunit of a melanoma cell line; the resulting frame-shift introduces an early stop codon. The dysfunctional TAP1 protein lacks ATP-binding, peptide-binding and peptide-translocation properties, which could be corrected by wild-type TAP1 gene transfer into these melanoma cells.

### 5.5.3
### Selective Loss or Down-regulation

The most common type of MHC class I alteration is represented by the selective loss or down-regulation of MHC class I allospecificities in malignant cells (Fig. 5.13). Although antigenic peptides are generated and transported into the ER, the trimeric complex cannot be formed and the peptides are not presented to CTLs. This type of

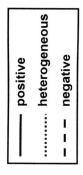

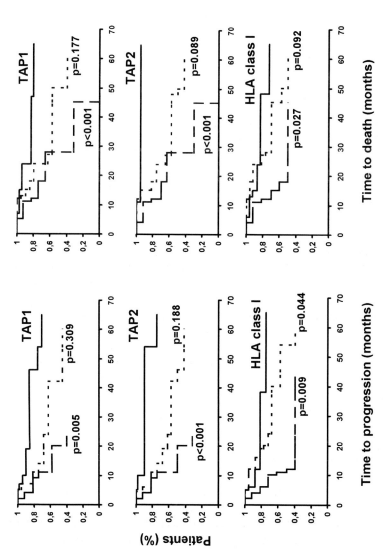

**Fig. 5.12** Correlation between the level of TAP and MHC class I expression with progression and survival time (according to Kageshita *et al.* [61]). Deficient MHC class I and TAP expression significantly correlates with the progression of disease as well as survival time.

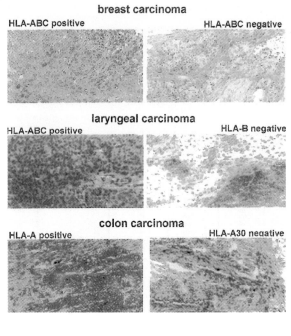

**breast carcinoma**

HLA-ABC positive · HLA-ABC negative

**laryngeal carcinoma**

HLA-ABC positive · HLA-B negative

**colon carcinoma**

HLA-A positive · HLA-A30 negative

**Fig. 5.13** Representative examples of defects in HLA class I antigen expression in surgically removed carcinoma lesions of distinct origin. Frozen tissue sections were stained in the immunoperoxidase reaction with respective anti-HLA class I mAbs. (Top panels) The lack of staining of the breast carcinoma lesions in the right top panel by the anti-HLA-A, -B and -C mAbs indicates a total HLA class I antigen loss in this lesion. (Middle panels) The lack of staining of the lesion with an anti-HLA-B mAb indicates a selective loss of the gene products of HLA-B loci. (Bottom panels) The lack of staining of the lesion with the anti-HLA-A30 mAb indicates selective loss of the HLA class I allospecificity. (see color plates page XXII)

MHC class I abnormalities might be missed if the different MHC molecules potentially expressed on the cell surface are not independently measured.

There exist distinct mechanisms resulting in allele- or locus-specific decrease or loss of MHC class I antigens. Loss of one MHC class I haplotype associated with LOH at chromosome 6p21 has been described in cell lines derived from melanoma, colon carcinoma, pancreatic carcinoma and cervical carcinoma lesions [33, 67–71] (Tab. 5.3). This altered MHC class I phenotype can be easily and reproducibly detected by microsatellite marker analysis using PCR amplification. A representative example is shown in Fig. 5.14 for a colon carcinoma cell line. This phenotype is caused by loss of variable portions of genomic DNA which is attributable to chromosomal segregation, non-dysjunction or mitotic recombination in the short arm of chromosome 6, where the MHC region has been mapped [72]. The frequency of haplotype loss in tumors derived from different tissues has not yet been evaluated in de-

**Tab. 5.3** HLA haplotype loss: LOH at 6p21

| Tumor cell line | Tumor | References |
| --- | --- | --- |
| FM55 | melanoma | 149 |
| FM37 | melanoma | |
| IMIM-PC2 | pancreatic carcinoma | 68 |
| NW145 | melanoma | 150 |
| OCM-3 | uveal melanoma | 154 |
| 877 | cervical carcinoma | 157 |
| CC-11 | cervical carcinoma | 155 |

**Fig. 5.14**   LOH in a colon carcinoma lesion. The electro-
pherogram profile obtained with the D6S311 microsatellite marker in lymphocyte (L), microdissected stroma
(S), tumor tissue (T) and microdissected tumor (DT)
shows that the signal obtained in one allele is reduced
and almost undetectable when DNA obtained from the
tumor and from the microdissected tumor, respectively,
is used.

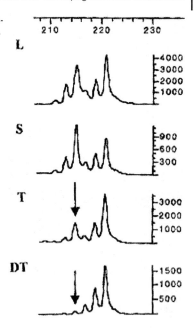

tail, although chromosomal loss has been identified in 14–17% of melanoma, colon
and laryngeal carcinoma, respectively. However, these results appear to be underesti-
mated since the heterogeneity of tumor tissues as well as its contamination with
stroma cells decreases the detection level of LOH.

Two mechanisms have been described to underlie the down-regulation of the gene
products of one HLA locus which appears to be more frequent for HLA-B than for
HLA-A antigens (Fig. 5.15A). An inverse association has been reported between
HLA locus antigen down-regulation and over-expression of various oncogenes, such
as c-*myc*, HER-2/*neu* and *ras* [73, 74], which interfere with the HLA locus transcription at the promoter level. An additional mechanism is represented by the loss of
transcription factor binding to HLA locus-specific regulatory elements as particularly
demonstrated in colon cancer cells [75].

Like the selective down-regulation of HLA-A or -B antigens in defined tumor types,
HLA class I allele-specific loss is not unique for malignant cells, since both of them
have also been found in normal cells [76]. The employment of a large series of mAbs
directed against specific alleles identified a MHC class I allele-specific loss in many
tumors with a frequency ranging from 15 to 51%, which is higher than other HLA
class I abnormalities (Fig. 5.15B). It is caused by mutations in the genes encoding
HLA class I HC including base pair insertions and base pair substitutions in exons
or introns and partial deletion as a consequence of chromosomal breakage or somatic recombination (Tab. 5.4). The available information is not sufficient to determine whether hot spot mutations are present in any of the HLA class I alleles or
whether the mutations occur randomly. Further studies are also required to determine whether mutations in HLA class I HC vary among malignant diseases.

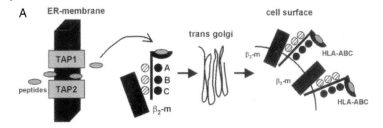

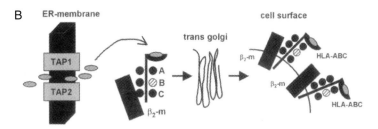

**Fig. 5.15** Selective (A) allelic- or (B) locus-specific HLA class I antigen down-regulation due to defects in the regulatory mechanisms controlling HLA class I antigen expression.

**Tab. 5.4** Allele-specific down-regulation or loss

| Tumor cell line | Tumor type | Molecular alterations | References |
|---|---|---|---|
| LS411 | colorectal carcinoma | chromosomal breakpoint in HLA A11 | 153 |
| CC11 | cervical carcinoma | G → T in exon 2 of HLA A24 | 156 |
| CSCC7 | | TGGG insertion at codon 32 in exon 2 of HLA-B15 | |
| 808 | | CAG → TAG in exon 3 of HLA-A2 | 157 |
| 778 | | G → C at the 3′ acceptor site of intron 1 of HLA-A2 | |
| | | 157 | |
| 624MEL28 | melanoma | base substitution at the 5′ donor site of intron 2 of HLA-A2 | 158 |

## 5.6
## MHC Class I Alterations: Impact on Immune Responses and Clinical Relevance

The functional significance of the MHC class I alterations described above will be discussed in this section. The loss of MHC class I surface expression causes escape from specific T cell-mediated antitumor responses directed against TAAs restricted by particular MHC class I molecules. The relevance of the down-regulation of MHC class I surface expression which directly correlates with the inadequate presentation of TAAs remains to be analyzed in terms of the frequency of occurrence *in vivo* and its effect on the natural history of the disease [77]. In addition, the role of the down-regulation of the MHC/peptide/epitope density for CTL-mediated recognition is controversially discussed. It has been postulated that as few as one peptide/MHC complex presented on a target is sufficient to elicit a potent CTL response [78]. However, the naturally occurring variation in the expression of TAAs and/or MHC class I surface molecules modulates the sensitivity of target cells to CTL-mediated lysis demonstrating a strictly quantitative relationship between MHC/antigen expression and CTL response [79]. This gradualness of heterogeneity suggests a potential mechanism for the progressive adjustment of tumor cells to a putative immunologically unfavorable environment.

It is generally accepted that MHC class I-deficient cells are susceptible to lysis by NK cells [80, 81] (see Fig. 5.5). The complementary interaction between loss of HLA class I expression and gain in NK cell sensitivity has been shown to be associated with the evolution of patients' immune responses over the course of several years demonstrating an increased sensitivity to NK cell-mediated lysis [39]. The level of MHC class I expression therefore influences the presentation and immunogenicity of CTL epitopes and the modulation of NK cell response. Thus, therapeutic approaches leading to the stimulation of the innate immunity in general and NK cell activity in particular may be of specific clinical significance for the treatment of MHC class I⁻ tumors. However, one has to consider that the loss of MHC class I molecules usually only occurs in a subset of the tumor due to its heterogeneity. A large fraction of tumor cells can exhibit total loss while a subpopulation might express normal levels of MHC class I antigens on the cell surface. In functional terms, this tumor would still be largely affected by the immune system.

The down-regulation of MHC class I surface antigens on tumors is often associated with the deficient expression of MHC class I APM components, in particular of the peptide transporter TAP. Animal experiments demonstrate that TAP over-expression in tumor cells can improve their immunogenicity as well as the host survival [82]. This has been attributed to an enhanced presentation of antigenic peptides. Targeting of TAP into tumor-burdened individuals may provide a possible method for anti-tumor immune therapy by controlling the occurrence of metastasis. Furthermore, TAP vaccines are independent of TAA expression and MHC polymorphism, both representing major problems for the induction of T cell-mediated immune responses.

The functional significance of the selective MHC class I allele loss has only been investigated in a few cases, and has mainly been described in mutant cells generated by mutagenesis and immune selection [83, 84]. Loss of a single HLA allele causes *in vitro* resistance of tumor cells to lysis by TAA-specific CTLs using the lost allele as restricting element [84, 85]. These allele-specific alterations of the MHC class I HC might reflect tumor adaptation to immune selection attributable to a dominant immune response restricted by a single MHC class I molecule, thereby explaining its high frequency [86]. The selection of HLA loss variants could severely affect the clinical outcome of patients as well as the design of immunotherapies. A combination of MHC class I allelic loss with the expression of HLA-C molecules (Fig. 5.16) which interact with the KIRs to maintain the inhibitory signal to NK cells is found in a minor-

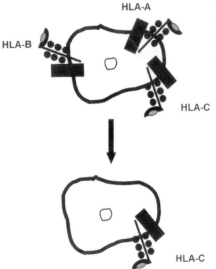

HLA-A

HLA-B

HLA-C

HLA-C

**Fig. 5.16**  HLA-C locus expression. This particular altered MHC class I phenotype expresses only HLA-C locus products. It is hypothesized that these tumor cells could escape from both T cell and NK cell-mediated cytotoxicity.

ity of colorectal (2.5%), laryngeal (5%) and breast carcinoma (9.5%) cells, respectively, thereby escaping not only from the CTL, but also from NK cell-mediated recognition [87].

To overcome the potential hurdle of allele-specific loss during immunotherapy, the induction of multispecific responses using a combination of peptides derived from TAAs will help to solve this problem. This strategy may counteract the ability of tumor cells with selective MHC class I allele loss to escape from immune recognition [88]. The biological significance of decreased MHC class I surface expression as a possible tumor escape mechanism from immune recognition is presently unclear, but is based on four different experimental approaches and observations: (1) CD8$^+$ cytotoxic T cells can recognize one MHC/peptide complex which is sufficient to lead to CTL-mediated tumor lysis; (2) the expression of MHC class I can often be up-regulated by IFN-γ which is commonly secreted by effector CTLs; (3) decreased levels of MHC class I expression render tumor cells more susceptible to NK cell-mediated lysis and (iv) the MHC class I-negative phenotype can be associated with poor survival [89]. However, a global down-regulation of MHC class I and TAP1 does not account for the ability of all tumors to evade the immune system. For example, impaired MHC class I antigen and TAP1 expression rarely occurs in NK/T cell lymphoma, suggesting that other immune escape mechanisms such as the production of IL-10 appear to suppress the local immune response [90].

There exist a number of studies demonstrating that IFN-γ induces MHC class I surface expression in a variety of human tumors of distinct histology which is at least partially due to an up-regulation of different components of the MHC class I APM. These data suggest that adjuvant IFN-γ immunotherapy may be of benefit for patients in the case of MHC class I$^-$ tumors. Local inflammation and immunization processes may induce or amplify the IFN-γ production of effector cells which could result in increases of MHC class I surface expression in regions distant from the inflammatory site.

However, some tumors are resistant to IFN-γ treatment. This can be due either to mutations in the IFN-γ receptor (R) or to deficiencies in components of the IFN-γ signal transduction pathway, e.g. the IFN-regulatory factors (IRFs [91, 92]; for further information, see Chapter 8). In addition to the IFNs, TNF-α has also been shown to affect the MHC class I antigen processing and presentation by coordinately modulating the expression of components of the MHC class I pathway. Thus, TNF-α may be useful when a concerted up-regulation of the MHC class I APM is required, but cannot be achieved by IFN-γ [93].

## 5.7
## The Role of MHC Class II Processing and Presentation in Tumors

The normal expression pattern of MHC class II genes is restricted to professional APCs, thymic epithelium and B cells. MHC class II induction can occur on most cell types through the exposure to various cytokines, in particular to IFN-γ [3]. The expression of MHC class II antigens on cells other than APCs can aid in the initiation and maintenance of an acute immune response.

Most human tumors do not express MHC class II molecules and the direct presentation pathway for activation of CD4$^+$ T cells is therefore not available. In general, CD4$^+$ T cell activation for these tumors depends exclusively on the indirect presentation via professional APCs. Limited CD4$^+$ T cell responses to such tumors may reflect the inefficiency of cross-priming. Immunization experiments using MHC class II-expressing tumor cells demonstrated that tumor cells are the predominant APCs *in vivo* for priming naïve CD4$^+$ T cells. Thus, their inclusion into cancer vaccines may enhance activation of tumor-reactive CD4$^+$ T cells [94].

### 5.7.1
### Frequency and Clinical Impact of MHC Class II Expression on Tumors

There is considerable evidence that the aberrant expression of MHC class II antigens and of the components involved in MHC class II antigen processing has pathophysiological consequences in malignant diseases. The constitutive or regulated expression of these proteins in tumors influences their immunity. The frequency of constitutive and/or IFN-γ-induced MHC class II expression varies between the different tumor types analyzed, but is usually associated with the co-expression of Ii and HLA-DM. One could distinguish three MHC class II phenotypes in human tumors: non-inducible, inducible and constitutive [95] (Fig. 5.17). It is generally assumed that the IFN-γ-inducible phenotype is normal, whereas the non-induced and constitutive MHC class II phenotypes are a result of neoplastic transformation.

The non-inducible MHC class II phenotype may represent a mutant cell line missing the required factors involved in the IFN-γ-mediated induction. Thus, it is questioned whether the tumor habors a mutation that prevents MHC class II inducibility,

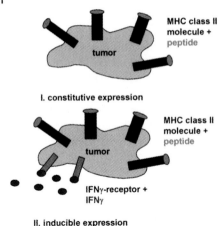

I. constitutive expression

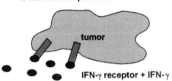

II. inducible expression

III. non-inducible expression

**Fig. 5.17** Possible pathway for the generation of an antitumor response dependent on the MHC class II expression of tumor cells (according to Blanck [95]). (I) The pathway which is directly affected by a tumor cell mutation leading to the generation of an antigenic, tumor-associated peptide. (II) The pathway which is directly affected by a tumor cell mutation due to inhibition of the $T_h1$ response or secretion of immunosuppressive cytokines. These mutations include defects in the retinoblastoma gene preventing MHC class II activation in response to IFN-γ. (III) The non-inducible expression could be caused by deficiencies in the IFN-γ signed transduction pathway. (see color plates page XXIII)

such as IRF1, or alternatively, whether the MHC class II inducibility could be inhibited by autocrine secretion of IL-10 or transforming growth factor (TGF)-β of the tumor cells [95]. The molecular basis of the constitutive MHC class II surface expression of tumor cells is unknown, but likely involves the inadequate activation of CIITA. High levels of constitutive MHC class II antigen expression were demonstrated in approximately 60% of nasopharyngeal tumors [96] and in a subset of malignant cells of Hodgkin's disease, termed Reed–Sternberg (HRS [97]).

The clinical impact of MHC class II antigen expression by malignant cells varies among tumors. Interestingly, there appears to exist an association between distinct MHC class II alleles and the development of some cancers, e.g. gastric carcinoma [98]. For some tumors, MHC class II antigen expression is associated with more aggressive malignancies and poor prognosis, e.g. in melanoma and osteosarcoma [99–101], whereas in others, such as squamous cell carcinoma, breast carcinoma, colorectal carcinoma, cervical carcinoma and laryngeal carcinoma, MHC class II expression directly correlates with a positive prognosis [102–106]. In breast carcinoma, MHC class II expression is further associated with the degree of differentiation. In addition, in melanoma, MHC class II antigens are not expressed in nevic cells, but can be induced by *ras*-mediated transformation of melanocytes and are frequently expressed by malignant cells [107].

5.7.2
**Molecular Mechanisms of Deficiencies in the MHC class II APM**

Qualitative differences in the MHC class II antigen-processing and -presentation pathway may be instrumental in shaping the CD4$^+$ T cell response directed against tumor cells (Fig. 5.18). Although multiple components of this pathway have been identified, their expression has not been analyzed systematically in human malignancies. Therefore, only limited information exists about defects in the MHC class II APM in human tumors especially concerning their functional significance. It is assumed that the timing and location of the MHC class II antigen expression is carefully controlled since aberrant expression of these molecules may lead to immune escape mechanisms of the tumor [108].

The transcription of the genes encoding the three MHC class II isotypes HLA-DR, -DP and -DQ is coordinately regulated by a set of conserved *cis*-acting promoter elements. One key regulator is the MHC class II transactivator CIITA, a non-DNA binding protein. CIITA expression is directly correlated with MHC class II surface expression and can be induced by IFN-γ. Thus, CIITA expression functions as a molecular switch for MHC class II gene regulation and is physiologically controlled during the cell cycle [109]. The lack of constitutive and/or IFN-γ-mediated CIITA expression has been detected in a number of tumor cells and may be attributable to dysregulation or structural alterations of CIITA. Defects in the allele locus which encodes the CIITA factor therefore result in deficient MHC class II surface expression. This mechanism has been shown in plasmocytoma, small cell lung carcinoma and hepatocarcinoma cells in which MHC class II antigen expression can be corrected by CIITA transfection [110–112]. In addition, defective CIITA expression is associated with lack of inducibility of class II antigen expression in many tumors and may at least partially be associated with the heterogeneity of MHC class II expression in tumors [111]. Furthermore, induction of MHC class II antigens requires retinoblastoma tumor suppressor gene [111]. Nitric oxide (NO) strongly inhibits the IFN-γ-stimulated expression of CIITA. This causes deficient expression of the family of genes regulated by CIITA, such as the Ii, HLA-DM and MHC class II molecules [113], suggesting that NO is an inhibitor of immune responses during malignant transformation by decreasing antigen presentation and subsequently CD4$^+$ T cell activation. The CIITA-mediated regulation of MHC class I surface expression is controversially discussed. In this case, CIITA controls the expression of the MHC class I HC and β$_2$-m, whereas the expression of components of the MHC class I APM, such as the peptide transporter TAP, are not affected [114]. Together, this transcription factor plays a crucial role in the design of both the MHC class I and II antigen-mediated immunotherapeutic approaches.

5.7.3
**Modulation of Immune Response by Altered MHC Class II Expression**

Alterations in the peptide repertoire presented by MHC class II molecules on tumor cells affect the generation of CD4$^+$ T cell response. Although HRS cells express all key effector molecules of APC, they fail to evoke an effective immune response. This paradox can be explained by the fact that a substantial number of MHC class II surface molecules are occupied by the non-immunogenic CLIP in HRS cells. This results in defective loading of these molecules with antigenic peptides and represents a further mechanism by which tumor cells can evade the immune system [97].

The impact of deficient HLA-DM expression on MHC class II antigen expression and peptide loading clearly depends on the MHC class II phenotype of the host. MHC class II$^+$, Ii$^-$, DM$^-$ tumor cells present a broader range of endogenous epitopes than MHC class II$^+$, Ii$^+$, DM$^+$ tumor cells [94]. The functional role of HLA-DO molecules in tumor antigen presentation has not yet been analyzed extensively. On the basis of immunohistological analyses in mice, HLA-DO-mediated effects may be limited to professional APCs. Recently, HLA-DO has been demonstrated to restrict the MHC class II peptide binding to the late endosomal compartments, thereby influencing the peptide repertoire presented to CD4$^+$ T cells. Furthermore, the tumor environment defined by locally secreted cytokines might also critically affect the coordinate regulation of the expression of molecules required for the MHC class II APM in a cell type-specific manner [115].

### 5.7.4
### MHC Class II Expression in Antitumor Response

Using animal models, the role of MHC class II in the antitumor response has been studied in syngeneic hosts. These experiments lead to the conclusion that MHC class II surface expression on tumor cells is able to vaccinate against parental MHC class II$^-$ cells (Fig. 5.18). Tumor cells expressing both MHC class II molecules as well as B7 co-stimulatory factors can stimulate a tumor-specific CD4$^+$ T cells and result in the eradication of pre-established invasive tumors. Co-expression of Ii with MHC class II antigens substantially reduces the antitumor efficacy of MHC class II-

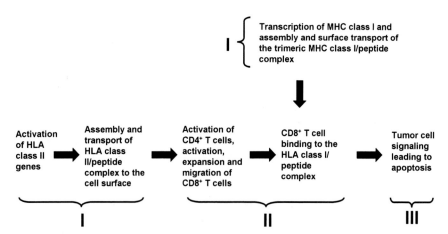

**Fig. 5.18** The different MHC class II phenotypes. There exist three distinct MHC class II phenotypes: constitutive MHC class II surface expression, IFN-γ-inducible MHC class I surface expression, and lack of both constitutive and IFN-γ-inducible MHC class I surface expression.

expressing tumor cells, which is consistent with the idea that endogenous TAAs are presented by exogenously expressed MHC class II molecules and that the Ii chain blocks the loading of the tumor antigen [97]. Furthermore, CIITA-transfected tumor cells are less efficient in generating antitumor immunity which could be mediated by the CIITA-facilitated activation of Ii expression. These results support the idea that tumor cell expression of MHC class II antigens under specific circumstances could lead to an antitumor immunity. However, these animal models raise the question about the differences in the development of human tumors. In the latter, IFN-γ can induce the Ii as well as CIITA. Mach et al. [116] demonstrated that antigen presentation requires both CIITA and IFN-γ treatment. Whether this is true for other cases may depend on the antigen required for MHC class II-dependent responses and the allele mediating the response. However, the identification of additional roles of MHC class II expression in the tumor development will depend on the characterization of a large series of MHC class II-presented TAAs or MHC class II-binding peptides as well as on the development of in vitro assays for TAA presentation to CD4+ T cells.

These results suggest that there exist a number of possible tumor cell defects that could account for the lack of tumor cell immunogenicity regarding HLA class II expression. These include the lack of certain MHC class II alleles to bind antigenic peptide in specific tumor types. If MHC class II expression can mediate tumor immunogenicity and MHC class II antigens are inducible or constitutively expressed in tumor cells, one can postulate that the impaired antitumor response is caused by deficiencies distinct from that of MHC class II antigen-processing and -presentation molecules. The molecular basis of constitutive expression of MHC class II in solid tumors is still unknown, but it likely involves the activation of CIITA which could be due to partial or total activation of the IFN-γ signaling pathway in these cells thereby resulting in the activation of CIITA.

## 5.8
### Role of IFN-γ in Immunosurveillance

IFN-γ is a pleiotropic cytokine which plays a central role in promoting immune responses directed against virus-infected or malignant transformed cells. It exerts its biological activities by interacting with the IFN-γR that is ubiquitiously expressed on most cell types. This directly leads to an activation of the janus tyrosine kinase (JAK)/signal transducers and activation of transcription (STAT) pathway [117]. STAT1 can be also activated by IFN-α and sodium butyrate [118]. The IRFs mediate the downstream effects of STAT1 activation. They belong to a large family of transcription factors. These molecules are important for the regulation of cell growth and transformation upon IFN treatment. IRF1 and IRF2 represent the best characterized family members and exert their biological activity by binding to the IRF element (IRF-E) which has been identified in the promoter of many IFN-inducible genes, including the MHC class I and II antigens, TAP1 and LMP2 as well as the transactivator CIITA [92, 121–123] (Fig. 5.19). IRF2 is the major activator of the IFN-

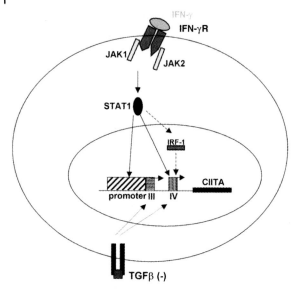

**Fig. 5.19** Model of the regulation of MHC class II genes by IFN-γ. The constitutive expression of CIITA is mediated by a proximal 5′ flanking sequence of the CIITA promoter III. In contrast, the induction of this promoter by IFN-γ is mediated by distal upstream sequences. Binding of IFN-γ to its receptor activates the JAK kinases which subsequently results in the phosphorylation of STAT1. STAT1 activation is accompanied by the activation of the CIITA promoter directly via STAT1 binding to sequences in this region. In addition, STAT1 activation induces the transcription of the CIITA promoter IV both by binding directly to sequences in this promoter or by inducing the transcription of IRF1 which is also required for the promoter activation. CIITA then activates the transcription of MHC class II antigens, the Ii and HLA-DM genes through common sequences located in the promoter regions of these genes. (see color plates page XXIV)

γ-inducible CIITA promoter type IV [123], but cooperates with IRF1 for the complete activation of CIITA [123]. This promoter is used by many cell types, including fibroblasts and endothelial cells [124].

## 5.8.1
### IFN-γ-dependent Immunosurveillance of Tumor Growth

The disruption of any step of IFN-γ signaling may result in an abrogation of the host antitumor response. Recently, the involvement of IFN-γ in tumor immunosurveillance has been studied in STAT1 as well as IFN-γR knockout mice using genetic or carcinogen-dependent tumorigenesis model systems [119, 120]. It has been demonstrated that the lack of IFN-γ sensitivity predisposes a murine host to enhance tumor development which leads to progressive tumor growth. These data suggest that IFN-γ plays a central role in promoting tumor surveillance. This could either be due to a direct effect of IFN-γ by enhancing MHC class I and/or II antigen processing or presentation on tumor cells or due to indirect effects of IFN-γ, such as activation of NK cells, macrophages and neutrophils, and antiangiostatic actions [163]. However, there also exist physiological alternative IFN-γR signaling pathways, but their consequences on the host antitumor response has still to be evaluated [125].

## 5.8.2
### Deficiencies in the IFN Signal Transduction Pathway

The deficient inducibility of components of the MHC class I and II antigen processing and presentation pathway can be due to either structural alterations of the IFNRs and factors involved in the modulation of IFN responses or dysregulation of components of the IFN signal transduction pathway.

Human tumors with mutations inactivating different components of the IFN-γ signal transduction pathway selectively become insensitive to IFN-γ treatment [120]. At present, only a few mutations in IRFs have been identified. Inactivation of IRF1 and IRF2 by point mutations or deletions was found in gastric cancer, leukemias and preleukemic myelodysplasias as well as pancreatic carcinomas, respectively [91, 126–128]. These structural alterations result in a markedly reduced DNA binding activity as well as transactivating capacity. The effects of these mutations on other IFN-regulated genes are unknown. Since only a few mutations have been identified so far, further studies will be necessary to determine the frequency of these mutations and their effect on tumor-related phenotypes, e.g. resistance to apoptosis, as well as whether they also occur in other tumor specimens [129].

The unresponsiveness to IFN could also be accounted to dysregulation of the JAK/STAT1 signaling. A link between defects in STAT1 phosphorylation or in the lack of binding activity to IFRs elements causing STAT1 protein deficiencies and the failure to up-regulate MHC class I surface expression has been demonstrated in MCA-induced tumors as well as gastric adenocarcinomas, respectively [130, 131].

## 5.9
### HLA-G Expression: an Immune Privilege for Malignant Cells?

Altered patterns of MHC class I surface expression in tumors have been shown to affect the capacity of CTL and NK cells to generate cytotoxic responses against tumor cells *in vitro* [26, 27]. The non-classical MHC class I antigens HLA-G and -E have recently been described as inhibitors of immune responses [43] as they inhibit CTL- as well as NK cell-mediated lysis. Furthermore, HLA-G plays a key role in establishing the feto-maternal tolerance during pregnancy. The potential impact of non-classical MHC class I antigen expression is currently under investigation. The data received so far suggest that the consequence of HLA-G expression in malignant cells is the escape of tumors from immunosurveillance.

5.9.1
### HLA-G Expression in Tumor Cells of Distinct Origin

Until now, there is limiting information available about HLA-G expression in human tumors. HLA-G expression has been investigated both at the mRNA and protein levels in a variety of tumor cell lines and surgically removed malignant lesions, especially in melanoma [43]. Both antisera and mAb have been utilized in immunohistochemical binding and immunochemical assays. Figure 5.20 shows a representative example of a flow cytometric staining of untreated and IFN-γ-treated RCC cells, but not of autologous renal epithelial cells utilizing the anti-HLA-G mAb MEM [30].

Results in the literature about the frequency of HLA-G expression by malignant cells are conflicting [132–137] (Tab. 5.5). High levels of HLA-G transcripts and/or proteins are found in tumor biopsies and cell lines derived from melanoma when compared to healthy skin or lymph nodes of the same patient [133]. In lung cancer, HLA-G ex-

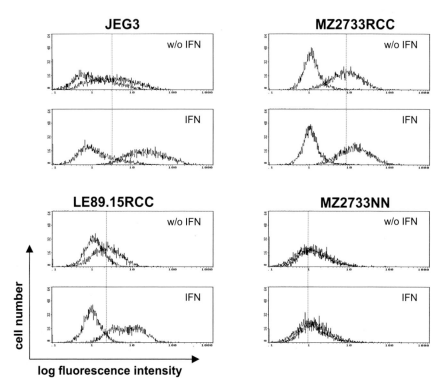

**Fig. 5.20** Differential HLA-G expression by RCC cells and by normal renal epithelial cells. The untreated and IFN-γ-treated RCC cell lines LE8915RC and MZ2733RCC as well as the cell line MZ2733NN derived from a normal renal epithelium were subjected to flow cytometric analysis using the anti-HLA-G-specific mAb MEM-G9 and a murine isotypic control antibody. The choriocarcinoma cell line JEG-3 served as a positive control. Results are expressed as histograms demonstrating constitutive and IFN-γ-mediated HLA-G expression in the cell lines JEG3, LE89.15RCC and MZ2733RCC, but not in the normal kidney cell line MZ2733NN.

**Tab. 5.5**  Expression of HLA-G in tumor cell lines of distinct origin

| Tumor | No. of cell lines analyzed | HLA-G expression |
|---|---|---|
| Breast carcinoma | 4 | none |
| Cervical carcinoma | 3 | none |
| Colon carcinoma | 6 | none |
| Head and neck carcinoma | 4 | none |
| Hepatocarcinoma | 4 | none |
| Lung carcinoma | 4 | none |
| Melanoma | 72 | 1 |
| Neuroblastoma | 7 | none |
| Ovarian carcinoma | 2 | none |
| RCC | 20 | 3 |
| B and T cell lymphoma | 19 | none |
| Histolytic lymphoma | 1 | 1 |
| Myelomonocytes | 9 | none |

pression also occurs at a high frequency. The HLA-G immunoreactivity is correlated with loss of MHC class I molecules and IL-10 production in these cells, thus suggesting an up-regulation of HLA-G by IL-10 [138].

In contrast, other authors show that HLA-G expression in tumors is extremely restricted [27, 139, 140]. HLA-G is not expressed on the cell surface of more than 70% cultured melanoma cell lines and in about 25% primary and metastatic lesions using polyclonal and monoclonal antibodies in a variety of assays. In addition, tumor cell lines of distinct origin, such as neuroblastoma, colon carcinoma, sarcoma, breast carcinoma and bladder carcinoma, lack HLA-G expression [140]. The conflicting information in the literature cannot be attributed to the specificity of antibodies used by various investigators, since at least some reagents were used in all studies [137]. Furthermore, it is unlikely that they reflect differences in the sensitivity of the assays used by the various investigators, since similar methodologies were utilized. Thus, differences in the characteristics of the cell lines and lesions analyzed appear to be most likely the source of conflicting results. It is also noteworthy that neither Garrido's group [136] nor Ferrone *et al.* (unpublished results) have detected HLA-G proteins in melanoma cell lines incubated *in vitro* with IFN-α, IFN-γ or TNF-α, although IFN-α induced HLA-G mRNA expression in at least one cell line. The lack of HLA-G translation in spite of the constitutive expression of transcripts of different sizes corresponding to various HLA-G isoforms has been found in several melanoma cell lines. These findings do not reflect structural abnormalities of HLA-G genes since sequencing of HLA-G transcripts from three melanoma cell lines detected no mutations. In view of the low HLA-G mRNA levels found in most of the melanoma cell lines analyzed, it is noteworthy that the lack of detection of HLA-G proteins does not reflect their expression by only a subpopulation of melanoma cells, since immunofluorescence staining of melanoma cell lines with anti-HLA-G mAb has not detected any HLA-G$^+$ cells in a minor subpopulation. Thus, impaired detection of HLA-G proteins in melanoma cell lines expressing HLA-G mRNA may be caused by protein levels too low for detection or by post-transcriptional down-regulation. These conflicting results are not unique for melanoma, since controversial findings have also been described in other types of malignancies [140].

### 5.9.2
### Clinical Impact of HLA-G Expression

In lung carcinoma, HLA-G protein expression correlated with both the histological tumor type and grade [138]. Paul *et al.* [133] reported HLA-G protein expression in cell lines and in biopsies derived from primary and metastatic melanoma lesions. Thus, HLA-G expression represents an early event in melanoma progression. HLA-G transcript levels in tumor regression sites were comparable to those in healthy skin, suggesting an association between HLA-G expression and disease progression. A similar conclusion has been reached by Wagner *et al.* [141] who investigated 10 patients with melanoma prior to treatment with high-dose IFN-α2 b. Immunohistochemical staining and SDS–PAGE analysis of antigens immunoprecipitated with a rabbit anti-HLA-G serum detected HLA-G antigens in five metastases all of which had lost classical HLA class I antigen expression. This phenotype was associated with relapse of the disease within the first six months of treatment. Wagner *et al.* [141] have suggested that the unresponsiveness to therapy with IFN-α2 b was caused by escape of melanoma cells from CTL recognition because of classical HLA class I antigen loss and by protection from NK cell recognition because of HLA-G expression.

### 5.9.3
### Induction of Tolerance by HLA-G Expression

Tumors with deficient MHC class I expression consequently become targets for NK cell-mediated lysis. Despite abnormalities in the surface expression of classical MHC class I antigens, most tumors grow *in vivo*, suggesting an additional escape of NK cell attack. The absence of a single HLA class I allele is sufficient for the activation of a particular NK cell population bearing the NK inhibitory receptor KIR. The non-classical HLA-G molecules inhibit NK lytic activity upon interaction with KIRs, thereby establishing a powerful mechanism of tumors to escape NK cell-mediated tumor immune surveillance. Thus, the role of HLA-G antigens in the interaction of CTLs and NK cells with target cells and the aberrant expression of these molecules by malignant cells have provided the impetus to characterize the expression of HLA-G antigens in malignant lesions and their clinical significance [43].

### 5.10
### Conclusions

The information we have reviewed clearly indicates that distinct molecular lesions underlie abnormalities in the expression of classical MHC class I as well as MHC class II antigens identified in malignant cells. Although the available information is still insufficient to draw definitive conclusions, it appears that mutations and/or dys-regulation can affect each step of the APMs which lead to abnormalities of MHC class I and/or II surface expression. Regulatory and structural defects appear to affect the components involved in the biosynthesis of the MHC class I and II complex with marked differences. For instance, defects in the regulation of TAP and CIITA are frequent, whereas sequence alterations in the components have only been rarely described. In contrast, structural defects appear to occur frequently in the $\beta_2$-m gene. Furthermore, it has to be considered that the frequency of mutations in various components of the MHC class I and II APMs varies significantly among various types of malignancies. These results suggest that a complete characterization of the molecular defects underlying abnormalities of the classical MHC class I and II APM in malignant diseases may suggest strategies to select and monitor patients to be treated with T cell-based immunotherapies, and to counteract the multiple escape mechanisms utilized by malignant cells.

The topic of expression of non-classical HLA class I antigens by malignant cells is in an early stage. The suggested role of these molecules in the immune escape of tumor cells is intriguing. However, the available information is still too limited and too conflicting to draw any conclusions at this time.

## Acknowledgments

We would like to thank J. Bukur (III. Department of Internal medicine, Mainz), Frederico Garrido and Teresa Cabrera (Granada, Spain) for kindly supplying Figs 5.14, 5.15 (F. G./T. C.) and 5.20 (J. B.), respectively, and I. Schmidt for help in preparing the manuscript. This work was partially supported by a grant from the Deutsche Forschungsgemeinschaft, SFB 432, project A5 (B. S.) and the Boehringer Ingelheim Fond.

## References

1 SCHWARTZ RH. *Adv Immunol* 1986; **38**: 31–201.

2 O'CALLAGHAN CA, BELL JI. *Immunol Rev* 1988; **163**: 129–138.

3 KAPPES D, STROMINGER JL. *Annu Rev Biochem* 1988; **57**: 991–1028.

4 VAN ENDERT PM. *Curr Opin Immunol* 1999; **11**: 82–88.

5 GROETTRUP M, SOZA A, KUCKELHORN U, KLOETZEL PM. *Immunol Today* 1996; **17**: 429–435.

6 YEWDELL JW. *Trends Cell Biol* 2001; **11**: 294–297.

7 MOMBURG F, HÄMMERLING HG. *Adv Immunol* 1998; **68**: 191–256.

8 BARNDEN MJ, PURCELL AW, GORMAN JJ, McCLUSKEY J. *J Immunol* 2000; **165**: 322–330.

9 HAMMOND C, HELENIUS A. *Curr Opin Cell Biol* 1995; **7**: 523–529.

10 SADASIVAN B, LEHNER PJ, ORTMANN B, SPIES T, CRESSWELL P. *Immunity* 1996; **5**: 103–114.

11 DIEDRICH G, BANGIA N, PAN M, CRESSWELL P. *J Immunol* 2001; **166**: 1703–1709.

12 PIETERS J. *Curr Biol Immunol* 1997; **9**: 89–96.

13 WANG RF. *Trends Immunol* 2001; **22**: 269–276.

14 Geuze HJ. *Immunol Today* 1998; **19**: 282–287.

15 Denzin LK, Cresswell P. *Cell* 1995; **82**: 155–165.

16 Kropshofer H, Arndt SO, Moldenhauer G, Hammerling GJ, Vogt AB. *Immunity* 1997; **6**: 293–302.

17 Kropshofer H, Vogt AB, Thery C, Armandola EA, Li BC, Moldenhauer G, Amigorena S, Hammerling GJ. *EMBO J* 1998; **17**: 2971–2981.

18 van Ham M, van Lith M, Lillemeier B, Tjin E, Grüneberg U, Rahman D, Pastoors L, van Meijgaarden K, Roucard C, Trowsdale J, Ottenhoff T, Pappin D, Neefjes J. *J Exp Med* 2000; **191**: 1127–1135.

19 Kirszenbaum M, Djoulah S, Hors J, Segall I, de Oliveira EB, Prost S, Dausset J, Carosella ED. *Hum Immunol* 1997; **53**: 140–147.

20 Carosella ED, Dausset J, Kirszenbaum M. *Immunol Today* 1996; **17**: 407–409.

21 Riteau B, Rouas-Freiss N, Menier C, Paul P, Dausset J, Carosella ED. *J Immunol* 2001; **166**: 5018–5026.

22 LeBouteiller P, Blaschitz A. *Immunol Rev* 1999; **167**: 233–244.

23 Diehl M, Münz C, Keilholz W, Stevanovic S, Holmes N, Loke YW, Rammensee HG. *Curr Biol* 1996; **6**: 305–314.

24 Le Gal F-A, Riteau B, Sedlik C, Khalil-Daher I, Menier C, Dausset J, Guillet J-G, Carosella ED, Rouas-Freiss N. *Int Immunol* 1999; **11**: 1351–1356.

25 Lopez-Botet M, Bellon T. *Curr Opin Immunol* 1999; **11**: 301–307.

26 Ferrone S, Marincola FM. *Immunol Today* 1995; **16**: 487–494.

27 Garrido F, Ruiz-Cabello F, Cabrera T, Perez-Villar JJ, López-Nevot MA, Duggan-Keen M, Stern PL. *Immunol Today* 1997; **18**: 89–95.

28 Algarra I, Cabrera T, Garrido F *Human Immunol* 2000; **61**: 65–73.

29 Sette A, Chesnut R, Fikes J. *Immunogenet* 2001; **53**: 255–263.

30 Fournel S, Huc X, Aguerre-Girr M, Solier C, Legros M, Praud-Brethenou C, Moussa M, Chaouat G, Berrebi A, Bensussan A, Lenfant F, Le Bouteiller P. *Tissue Antigens* 2000; **55**: 510–518.

31 Diederichsen AC, Hansen TP, Nielsen O, Fenger C, Jensenius JC, Christensen PB, Kristensen T, Zeuthen J. *Int J Cancer* 1998; **79**: 283–287.

32 Tait BD. *Hum Immunol* 2000; **61**: 158–165.

33 Koopmann LA, Corver WE, van den Slik AR, Gipyhart MJ, Fleuren GJ. *J Exp Med* 2000; **191**: 961–975.

34 Parmiani G. *Keio J Med* 2001; **50**: 86–90.

35 Rosenberg S, Yang JC, Douglas J, Schwartzentruber PH, Marincola FM, Topalian SL, Restifo NP, Dudley ME, Schwarz SL Spiess PJ, Wunderlich JR, Parkhurst MR, Kawakami Y, Seipp CA, Einhorn JH, White DE. *Nat Med* 1998; **4**: 321–327.

36 Rosenberg SA, Zhai Y, Yang JC, Schwartzentruber DJ, Hwu P, Marincola FM, Topalian S, Restifo N, Seipp CA, Einhorn JH, Roberts B, White DE. *J Natl Cancer Inst* 1998; **90**: 1894–1900.

37 Armstrong TD, Clements VK, Martin BK, Ting JP, Ostrand-Rosenberg S. *Proc Natl Acad Sci USA* 1997; **94**: 6886–6891.

38 Schultze JL, Maecker B, von Bergwelt-Baildon MS, Anderson KS, Vonderheide RH. *Vox Sanguinis* 2001; **80**: 81–89.

39 Coulie PG, Ikeda H, Baurain JF, Chiari R. *Adv Cancer Res* 1999; **76**: 213–242.

40 Rees RC, Mian S. *Cancer Immunol Immunother* 1999; **48**: 374–381.

41 Ruiz-Cabello F Garrido F. *Immunol Today* 1998; **19**: 539–542.

42 Marincola FM, Jaffee EM, Hicklin DJ, Ferrone S. *Adv Immunol* 2000; **74**: 181–273.

43 Carosella ED, Rouas-Freiss N, Paul P, Dausset J. *Immunol Today* 1999; **20**: 60–62.

44 Algarra I, Collado A, Garrido F. *Int J Clin Lab Res* 1997; **27**: 95–102.

45 Goodfellow PN, Jones EA, Van Heyningen V, Solomon E, Bobrow M, Miggiano V, Bodmer WF. *Nature* 1975; **254**: 267–269.

46 Aviv A, Aviv H. *Hum Genet* 1998; **103**: 2–4.

47 D'Urso CM, Wang Z, Cao Y, Tatake R, Zeff RA, Ferrone S. *J Clin Invest* 1991; **87**: 284–292.

48 Wang Z, Cao Y, Albino AP, Zeff RA, Houghton A, Ferrone S. *J Clin Invest* 1993; **91**: 684–692.

49 Hicklin DJ, Wang Z, Arienti F, Rivoltini L, Parmiani G, Ferrone S. *J Clin Invest* 1998; **101**: 2720–2729.

50 Pérez B, Benitez R, Fernández MA, Oliva MR, Soto JL, Serrano S, López Nevot MA, Garrido F. *Tissue Antigens* 1999; **53**: 569–572.

51 Branch P, Bicknell DC, Rowan A, Bodmer WF, Karran P. *Nat Genet* 1995; **9**: 231–232.

52 Henseling U, Schmidt W, Scholer HR, Gruss P, Hatzopoulos AK. *Mol Cell Biol* 1990; **10**: 4100–4109.

53 Blanchet O, Bourge JF, Zinszner H, Israel A, Kourilsky P, Dausset J, Degos L, Paul P. *Proc Natl Acad Sci USA* 1992; **89**: 3488–3492.

54 Seliger B, Maeurer MJ, Ferrone S. *Immunol Today* 2000; **21**: 455–464.

55 Dahlmann B, Ruppert T, Kuehn L, Merforth S, Kloetzel PM. *J Mol Biol* 2000; **303**: 643–653.

56 Theobald M, Ruppert T, Kuckelhorn U, Hernandez J, Haussler A, Ferreira EA, Liewer U, Biggs J, Levine AJ, Huber C, Koszinowski UH, Klötzel PM, Sherman LA. *J Exp Med* 1998; **188**: 1017–1028.

57 Beckmann NJ, van Veelen PA, van Hall T, Neisig A, Sijts A, Camps M, Kloetzel PM, Neefjes JJ, Melief CJ, Ossendorp F. *J Immunol* 2000; **164**: 1898–1905.

58 Castilleja A, Ward NE, O'Brian CA, Swearingen II B, Swan E, Gillogly MA, Murray JL, Kudelka AP, Gershenson DM, Ioannides CG. *Mol Cell Biochem* 2001; **217**: 21–33.

59 Seliger B, Schreiber K, Delp K, Meissner M, Hammers S, Reichert T, Pawlischko K, Tampé R, Huber C. *Tissue Antigens* 2001; **57**: 39–45.

60 Matsui M, Machida S, Tomiyama H, Takiguchi M, Akatsuka T. *Biochem Biophys Res Commun* 2001; **285**: 508–517.

61 Kageshita T, Hirai S, Ono T, Hicklin DJ, Ferrone S. *Am J Pathol* 1999; **154**: 745–754.

62 Cresswell AC, Sisley K, Laws D, Parsons MA, Rennie IG, Murray AK. *Melanoma Res* 2001; **11**: 275–281.

63 Murray JL, Hudson JM, Ross MI, Zhang HZ, Ionnides CG. *J Immunother* 2000; **23**: 28–35.

64 Kamarashev J, Ferrone S, Seifert B, Boni R, Nestle FO Burg G, Dummer R. *Int J Cancer* 2001; **95**: 23–28.

65 Dovhey SE, Ghosh NS, Wright KL. *Cancer Res* 2000; **60**: 5789–5796.

66 Chen HL, Gabrilovich D, Tampé R, Girgis KR, Nadaf S, Carbone DP. *Nat Genet* 1996; **13**: 210–213.

67 Marincola FM, Shamamian P, Alexander RB, Gnarra JR, Turetskaya RL, Nedospasov SA, Simonis TB, Taubenberger JK, Yannelli J, Mixon A. *J Immunol* 1994; **153**: 1225–1237.

68 Torres MJ, Ruiz-Cabello F, Skoudy A, Berrozpe G, Jimenez P, Serrano A, Real FX, Garrido F. *Tissue Antigens* 1996; **47**: 372–381.

69 Jimenez P, Canton J, Collado A, Cabrera T, Serranom A Realm L M Garcia A, Ruiz-Cabello F, Garrido F. *Int J Cancer* 1999; **83**: 91–97.

70 Jimenez P, Canton J, Concha A, Cabrera T, Fernandez M, Real LM, Garcia A, Serrano A, Garrido F, Ruiz-Cabello F. *Cancer Immunol Immunother* 2000; **48**: 684–690.

71 Ramal LM, Maleno I, Cabrera T, Collado A, Ferron A, López-Nevot MA, Garrido F. *Hum Immunol* 2000; **61**: 1001–1012.

72 Francke U, Pellegrino MA. *Proc Natl Acad Sci USA* 1977; **74**: 1147–1151.

73 Versteeg R, Noordermeer IA, Kruse-Wolters M, Ruiter DJ, Schrier PI. *EMBO J* 1988; **7**: 1023–10229.

74 Delp K, Momburg F, Hilmes C, Huber C, Seliger B. *Bone Marrow Transplant* 2000; **25**: S88–S95.

75 Soong TW, Hui KM. *J Immunol* 1992; **149**: 2008–2020.

76 Elsner HA, Drabek J, Rebmann V, Ambruzova Z, Grosse-Wilde H, Blaszczyk R. *Tissue Antigens* 2001; **57**: 369–372.

**77** RIKER AI, KAMMULA US, PANELLI MC,
WANG E, OHNMACHT GA, STEINBERG
SM, ROSENBERG SA, MARINCOLA FM.
*Int J Cancer* 2000; **86**: 818–826.

**78** SYKULEV Y, JOO M, VIRTURINA I, TSO-
MIDES TJ, EISEN HN. *Immunity* 1996;
4: 565–571.

**79** CORMIER JN, PANELLI MC, HACKETT
JA, BETTINOTTI MP, MIXON A, WUN-
DERLICH J, PARKER LL, RESTIFO NP,
FERRONE S, MARINCOLA FM. *Int J Can-
cer* 1999; **80**: 781–790.

**80** LJUNGGREN HG, KÄRRE K. *J Exp Med*
1985; **162**: 1745–1759.

**81** OHNMACHT GA, MARINCOLA FM. *J Cell
Physiol* 2000; **182**: 332–338.

**82** ALIMONTI J, ZHANG Q J, GABAT-
HULER R, REID G, CHEN SS, JEFFRIES
WA. *Nat Med* 2000; **18**: 515–520.

**83** ZEMMOUR J, LITTLE AM, SCHENDEL DJ,
PARHAM P. *J Immunol* 1992; **148**: 1941–
1948.

**84** WANG Z, SELIGER B, MIKE N, MOM-
BURG F, KNUTH A, FERRONE S. *Cancer
Res* 1998; **58**: 2149–2157.

**85** WÖLFEL T, KLEHMANN E, MÜLLER C,
SCHÜTT KH, MEYER-ZUM-BÜSCHEN-
FELDE KH, KNUTH A. *J Exp Med* 1989;
**170**: 797–810.

**86** LEHMANN F, MARCHAND M, HAINAUT P,
POUILLART P, SASTRE H, IKEDA H,
BOON T, COULIE PG. *Eur J Immunol*
1995; **25**: 340–347.

**87** CABRERA T, FERNANDEZ MA, SIERRA A,
GARRIDO A, HERRUZZO A, ESCOBEDO A,
FABRA A, GARRIDO F. *Hum Immunol*
1996; **50**: 127–134.

**88** WANG Z, MARINCOLA FM, RIVOLTINI L,
PERMIANI G, FERRONE S. *J Exp Med*
1999; **190**: 205–213.

**89** ZIA A, SCHILDBERG FW, FUNKE I. *Int J
Cancer* 2001; **93**: 566–570.

**90** SHEN L, CHIANG AK, LIU WP, LI GD,
LIANG RH, SRIVASTAVA G. *Int J Cancer*
2001; **92**: 692–696.

**91** HARADA H, KONDO T, OGAWA S, TA-
MURA T, KITAWAGA M, TANAKA N,
LAMPHIER MS, HIRAI H, TANIGUCHI T.
*Oncogene* 1994; **9**: 3313–3320.

**92** FUJITA T, SAKAKIBARA J, SUDO Y, MIYA-
MATO M, KIMURA Y, TANIGUCHI T.
*EMBO J* 1988; **7**: 3397–3405.

**93** HALLERMALM K, SEKI K, WEI C, CAS-
TELLI C, RIVOLTINI L, KIESSLING R, LE-
VITSKAYA J. *Blood* 2001; **98**: 1108–1115.

**94** QI L, ROJAS J-M, OSTRAND-ROSEN-
BERG S. *J Immunol* 2000; **165**: 5451–
5461.

**95** BLANCK G. *Microbe Infect* 1999; **1**: 913–
918.

**96** YAO Y, MINTER HA, CHEN X, REYNOLDS
GM, BROMLEY M, ARRAND JR. *Int J
Cancer* 2000; **88**: 949–955.

**97** BOSSHART H, JARRETT RF. *Blood* 1998;
**7**: 2252–2259.

**98** MAGNUSSON PKE, EUROTH H, ERIKS-
SON I, HELD M, NYREN O, ENGSTAN
HANSSON LE, GYLLENSTEIN UB. *Cancer
Res* 2001; **61**: 2684–2689.

**99** MORETTI S, PINZI C, BERTI E, SPALLAN-
ZANI A, CHIARUGI A, BODDI V, REALI
UM, GIANNOTTI B. *Melanoma Res* 1997;
**7**: 313–321.

**100** CONCHA A, ESTEBAN F, CABRERA T,
RUIZ-CABELLO F, GARRIDO F. *Semin Oncol* 1991; **2**: 47–54.

**101** TRIEB K, LECHLEITNER T, LANG S,
WINDHAGER R, KOTZ R, DIRNHOFER S.
*Pathol Res Pract* 1998; **194**: 679–684.

**102** CROMME FV, VON BOMMEL PF, WALBOO-
MERS JM, GALLEE MP, STERN PL, KENE-
MANS P, HELMERHORST TJ, STUKART MJ,
MEIJER CJ. *Br J Cancer* 1994; **69**: 1176–
1181.

**103** MATSUSHITA K, TAKENOUCHI T, KOBAYA-
SHI S, HAYASHI H, OKUYAMA K,
OCHIAI T, MIKATA A, ISONO K. *Br J
Cancer* 1996; **73**: 644–648.

**104** NORHEIM ANDERSEN S, BREIVIK J, LO-
VIG T, MELING GI, GAUDERNACK G,
CLAUSEN OP, SCHJOLBERG A, FAUSA O,
LANGMARK F, LUND E, ROGNUM TO.
*Br J Cancer* 1996; **74**: 99–108.

**105** SIKORSKA B, DANILEWICZ M, WAGROWS-
KA-DANILEWICZ M. *APMIS* 1999; **107**:
383–388.

**106** BRUNNER C, GOKEL J, RIETHMÜLLER G,
JOHNSON J. *Eur J Cancer* 1991; **27**: 411–
416.

**107** ALBINO AP, NANUS DM, MENTLE IR,
CORDON-CARDO C, MCNUTT NS, BRESS-
LER J, ANDREEFF M. *Oncogene* 1992; **7**:
2315–2321.

**108** MORRIS AC, SPANGLER WE, BOSS JM.
*J Immunol* 2000; **164**: 4143–4149.

109 Xaus J, Comalada M, Barrachina M, Herrero C, Gonalons E, Soler C, Lloberas J, Celada A. *J Immunol* 2000; **165**: 6364–6371.

110 Yazawa T, Kamma H, Fujiwara M, Matsui M, Horiguchi H, Satoh H, Fujimoto M, Yokoyama K, Ogata T. *J Pathol* 1999; **187**: 191–199.

111 Lu Y, Boss JM, Hu SX, Xu HJ, Blanck G. *J Immunol* 1996; **156**: 2495–2502.

112 Sartoris S, Valle MT, De Lerma Barbaro A, Tosi G, Cestari T, D'Agostino A, Megiovanni AM, Manca F, Accolla RS. *J Immunol* 1998; **161**: 814–820.

113 Kielar ML, Sicher SC, Penfield JG, Jeyarajah DR, Lu CY. *Inflammation* 2000; **24**: 431–445.

114 van den Elsen P, Peijnenburg A, van Eggermond MCJA, Gobin SJP. *Immunol Today* 1998; **19**: 308–312.

115 Walter W, Lingnau K, Schmitt E, Loos M, Maeurer MJ. *Br J Cancer* 2000; **83**: 1192–1201.

116 Mach B, Steimle V, Martinez-Soria E, Reith W. *Annu Rev Immunol* 1996; **14**: 301–331.

117 Bach EA, Aguet M, Schreiber RD. *Annu Rev Immunol* 1997; **15**: 749–797.

118 Hung WC, Chuang LY. *Br J Cancer* 1999; **80**: 705–710.

119 Dighe AS, Richards E, Old LJ, Schreiber RD. *Immunity* 1994; **1**: 447–456.

120 Kaplan DH, Shankaran V, Dighe AS, Stockert E, Aguet M, Old LJ, Schreiber RD. *Proc Natl Acad Sci USA* 1998; **95**: 7556–7561.

121 Blanar M, Baldwin ASJ, Flavell RA, Sharpe PA. *EMBO J* 1989; **8**: 1139–1144.

122 Wright KL White LC, Kelly A, Beck S, Trowsdale JJ, Ting JPY. *J Exp Med* 1995; **181**: 1459–1571.

123 Xi H, Eason DD, Ghosh D, Dovhey S, Wright KL, Blanck G. *Oncogene* 1999; **18**: 5889–5903.

124 Muhlethaler-Mottet A, Otten LA, Steimle V, Mach B. *EMBO J* 1997; **16**: 2851–2860.

125 Gil P, Bohn E, O'Guin AK, Ramana CV, Levine B, Stark GR, Virgin HW, Schreiber RD. *Proc Natl Acad Sci USA* 2001; **98**: 6680–6685.

126 Nozawa H, Oda E, Ueda S, Tamura G, Maesawa C, Muto T, Taniguchi T, Tanaka N. *Int J Cancer* 1998; **77**: 522–527.

127 Willman CL, Sever CE, Pallvicini MG, Harada H, Tanaka N, Slovak ML, Yamamoto H, Harada K, Meeker TC, List AF Taniguchi T. *Science* 1995; **259**: 968–971.

128 Xi H, Blanck G. *Int J Cancer* 2001; **87**: 803–808.

129 Lowney JK, Boucher LD, Swanson PE, Doherty GM. *Ann Surg Oncol* 1999; **6**: 604–608.

130 Svane IM, Engel AM, Nielsen M, Werdelin O. *Scand J Immunol* 1997; **46**: 379–387.

131 Abril E, Real LM, Serrano A, Jiminez P, Garcia A, Canton J, Trigo I, Garrido F, Ruiz-Cabello F. *Cancer Immunol Immunother* 1998; **47**: 113–120.

132 Paul P, Rouas-Freiss N, Khalil-Daher I, Moreau P, Riteau B, Le Gal FA, Avril MF, Dausset J, Guillet JG, Carosella ED. *Proc Natl Acad Sci USA* 1998; **95**: 4510–4515.

133 Paul P, Cabestre FA, Le Gal FA, Khalil-Daher I, Le Danff C, Schmid M, Mercier S, Avril MF, Dausset J, Guillet JG, Carosella ED. *Cancer Res* 1999; **59**: 1954–1960.

134 Rouas-Freiss N, Khalil-Daher I, Riteau B, Menier C, Paul P, Dausset J, Carosella ED. *Semin Cancer Biol* 1999; **9**: 3–12.

135 Fukushima Y, Oshika Y, Nakamura M, Tokunaga T, Hatanaka H, Abe Y, Yamazaki H, Kijima H, Ueyama Y, Tamaoki N. *Int J Mol Med* 1998; **2**: 349–351.

136 Real LM, Cabrera T, Collado A, Jimenez P, Garcia A, Ruiz-Cabello F, Garrido F. *Int J Cancer* 1999; **81**: 512–518.

137 Davies B, Hilby S, Gardner L, Loke YW, King A. *Am J Reprod Immunol* 2001; **45**: 103–107.

138 Urosevic M, Kurrer MO, Kamarashev J, Mueller B, Weder W, Burg G, Stabel RA, Dummer R, Trojan A. *Am J Pathol* 2001; **159**: 817–824.

**139** FRUMENTO G, FRANCHELLO S, PALMI-SANO GL, NICOTRA MR, GIACOMINI P, LOKE YW, GERAGTHY D, MAIO M, MANZO C, NATALI PG, FERRARA GB. *Tissue Antigens* 2000; **56**: 30–37.

**140** POLAKOVA K, RUSS G. *Neoplasma* 2000; **47**: 342–348.

**141** WAGNER SN, REBMANN V, WILLERS CP, GROSSE-WILDE H, GOOS M. *Lancet* 2000; **356**: 220–221.

**142** TROWSDALE J, RAGOUSSIS J, CAMPBELL RD. *Immunol Today* 1991; **12**: 443–446.

**143** HERBERG JA, SGOUROS J, JONES T, CO-PEMAN J, HUMPHRAY SJ, SHEER D, CRESSWELL P, BECK S, TROWSDALE J. *Eur J Immunol* 1998; **28**: 459–467.

**144** BENITEZ R, GODELAINE D, LÓPEZ-NEVOT MA, BRASSEUR F, JIMÉNEZ P, MARC-HAND M, OLIVA MR, VAN BAREN N, CABRERA T, ANDRY G, LANDRY C, RUIZ-CABELLO F, BOON T, GARRIDO F. *Tissue Antigens* 1998; **52**: 520–529.

**145** BICKNELL DC, ROWAN A, BODMER WF. *Proc Natl Acad Sci USA* 1994; **91**: 4751–4755.

**146** BROWNING M, PETRONZELLI F, BICK-NELL D, KRAUSA P, ROWAN A, TONKS S, MURRAY N, BODMER J, BODMER W. *Tissue Antigens* 1996; **47**: 364–371.

**147** ROSA F, BERISSI H, WEINSSENBACH J, MAROTEAUX L, FELLOUS M, REVEL M. *EMBO J* 1983; **2**: 239–243.

**148** CHEN HL, GABRILOVICH D, VIRMANI A RATNANI I, GIRGIS KR, NADAF-RAHROV S, FERNÁNDEZ-VIÑA M, CAR-BONE P. *Int J Cancer* 1996; **67**: 756–763.

**149** REAL LM, JIMÉNEZ P, CANTÓN J, KIR-KIN A, GARCÍA A, ABRIL E, ZEUTHEN J, RUIZ-CABELLO F, GARRIDO F. *Int J Cancer* 1998; **75**: 317–323.

**150** MÉNDEZ R, SERRANO A, JÄGER E, MALENO I, RUIZ-CABELLO F, KNUTH A, GARRIDO F. *Tissue Antigens*, 2001; **57**: 508–519.

**151** SANDA MG, RESTIFO NP, WALSH JC, KA-WAKAMI Y, NELSON WG, PARDOLL DM,

SIMONS JW. *J Natl Cancer Inst* 1995; **87**: 280–285.

**152** RESTIFO NP, ESQUIVEL F, KAWAKAMI Y, YEWDELL JW, MULÉ JJ, ROSENBERG SA, BENNINK JR. *J Exp Med* 1993; **177**: 265–272.

**153** BROWNING MJ, KRAUSA P, ROWAN A, HILL AB, BICKNELL DC, BODMER JG, BODMER WF. *J Immunother* 1993; **14**: 163–168.

**154** HURKS HM, METZELAAR-BLOK JA, MULDER A, CLAAS FH, JAGER MJ. *Int J Cancer* 2000; **85**: 697–702.

**155** KOOPMAN LA, MULDER A, CORVER WE, ANHOLTS JD, GIPHART MJ, CLAAS FH, FLEUREN GJ. *Tissue Antigens* 1998; **51**: 623–636.

**156** KOOPMAN LA, VAN DER SILK AR, GIP-HART MJ, FLEUREN GJ. *J Natl Cancer Inst* 1999; **91**: 1669–1677.

**157** BRADY CS, BARTHOLOMEW JS, BURT DJ, DUGGAN-KEEN GLENVILLE S, TELFORD N, LITTLE AM, DAVIDSON JA, JIMÉNEZ P, RUIZ-CABELLO F, GARRIDO F, STERN PL. *Tissue Antigens* 2000; **55**: 401–411.

**158** WANG Z, MARINCOLA FM, RIVOLTINI L, PARMIANI G, FERRONE S. *J Exp Med* 1999; **190**: 205–215.

**159** GATTONI-CELLI S, KIRSCH K, TIMPANE R, ISSELBACHER KJ. *Cancer Res* 1992; **52**: 1201–1204.

**160** SELIGER B, HOHNE A, JUNG D, KALL-FELZ M, KNUTH A, JAEGER E, BERN-HARD H, MOMBURG F, TAMPE R, HUBER C. *Exp Hematol* 1997; **25**: 608–614.

**161** SCHRIER PI, VERSTEEG R, PELTENBURG LT, PLOMP AC, VAN'T VEER LJ, KRUSE-WOLTERS KM. *Semin Cancer Biol* 1991; **2**: 73–83.

**162** SELIGER B, RITZ U, ABELE R, BOCK M, TAMPE R, SUTTER G, DREXLER I, HU-BER C, FERRPME S. *Cancer Res* 2001; **24**: 8647–50.

**163** QIN Z, BLANKENSTEIN T. *Immunity* 2000; **6**: 677–86.

# 6
# Immune Cells in the Tumor Microenvironment
Theresa L. Whiteside

## 6.1
## Introduction

Tumors create a unique microenvironment, in which all cells appear to be devoted to one purpose, i.e. that of supporting and promoting tumor progression. Although immune and inflammatory cells are frequently a component of this microenvironment, their functional status appears to be different from that of leukocytes infiltrating inflammatory sites in non-malignant tissues. Also, effects of the tumor microenvironment seem to extend beyond the tumor and systemic changes in the immune cell responses have been observed in tumor-bearing hosts. Over the years, speculations about the role of tumor-infiltrating immune cells in promoting or controlling tumor growth have been replaced by more solid information based on results of increasingly sophisticated *in situ* analyses. In this chapter, recent progress in our understanding of the immune cell interactions with the tumor will be reviewed. The complexity of these interactions and the existence of multiple ingenious ways in which tumors manage to disarm the host immune system indicate that novel approaches are necessary to immune therapies targeting human cancer.

## 6.2
## The Immune System and Tumor Progression

In man, tumor development from a single transformed cell to a clone of malignant cells forming a tumor is a multi-step process [1]. It involves multiple genetic changes, which occur in the progeny of the transformed cell over many years, accumulate and result in the establishment of the malignant phenotype characterized by uncontrolled growth [1]. The cumulative effect of these changes is to assure survival of the tumor at the expense of surrounding normal tissue cells. Thus, the tumor microenvironment within a tissue becomes modified in the course of tumor development, largely to meet its requirements and sustain its growth. Among the tissue cells surrounding the tumor and forming a scaffold supporting its expansion, cells of the hematopoietic system, lymphocytes, macrophages and granulocytes are frequently found. While the presence of the immune cells in the tumor microenvironment has been generally taken as a sign that the tumor is not ignored by the host immune system, it is important to point out that the earliest stages of tumor progression defined morphologically, i. e. hyperplasias and dysplasias, appear to be invisible to the immune system. There may be at least two explanations for this lack of the visible involvement of immune cells in the earliest phase of tumor growth: (i) the genetic modification in the tumor cell does not result in the phenotypic change at its surface and remains "silent" or (ii) the genetic change is noted, the immune response is made and the genetically unstable tumor under immune pressure develops immunoresistant variants, the phenomenon referred to as "immune selection". The immunoselection alternative appears to fit with the immune surveillance theory introduced some years ago by F. M. Burnett and others, which defined the immune system as the primary mechanism for elimination of transformed cells [2, 3]. In the modern re-interpretation, the immune surveillance hypothesis emphasizes the ability of the immune system to detect tumor cells and to destroy them. Thus, it is currently accepted that tumors are not ignored by the host immune system. On the other hand, it is also clear that tumors are not passive targets for immune intervention. Modern immune surveillance theory is based on the premise that interactions between the tumor and immune cells or their soluble products are complex, bi-directional and often result in the demise of immune rather than tumor cells.

With the identification of multiple tumor-associated antigens (TAA), which induce either humoral or cellular immune response or both, a scientifically justifiable rationale for the testing of TAA-specific immunotherapies has been obtained [4–6]. Yet, relatively modest clinical responses to these therapeutic interventions in recent years beg the question of why it has been so difficult to induce and maintain tumor-specific responses in man. In an attempt to answer this question, it becomes necessary to consider the interplay between the tumor and immune cells that takes place in the tumor microenvironment during tumor progression. Figure 6.1 is a pictorial attempt to explain some of these interactions in comparison to events that occur during the infection by an exogenous pathogen. This comparison contrasts the vigorous cellular and antibody responses generated to viral or bacterial antigens (Fig. 6.1A) with a relatively weak immune responses to TAA (Fig. 6.1B). At least one reason for the lack of robust immune responses to the tumor is the absence of a "danger signal" in the tumor microenvironment [7, 8]. The immune system perceives infections as "danger" and the tumor as "self". It responds vigorously to contain the external danger introduced by a pathogen and only weakly, if at all, to TAA, which are largely self-antigens or altered self-antigens (Fig. 6.1). Tolerance to self that needs to be overcome for a full-scale immune response to TAA is one, but not the only, detriment to the generation of effective anti-tumor immune responses [9]. The nature of the tumor microenvironment characterized by the presence of immunosuppressive factors, and by the excess of antigens produced and released by the growing tumor is clearly not the optimal venue for the immune cells. However, the immune response to the pathogens or TAA takes place in the lymph nodes draining the infected tissue or the tumor and not in the tumor microenvironment. It is, therefore, reasonable to postulate that effects of the pathogen and the tumor alike are not only local but also systemic, affecting the host immune system as a whole. As discussed below, this appears to be the case.

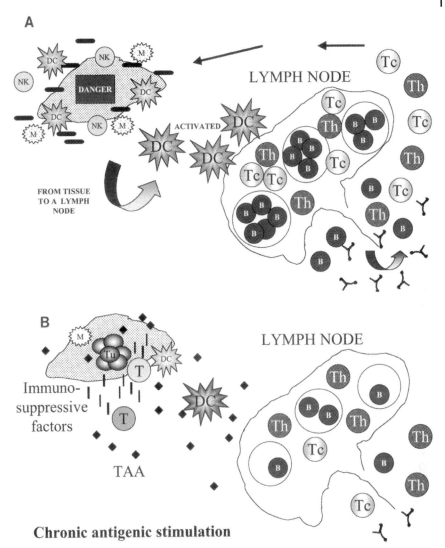

**Fig. 6.1** Schematic representations of immune responses to a pathogen (A), which presents a danger signal or to a tumor (B), which presents largely self-epitopes to the immune system and also produces and releases iimmunoinhibitory factors. In the absence of the "danger signal" a weak immune response is generated.

## 6.3
### Immune Cells in the Tumor Microenvironment

Pathologists have long ago called attention to the fact that human tumors are often surrounded by as well as infiltrated with mononuclear cells [10, 11]. The role of tumor-infiltrating lymphocytes (TIL) in tumor progression remains a highly controver-

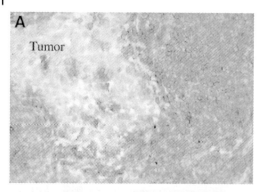

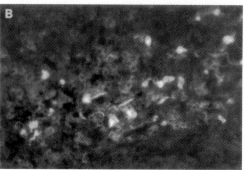

**Fig. 6.2** T lymphocytes in the tumor microenvironment. In (A), a mass of HLA-DR[+] T cells surrounds the tumor. Immunoperoxidase staining of the biopsy obtained from a patient with head and neck cancer. Original magnification: × 400. In (B), a cluster of CD8[+] T cells (red) infiltrating a human head and neck cancer. Apoptotic T cells (TUNEL[+] whitish) are evident among the CD8[+] T cells. A TUNEL reagent was used in combination with immunoperoxidase staining. Original magnification: × 400. Dr T. E. Reichert, U. Mainz, Germany contributed Fig. 2(B). (see color plates page XXV)

sial issue, with evidence ushered in support of as well as against the TIL involvement in the control of tumor growth [12]. Figure 6.2(A) depicts the tumor surrounded by a mass of lymphocytes. In an effort to summarize the body of available literature, it is necessary to stress that not all tumors are similarly well infiltrated or surrounded by immune cells, and that both the size and the composition of tumor infiltrates vary widely even among the tumors of the same histologic type. The diagram shown in Fig. 6.3 indicates that cells mediating innate as well as adaptive immunity may be present at the tumor site. Further, a variety of soluble products, including cytokines and antibodies, may be released by these cells in response to non-specific or tumor-

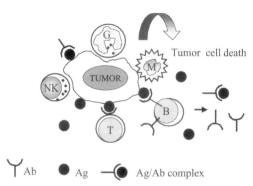

**Fig. 6.3** Diagram depicting interactions of various immune cells with the tumor. In the presence of immune cells, the tumor is expected to fail. Instead, it usually continues to progress.

specific signals in the microenvironment. Theoretically, it is the anti-tumor effects of these products as well as direct interactions of the immune cells with the tumor that should lead to its demise. In most cases, however, the tumor grows progressively and metastasizes, largely because it evolves strategies to escape the immune intervention and to debilitate the immune system ([13] and see below).

Among the various cells present at the tumor site, T cells have received the most attention. This may be because some early histologic and immunohistologic studies indicated that not only prognosis but also survival of patients with solid tumors correlated positively with the size of the lymphocytic infiltrates [14, 15]. These infiltrates were later shown to consist largely of CD3$^+$ cells, which proliferated *ex vivo* in the presence of interleukin (IL)-2 [16]. In fact, TIL isolated from human tumors and expanded *ex vivo* in IL-2 were used for adoptive immunotherapy of patients with advanced malignancies by Rosenberg and others [17]. The results suggested that adoptively transferred TIL could exert anti-tumor effects, although only 15–20% of patients with advanced cancers who received this therapy had objective clinical responses [17]. A number of subsequent immunohistologic studies attempting to relate the number of TIL to prognosis or survival of patients with cancer failed to confirm the early results (reviewed in [18]). With more recent advances in methodologies allowing not only for the phenotypic but also functional *in situ* analysis, characteristics of TIL in human solid tumors became defined and the role of TIL in tumor progression was, in part, clarified.

## 6.4.
### Phenotypic and Functional Characteristics of Immune Cells Present at the Tumor Site

Immune cell infiltrates in the tumor microenvironment are largely composed of T lymphocytes (reviewed in [18]). In various tumor types, macrophages, dendritic cells (DCs) and B cells are represented with different frequencies. Characteristics of these immune cells present at the tumor site are briefly summarized below.

### 6.4.1.
### T Cells

T cells [CD3$^+$ T cell receptor (TCR)$^+$] found in the tumor microenvironment appear morphologically as small lymphocytes. The hypothesis that TIL-T represent autotumor-specific T cells has been debated for a long time and there is evidence in support of clonal TCR V$_\beta$ restriction of freshly isolated TIL as well as for their ability to recognize autologous tumor cells in some cases [19, 20]. The phenotypic analysis of T cells in human tumors shows that TIL-T are memory lymphocytes expressing either CD8 or CD4 markers, although the CD4/CD8 ratio may be highly variable from one tumor to another [18]. In several studies, the CD4/CD8 ratio was found to be reduced as a result of enrichment in CD8$^+$ T cells [21, 22], in contrast with non-malignant inflammatory infiltrates, which consist largely of CD4$^+$ T cells. Furthermore, some reports have linked a high tumor content of CD8$^+$ T cells with a better prognosis [15], although no consistent data supporting this finding had been obtained. The phenotypic and functional characteristics of T cells found in human tumors are listed in Tab. 6.1. In considering properties of these cells, the first striking observation was that a vast majority of TIL-T expressed phenotypic markers of activation, i.e. were HLA-DR$^+$ and often also CD25$^+$ (reviewed in [18]). By this criterion, TIL-T are in the state of activation, ready for elimination of suitable targets. However, when proliferative and anti-tumor functions of freshly isolated TIL-T were evaluated in conventional *ex vivo* assays, it appeared that they were significantly depressed compared with equivalent functions of normal T cells [23]. The cytokine profile of these cells was also different from that of normal activated T cells in that either no or little type 1 cytokines [IL-2, interferon (IFN)-$\gamma$] were produced by TIL-T, but instead they appeared to preferentially secrete down-regulatory cytokines, IL-10 and transforming growth factor (TGF)-$\beta$ [24]. These data suggested that TIL-T expressing an activation phenotype were, in fact, functionally compromised. The loss of function was not an all-or-none phenomenon, as some TIL-T retained substantial levels of effector cell function, while others, particularly those isolated from advanced cancers and from metastatic lesions, often had none. This pattern of functional defects seemed to be related to the tumor burden and was consistent with tumor-induced immunosuppression [25]. More recent *in situ* studies of signaling molecules in TIL-T confirm these earlier observations by demonstrating that expression of the TCR-associated $\zeta$ chain as well as that of the transcription factor regulating expression of a number of immune and inflammatory genes, NF-$\kappa$B, is significantly decreased in TIL-T compared to their expression in T cells obtained from the peripheral circulation of normal donors [26, 27]. In a study comprising over 130 cases of human oral cell carcinomas, expression of $\zeta$ in TIL-T was found to be an independent and highly statistically significant biomarker of prognosis and survival in patients with stage III and IV disease [28]. The patients with tumors infiltrated by T cells with low or absent $\zeta$ expression had significantly shorter 5-year survival compared to the patients with tumors infiltrated by T cells with normal $\zeta$ expression [28]. Stimulus-dependent activation of NF$\kappa$B was found to be impaired in T cells of patients with renal cell carcinoma (RCC). In some patients, the primary defect was the failure of the transactivating complex RelA/NF-$\kappa$B1 (p50) to accumulate in the nucleus following T cell activation due to a defect in phosphorylation and degradation of the inhibitor I$\kappa$B$\alpha$ [29, 30]. In other patients, NF-$\kappa$B activation was defective despite normal stimulus-dependent degradation of I$\kappa$B$\alpha$ [31]. In both situations, this defective state could be induced by exposure of normal T cells to supernatants of RCC and the soluble product responsible was identified as an RCC-derived ganglioside [31]. Impaired NF-$\kappa$B activity may contribute to reduced T cell function seen in TIL-T present in RCC, since this transcription factor controls expression of a number of genes encoding cytokines, their receptors and other membrane regulatory molecules essential for T cell activation [32, 33]. It is important to note that defects in function of the $\zeta$ chain and activation of NF-$\kappa$B are observed in TIL-T as well as circulating T cells of patients with cancer [34, 35]. These signaling defects in T cells are both local and systemic and may be related to the tumor burden. Taken together, functional studies of TIL-T obtained from a variety of human solid tumors in many different laboratories indicate that these cells are func-

**Tab. 6.1** Morphologic, phenotypic and functional characteristics of TIL found in human solid tumors

| 1. Morphology | small to large lymphocytes |
|---|---|
| 2. Phenotype | CD3$^+$TCR$\alpha$/$\beta^+$ T cells; few (<5%) CD3$^-$CD56$^+$ NK cells |
| | mix of CD4$^+$and CD8$^+$ cells; high proportions of CD8$^+$ cells reported in some tumors |
| | variable CD4/CD8 ratio |
| | increased proportions of double-negative (CD4$^-$CD8$^-$) T cells |
| | largely CD45RO$^+$ memory cells |
| | express activation markers (CD25, HLA-DR) |
| | nearly all are CD95$^+$ |
| 3. Clonality | oligoclonal as determined by TCR V$_\beta$ gene expression |
| 4. Function | low or absent $\zeta$ chain expression: inefficient TCR signaling |
| | suppressed NF-$\kappa$B activation |
| | depressed locomotion, proliferation, cytotoxicity |
| | cytokine profile: no/little IL-2 or IFN-$\gamma$ production; excess of IL-10 or TGF-$\beta$ |
| | *in vitro* response to IL-2 variable, but more depressed in TIL recovered from metastatic than primary lesions |
| | increased levels of caspase-3 activity |
| | apoptosis of CD8$^+$ T cells (TUNEL$^+$) |

tionally incompetent, possibly because of the inhibitory effects of the tumor microenvironment. In addition, it appears that the lack of functions in TIL-T rather than the number or phenotype of T cells infiltrating the tumor may be important in predicting patient survival.

### 6.4.2
### Natural Killer (NK) Cells

NK cells (CD3$^-$CD56$^+$CD16$^+$) mediate innate immunity. Characteristically, they contain perforin- and granzyme-rich granules, and are able to lyse NK-sensitive tumor targets without prior sensitization (reviewed in [36]). Furthermore, NK cells express Fc$\gamma$RIII and are largely responsible for mediating antibody-dependent cellular cytotoxicity (ADCC) [36]. Recent data suggest that NK cells constitutively express several ligands of the tumor necrosis factor (TNF) family and can induce apoptosis in a broad variety of tumor cell targets [37]. This apoptotic mechanism of tumor cell elimination may be of a greater biologic importance than secretory, granule-mediated killing, largely because most tumor cells express receptors for the TNF family ligands and are sensitive to death by apoptosis [37]. Macrophages and DCs present in the tumor microenvironment phagocytose apoptotic tumor cells and process them for subsequent presentation to T cells, thereby promoting cellular and humoral antitumor responses. Circulating NK cells as well as those found in tissues are not only cytotoxic effector cells, but might also be able to significantly contribute to driving immune responses to TAA [38, 39]. Thus, NK cells appear to be well equipped for interfering with the processes of tumor growth and metastasis. They are able to discriminate between normal and abnormal cells, mainly because they express receptors which enable them to survey the target for the presence of class I MHC molecules [40]. These receptors are of two types: killer inhibitory receptors (KIRs) and killer activating receptors (KARs) [41, 42]. NK cell functions and their interactions with other cells or the extracellular matrix (ECM) molecules are regulated through these receptors and Fcγ receptors (FcγRs).

NK cells are strategically distributed throughout body fluids and tissues. Studies of NK cell localization in human tissues have been difficult, however, because immunostaining for NK cells has not been reliable. The anti-NK cell antibodies which work well in flow cytometry are not useful for phenotyping in tissues, especially in paraffin-embedded human specimens [43]. Antibodies specific for perforin or granzymes are more reliable immunostaining reagents, with a caveat that activated cells other than NK cells may be enriched in granules containing these components. Therefore, much of the information about NK cell distribution in human tissues, including tumors, is derived from studies performed with freshly isolated NK cells using flow cytometry for phenotyping and $^{51}$Cr-release assays with K562 as targets, which measure the capability of these effector cells to induce secretory or necrotic killing [37]. Tissues that are known to contain the largest proportions of activated NK cells include the liver, lungs and the placenta during pregnancy [36, 43]. Lymphocytic infiltrates associated with infections in these organs contain numerous activated NK cells [44]. Importantly, however, hepatocellular carcinomas, colon tumors metastatic to liver, lung cancers or ovarian carcinomas are not found to be enriched in NK cells [43]. In general, few NK cells have been observed in lymphocytic infiltrates of human solid tumors and particularly of advanced lesions, although they may be a more prominent component of early lesions or tumors associated with viral infections, such as the cervical carcinoma [18, 36]. The presence of NK cells in inflammatory but not neoplastic conditions suggests either that their primary biologic role is elimination of infectious targets rather than tumor cells [45] or that the tumor microenvironment preferentially induces their demise. The available evidence appears to point to the latter possibility. Indeed, it has been observed that NK cells purified from ascites of women with ovarian carcinoma have profoundly depressed responses to IL-2 (Fig. 6.4) [46] and express low levels of message for IFN-_ but significantly increased levels of mRNA for IL-10 compared to normal circulating NK cells (Fig. 6.5). Furthermore, relative to normal NK cells, decreased or absent expression of the ζ chain, associated in NK cells with FcγRIII, was observed in NK cells obtained from ovarian ascites as well as in circulating NK cells of patients with several types of cancer, including melanoma (Fig. 6.6). Our recent studies suggest that among circulating NK cells in patients with breast cancer, a subset of CD56$^{bright}$CD16$^{dim}$ NK cells, which represents about 95% of all NK cells and is responsible for effector functions, preferentially binds Annexin V and thus is primed for apoptosis (unpublished data). These patients also had significantly lower NK activity than the age- and sex-matched healthy controls tested in parallel, an indication that Annexin-binding NK cells were indeed functionally impaired. These and other recent observations suggest that endogenous circulating or tissue-resident NK cells have the potential to play a role in tumor surveillance and control of metastasis dissemination. However, once the tumor is established, it might subvert anti-tumor functions of NK cells, especially in

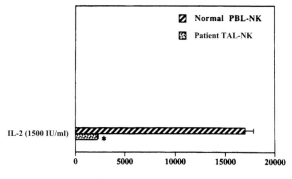

**Fig. 6.4** Proliferative responses of tumor-associated NK cells as compared to NK cells isolated from normal peripheral blood mononuclear cells. The [³H]thymidine uptake was determined after a 3-day culture in the presence of IL-2. The results are mean c.p.m. counts ± SD of cell cultures established with cells of four patients and four normal donors. The asterisk indicates a significantly reduced proliferation of TAL-NK cells as compared to that of normal NK cells ($p < 0.001$). Reproduced with permission from Lai *et al.* [46]. © AACR.

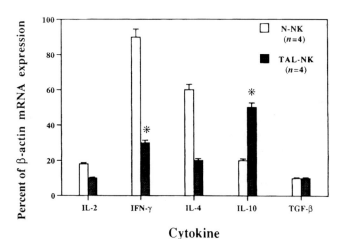

**Fig. 6.5** Expression of cytokine genes in ovarian tumor-associated NK cells (TAL-NK) as compared with normal peripheral blood lymphocyte NK cells. The data are means ± SEM of the ratio between a cytokine mRNA expression and β-actin. Hot RT-PCR assays were performed and cytokine mRNA expression relative to that of β-actin was calculated after measuring levels of ³²P in a Phosphorimager. The asterisks indicate significant differences ($p < 0.01$) between experimental and control specimens. Reproduced with permission from Rabinowich *et al. Int. J. Cancer* 1996; **68**: 276–284. © Wiley-Liss, Inc.

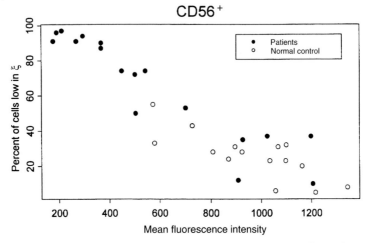

**Fig. 6.6** Correlations between the percent of CD3⁻CD56⁺ NK cells expressing low ζ versus mean fluorescence index (MFI) for ζ. The percentage of NK cells with low ζ expression in the circulation of 17 patients with melanoma or 15 normal controls was obtained by taking the mean of MFI established for all normal controls – 2 SD as the cut-off point for calculating cell frequencies. The correlation for NK cells was negative ($r = 0.92$; $p < 0.0001$) and the patients had significantly higher percentages of NK cells with low æ than normal controls. Reproduced with permission from Dworacki *et al.* [98]. © AACR.

the subsets of NK cells found at the sites of metastasis and those responsible for cytotoxic functions.

NK cells constitutively express IL-2 receptor and are able to rapidly respond to IL-2 stimulation [47]. Subsets of IL-2-activated NK cells such as A-NK cells, for example, are potent anti-tumor effector cells which have been used for therapy of cancer in animal models of tumor growth [48] and in human clinical trials of patients with cancer [49]. Studies in pre-clinical tumor models in mice suggest that genetically modified tumors secreting IL-2 become infiltrated by NK cells and rejected, in contrast to mock-transfected tumors, which harbor few NK cells and grow progressively [50]. In these experiments performed in nude mice, IL-2 secreted locally by implanted tumor cells was able to mobilize and activate endogenous NK cells, which in the absence of T cells were able to induce tumor regression [50]. Although this model of tumor growth in immunodeficient mice is obviously limited in its therapeutic implications, it serves to confirm *in vitro* data, which indicate that IL-2-activated NK cells are potentially effective in controlling tumor growth, even when T cells are not present. Another lesson learned from these experiments is that the lack of IL-2 may be a determining factor in the relative paucity of NK cells in the tumor microenvironment. Indeed, it has been shown that human tumors are depleted of IL-2 and IFN-γ, and this would make it difficult, if not impossible, to sustain any substantial level of anti-tumor activity in NK or any other lymphoid cells found at the site [51].

6.4.3.
## DCs

DCs (*Lin⁻*CD80⁺CD86⁺HLA-DR⁺) are the most potent antigen-presenting cells (APCs). DCs are a heterogeneous population of highly motile cells that originate from the precursors in the bone marrow and migrate through the blood stream to peripheral non-lymphoid tissues, capturing antigens. Antigen presentation to T cells by DCs takes place in the lymph nodes or other T cell-rich areas of secondary lymphoid organs [52]. DCs are present in tumors, often in substantial numbers [53]. In tumor-bearing hosts, DCs are responsible for the uptake, processing and cross-presentation of TAA to naïve or memory T cells, thus playing a crucial role in the generation of tumor-specific effector T cells. Because anti-tumor immune responses are inefficient in tumor-bearing individuals, it has been suggested that DCs are also subverted by the tumor. Considerable evidence in support of this hypothesis is available. Phenotypic and functional alterations in DCs infiltrating human tumors as well as DCs recovered from the peripheral circulation of patients with cancer have been reported [54, 55]. The cytokine profile of DCs varies depending on the nature of the microenvironment they infiltrate [52]. Tumor-associated DC (TADCs) appear to be at a particular disadvantage, because tumors or tumor-derived factors have been shown to induce DC apoptosis or impair their maturation [56, 57]. Co-culture of murine or human DCs (obtained from isolated CD34⁺ precursors or plastic-adherent mononuclear cells) with a variety of tumor cell lines for 4–48 h resulted in apoptotic death of DCs, as verified by morphology, TUNEL assays, Annexin binding, caspase activation and DNA laddering [58]. Tumor cells induced DC apoptosis by direct contact or through release of soluble factors. Furthermore, TADC isolated from tumors contained a high proportion of apoptotic cells [58]. Tumor-induced apoptosis of DC was inhibited in the presence of IL-12 and IL-15, an indication that cytokines might regulate DC generation and survival. In fact, these cytokines were shown to stimulate expression of Bcl-2 and Bcl-X$_L$ in DCs and to protect them from tumor-induced apoptosis [59]. Experiments performed by Shurin and colleagues further demonstrated that tumor-derived factors, e.g. gangliosides, inhibited DC generation and their function *in vitro* [60]. This suppressive effect of gangliosides on DCs was found to be mediated by tumor-derived vascular endothelial growth factor (VEGF), a known anti-dendropoietic factor [57]. Importantly, cytokines (IL-12, IL-15 and FLT3L) were found to promote DC generation and their functions by exerting a protective anti-apoptotic effect, while tumor-derived factors caused apoptosis in mature DCs and inhibited differentiation of hematopoietic precursors into DCs. These studies underscore the role of the microenvironment in shaping the functional potential of DCs and perhaps other immune cells.

The DC compartment is comprised of subpopulations of morphologically and functionally distinct cells, depending on their hematopoietic origin, maturation stage or tissue localization [61]. The two main subpopulations are myeloid-derived DCs (DC1) and lymphoid-derived DCs (DC2). While in man this distinction is somewhat blurred, many phenotypic and functional differences exist between monocyte-derived CD11c⁺ DC and CD11c⁻CD123⁺ (IL-3 receptor α^high) lymphoid-derived DC

[61]. Furthermore, a division of labor exists among DCs, in that immature CD83⁻ DC are primarily responsible for antigen uptake, while mature CD83⁺ DC are excellent APCs [61]. Several reports showed that DC obtained from peripheral blood mononuclear cells of patients with cancer had lower than normal expression of HLA-DR and co-stimulatory molecules, and had depressed stimulatory activity [54, 62]. Our own recent studies in patients with head and neck cancer indicated that while the percentage of total LIN-DR⁺ DC was comparable in the circulation of patients and controls (1.6 versus 1.5%), DR expression on individual DCs was clearly decreased in patients relative to that in control DC [63]. When we determined the proportions of LIN-DR⁺CD123⁺ versus LIN-DR⁺CD11c⁺ subsets of DCs in the circulation by multicolor flow cytometry, we found that myeloid-derived DCs were significantly depleted in patients compared to controls [63]. After tumor surgery, significant normalization of the proportion of myeloid DCs was observed. These data suggest that an imbalance in DC subsets and the paucity of co-stimulatory molecules on DC are consequences of the malignancy, and mechanisms responsible for these alterations are under investigation.

The data on functional impairments of TADC have to be balanced by numerous reports in the literature, which suggest that the presence of DCs in tumors is associated with improved prognosis [64, 65]. DC infiltrations into tumors have been associated with significantly prolonged patient survival, and reduced incidence of recurrent or metastatic disease in patients with bladder, lung, laryngeal, oral, gastric and nasopharyngeal carcinomas [66–72]. In contrast, patients with lesions reported to be scarcely infiltrated with DC had a relatively poor prognosis [73]. Fewer DC were observed in metastatic than primary lesions [74]. In a recent study, we demonstrated that the number of S-100⁺ DC present in the tumor was by far the strongest independent predictor of overall survival as well as disease-free survival and time to recurrence in 132 patients with oral carcinoma, compared with such well-established prognostic factors as disease stage or lymph node involvement [65]. Another striking observation we made concerns the relationship between the number of DC in the tumor and expression of the TCR-associated $\zeta$ chain in TIL. The paucity of DC in the tumor was significantly related to the loss of $\zeta$ expression in TIL and these two factors had a highly significant effect on patient overall survival. As illustrated in Fig. 6.7, the poorest survival and the greatest risk was observed in patients with tumors that had small number of DC and little or no $\zeta$ expression in TIL ($p = 2.4 \times 10^{-8}$). These data suggest that both the number of DC and the presence of functionally unimpaired T cells in the tumor microenvironment are important for overall survival of patients with cancer. Interactions of DC and T cells in the tumor appear to sustain TCR-mediated, and presumably tumor-directed, functions of the T cells infiltrating the same area. It is possible that DC protect T cells from tumor-induced immune suppression, although the mechanism responsible for such protection remains unknown.

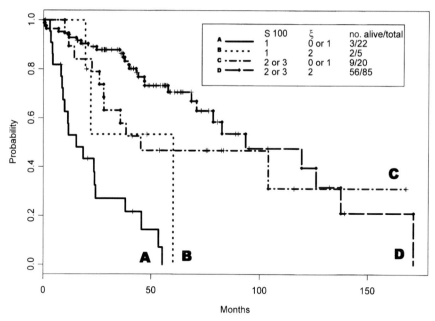

| | S 100 | ξ | no. alive/total |
|---|---|---|---|
| A ——— | 1 | 0 or 1 | 3/22 |
| B ······ | 1 | 2 | 2/5 |
| C ·—·— | 2 or 3 | 0 or 1 | 9/20 |
| D ——— | 2 or 3 | 2 | 56/85 |

**Fig. 6.7** Kaplan–Meier survival curves generated by multivariate analysis. Overall survival of 132 patients with oral carcinoma according to the S-100 expression on tumor-infiltrating DC and ξ chain expression in TIL. The numbers of DC were determined by microscopic counts of immunostained tumor sections: 1 = low numbers of S-100⁺ DC; 2 = intermediate numbers of S-100⁺ DC; 3 = high numbers of S-100⁺DC. TIL were defined based on immunocytochemistry as follows: 0 or 1 = cells with no or low ξ expression; and 2 = cells with normal ξ expression. Lines A–D identify groups of patients assigned to each category as indicated in the inset. Reproduced with permission from Reichert *et al. Cancer* 2001; **91**: 2136–2147. © American Cancer Society/Wiley-Liss, Inc.

## 6.4.4
## Macrophages

Macrophages (CD14⁺) are commonly found in human tumors and are referred to as tumor-associated macrophages (TAM). While normal macrophages are APCs which play an important role in control of infections, TAM are re-programmed to inhibit lymphocyte functions through a release of specific cytokines, prostaglandins or reactive oxygen metabolites (ROM). It is hypothesized that re-programming of TAM occurs in the tumor microenvironment as a result of tumor-driven activation [75]. Evidence has accumulated indicating that invasiveness of tumors, e. g. human primary colon carcinomas, is directly related to the number of TAM detected in the tumor [76]. In invasive breast cancer, an increased TAM count is an independent predictor of reduced relapse-free survival as well as reduced overall survival [77]. The available data support the active role of TAM in tumor-induced immunosuppression, on the one hand, and in the promotion of tumor growth, on the other. The mechanisms that contribute to TAM-mediated inhibition of immune cells are probably numerous, but much attention has been recently devoted to the role of NADPH-dependent ROM, such as superoxide anion or hydrogen peroxide, as potential inhibitors of TIL [78]. T cell proliferation and NK-mediated anti-tumor cytotoxicity are profoundly inhibited by macrophage-derived ROM *in vitro* [79]. T and NK cells isolated from human tumors have a decreased expression of CD3ζ and FcγRIII-associated ζ, respectively, and this down-modulation of ζ, a critical signal-transducing molecule, is apparently induced by ROM produced by TAM [78]. The changes observed in TIL – a loss of normal ζ expression accompanied by a decreased ability to proliferate and subsequent apoptotic cell death – correspond to similar changes induced in T and NK cells co-cultured with activated macrophages [79]. Removal of macrophages from these cultures restores T and NK cell functions [79]. The overall conclusion from these studies is that iimmunoinhibitory activities of TAM, whether due to oxidative stress or to release of inhibitory cytokines, such as IL-10, contribute to making the tumor microenvironment a particularly unfriendly milieu for immune cells [80].

### 6.4.5
### B Cells

B cells (CD19⁺CD20⁺) are uncommon components of human solid tumors. While anti-tumor antibodies are frequently detected in the circulation of cancer patients, these antibodies are made and secreted by plasma cells situated in the tumor draining lymph nodes, spleen or other lymphoid tissues. In some carcinomas, plasma cells may be present and, occasionally, represent a substantial infiltrating element [81]. The significance of their presence at the tumor site or their prognostic importance is unknown, although it might be that the ability to make antibodies *in situ* may be an important aspect of host defense.

In aggregate, functional assessments of tumor-associated cells responsible for mediating anti-tumor immune responses indicate that these cells may not be able to function optimally or, as is the case with TAM, are stimulated to perform inhibitory functions. The degree of impairment of immune cells in the tumor microenvironment differs widely in individual tumors. While the inhibitory effects are strongest in the tumor, they extend to include the peripheral immune system. As a result, both local and systemic anti-tumor immunity is impaired in patients with cancer. It is important to note that these patients generally have normal immune responses to recall antigens and can mount normal primary responses, except for those with terminal cancers. The possible mechanisms involved in selective and persistent inhibition of anti-tumor immune responses in patients with cancer are discussed below.

### 6.5
### Mechanisms Linked to Dysfunction of Immune Cells in Cancer

In considering cellular interactions that take place in the tumor microenvironment, three obvious candidates responsible for inhibition of immune responses emerge. First is the tumor itself, and there is convincing evidence demonstrating that co-in-

**Tab. 6.2** Molecularly defined immunoinhibitory factors produced by human tumors[a]

| | |
|---|---|
| 1. TNF family ligands | induce apoptosis via the TNF family receptors |
|    FasL | Fas |
|    TRAIL | TRAIL-R |
|    TNF | TNF-R1 |
| 2. Cytokines | |
|    TGF-β | inhibits perforin and granzyme mRNA expression; inhibits lymphocyte proliferation |
|    IL-10 | inhibits cytokine production, including that of IL-12 |
|    granulocyte macrophage colony stimulating factor | promotes expansion of immunosuppressive tumor-associated macrophages [119] |
|    ZIP (ζ-inhibitory protein) | mediates degradation of ζ or inhibits its mRNA expression [120] |
| 3. Small molecules | |
|    prostaglandin $E_2$ | inhibits leukocyte functions via increased cAMP |
|    epinephrine | inhibits leukocyte functions via increased cAMP |
|    ROM | inhibits leukocyte functions via superoxide generation |
| 4. Viral-related products | |
|    p15E (CKS-17, synthetic peptide) | inhibits production of type I cytokines, up-regulates IL-10 synthesis |
|    EBI-3 (homologue of IL-12 p40) | inhibits IL-12 production |
| 5. Tumor-associated gangliosides | inhibit IL-2-dependent lymphocyte proliferation, induce apoptotic signals, suppress NF-κB activation, interfere with DC generation |

[a] This partial listing of tumor-associated immunoinhibitory factors has been modified from a review by Whiteside and Rabinowich [13]. It demonstrates the diversity of mechanisms that human tumors are known to have evolved in order to incapacitate the host immune system.

cubation of activated T cells with tumor cells induces signaling defects, impaired functions and apoptosis [13, 35]. Table 6.2 is a partial list of tumor-derived factors that have been described to exert immunosuppressive effects. Second, TAM or TADC upon ingesting apoptotic or necrotic tumor cells or activated by TAA–antibody complexes may be a source of oxidative radicals, immunosuppressive cytokines or suppressive small molecules, as described above. Third, subsets of TIL could become activated and exercise suppressive functions with respect to other T cells present in the microenvironment. It is possible, even likely, that all three scenarios are simultaneously enacted in tumors. Their interplay may vary, depending on the local conditions. It is certain, however, that this interplay leads to sustained local and systemic suppression of anti-tumor immune cells in tumor-bearing hosts. A mechanism that may be common to all three, and is certainly utilized by tumors and T lymphocytes involves the apoptosis-inducing members of the TNA family of receptors and ligands.

6.5.1
**The CD95–CD95 Ligand (CD95L) Pathway**

The CD95–CD95L pathway has been implicated in tumor-mediated apoptosis of immune cells, contributing to immune privilege of tumors [82]. CD95L ([Fas ligand (FasL)] is expressed on the surface of a wide variety of tumor cells [83–88], and mRNA for FasL has been detected in cultured tumor cells and in tumor tissues by *in situ* hybridization (reviewed in [89]). A controversy that developed in respect to FasL expression in tumor cells can perhaps be explained based on its well-documented cleavage into soluble fragments by membrane associated matrix metalloproteinases (MMPs), resulting in its removal from the cell surface of tumors [90, 91]. Also, mRNA expression of FasL may be weak in some tumors, perhaps because of its very rapid turnover, which implies that many cycles of amplification may be necessary for its detection by reverse transcription-polymerase chain reaction (RT-PCR). As these mechanisms are likely to differ in magnitude in various tumor cells, depending on the cellular MMP profile, surface expression of FasL is a highly variable trait in these cells. Nevertheless, *in situ* studies indicate that a substantial proportion of T cells undergo apoptosis at the tumor site [26]. Furthermore, we observed that $CD8^+$ T cells present in the tumor are particularly sensitive to apoptosis (see Fig. 6.2B). Functional *in vitro* studies as well as immunohistology *in situ* indicate that FasL expressed in tumors is able to induce apoptosis of lymphocytes [83, 85]. The presence and numbers of apoptotic TIL in the tumor appear to correlate with FasL expression on the tumor cells [83, 85]. A number of recent studies have correlated the level of FasL expression on tumor cells to poor prognosis and survival in patients with cancer [92–94]. In addition to the ability of such tumor cells to induce immune cell apoptosis, expression of FasL might also provide them with an advantage in metastasizing and colonizing distant organs, for example, liver [95]. *In vitro*, co-culture of $FasL^+$ tumor cells with activated $Fas^+$ T lymphocytes was shown to induce lymphocyte apoptosis, which could be blocked in the presence of anti-FasL antibodies or Fas–Fc constructs as well as anti-Fas antibodies and caspase inhibitors [85]. Tumor cell lines stably transduced with the FasL gene, so that they not only expressed but also secreted FasL and their supernatants rapidly induced apoptosis of $Fas^+$ T cells [85, 96]. These co-culture experiments were criticized as inconclusive, because of the possibility that apoptosis of T cells was not induced by the tumor, but by fratricidal death of the T cells activated in the presence of the tumor [97]. However, using a variety of anti-FasL antibodies and amplification strategies, we do not detect FasL expression on T cells co-incubated with the tumor or on the surface of T lymphocytes freshly isolated from the circulation of patients with cancer [85, 98]. We, therefore, attribute the observed apoptosis to the effects mediated by the tumor and refer to it as tumor-induced cell death (TICD). It is possible that lymphocytes are also dying in consequence of their activation in the tumor microenvironment by activation-induced cell death (AICD). In any event, it is the presence of the tumor that brings about the demise of immune cells. It is also important to remember that not only T cells but also DC and macrophages are susceptible to apoptosis in the tumor microenvironment, which is distinctly anti-inflammatory [59].

6.5.2
**T Lymphocyte Apoptosis in Patients with Cancer**

Lymphocytes in the circulation of patients with cancer have been observed to express Fas and bind Annexin V. As many as 95% of circulating T cells express Fas in some patients and $Fas^+CD3^+$ cells have been shown to preferentially bind Annexin V [99, 100]. These T cells also have high levels of caspase-3 activity and reduced or absent expression of the TCR-associated $\zeta$ protein [98–100]. The significantly elevated proportions of T cells with this pre-apoptotic profile in the circulation of patients with cancer relative to healthy controls suggest that a rapid turnover of T cells occurs in these patients. As the patients with cancer are generally not lymphopenic, it has to be assumed that new lymphocytes are being recruited from the precursors in the bone marrow to replace those undergoing apoptosis. We recently found that $CD3^+CD8^+$ T cells as well as $CD3^+CD8^+CD28^-$ and $CD3^+$ $CD8^+CD45RO^-CD27^-$ sub-populations of "effector" T cells contained especially high proportions of $\zeta^{low}$ or Annexin-binding cells in patients with cancer, an indication that these subsets were preferentially targeted for apoptosis ([100] and unpublished data). Preliminary results suggest that consumption of sFasL and its binding to Fas expressed by these T cells may be, in part, responsible for the high proportions of dying T cells seen in the circulation, because sFasL levels in the patients' sera were found to be significantly decreased relative to those in the sera of normal age- and sex-matched controls (unpublished data). Also, there appears to be a significant association between the frequency of circulating T cells with the pre-apoptotic phenotype and disease activity, with the highest proportions of Annexin-binding, $Fas^+$ T cells and lowest sFasL serum levels seen in the patients with active disease. In aggregate, these results suggest to us that in tumor-bearing hosts, effects of the tumor microenvironment extend far beyond the tumor, and that the presence of tumor has profound effects on lymphocyte homeostasis, kinetics of recirculation and levels of activation.

6.5.3
**Tumor Sensitivity to FasL-Mediated Signals**

Expression of FasL as well as Fas on the surface of tumor cells implies that tumors might be sensitive to Fas–FasL-mediated apoptosis. Most human tumors express more Fas than FasL on the cell surface, as determined by *in situ* immunostaining [101]. However, using tumor cell lines, we failed to observe any correlation between the level of Fas expression and tumor cell sensitivity to FasL-mediated apoptosis [101]. It appears that Fas, although expressed on tumor cells, is not a functional receptor in many cases. The mechanisms responsible for resistance of human tumors to FasL-mediated apoptosis may vary, but in most cases they involve overexpression of one or another of apoptosis-inhibitory proteins [102]. One of the more extensively studied inhibitors of the Fas–FasL pathway, cFLIP, interacts with FADD in the DISC complex, preventing cleavage of pro-caspase 8 and blocking the apoptotic cascade [102]. Another inhibitor, which may be overexpressed in some tumor cells, is a Fas-associated phosphatase named FAP-1 [103]. In addition to utilizing these natural inhibitors, tumors may down-regulate Fas and thus avoid FasL-mediated death. On balance, Fas$^+$-activated T cells appear to be much more sensitive to FasL-mediated apoptosis than tumor cells, which have devised multiple ways of protecting themselves and surviving.

### 6.5.4
### A Dual Biologic Role of FasL

FasL is a death-inducing as well as pro-inflammatory molecule [104]. *In vivo* experiments, in which tumor cells transfected with FasL cDNA and expressing FasL were implanted in animals demonstrated that, contrary to expectations, such cells were rapidly rejected and that the rejection was mediated by granulocytes accumulating at the site of tumor implantation [105]. In an elegant series of experiments, Nabel and colleagues showed that in mice injected subcutaneously with genetically modified CT26-CD95L tumor cells, infiltrating neutrophils eliminated the tumor. However, the same CT26-CD95L cells survived in the intraocular site, because of the presence in this location of TGF-β, which inhibited p38 MAP kinase activity in neutrophils and thus disabled their anti-tumor functions. Neutrophils, which accumulated at the site in response to FasL, were thus unable to exercise their anti-tumor effects in the presence of TGF-β, with the net result of promoting tumor growth by disabling the effector cells [106]. Thus, TGF-β was able to override the pro-inflammatory effects of FasL, an indication that cytokines produced in the tumor microenvironment can regulate immunosuppressive versus pro-inflammatory activity of this ligand. This "contextual" regulation of FasL activity strongly suggests that the final outcome of interactions between tumor and immune cells depends on the tumor microenvironment. It is, therefore, not in the least surprising that conflicting results emerge from various studies probing these interactions. Furthermore, the diversity of pathways that might be employed by the tumor in the process of evasion from the host immune system (see Tab. 6.2) emphasizes the likelihood of individual differences between tumors of the same type in their interactions with immune cells. In such a case, cellular and molecular events mediated by the same receptor–ligand pair might be quite distinct or even opposite in the particular microenvironment. The consequences of this diversity, as manifested by a successful escape of the tumor from immune control, will not be easy to deal with from the clinical point of view.

### 6.5.5
### Contributions of other Pathways to Lymphocyte Demise in Cancer

In this review, I have focused on the Fas–FasL pathway to illustrate one of the many possible mechanisms implicated in mediating death of immune cells in the tumor microenvironment. It is, of course, highly likely that the other TNF family members play an equally important role in tumor-effector cell interactions. The *TRAIL–TRAIL receptor* pathway in melanoma, for example, has been studied by several investigators, largely, however, in respect to tumor cell resistance or sensitivity to apoptosis [107, 108]. There is evidence indicating that TRAIL and other TNF family death-inducing ligands and receptors for these ligands are expressed by both human tumor cells and lymphoid effector cells [109, 110]. The ability of activated lymphocytes to cross-link the death receptors on tumor cells, thus bringing about death of the target, has been demonstrated in *ex vivo* experiments [110]. The most efficient apoptosis of target cells occurs when at least three different TNF family ligands act in concert, allowing for delivery of a strong apoptotic signal [110]. At the same time, tumor cells, which also express a broad panopoly of membrane-associated TNF family ligands, have the potential of inducing apoptosis in immune cells by a comparable mechanism acting in a reverse direction. The end-point of this interaction is death of one or the other party, depending on the microenvironmental factors which regulate not only the number of immune cells at the site but also levels of expression of the relevant receptors and ligands.

Not all effector–tumor cell interactions are mediated by the TNF family of receptors and ligands. Thus, there is considerable interest in and convincing evidence for the mechanism involving activation of macrophages or granulocytes in cancer patients either *in situ* or in the circulation, respectively, and oxidative stress mediated by hydrogen peroxide they produce [111, 112]. Release by an oxidative burst of ROM from these cells is thought to lead to $\zeta$ degradation in T and NK cells and to the inhibition of their functions, including NF-$\kappa$B activation, and alteration in the cytokine production profile by these immune cells [112, 113].

Finally, the highly controversial but slowly and grudgingly acknowledged mechanism of the production of immunoinhibitory factors by the tumor has to be factored in (see Tab. 6.1). The controversy largely has to do with biochemical purification and cloning of the purported inhibitory factors. The situation resembles that in the cytokine field a dozen or so years ago, when soluble, unpurified and uncharacterized soluble factors were being introduced as regulators of multiple cellular interactions. Today, several of these cytokines and a handful of cloned soluble factors are known to be produced by the tumor, and to regulate not only tumor growth but also its relationship with immune cells (reviewed in [13]). The increasingly important role in these cellular interactions of metalloproteinases and their inhibitors, TIMP(s), cannot be overemphasized [114]. However, the major question of who controls these mechanisms (the tumor or the immune system) has not yet been answered. Hence, there is enormous interest in the mechanisms exercised by these interacting systems in patients with cancer and much controversy still surrounds the accumulating evidence that the tumor may be masterminding the outcome in its favor.

## 6.6
## Conclusions

T lymphocytes present at the tumor site or in the circulation of patients with cancer have depressed functions and are more sensitive to apoptosis than their counterparts in non-cancer lesions or in the circulation of healthy donors. Evidence is emerging that subsets of CD3$^+$CD8$^+$ anti-tumor effector cells may be selectively or preferentially destined to die in cancer patients. However, a controversy has developed in respect to the mechanism of effector cell death in cancer patients. To a large extent, this controversy exists because of a current incomplete understanding of molecular pathways that lead to death of certain but not other subsets of lymphocytes found in the tumor microenvironment. In addition, the existing animal models of tumor growth appear to be inadequate for clarification of these phenomena, for a simple reason that murine tumors appear to be much less immunosuppressive than human tumors. It is also necessary to recall that a wide variety of signals can induce apoptosis in immune effector cells, including drugs, cytokines, irradiation, low pH, oxygen intermediates, stress and others [115]. Caspase activation can be induced in hematopoietic cells independent of the expression of death receptors [116]. As reviewed above, a broad variety of tumor-derived factors have been identified as contributors to functional impairment and death of immune cells in tumor-bearing hosts. In this context, it seems reasonable to coin the term TICD to more accurately define a general phenomenon of immune cell demise in the tumor microenvironment. This definition is broad enough to include AICD of lymphocytes, which upon reaching a certain stage of activation commit suicide or murder other lymphocytes [117]. It also includes a possibility of the direct engagement of death receptors on immune cells by the corresponding ligands expressed on tumor cells. Further, it recognizes the fact that chronic antigenic stimulation existing in the presence of the tumor probably plays a major role in shaping responses of immune cells. Operationally, therefore, tumor-specific T cells in the tumor-bearing host are dying of AICD, which is initiated or staged by the tumor.

Given the existing evidence for dysfunction and death of T cells in the tumor-bearing hosts, it is necessary to identify and evaluate therapeutically promising strategies for protection of immune cells in the tumor microenvironment. Preliminary studies suggest that cytokines or DC-based vaccines might be able to offer such protection from apoptosis to immune effector cells. Although therapy with cytokines, IL-2, IFNs or IL-12, has been used by numerous investigators to treat malignancies in recent years (reviewed in [118]), it has never been specifically directed toward preventing death of immune effector cells. On the contrary, the rationale behind cytokine-based therapy has been up-regulation of anti-tumor functions of immune effector cells, especially T cells specific for the tumor. In retrospect, it seems that attempts to up-regulate functions of cells that are dying in the tumor microenvironment are not likely to succeed. A new strategy for cytokine delivery and perhaps new cytokines are necessary to rescue the dying cells or, better, to protect them from death-inducing signals. It is hoped that in the future, this long-neglected aspect of immunotherapy will receive the attention of both basic and clinical investigators. There is a certain degree of urgency associated with the implementation of new strategies for immunotherapy of cancer in view of extensive vaccination efforts on-going world wide in patients with malignancies. These clinical trials, largely conducted with patients who have advanced disease, are not likely to succeed if only a proportion of the vaccine-induced, tumor-specific effector cells survive *in vivo*. To avoid likely disappointments, it will be necessary in the future to combine anti-tumor vaccines with therapies providing protection of activated T cells from tumor-induced apoptosis.

## References

1 L. Zhang, W. Zhou, V. E. Velculescu, et al. *Science* 1997; **276**: 1268–1272.

2 F. M. Burnett. *Prog. Exp. Tumor Res.* 1970; **13**: 1–27.

3 G. Klein. *Harvey Lect.* 1975; **69**: 71.

4 T. Boon, J.-C. Cerottini, B. Van den Eynde, P. Van der Bruggen and A. Van Pel. *Annu. Rev. Immunol.* 1994; **12**: 337–365.

5 B. J. Van den Eynde and P. Van der Bruggen. *Curr. Opin. Immunol.* 1997; **9**: 684–693.

6 Y. Kawakami, S. Eliyahu, C. Jennings, et al. *J. Immunol.* 1995; **154**: 3961–3968.

7 P. Matzinger. *Annu. Rev. Immunol.* 1994; **12**: 991–1045.

8 P. Matzinger. *Immunology* 1998; **10**: 399–415.

9 C. A. Janeway. *Immunol. Today* 1992; **13**: 11–16.

10 H. L. Ioachim. *J Natl Cancer Inst* 1979; **57**: 465–475.

11 J. C. E. Underwood. *Br. J. Cancer* 1974; **30**: 538–548.

12 B. M. Vose and M. Moore. *Semin. Hematol.* 1985; **22**: 27–40.

13 T. L. Whiteside and H. Rabinowich. *Cancer Immunol. Immunother.* 1998; **46**: 175–184.

14 J. L. Svennevig, O. C. Lunde, J. Holter and D. Bjorgsvik. *Br. J. Cancer* 1984; **49**: 375–377.

15 G. Wolf, J. Hudson, K. Peterson, H. Miller and K. D. McClatchey. *Otolaryngol Head Neck Surg.* 1986; **95**: 145–152.

16 K. Itoh, A. B. Tilden and C. M. Balch. *Cancer Res.* 1986; **46**: 3011–3017.

17 S. A. Rosenberg, B. S. Packard, P. M. Aebersold, et al. *N Engl J Med* 1988; **319**: 1676–1680.

18 T. L. Whiteside. *Tumor Infiltrating Lymphocytes in Human Malignancies.* R. G. Landes, Austin, TX 1993.

19 E. Weidmann, E. M. Elder, M. Trucco, M. T. Lotze and T. L. Whiteside. *Int. J. Cancer* 1993; **54**: 383–390.

20 B. Mukherji, A. Guha, N. G. Chakraborty, et al. *J. Exp. Med.* 1989; **169**: 1961–1976.

21 T. L. Whiteside. *Biotherapy* 1992; **5**: 47–61.

22 P. Whitford, E. A. Mallon, W. D. George and A. M. Campbell. *Br. J. Cancer* 1990; **62**: 971–975.

23 S. Miescher, T. L. Whiteside, L. Moretta and V. Von Fliedner. *J. Immunol.* 1987; **138**: 4004–4011.

24 D. Vitolo, A. Kanbour, J. T. Johnson, R. B. Herberman and T. L. Whiteside. *Eur. J. Cancer* 1993; **3**: 371–377.

25 T. L. Whiteside, L. M. Jost and R. B. Herberman. *Crit. Rev. Oncol./Hematol.* 1992; **12**: 25–47.

26 T. E. Reichert, H. Rabinowich, J. T. Johnson and T. L. Whiteside. *J. Immunother.* 1998; **21**: 295–306.

27 X. Li, J. Liu, J. K. Park, et al. *Cancer Res.* 1994; **54**: 5424–5429.

28 T. E. Reichert, E. Day, E. M. Wagner and T. L. Whiteside. *Cancer Res.* 1998; **58**: 5344–5347.

29 R. G. Uzzo, P. Rayman, V. Kolenko, et al. *J. Clin Invest.* 1999; **104**: 769–776.

30 W. Ling, P. Rayman, R. G. Uzzo, et al. *Blood*, 1998; **92**: 1334–1341.

31 R. G. Uzzo, P. E. Clark, P. Rayman, et al. *J. Natl Cancer Inst.* 1999; **91**: 718–721.

32 P. A. Baeuerle and D. Baltimore. *Cell* 1996; **87**: 13–20.

33 M. J. May and S. Ghosh. *Immunol. Today* 1998; **19**: 80–88.

34 I. Kuss, T. Saito, J. T. Johnson and T. L. Whiteside. *Clin. Cancer Res.* 1999; **5**: 329–334.

35 T. L. Whiteside. *Cancer Immunol. Immunother.* 1999; **48**: 346–352.

36 T. L. Whiteside, N. L. Vujanovic and R. B. Herberman. *Curr. Topics Microbiol. Immunol.* 1998; **230**: 221–244.

37 N. L. Vujanovic, S. Nagashima, R. B. Herberman and T. L. Whiteside. *J. Immunol.* 1996; **157**: 1117–1126.

38 B. J. Chambers and H-G. Ljunggren. In M. T. Lotze and A. W. Thomson (eds), *Dendritic Cells: Biology and Clinical Applications.* Academic Press, New York 1999: 257–265.

39 Y.-.I SON, R. M. DALLAL, R. B. MAIL-
LIARD, *et al. Cancer Res.* 2001; **61**: 884–
888.

40 K. KARRE. *Science* 1995; **267**: 978–979.

41 W. M. YOKOYAMA. *Curr. Opin. Immunol.*
1998; **10**: 298–305.

42 D. N. BURSHTYN and E. O. LONG. *Trends
Cell Biol.* 1997; **7**: 473–478.

43 N. L. VUJANOVIC, P. BASSE, R. B. HER-
BERMAN and T. L. WHITESIDE. *Meth-
ods:A Companion to Methods Enzymol.*
1996; **9**: 394–408.

44 K. HATA, D. H. VAN THIEL, R. B. HER-
BERMAN and T. L. WHITESIDE. *Hepatol-
ogy* 1992; **15**: 816–823.

45 C. BIRON. *Curr. Opin. Immunol.* 1997;
**9**: 24–34.

46 P. LAI, H. RABINOWICH, P. A. CROWLEY-
NOWICK, M. C. BELL, G. MANTOVANI
and T. L. WHITESIDE. *Clin. Cancer Res.*
1996; **2**: 161–173.

47 M. A. CALIGIURI, A. ZMUIDZINAS,
T. MANLEY, H. LEVINE, K. A. SMITH and
J. RITZ. *J. Exp. Med.* 1990; **171**: 1509–
1513.

48 P. BASSE, R. B. HERBERMAN, U. NANN-
MARK, *et al. J. Exp. Med.* 1991; **174**:
479–488.

49 J. LISTER, W. B. RYBKA, A. D. DONNEN-
BERG, *et al. Clin. Cancer Res.* 1995; **1**:
607–614.

50 S. NAGASHIMA, T. E. REICHERT, Y. KA-
SHII, Y. SUMINAMI, K. CHIKAMATSU and
T. L. WHITESIDE. *Cancer Gene Ther.*
1997; **4**: 366–376.

51 C. B. LOPEZ, T. D. RAO, H. FEINER,
R. SHAPIRO, J. R. MARKS and A. FREY.
*Cell Immunol.* 1998; **190**: 141–155.

52 J. BANCHEREAU and R. STEINMEIN.
*Nature* 1998; **392**: 245–252.

53 M. THURNHER, C. RADMAYAR, R. RA-
MONER, *et al. Int. J. Cancer,* 1996; **67**: 1– 7.

54 D. I. GABRILOVICH, J. CORAK, I. F. CIER-
NIK, D. KAVANAUGH and D. P. CAR-
BONE. *Clin. Cancer Res.* 1997; **3**: 483–
490.

55 B. ALMAND, J. R. RESSER, B. LINDMAN,
*et al. Clin. Cancer Res.* 2000; **6**: 1755–
1766.

56 M. R. SHURIN, *J. Leuk. Biol. Suppl.*
1998; **2**: 13.

57 D. I. GABRILOVICH, H. L. CHEN and
K. R. GIRGIS, *et al. Nat. Med.* 1996; **2**:
1096–1103.

58 C. ESCHE, A. LOCKSHIN and G. V.
SHURIN, *et al. J. Leuk. Biol.* 1999; **66**:
336–344.

59 M. R. SHURIN, C. ESCHE, A. LOCKSHIN
and M. T. LOTZE. IN M. T. LOTZE, A. W.
THOMSON (EDS), *Dendritic Cells: Biology
and Clinical Applications.* Academic
Press, New York 1999: 673–692.

60 G. V. SHURIN, M. R. SHURIN, S. BY-
KOVSKAJA, *et al. Cancer Res.* 2001; **61**:
363–369.

61 J. BANCHEREAU, F. BRIERE, C. CAUX,
*et al. Annu. Rev. Immunol.* 2000; **18**:
767–811.

62 F. O. NESTLE, G. BURG, J. FAH,
T. WRONE-SMITH and B. J. NICKOLOFF.
*Am. J. Pathol.* 1997; **150**: 641–651.

63 T. K. HOFFMANN, J. MULLER-BERGHAUS,
J. T. JOHNSON, W. J. STORKUS and
T. L. WHITESIDE. *Clin. Cancer Res.* 2002;
in press.

64 Y. BECKER. *In Vivo* 1993; **7**: 187–191.

65 T. E. REICHERT, C. SCHEUER, R. DAY,
W. WAGNER and T. L. WHITESIDE. *Cancer* 2001; **91**: 2136–2147.

66 Y. KOTERA, J. D. FONTENOT, G. PECHER,
R. S. METZGAR and O. J. FINN. *Cancer
Res.* 1994; **54**: 2856–2860.

67 J. ALLISON, H. M. GEORGIOU, A. STRAS-
SER and D. L. VAUX. *Proc. Natl Acad. Sci.
USA* 1997; **94**: 3943–3947.

68 K. SEINO, N. KAYAGAKI, K. OKUMURA
and H. YAGITA. *Nat. Med.* 1997; **3**: 165–
170.

69 T. S. GRIFFITH, T. BRUNNER, S. M.
FLETCHER, D. R. GREEN and T. A. FER-
GUSON. *Science* 1995; **270**: 1189–1192.

70 T. S. GRIFFITH and T. A. FERGUSON.
*Immunol. Today* 1997; **18**: 240–244.

71 B. R. GASTMAN, Y. ATARASHI, T. E.
REICHERT, *et al. Cancer Res.* 1999; **59**:
5356–5364.

72 P. SAAS, P. R. WALKER, M. HAHNE, *et al.
J. Clin Invest.* 1997; **99**: 1173–1178.

73 S. TSUJITANI, Y. KAKEJI, A. WATANABE,
S. KOHNOE, Y. MAEHARA and K. SUGI-
MACHI. *Cancer* 1990; **66**: 2012–2016.

74 G. F. MURPHY, A. RADU, M. KAMINER
and D. BERG. *J. Invest. Dermatol.* 1993;
**100**: 335 S.

75 B. AL-SARIREH and O. EREMIN. *J. R. Coll.
Surg. Edinb.* 2000; **45**: 1–16.

76 C. ALLEN and N. HOGG. *Immunology*
1985; **55**: 289–299.

77 R. D. Leek, C. E. Lewis, R. Whitehouse, M. Greenall, J. Clarke and A. L. Harris. *Cancer Res.* 1996; **56**: 4625–4629.

78 R. Kiessling, K. Kono, M. Petersson and K. Wasserman. *Semin. Immunopathol.* 1996; **18**: 227–242.

79 M. Hansson, A. Asea, U. Ericsson, S. Hermodsson and K. Hellstrand. *J. Immunol.* 1996; **156**: 42–47.

80 P. Allavena, L. Piemonti, D. Longoni, *et al. Eur. J. Immunol.* 1998; **28**: 359–369.

81 M. J. Kornstein, J. S. Brooks and D. E. Elder. *Cancer Res.* 1983; **43**: 2749–2753.

82 J. O'Connell, G. D. O'Sullivan, J. K. Collins and F. Shanahan. *J. Exp. Med.* 1996; **184**: 1075–1082.

83 M. W. Bennett, J. O'Connell, G. C. O'Sullivan, *et al. J. Immunol.* 1998; **160**: 5669–5675.

84 K. Shiraki, N. Tsuji, T. Shioda, K. J. Isselbacher and H. Takahashi. *Proc. Natl Acad. Sci. USA* 1997; **94**: 6420–6425.

85 B. R. Gastman, Y. Atarashi, T. E. Reichert, *et al. Cancer Res.* 1999; **59**: 5356–5364.

86 G. A. Niehans, T. Brunner, S. P. Frizelle, *et al. Cancer Res.* 1997; **57**: 1007–1012.

87 N. Mitsiades, V. Poulaki, G. Mastorakos, *et al. J. Clin. Endocrinol Met.* 1999; **84**: 2924–2932.

88 M. Hahne, D. Rimoldi, M. Schroter, *et al. Science* 1996; **274**: 1363–1366.

89 T. L. Whiteside. *Semin. Cancer Biol.* 2002; **12**: 43–50.

90 N. Mitsiades, V. Poulaki, V. Kotoula, A. Leone and M. Tsokos. *Am. J. Pathol.* 1998; **153**: 1947–1956.

91 N. Kayagaki, A. Kawasaki, T. Ebata, *et al. J. Exp. Med.* 1995; **182**: 1777.

92 S. Munakata, T. Enomoto, M. Tsujimoto, *et al. Br. J. Cancer,* 2000; **82**: 1446–1452.

93 T. Reimer, C. Herrnring, D. Koczan, *et al. Cancer Res.* 2000; **60**: 822–828.

94 M. Mottolese, S. Buglioni, C. Bracalenti, *et al. Int. J. Cancer* 2000; **89**: 127–132.

95 K. F. Yoong, S. C. Afford, S. Randhawa, S. G. Hubscher and

D. H. Adams. *Am. J. Pathol.* 1999; **154**: 693–703.

96 Y. Atarashi, H. Kanaya and T. L. Whiteside. *J. Immunol. Methods* 1999; **233**: 179–182.

97 N. Restifo. *Nat. Med.* 2000; **6**: 493–495.

98 G. Dworacki, N. Meidenbauer, I. Kuss, *et al. Clin. Cancer Res.* 2001; **7**: 947s–957s.

99 T. Saito, G. Dworacki, W. Gooding, M. T. Lotze and T. L. Whiteside. *Clin. Cancer Res.* 2000; **6**: 1351–1364.

100 T. K. Hoffmann, G. Dworacki, T. Tsukishiro, *et al. Clin. Cancer Res.* 2001; in press..

101 Y. Atarashi, H. Rabinowich, S. Sato and T. L. Whiteside. *Proc. Am. Ass. Cancer Res.* 2000; **41**: 557.

102 J. Tschopp, M. Irmler and M. Thome. *Curr. Opin. Immunol.* 1998; **10**: 552–558.

103 T. Sato, S. Trie, S. Kitada and J. C. Reed. *Science* 1995; **268**: 411–415.

104 A. M. Holbaum, S. Moe and A. Marshak-Rothstein. *J. Exp. Med.* 2000; **191**: 1209–1219.

105 H. Arai, D. Gordon, E. G. Nabel and G. J. Nabel. *Proc. Natl Acad. Sci. USA* 1997; **94**: 13862–13867.

106 J. J. Chen, Y. Sun and G. J. Nabel. *Science* 1998; **282**: 1714–1717.

107 X. D. Zhang, A. V. Franco, T. Nguyen, C. P. Gray and P. Hersey. *J. Immunol.* 2000; **164**: 3961–3970.

108 T. S. Griffith, C. T. Rauch, P. J. Smolak, *et al. J. Immunol.* 1999; **162**: 2597–2605.

109 A. Ashkenazi and V. M. Dixit. *Curr. Opin. Cell Biol.* 1999; **11**: 255–260.

110 Y. Kashii, R. Giorda, R. B. Herberman, T. L. Whiteside and N. L. Vujanovic. *J. Immunol.* 1999; **163**: 5358–5366.

111 J. Schmielau and O. J. Finn. *Cancer Res.* 2001; **61**: 4756–4760.

112 K. Kono, F. Salazar-Onfray, M. Patersson, *et al. Eur. J. Immunol.* 1996; **26**: 1308–1313

113 K. J. Malmberg, V. Arulampalam, F. Ichihara, *et al. J. Immunol.* 2001; **167**: 2595–2601.

114 M. Wang, Y. Hu, I. Shima and M. E. Stearns. *Oncol. Res.* 1998; **10**: 219–233.

**115** S. W. SMITH and B. A. OSBORNE. *J. NIH Res.* 1997; **9**: 33–37.

**116** N. A. THOENBERRY and Y. LAZEBRIK. *Science* 1998; **281**: 1312–1316.

**117** M. LENARDO, F. K-M. CHAN, F. HORNUNG, *et al. Annu. Rev. Immunol.* 1999; **17**: 221–253.

**118** F. G. HALUSKA and P. S. MULTANI. *Cancer Chemother. Biol. Response Modif.* 1999; **18**: 470–488.

**119** M. R. I. YOUNG, A. SCHMIDT-PAK and M. A. WRIGHT, *et al. Clin. Cancer Res.* 1995; **1**: 95–130.

**120** D. D. TAYLOR, D. P. BENDER, C. GERCEL-TAYLOR, J. STANSON and T. L. WHITESIDE. *Br. J. Cancer* 2001; **84**: 1624–1629.

# 7
# Immunosuppresive Factors in Cancer
Richard Bucala and Christine N. Metz

## 7.1    Introduction

Tumors have paradoxical effects on the host immune system: they stimulate immune cells and they suppress immune cells. When host immunostimulation is effective, tumor cells are destroyed. However, tumors produce several suppressive cytokines and other factors that subvert the host antitumor immune response. These immunosuppressive factors function by repressing the host antitumor immune cells and/or by promoting host immunosuppressor cell activity. Suppression of the host antitumor immune response occurs by preventing tumor recognition by immune cells and/or by inhibiting immune cell-mediated tumor killing. An accurate identification and understanding of the immunosuppressive factors that contribute to the host antitumor immune response is critical for the effective treatment of cancer patients, whether by conventional treatments or by newly developed immunotherapeutic strategies. In this chapter, we will discuss the effects of tumor-derived suppressive cytokines, factors, and shed antigens on host immune cells (summarized in Tab. 7.1) and on tumor cells. In addition, we will address the implications for the inhibition of these immunosuppressive agents during cancer treatment.

## 7.1
### Transforming Growth Factor (TGF)-$\beta$

TGF-$\beta$ was originally described for its ability to induce NRK rat kidney fibroblasts to form large colonies in soft agar in the presence of epidermal growth factor [1, 2]. Since its discovery, TGF-$\beta$ has been shown to play a role in cell growth, differentiation and transformation, and to modulate the host immune response to tumor growth and metastases. The TGF-$\beta$ superfamily consists of TGF-$\beta$1, -$\beta$2 and -$\beta$3, as well as an additional 40 different TGF-$\beta$-related proteins (reviewed in [3]). The three mammalian isoforms (TGF-$\beta$1, -2 and -3) are synthesized as pre-pro-TGF-$\beta$ polypeptides that contain a signal sequence, the pro-region [latency associated peptide (LAP)] and mature TGF-$\beta$ (N-terminal region). The majority of TGF-$\beta$ is secreted as an inactive complex associated with a second gene product known as the "latent

**Tab. 7.1** Effects of tumor-derived molecules on the host antitumor immune response

| Factor | Monocytes/macrophages | Dendritic cells | T lymphocytes | Natural killer cells (NK)/lymphokine activated killer (LAK) |
|---|---|---|---|---|
| TGF-β | ↓ mac production<br>↓ cytokine and NO production<br>↓ mac proliferation<br>'deactivates' macs | ↓ DC maturation<br>↓ DC activity<br>alters DC chemotaxis | ↓ T cell lytic activity<br>↓ $T_h$1 cytokine release<br>↓ T cell proliferation<br>↓ T cell differentiation<br>↓/↑ T cell apoptosis<br>indirect and direct effects | ↓ NK cytokine production<br>↓ NK proliferation<br>↓ NK cytolytic activity<br>↓ LAK production<br>↓ LAK cytotoxic activity |
| IL-10 | ↓ cytokine synthesis by macs<br>↑ $PGE_2$ production<br>↓ NO production by macs<br>↓ MHC class II exprn<br>↓ co-stimulatory molecule exprm | ↓ DC ability to stimulate T cell responses<br>↓ DC migration<br>↓ DC accumulation<br>alters DC maturation<br>↓ DC apoptosis | ↑ $T_h$1 cytokine production<br>↓ AG-induced $CD4^+$ proliferation<br>↓/↑ T cell cytolytic responses<br>induces $CD4^+$ T cell anergy<br>↑/↓ CTL activity<br>↑ $CD8^+$ T cell proliferation<br>↑ $CD8^+$ T cell outgrowth<br>indirect and direct effects | ↑ IL-2 induced NK proliferation<br>↑ NK cytokine production<br>↑ NK cytoxicity |
| MIF | ↓ macrophage migration<br>associated with ↑ mac activation<br>↑ COX-2/$PGE_2$ production<br>↑ TNF production by macs<br>↓ antitumor activity of macs | | mediates T cell activation<br>↓ presence of intra-tumoral T cells<br>associated with ↓ CTL activity | ↓ NK activity |
| $PGE_2$ | | | ↑ T cell proliferation<br>↓ Th1 cytokine production<br>↓ T cell migration<br>↓ T cell activation<br>↓ CTL generation/activity<br>↑ T cell anergy<br>required for CTL induction<br>required for T cell differentiation | ↓ NK activity<br>↓ LAK activity |
| Polyamines | ↓ NO production by macs<br>↓ cytokine production by macs<br>↓ mac phagocytosis | | | ↓ NK activity |
| Shed tumor antigen: MUC | | | ↓ effectiveness of CTL response<br>↓ T cell proliferation<br>↓ cytokine production by T cells<br>↓ T cell activation | |

See text for details and references.

TGF-β binding protein". Thus, activation of the TGF-β complex is a key regulatory step for controlling its activity. The biological effects of TGF-β1, -2 and -3 are mediated through the same high-affinity serine-threonine kinase type I and II receptors, followed by downstream signaling intermediates known as Smad proteins (reviewed in [4]).

## 7.1.1
## Sources of TGF-β

Almost all cells in culture can be stimulated to secrete TGF-β, including activated (not resting) macrophages [3], T cells [5], B cells [6], natural killer (NK) cells [7], as well as numerous tumor cell types including pancreatic [8], prostate [9, 10], lung [11], colon [12], melanoma [13] and breast carcinomas (reviewed in [14]). Elevated levels of TGF-β in serum negatively correlate with cancer progression and reduced survival for many cancers (reviewed in [15]), including nasopharyngeal [16], colorectal [17], cervical [18], prostatic [9] and gastric carcinomas [19].

Although TGF-β has been shown to inhibit MHC class II expression on tumor cells, most tumor cells resist the tumor suppressor and growth inhibitory effects of TGF-β. Tumor cells are rendered insensitive to the suppressive effects of TGF-β by: (1) receptor down-regulation [20–22], (2) inactivating mutations within the TGF-β receptor [23–25] and/or (3) anomalies in the post-receptor TGF-β signaling pathway including the Smad proteins [21, 26, 27]. By contrast, TGF-β has profound direct effects on immune cells expressing TGF-β receptors and indirect effects on downstream cellular mediators.

## 7.1.2
## Effects of TGF-β

### 7.1.2.1   Effects of TGF-β on monocytes/macrophages

Macrophages are important cellular mediators of the host immune response to tumors. Macrophages produce cytotoxic molecules, such as tumor necrosis factor (TNF)-α and nitric oxide (NO) that kill tumor cells and serve as antigen-presenting cells. Thus, macrophages function as cellular mediators of both T and NK cell antitumor activities. The suppressive effects of TGF-β on monocytes/macrophages are complex, and depend on their origin, differentiation state and cytokine milieu. TGF-β has been shown to block colony stimulating factor-1-dependent proliferation of bone marrow precursor cells [28] and hence, *macrophage production*, as well as inhibit lipoprotein (a)-induced *macrophage proliferation* [29]. Tumor-derived TGF-β is well known for its ability to 'deactivate' tissue macrophages that express high levels of TGF-βR1 and TGF-βR2 (reviewed in [30]). TGF-β *suppresses the antitumor cytolytic activity* of bone marrow-derived macrophages already activated with interferon (IFN)-γ and lipopolysaccharide [31]. *TGF-β inhibits cytokine (TNF-α) and NO production by macrophages* [32–34], an effect reversed by antisense oligonucleotides to TGF-β [35]. Finally, *macrophages rendered dysfunctional by TGF-2;b have powerful inhibitory effects on the development of the host T cell-mediated antitumor immune response.*

### 7.1.2.2 Effects of TGF-β on T lymphocytes

Multiple T cell types, including CD4$^+$, CD8$^+$ cytolytic T lymphocytes (CTLs) and tumor-infiltrating lymphocytes (TILs), function as key cellular mediators of the host immune response to tumors. TGF-β directly *suppresses T lymphocyte activity.* TGF-β reduces pore-forming protein expression in human peripheral CD8$^+$ T cells [36], and inhibits the cytolytic activity of anti-CD3 stimulated CD8$^+$ T cells [37] and of CTLs directed against fresh tumor targets [38]. Furthermore, TGF-β *inhibits the generation of CTLs in vitro* [38]. Similar to its effect on macrophages, *TGF-β suppresses cytokine release by T lymphocytes,* including IFN-γ, TNF-α, interleukin (IL)-2, IL-6, IL-4 and IL-5 [39–41], which further represses their antitumor activity.

The effects of TGF-β on T cell immune responses are dependent on numerous factors, including T cell type and activation status. Recently, Ludviksson *et al.* examined the effect of TGF-β on T cells (stimulated versus non-stimulated) exhibiting a defined phenotype [CD4$^+$ versus CD8$^+$ and T helper ($T_h$) 1 versus $T_h$2] and a defined maturational stage (naïve versus memory T cells) [42]. They found that:

1. *TGF-β inhibits both the proliferation and differentiation of $T_h$1 and $T_h$2 cells,* even when TGF-β is present during primary stimulation.
2. *CD4$^+$ T cells primed in the presence of TGF-β exhibit reduced immune responses* induced by receptor cross-linking and/or by specific antigen stimulation which is independent of co-stimulatory molecule and IL-2 expression.
3. The presence of TGF-β during primary T cell stimulation has a long-lasting or "imprinting" effect.
4. The immunosuppressive effects of TGF-β on T cells cannot be reversed with IL-2.
5. *TGF-β directly suppresses memory $T_h$1 cytokine production* by down-regulating the IL-12 receptor β2 chain on T cells, while TGF-β has no effect on memory $T_h$2 cytokine production.

Therefore, tumor-derived TGF-β assists in the escape of tumors from the host cell-mediated immune response by *suppressing the host $T_h$1 response and promoting an ineffective $T_h$2 response.*

Similar to its many other activities, the effect of TGF-β on *T cell proliferation* is dependent on the cell population and activation status. In early studies, Kehrl *et al.* reported that *TGF-β inhibits T cell proliferation* [43]. The addition of TGF-β to mixed lymphocyte tumor cultures results in a decrease in the number of effector CD8$^+$ CTLs by inhibiting their proliferation [44]. Similarly, TGF-β inhibits the proliferation of intraepithelial CD8$^+$ lymphocytes following activation [45]. By contrast, when naive T cells are activated in the presence of TGF-β, they proliferate and secrete IL-2 [46]. The antiproliferative effect of TGF-β has been attributed to down-regulation of the IL-2 receptor [43, 47] and the inhibition of IL-2 and IL-12-mediated proliferation signals [48, 49]. IL-2 and IL-12 are immunostimulating cytokines capable of inducing cytokine production, enhancing cytolytic activity and promoting T cell proliferation. There are two opposing reports describing the mechanism by which TGF-β inhibits IL-12-mediated proliferation. Bright *et al.* showed that TGF-β blocks IL-12 induced phosphorylation and activation of the Jak-2, Tyk-2 kinases and STAT3 and 4 transcription factors in activated lymphocytes [50]. By contrast, Sudarshan *et al.* reported that TGF-β does not block cytokine (IL-12 and IL-2) induced Janus tyrosine kinase (JAK) and signal transducers and activators of transcription (STAT) phosphorylation in T cells [51]. Thus, the mechanism by which TGF-β inhibits IL-1- induced T cell proliferation is not clear and may depend on many factors.

Numerous conflicting reports of the effects of TGF-β on *T cell apoptosis* have been described. TGF-β has been found to *induce T cell apoptosis* [50, 52, 53] and to *prevent T cell apoptosis* [54–59]. These conflicting reports suggest that multiple factors (microenvironment, origin, as well as differentiation and activation states) influence the T cell apoptotic response to TGF-β. TGF-β has been reported to promote apoptosis in T cells independent of the IL-2/IL-2 receptor pathway [52] and through the activation of caspase-like proteases in activated murine T cells [59]. By contrast, TGF-β when present during the course of T cell activation *inhibits activation-induced cell death (AICD) and Fas-mediated apoptosis* [54]. AICD by T cells is one mechanism for controlling the size and the duration of the primary immune response. Further studies show that *TGF-β prevents apoptosis in memory T$_h$1 CD4$^+$ T cells* [42]. Genestier *et al.* have shown that the addition of TGF-β to human T cells and T cell hybridomas significantly reduced apoptosis after activation by anti-CD3 [58]. TGF-β blockade of T cell apoptosis was associated with decreased Fas ligand expression and not Fas signaling. These findings suggest that TGF-β, when present at the right time, functions as a "viability factor" allowing the clonal expansion of effector T cells and the generation of long-lived memory T cells during the immune response. More recently, Sillett *et al.* demonstrated the importance of the timing of TGF-β administration for inducing T cell apoptosis *in vitro* [60]. TGF-β, when added at the initiation of T cell mitogenesis did not induce T cell apoptosis, whereas TGF-β added post-activation enhanced apoptosis in T cells independent of Bcl family members.

### 7.1.2.3 Effects of TGF-β on NK and lymphokine-activated killer (LAK) activity

NK cells are a subset of bone marrow-derived immune cells that proliferate in response to viral and cellular invasion. Once activated, NK cells directly kill tumor cells, but do not require matching of MHC molecules between effector and target cells. Overall, *TGF-β has an inhibitory effect on peripheral blood NK cells* [7]. TGF-β *inhibits NK proliferation, cytokine production [IFN-γ, TNF-α and granulocyte macrophage colony stimulating factor (GM-CSF)], NK activation and NK cytotoxicity.* [7, 61].

NK cells represent the main precursors of LAK activity. *TGF-β inhibits the induction of LAK cell activity* in vitro [62–64] and *suppresses the production and the antitumor cytotoxic activity of LAKs* [38, 39].

### 7.1.2.4 Effects of TGF-β on dendritic cells (DCs)

DCs are critical immune cells responsible for innate and adaptive immunity during tumor killing (reviewed in [65, 66]). DCs initiate and regulate both cell-mediated and humoral responses. Immature DCs express abundant intracellular levels of MHC class I and II molecules which bind specific tumor antigens. Once matured, DCs display the MHC bound antigen on their surface together with multiple co-stimulatory molecules (CD40, CD50, CD54, CD58, CD80, CD83 and CD86) and potently activate resting or naive CD4[+] and CD8[+] T cells to promote their differentiation into functional helper and effector (tumor killing) T cells. Thus, the most important function of DCs is to sensitize the immune system to specific antigens. Because DCs are 10–100 times more potent antigen-presenting cells than cells and monocytes/macrophages, much work has focused on their use to stimulate immunity against cancer (reviewed in [65]).

*TGF-β is immunosuppressive to DCs* by its ability to *block the GM-CSF-induced maturation* [defined as CD86 and MHC class II expression and mixed lymphocyte reaction (MLR)-stimulating activity] of DCs from mouse bone marrow progenitor cells [67]. In addition, *TGF-β over-expressing murine bone marrow-derived DCs exhibit lower allogeneic T cell stimulatory activity* (assessed by MLR and CTL assays than non-transduced cells) [68]. Thus, TGF-β suppresses important DC activities required during host antitumor responses.

DCs must localize, presumably from the bone marrow to the tumor site where specific antigens are present, and then antigen-loaded DCs must migrate to lymphoid tissue to function optimally as antigen-presenting cells. However, little is known about the directed migration of DCs *in vivo*. Recent studies show that *TGF-β reversibly regulates human DC chemotaxis* in vitro [69]. TGF-β enhances the expression of CCR1, CCR3, CCR5 and CXCR4 on immature DCs, and promotes their chemotaxis *in vitro*. However, the transcriptional expression of CCR7 by mature DCs is suppressed by TGF-β. Therefore, *TGF-β might promote the migration immature DCs, but inhibit the localization of mature DCs to the lymphoid organs during the host immune response to tumors.*

### 7.1.3
### Inhibition of TGF-β: Implications for Therapy

Numerous methods for inhibiting the immunosuppressive effects of TGF-β during tumor growth in experimental models have been described. The biological activity of mature TGF-β can be controlled by suppressing the production of TGF-β or by inhibiting the activity of mature TGF-β and/or by altering its interaction with TGF-β receptors on immune cells. Examples of direct inhibition of TGF-β activity/production during tumor growth to improve the host immune response include: soluble TGF-β receptors [70], non-signaling TGF-β binding proteins such as decorin [71–73] and $\alpha_2$-macroglobulin [74], neutralizing anti-TGF-β antibodies [75–77] and antisense oligonucleotides [78–80]. Interestingly, numerous cytotoxic agents also inhibit TGF-β secretion by malignant glioma cell lines [81]. In addition, TGF-β immunoneutralization significantly enhances the sensitivity of human breast carcinoma cells to cisplatin-mediated cytotoxicity *in vitro* [77], suggesting that TGF-β blockade during chemotherapy treatment may promote tumor cell killing.

Although there are a few reports describing the secretion of biologically active TGF-β, the majority of TGF-β is secreted as a latent complex. This latent TGF-β complex is then activated to release mature TGF-β consisting of two identical disulfide-linked polypeptide homodimers (reviewed in [82, 83]). Therefore, *activation of the latent TGF-β complex appears to be the major regulator of TGF-β activity* in vivo. Activation of latent

TGF-β occurs by both *proteolysis* including subtilisin-like proprotein convertases, such as furin [84], plasmin, tissue and urokinase plasminogen activator [85] and transgluta-minase [86, 87], and by *non-proteolytic* mechanisms, such as thrombospondin [88–91] and by mannose-6-phosphate/insulin growth factor II receptor interactions [92].

Recent investigations highlight the importance of TGF-β activation by subtilisin-like convertases, such as furin [84, 93]. Like TGF-β, furin is ubiquitously expressed. Recent studies show that the formation of active TGF-β by glioma cells *in vitro* can be blocked by agents that specifically inhibit the enzymatic activity of furin [94]. *Thus, the development of agents that block the activation of the latent TGF-β complex may represent a new class of anti-immunosuppressive agents for the treatment of cancer.*

Although much is known about the specific suppressive effects of TGF-β on immune cells *in vitro*, the precise role of TGF-β in host immunosuppression during tumor growth *in vivo* is not well understood. Obviously numerous factors play a role in the host immune response to TGF-β during tumor growth and TGF-β is not always associated with immunosuppressive activities, e.g. (1) high expression of TGF-β is not always associated with a poor prognostic outcome [95, 96], (2) over-expression of TGF-β in experimental models does not always lead to tumor formation and immunosuppression [97] and (3) the host response to tumors over-expressing TGF-β can vary depending on the site of tumor implantation [98]. However, most researchers and clinicians would agree that further studies investigating the potential use of TGF-β inhibitors to reduce cancer-induced immunosuppression are justified.

## 7.2
## IL-10

Human IL-10 is a homodimeric 17–20 kDa glycoprotein exhibiting a high degree of homology with the non-glycosylated mouse IL-10 (reviewed in [99]). Unlike TGF-β, it is synthesized and released as an active cytokine. It signals through the IL-10 receptor, a member of the IFN receptor family (reviewed in [99]). The IL-10 receptor, which is expressed on numerous immune cells, is composed of two subunits: IL-10 receptor 1 (ligand binding subunit) and IL-10 receptor 2 (signaling subunit).

### 7.2.1
### Sources of IL-10

IL-10 was originally identified as a product of $T_h2$ cells in response to antigen stimulation in the presence of antigen-presenting cells [100]. IL-10 is expressed by other immune cells including: naive and memory T cells, B cells, and monocytes (reviewed in [99]), as well as tumor (melanoma)-infiltrating T cells [101, 102], NK cells [103] and peritoneal monocytes present in the malignant ascites of ovarian cancer patients [104]. Many solid tumors express IL-10 *in vitro* and *in vivo* including lung tumor nodules [105], melanoma [106] and gliomas [107]. In addition, leukemic tumors originating from the peripheral and bone marrow (including T and B cells) [108], including Hodgkin's [109] as well as non-Hodgkin's lymphomas [110], express high levels of IL-10. The general effect of IL-10 on tumor cells themselves is protective. Pretreatment of tumor target cells with IL-10 defends them from allo-specific CTL lysis [111, 112]. In addition, IL-10 treatment of tumor cells down-regulates their expression of the NK target molecule structure which mediates NK cell-mediated antitumor cytotoxicity and, thus, protects them from NK cell-induced lysis [113]. Furthermore, very recent studies demonstrated that tumor cells use IL-10 as an anti-apoptotic factor to protect themselves against cytotoxic drugs [114]. However, tumor cells also secrete IL-10 to manipulate the host antitumor immune response.

Elevated serum IL-10 is considered a negative prognostic indicator for numerous cancers including Hodgkin's disease [115–117], metastatic melanoma [118] and pancreatic cancer [8]. Circulating IL-10 often serves as a potential marker for (1) the progression from adenoma to carcinoma, (2) metastastic disease and (3) the degree of malignancy [106, 119, 120]. Based on the significant relationship between serum IL-10 levels and the time to treatment failure and overall survival, IL-10 appears to be an important indicator for monitoring disease progression in cancer patients (reviewed in [121]). Although IL-10 exhibits some "anti-angiogenic activity" [122, 123], it has been shown to promote tumor growth by significantly suppressing the host immune response.

### 7.2.2
### Effects of IL-10

#### 7.2.2.1 Effects of IL-10 on monocytes/macrophages
IL-10 was first described as "cytokine synthesis inhibitory factor". *IL-10 inhibits cytokine synthesis* (IL-1, IL-6, IL-8 and IL-12) *by monocytes/macrophages* induced by lipopolysaccharide [124, 125]. In addition, *IL-10 regulates the production of another potent immunosuppressive agent, prostaglandin,* by macrophages [126] and *inhibits NO production and the cytotoxic activity* of monocytes/macrophages [127, 128].

IL-10 *reduces the antigen-presenting capacity of certain classes of macrophages* by multiple mechanisms. *IL-10 suppresses cell surface MHC class II expression* by macrophages [129], in part by inhibiting the transport of peptide-loaded MHC molecules to the plasma membrane [130]. *IL-10 also inhibits the surface expression of CD80 and CD86,* as well as other important co-stimulatory molecules [131, 132]. In summary, by manipulating cytokine production by macrophages and the expression of important cell surface molecules, IL-10 reduces the cytotoxic activity and antigen-presenting capacity of macrophages to specific T cells and, thus, suppresses the host antitumor immune response. Furthermore, macrophages obtained from tumor-bearing hosts are more susceptible to the immunosuppressive activities of IL-10 and less sensitive to immunostimulatory factors necessary to mount an effect antitumor response [133].

#### 7.2.2.2 Effects of IL-10 on T lymphocytes
IL-10 *directly* affects T cells by interacting with membrane associated IL-10 receptors and *indirectly* through the suppressive effects of IL-10 on antigen-presenting cells. Similar to its effect on monocytes/macrophages, IL-10 directly inhibits cytokine production by T cells. *IL-10 inhibits type I cytokine (IL-2 and TNF-α) production* by stimu-

lated CD4$^+$ T cells [134, 135]. By contrast, IL-10 does not inhibit IFN-$\gamma$ secretion by CD8$^+$ T cells in response to tumor stimulation *in vivo* [136].

However, most often the inhibitory effects of IL-10 on T cells are mediated indirectly through its effect on antigen-presenting cell functions. *IL-10 suppresses antigen-induced CD4$^+$ T cell proliferation* [129, 134, 135]. Similarly, Steinbrink *et al.* report that *IL-10 treatment of DCs cells induces alloantigen-specific anergy in both CD4$^+$ and CD8$^+$ T cells* [137, 138]. *IL-10 induces T cell anergy* (unresponsiveness) when present during antigen-specific activation [139]. IL-10-induced CD4$^+$ T cell anergy can be reversed by IL-2 administration or receptor cross-linking (anti-CD3/anti-CD28) [139], as well as by immunization with mature DCs [140].

The effects of IL-10 on the host antitumor CD8$^+$ CTL responses are somewhat contradictory. IL-10 has been reported to exhibit both immunosuppressive and immunostimulatory effects on CD8$^+$ T cells *in vitro* and *in vivo*. *IL-10 inhibits proliferative and cytotoxic T cell responses* generated in primary MLRs *in vitro* [141]. *In vivo*, IL-10 has been shown to *repress CTL activity* directly [142] (by inhibiting granzyme B expression [143]) and indirectly (by inhibiting the generation of functional CTLs [144]). IL-2 or IFN-$\gamma$restores the IL-10-suppressed CTL alloreactivity if administered at the time of tumor challenge, suggesting that the immunosuppressive effect of IL-10 can be blocked by T$_h$1-type cytokines. In accordance with the immunosuppressive effects of IL-10 on host CTLs, Sharma *et al.* examined the growth of Lewis lung tumors in mice engineered to over-express T cell-derived IL-10 [145]. *Over-expression of IL-10 significantly enhanced tumor growth associated with decreased cytokine production by T cells (IL-2 and IFN-$\gamma$), and suppressed cytolytic activity of CD8$^+$ T cells.* Furthermore, these mice produced dysfunctional splenic antigen-presenting cells that expressed significantly reduced cell surface levels of MHC class I, CD80, CD86 and CD11c molecules. These dysfunctional antigen-presenting cells could not support MLRs or promote antitumor CTL induction. Furthermore, DCs obtained from the IL-10 transgenic mice fail to induce antitumor CD8$^+$ T cell reactivity *in vivo* following exposure to tumor-specific peptides. This finding supports previous work showing that IL-10 treatment of DCs reduced their allostimulatory activity for CD8$^+$ T cells and induced alloantigen-specific anergy in CD8$^+$ T cells [137].

By contrast, IL-10 has been shown to stimulate the host immune system and contribute to limited tumor growth and metastases [146, 147]. *IL-10 enhances cellular recruitment* [148], *promotes CD8$^+$ T cell proliferation* [139, 149], *augments the outgrowth of CTL precursor cells* [150, 151] and *enhances cytolytic activity* [152]. *In vivo*, anti-IL-10 reduced the host primary CTL response in mice following immunization with B7-1$^+$ P815 tumor cells, *suggesting the important role of IL-10 in the host antitumor CTL response* [153]. In accordance with the reported immunostimulating properties of IL-10, Groux *et al.* report the enhanced CTL response in IL-10 transgenic mice [154]. Mice engineered to over-express IL-10 in antigen-presenting cells under the control of the MHC class II Ea promoter exhibited a biphasic pattern of tumor growth in which the tumors grew rapidly during the first 2 weeks and then completely regressed. Thus, *the effects of IL-10 on the host CTL response is complex*; T cell-derived IL-10 may function as an immunosuppressive factor, whereas antigen-presenting cell-derived IL-10 might act as an immunostimulating factor.

### 7.2.2.3  **Effects of IL-10 on NK cells**

Overall, *IL-10 exerts an immunostimulatory effect on NK cells*. NK cells exhibit low level IL-10 receptor expression and treatment of NK cells with *IL-10 potentiates NK cytokine production and enhances NK cytotoxicity* toward NK-resistant tumors *in vitro* [155]. Furthermore, IL-10 alone has no effect on NK proliferation, but *IL-10 augments IL-2 induced NK proliferation* [155]. These *in vitro* findings have been confirmed *by in vivo* studies. In experimental tumor models, IL-10 injection or IL-10-secreting tumor cells inhibit tumor metastases by an NK-dependent mechanism [147, 156, 157]. Thus, unlike the majority of the host immune system that is stimulated by IL-10 blockade during cancer therapy, NK cell production and activity is reduced by IL-10 inhibition.

### 7.2.2.4  **Effects of IL-10 on DCs**

DCs are central cellular inducers of the host antitumor immune response because of their potent antigen-presenting capacity and T cell co-stimulatory abilities. The majority of published studies support the immunosuppressive effects of IL-10 on DCs. *IL-10 treatment of DCs reduces their capacity to stimulate CD4$^+$ and CD8$^+$ T cell responses and promote T cell anergy* [137, 138]. Tumor expression of IL-10 has been shown to *prevent the migration and accumulation of DCs* within tumors, thus suppressing GM-CSF-induced antitumor responses [158].

The functional activities of DCs during cancer and cancer immunotherapy depend on their state of maturation. *In vitro*, exogenous *IL-10 inhibits the generation of mature monocyte-derived DCs* in response to GM-CSF and IL-4 [159], and *promotes the differentiation of immature DCs* into macrophage-like cells with decreased MHC class II expression and suppressed phagocytosic capacity exhibiting no IL-12 expression [159–161]. A similar reduction of MHC class II and co-stimulatory molecule expression was observed in IL-10-transduced DCs when compared to control gene-modified DCs [162]. These IL-10-transduced DCs cannot induce T cell proliferation; however, they can augment CTL generation and NK cell activity. A very recent study by Corinti *et al.* found that autocrine production of IL-10 by DCs prevents their spontaneous maturation of monocyte-derived DCs and treatment of immature DCs with anti-IL10 antibody enhances the expression of MHC and co-stimulatory molecules (CD80, CD83 and CD86) and cytokines (TNF-α and IL-12) [163]. Thus, IL-10 appears to exhibit complex and multifunctional activities on DCs of the immune system.

Finally, *IL-10 induces spontaneous DC apoptosis* [164]. Thus, the immunosuppressive effects of IL-10 on DC generation, activity, migration and survival may limit the effectiveness of DC-based antitumor vaccines that are being used in clinical trials for the treatment of various forms of cancer. An improved understanding of the regulators of tumor-derived IL-10 expression and the development of appropriate anti-IL-10 strategies may improve DC trial outcomes.

### 7.2.3
**Inhibition of IL-10: Implications for Therapy**

Although not as well developed as anti-TGF-β strategies, several IL-10 inhibitory treatments have been considered for the improvement of the host immune response during tumor growth *in vivo*. These include neutralizing IL-10 antibodies [165, 166], anti-IL-10 receptor antibodies [104], IL-10 antisense strategies [158, 167], drugs [168] and the removal of IL-10-producing suppressor T cells [169]. However, not all studies report improved host antitumor immune responses following IL-10 inhibition or depletion. *In vivo*, IL-10 gene-transfected melanoma [146] and mammary adenocarcinoma cells [170] significantly reduced the tumorigenic and metastatic potential of these cells in mice and appear to be anti-angiogenic. Similarly, injection of IL-10 resulted in the inhibition of both B16-F10 melanoma metastases and spontaneous melanoma development in experimental models [147]. The antitumor activity of IL-10, in part, is mediated via IFN-γ (inducible NO synthase and NO) [171]. Thus, an improved understanding of the role of IL-10 inhibition on host immunosuppression during cancer therapies is warranted.

### 7.2.3.1 Antibodies

Anti-IL-10 antibodies have been shown to up-regulate anticancer autoreactive T cell responses by inhibiting macrophage suppressor activity *in vitro* [165]. Anti-IL-10 promotes survival in tumor-bearing mice, and enhances host CTL activity *in vivo*, as well as the production of IL-2, IL-12 and IFN-γ by host spleen cells [166]. Recently, Loercher *et al.* showed that anti-IL-10 receptor antibodies block the inhibition of phytohemagglutinin-stimulated T cell proliferation induced by IL-10-secreting peritoneal monocytes obtained from ovarian cancer patients [104]. This finding suggests that inhibition of IL-10 signaling in immune cells might promote the production of anti-tumor T cells.

### 7.2.3.2 Drugs

Cyclophosphamide (low dose) has been used during active specific immunotherapy in patients with advanced melanoma and other metastatic cancers [172, 173]. The principle of using cyclophosphamide is to selectively reduce suppressor cell activity and to inhibit the production of suppressive factors such as TGF-β, IL-10 and NO while promoting antitumor immunity during tumor vaccine strategies [168]. A recent study by Matar *et al.* showed that low-dose cyclophosphamide treatment in lymphoma-bearing rats exhibiting an impaired lymphocyte proliferative response led to a decrease in IL-10 production by T cells and, consequently, a shift in the immune response from suppression toward immunopotentiation [174]. This state of immunostimulation was accompanied by reduced tumor growth and metastases in cyclophosphamide treated animals.

### 7.2.3.3 Removal of the source of IL-10

γδ T cells accumulate in early tumor lesions and spleens of tumor-bearing animals and express both TGF-β and IL-10. Therefore, depletion of these suppressor cells might lead to enhanced antitumor immune responses. Seo *et al.* recently demonstrated that lysis of tumor-associated γδ cells using a daunomycin-conjugated anti-γδ antibodies improved host tumor-specific NK and CTL responses, and resulted in tumor regression in an experimental tumor model [169]

**7.3**
**Macrophage Migration Inhibitory Factor (MIF)**

MIF was originally described in the 1960s as a product of activated T cells that inhibited the random migration of guinea pig macrophages [175, 176]. Later studies revealed the critical role of MIF in the host inflammatory response to endotoxin [177, 178]. Over the past decade, a large body of work described a role for MIF in the regulation of host inflammatory responses (reviewed in [179, 180]). Inhibition of MIF using neutralizing antibodies significantly reduces the severity of inflammatory diseases including arthritis [181–183], peritonitis [184] and glomerulonephritis [185]. In addition to its pro-inflammatory activity, our laboratory and others have identified the role of MIF as an immunomodulatory factor in T cell activation and antigen-specific T cell responses *in vitro* and *in vivo* [186, 187].

It is now known that numerous cell types found in most organs constitutively express MIF, including immune cells (reviewed in [179, 180]). However, the expression of MIF is significantly higher in tumor cells than normal cells [188–192]. Furthermore, enhanced tumor MIF expression positively correlates with a more invasive phenotype [189]. More recent studies suggest a role for MIF in positively regulating cellular proliferation [193–197].

The identification of the potential growth-promoting function of MIF led us to examine the effect of MIF neutralization on tumor growth *in vivo*. We found that MIF blockade significantly inhibited tumor growth and tumor-associated angiogenesis [198]. Similar observations demonstrating the growth promoting and pro-angiogenic functions of MIF were reported by other groups using experimental models of melanoma [199] and colon adenocarcinoma [200]. However, no direct effect of MIF on tumor cell proliferation has been reported.

Recent studies demonstrate the role of MIF in inhibiting NK-mediated lysis of endothelial cells [201] and uveal melanoma cells [202]. These studies suggest that tumor cells may secrete high levels of MIF to protect themselves from host NK-mediated destruction. More recently, our laboratory examined the effect of MIF neutralization on CTL responses during tumor growth. Using the ovalbumin-specific EG7 tumor cell model, we found that MIF immunoneutralization delays tumor growth, and was associated with increased CTL activity, an accumulation of intra-tumoral CD8[+] T cells, enhanced tumor-associated apoptosis and increased CD8[+] T cell migration to the tumor [203]. These observations are important because cell-mediated tumor destruction relies on a rapid, extensive and sustained infiltration of killer T cells [204–207]. Thus, we hypothesize that tumor-derived MIF promotes host immune suppression and prevents tumor destruction. More interestingly, these observations also raise the possibility that additional unidentified immunosuppressive factors might exist.

**7.4**
**Prostaglandin (PG) E$_2$**

PGE$_2$ is a powerful lipid mediator that influences inflammation, promotes tumor growth and suppresses the host antitumor immune response. PGE$_2$ belongs to a family of eicosanoids that are derived from n-3 and n-6 polyunsaturated fatty acids. Its synthesis is regulated by a series of steps following the cyclooxygenation of arachidonic acid by two key regulatory enzymes, cyclooxygenase (COX)-1 and -2 (reviewed in [208]). COX-1 is constitutively expressed, whereas the inducible COX-2 ("oncogene-responsive COX") is over-expressed by many tumors [209–211].

**7.4.1**
**Sources of PGE$_2$**

PGE$_2$ is expressed by numerous tissues and cell types, including breast fibroblasts [212], colonic muscle cells and mucosa [213], peritoneal mesothelial cells [214], vascular endothelial cells [215] and macrophages [216, 217], as well as many tumors and tumor cell lines including, prostate [218], squamous cell carcinoma of the head and neck [219], and mammary epithelial cells [220]. PGE$_2$ expression by macrophages can be induced by tumor cell factors [221] and in tumor-bearing mice [222]. PGE$_2$ expression often correlates with prognosis in cancer patients [223].

PGE$_2$ promotes tumor cell proliferation [224], enhances tumor cell invasiveness [218] and down-regulates MHC class II expression by tumor cells [225]. In addition to its effects of tumor cell growth, invasiveness and metastatic potential, PGE$_2$ has been shown to promote host immunosuppression during tumor progression.

**7.4.2**
**Effects of PGE$_2$**

**7.4.2.1 Effects of PGE$_2$ on monocytes/macrophages**
Host antitumor macrophage activity inversely correlates with PGE$_2$ expression [226]. Although host macrophages are considered to be the major source of PGE$_2$ during tumor growth, they express PGE$_2$ receptors [227] and thus, can be rendered dysfunctional by PGE$_2$. Similar to IL-10, *PGE$_2$ inhibits T$_h$1 cytokine synthesis (TNF-α) by macrophages while promoting ineffective T$_h$2 cytokine production* (IL-10) [228]. This ineffective shift in the host antitumor activity toward a T$_h$2 response by PGE$_2$ during tumor growth encourages host immunosuppression.

**7.4.2.2 Effects of PGE$_2$ on T lymphocytes**
*PGE$_2$ is immunosuppressive to various types of T cells through its inhibitory effects on proliferation, cytokine production, migration and effector activity* (reviewed in [229, 230]). Very early studies showed that immunization with PGE$_2$ significantly reduced tumor-induced immunosuppression (as measured by spleen cell proliferation assays) in mice [231, 232], suggesting the role of PGE$_2$ in *suppressing T cell proliferation*. Further studies using experimental tumor models and anti-PGE$_2$ antibodies demon-

strated the role of $PGE_2$ in *suppressing polyclonal T cell activation and CTL generation* following MLRs by splenic T cells [233]. $PGE_2$ treatment of stimulated peripheral blood lymphocytes and $CD4^+$ T cells *decreases IL-2 and IFN-γ production and promotes IL-10 production* [234, 235]. However, $CD8^+$ T cell effector functions are reported to be more sensitive to the suppressive effects of $PGE_2$ than $CD4^+$ T cells [236]. $PGE_2$ inhibits T cell migration [237], promotes T cell anergy [238], and suppresses $CD8^+$ CTL activity *in vitro* and *in vivo* [239–242].

### 7.4.2.3 Effects of $PGE_2$ on NK cells and LAK activity

Similar to its immunosuppressive effects on CTLs, $PGE_2$ *has been reported to inhibit NK activity* [233, 243–246] *and LAK cell activity* [233]. These findings correlate with reports that NK activity inversely correlates with monocyte-derived $PGE_2$ levels, and that removal of monocytes from the PBMCs of patients with breast cancer restored NK and LAK levels when compared to healthy controls [247].

### 7.4.3
### Inhibition of $PGE_2$: Implications for Therapy

Slowed tumor growth and the inhibition of metastases has been observed by *in vivo* blockade of $PGE_2$ activity using $PGE_2$ immunization [248], anti-$PGE_2$ antibodies [249] and inhibition of $PGE_2$ production using COX inhibitors [244, 250–254]. Inhibition of $COX_2$ (and thus $PGE_2$ production) in an experimental tumor model using the Lewis lung carcinoma cell line results in a significant decrease in IL-10 production together with a significant increase in IL-12 secretion, thus restoring host antitumor reactivity [253]. Similar findings have been observed in COX knockout mice [255, 256].

The precise mechanisms by which COX inhibitors slow tumor growth are not well understood. A very recent study by Specht *et al.* revealed that COX inhibitors enhance the host CTL responses in an experimental tumor model [252]. More interestingly, human epidemiological studies suggest the antineoplastic activities of COX inhibitors [257–259]. However, COX inhibitors also have been associated with the inhibition of angiogenesis (reviewed in [260]) and tumor growth and telomerase elongation activity in tumor cells [254].

### 7.5
### Polyamines

Polyamines (putrecine, spermine and spermadine) are natural occurring small organic cations. Polyamines are critical for both cell proliferation and differentiation (reviewed in [261]). Much of our knowledge of polyamine bioactivity stems from the use of inhibitors of polyamine biosynthesis (see below).

## 7.5.1
## Sources of Polyamines

Polyamines are found in all in all living cells. Polyamine levels (urine, serum and red blood cell) have been correlated with stage of malignancy and tumor burden [262, 263]. In addition, because dying tumor cells release high levels of polyamines, circulating polyamine levels have been proposed to serve as indicators of the success of chemotherapeutic agents [264–266]. In addition, food is a significant exogenous source of polyamines [267].

Polyamine biosynthesis can be selectively blocked by d,l-2-(difluoromethyl)ornithine (DFMO). DFMO is an irreversible inhibitor of ornithine decarboxylase (ODC) which mediates the first step in polyamine synthesis [268]. DFMO depletes the cells of intracellular putrescine and spermidine (but not spermine), and inhibits cell proliferation without cell death [269]. DFMO treatment is associated with weight loss and toxicity, and therefore led to the development of less toxic polyamine analogs. Polyamine analogs such as $N^1,N^8$-bis(ethyl)spermidine [270] are reported to rapidly deplete intracellular polyamines and induce cell death. Because exogenous polyamines found in food also contribute to the polyamine status of an individual, blockade of endogenous and exogenous (polyamine-deficient diet) is sometimes required to identify the role of polyamines on host immunosuppression during tumor growth [267].

Inhibitors of polyamine biosynthesis have been shown to inhibit tumor growth and metastases *in vivo* [271–276]. Interestingly, these inhibitors prevent the growth and metastases in experimental models of B16 melanoma and Lewis lung carcinoma when the tumor cells are s.c. implanted, but not when tumor cells are i.v. injected [273]. Much of the antitumor activity of ODC inhibitors has been attributed to their antiproliferative activity [277–281]. However, polyamines also appear to play a role in the differentiation of tumor cells [282], protease expression [283], invasiveness [284], protection against apoptosis [285, 286], malignant transformation [284, 287–290] and tumor-associated angiogenesis [291, 292]. Inhibitors of polyamines biosynthesis prevents proliferation of normal and tumor cells *in vitro,* including small cell lung carcinoma [278], mammary tumor cells [281] and melanoma cells [282]. However, tumor cells may be more dependent on polyamines for proliferation than normal host cells due to their increased proliferative rate (reviewed in [293]). In addition to their numerous effects on tumor cells, polyamines serve as suppressors of the host immune system.

## 7.5.2
## Effects of Polyamines

### 7.5.2.1  Effects of polyamines on monocytes/macrophages
*Polyamines are associated with numerous functional activities of macrophages/monocytes that may contribute to host immunosuppression during tumor growth.* Inhibitors of polyamines biosynthesis inhibit TNF-α-mediated macrophage activation [294], and the respiratory burst of macrophages [295], whereas polyamines block both NO [296, 297] and cytokine synthesis [298] by macrophages. In addition, a negative correlation

between total polyamine levels and monocyte phagocytosis has been reported in patients with colorectal cancer [299]. Accordingly, treatment of tumor-bearing animals with polyamine deprivation combined with low-dose cyclophosphamide resulted in a synergistic inhibition of tumor growth and metastasis associated with enhanced macrophage tumoricidal activities [300].

### 7.5.2.2 Effects of polyamines on T lymphocytes

Polyamine synthesis is required for the induction of CTLs and IL-2 responsiveness [301–303]. CTL differentiation is more affected by the inhibition of polyamine biosynthesis than CTL proliferation [304]. *These data suggest that polyamines are immunostimulating for T cells.* In addition, polyamine deprivation in animals grafted with Lewis lung carcinoma tumors reverses tumor-induced immunosuppression (decreased splenic IL-2 production, and depressed levels of CD4$^+$ and CD8$^+$ T cell populations), but is not associated with any changes in host CTL activity [305].

### 7.5.2.3 Effects of polyamines on NK cells

Inhibition of polyamine biosynthesis and polyamine deprivation *in vivo* is associated with decreased tumor growth and metastases and significantly enhanced NK cytotoxic activity [267, 306]. Thus, *polyamines are inhibitory for NK cells.*

### 7.5.3
### Inhibition of Polyamine Biosynthesis: Implications for Therapy

As described above, inhibitors of ODC, polyamine analogs and polyamine-deficient diets have been used in animal models to suppress polyamine levels. Both ODC inhibitors and polyamine analogs have been useful in identifying the role of polyamines on tumor growth and host immunosuppression. However, polyamine inhibition as a target for cancer treatment is very complicated due to the ubiquitous expression of polyamines and the contribution of food sources to an individual's polyamine status, as well as the critical role of polyamines on the proliferation and survival of both normal and cancer cells. Future studies are required to identify mechanism(s) to target polyamine inhibitors to neoplastic cells thereby improving the therapeutic index of these inhibitors.

### 7.6
### Tumor-Shed Immunosuppressive Molecules

In addition to tumor-secreted immunosuppressive cytokines and other intracellular-derived factors, tumors shed many antigens believed to exert immunosuppressive effects. The most well-characterized immunosuppressive antigens shed from tumors are the mucins. Mucins are high molecular weight glycoproteins present on most secretory epithelial tissues. However, most human epithelial tumors over-express aberrantly glycosylated mucins referred to as MUC-1 and -2 (reviewed in [307, 308]). MUC-1 has been employed as an immunotherapeutic target for cancer patients because of its ability to induce both anti-MUC-1 antibodies and CTL responses (reviewed in [309, 310]). However, soluble MUC-1 and -2 have been shown to be immunosuppressive tumor antigens. Accordingly, high serum levels of MUC-1 correlate with poor survival and enhanced metastatic disease for adenocarcinoma (breast, ovarian, pancreatic and colorectal) following active specific immunotherapy [311, 312]. Therefore, the release of MUC antigens from the surface of tumor cells might promote tumorigenesis and subvert the host immune system by two mechanisms: (1) *release of MUC-1 by tumor cells would inhibit the effectiveness of the host anti-MUC-specific CTL response* due to the down-regulation of specific tumor antigen expression and (2) release of tumor-associated MUC-1 molecules might have *direct immunosuppressive effects on the host immune system*. Mucins have been shown to *inhibit T cell proliferation* which can be reversed by IL-2 [313], *suppress IL-2* [314] and *IFN-γ production* by CD4$^+$ T cells [314], and *negatively regulate T cell activation* at the resting stage [315].

Similarly, the soluble forms of annexin II and carcinoembryonic antigen (CEA), additional tumor-shed antigens, appear to function as immunosuppressive factors. Annexin is a membrane-associated glycoprotein expressed by normal and tumor cells [316, 317]. Annexin II expression has been correlated with higher grade tumors [318, 319] and poor prognosis in cancer patients [320]. In its soluble form, *annexin II inhibits T cell proliferation* [321], and *suppresses IgG and IgM secretion from mononuclear cells* [322]. CEA is another example of a "tumor antigen" currently being evaluated for use in anticancer immunotherapeutic strategies. CEA is frequently present on colorectal tumors and circulating CEA levels correlate with poor survival rates [323]. *The shedding of CEA* from the surface of tumor cells has been proposed to serve as an *immunosuppressive factor for LAK cytotoxic activity* [324], *as well as NK and T$_h$1 cells* [325]. Thus, multiple shed tumor-associated antigens may function as immunosuppressive agents.

## 7.7
## Conclusion

Unfortunately, the struggle between the host and the tumor often results in defeat for the host. Tumors escape the host's innate and acquired antitumor immune response through multiple and complex mechanisms. In many cases, tumors release factors including cytokines, lipids, polyamines and/or tumor-related antigens that suppress the host immune response, and at the same time stimulate tumor growth and survival. Much is known regarding how single tumor-derived suppressive factors impair various immune cell subtypes. However, the reported immunosuppressive effects of numerous factors are often inconsistent. These inconsistencies suggest that the effects of immunosuppressive factors on the host antitumor immune response depend on many factors, including the tumor type, tumor location, cytokine milieu, timing of the appearance of the suppressive factor, as well as the origin and state of activation of the specific immune cells. In addition, we do not understand how multiple tumor-derived immunosuppressive factors interact with immune cells to subvert the host immune system *in vivo*. Furthermore, it is unlikely that we have identified all of the tumor-derived immunosuppressive factors. Thus, more extensive studies are required to improve our understanding of how tumors suppress the host immune response. This information will be invaluable for the future development of improved therapeutics designed to block tumor-associated host immunosuppression in cancer patients and to improve host antitumor immunity using conventional cancer treatments and novel immunotherapeutic approaches.

**References**

1 ASSOIAN, R. K., C. A. FROLIK, A. B. RO-BERTS, D. M. MILLER and M. B. SPORN. 1984. Transforming growth factor-β controls receptor levels for epidermal growth factor in NRK fibroblasts. *Cell* **36**: 35.

2 ROBERTS, A. B., M. A. ANZANO, L. C. LAMB, J. M. SMITH and M. B. SPORN. 1984. Antagonistic actions of retinoic acid and dexamethasone on anchorage-independent growth and epidermal growth factor binding of normal rat kidney cells. *Cancer Res.* **44**: 1635.

3 FLANDERS, K. C. and A. B. ROBERTS. 2000. TGF-β. In: M. Feldmann, S. Durum, N. Nicola, J. Vilchek and T. Hiran (eds), *Cytokine Reference*. Academic Press, New York, p. 719.

4 MASSAGUE, J. 2000. How cells read TGF-β signals. *Nat. Rev. Mol. Cell Biol* **1**: 169.

5 FOX, F. E., H. C. FORD, R. DOUGLAS, S. CHERIAN and P. C. NOWELL. 1993. Evidence that TGF-β can inhibit human T-lymphocyte proliferation through paracrine and autocrine mechanisms. *Cell. Immunol.* **150**: 45.

6 KEHRL, J. H., A. B. ROBERTS, L. M. WAKEFIELD, S. JAKOWLEW, M. B. SPORN and A. S. FAUCI. 1986. Transforming growth factor β is an important immunomodulatory protein for human B lymphocytes. *J. Immunol.* **137**: 3855.

7 BELLONE, G., M. ASTE-AMEZAGA, G. TRINCHIERI and U. RODECK. 1995. Regulation of NK cell functions by TGF-β1. *J. Immunol.* **155**: 1066.

8 VON BERNSTORFF, W., M. VOSS, S. FREICHEL, A. SCHMID, I. VOGEL, C. JOHNK, D. HENNE-BRUNS, B. KREMER and H. KALTHOFF. 2001. Systemic and local immunosuppression in pancreatic cancer patients. *Clin. Cancer Res.* **7**: 925s.

9 STRAVODIMOS, K., C. CONSTANTINIDES, T. MANOUSAKAS, C. PAVLAKI, D. PANTAZOPOULOS, A. GIANNOPOULOS and C. DIMOPOULOS. 2000. Immunohistochemical expression of transforming growth factor β1 and nm-23 H1 antioncogene in prostate cancer: divergent correlation with clinicopathological parameters. *Anticancer Res.* **20**: 3823.

10 CARDILLO, M. R., E. PETRANGELI, L. PERRACCHIO, L. SALVATORI, L. RAVENNA and F. DI SILVERIO. 2000. Transforming growth factor-β expression in prostate neoplasia. *Anal. Quant. Cytol. Histol.* **22**: 1.

11 KANG, Y., M. A. PRENTICE, J. M. MARIANO, S. DAVARYA, R. I. LINNOILA, T. W. MOODY, L. M. WAKEFIELD and S. B. JAKOWLEW. 2000. Transforming growth factor-β1 and its receptors in human lung cancer and mouse lung carcinogenesis. *Exp. Lung Res.* **26**: 685.

12 BELLONE, G., A. CARBONE, D. TIBAUDI, F. MAURI, I. FERRERO, C. SMIRNE, F. SUMAN, C. RIVETTI, G. MIGLIARETTI, M. CAMANDONA, G. PALESTRO, G. EMANUELLI and U. RODECK. 2001. Differential expression of transforming growth factors-β1, -β2 and -β3 in human colon carcinoma. *Eur. J. Cancer* **37**: 224.

13 MORETTI, S., C. PINZI, A. SPALLANZANI, E. BERTI, A. CHIARUGI, S. MAZZOLI, M. FABIANI, C. VALLECCHI and M. HERLYN. 1999. Immunohistochemical evidence of cytokine networks during progression of human melanocytic lesions. *Int. J. Cancer* **84**: 160.

14 KOLI, K. M. and C. L. ARTEAGA. 1996. Complex role of tumor cell transforming growth factor (TGF)-βs on breast carcinoma progression. *J. Mammary Gland. Biol. Neoplasia* **1**: 373.

**15** GOLD, L. I. 1999. The role for transforming growth factor-β (TGF-β) in human cancer. *Crit. Rev. Oncogenes* **10**: 303.

**16** XU, J., J. MENEZES, U. PRASAD and A. AHMAD. 1999. Elevated serum levels of transforming growth factor β1 in Epstein–Barr virus-associated nasopharyngeal carcinoma patients. *Int. J. Cancer* **84**: 396.

**17** SHIM, K. S., K. H. KIM, W. S. HAN and E. B. PARK. 1999. Elevated serum levels of transforming growth factor-β1 in patients with colorectal carcinoma: its association with tumor progression and its significant decrease after curative surgical resection. *Cancer* **85**: 554.

**18** CHOPRA, V., T. V. DINH and E. V. HANNIGAN. 1998. Circulating serum levels of cytokines and angiogenic factors in patients with cervical cancer. *Cancer Invest.* **16**: 152.

**19** SAITO, H., S. TSUJITANI, S. OKA, A. KONDO, M. IKEGUCHI, M. MAETA and N. KAIBARA. 2000. An elevated serum level of transforming growth factor-β 1 (TGF-β1) significantly correlated with lymph node metastasis and poor prognosis in patients with gastric carcinoma. *Anticancer Res.* **20**: 4489.

**20** PATERSON, I. C., J. B. MATTHEWS, S. HUNTLEY, C. M. ROBINSON, M. FAHEY, E. K. PARKINSON and S. S. PRIME. 2001. Decreased expression of TGF-β cell surface receptors during progression of human oral squamous cell carcinoma. *J. Pathol.* **193**: 458.

**21** WEST, J., T. MUNOZ-ANTONIA, J. G. JOHNSON, D. KLOTCH and C. A. MURO-CACHO. 2000. Transforming growth factor-β type II receptors and smad proteins in follicular thyroid tumors. *Laryngoscope* **110**: 1323.

**22** FUJIWARA, K., H. IKEDA and T. YOSHIMOTO. 1998. Abnormalities in expression of genes, mRNA and proteins of transforming growth factor-β receptor type I and type II in human pituitary adenomas. *Clin. Neuropathol.* **17**: 19.

**23** GARRIGUE-ANTAR, L., T. MUNOZ-ANTONIA, S. J. ANTONIA, J. GESMONDE, V. F. VELLUCCI and M. REISS. 1995. Missense mutations of the transforming growth factor β type II receptor in human head and neck squamous carcinoma cells. *Cancer Res.* **55**: 3982.

**24** LUCKE, C. D., A. PHILPOTT, J. C. METCALFE, A. M. THOMPSON, L. HUGHES-DAVIES, P. R. KEMP and R. HESKETH. 2001. Inhibiting mutations in the transforming growth factor β type 2 receptor in recurrent human breast cancer. *Cancer Res.* **61**: 482.

**25** KIM, S. J., Y. H. IM, S. D. MARKOWITZ and Y. J. BANG. 2000. Molecular mechanisms of inactivation of TGF-β receptors during carcinogenesis. *Cytokine Growth Factor Rev.* **11**: 159.

**26** IMAI, Y., M. KUROKAWA, K. IZUTSU, A. HANGAISHI, K. MAKI, S. OGAWA, S. CHIBA, K. MITANI and H. HIRAI. 2001. Mutations of the Smad4 gene in acute myelogeneous leukemia and their functional implications in leukemogenesis. *Oncogene* **20**: 88.

**27** HU, W., W. WU, M. A. NASH, R. S. FREEDMAN, J. J. KAVANAGH and C. F. VERSCHRAEGEN. 2000. Anomalies of the TGF-β postreceptor signaling pathway in ovarian cancer cell lines. *Anticancer Res.* **20**: 729.

**28** STRASSMANN, G., M. D. COLE and W. NEWMAN. 1988. Regulation of colony-stimulating factor 1-dependent macrophage precursor proliferation by type β transforming growth factor. *J. Immunol.* **140**: 2645.

**29** SATO, Y., S. KOBORI, M. SAKAI, T. YANO, T. HIGASHI, T. MATSUMURA, W. MORIKAWA, T. TERANO, A. MIYAZAKI, S. HORIUCHI and M. SHICHIRI. 1996. Lipoprotein(s) induces cell growth in rat peritoneal macrophages through inhibition of transforming growth factor-β activation. *Atherosclerosis* **125**: 15.

**30** LETTERIO, J. J. and A. B. ROBERTS. 1998. Regulation of immune responses by TGF-β. *Annu. Rev. Immunol.* **16**: 137.

**31** PINSON, D. M., R. D. LECLAIRE, R. B. LORSBACH, M. J. PARMELY and S. W. RUSSELL. 1992. Regulation by transforming growth factor-β1 of expression and function of the receptor for IFN-γ on mouse macrophages. *J. Immunol.* **149**: 2028.

**32** DING, A., C. F. NATHAN, J. GRAYCAR, R. DERYNCK, D. J. STUEHR and S. SRIMAL. 1990. Macrophage deactivating factor and transforming growth factors-β1, -β2 and -β3 inhibit induction of macrophage nitrogen oxide synthesis by IFN-γ. *J. Immunol.* **145**: 940.

**33** ALLEVA, D. G., C. J. BURGER and K. D. ELGERT. 1994. Tumor-induced regulation of suppressor macrophage nitric oxide and TNF-α production. Role of tumor-derived IL-10, TGF-β and prostaglandin E$_2$. *J. Immunol.* **153**: 1674.

**34** MAEDA, H., S. TSURU and A. SHIRAISHI. 1994. Improvement of macrophage dysfunction by administration of anti-transforming growth factor-β antibody in EL4-bearing hosts. *Jpn J. Cancer Res.* **85**: 1137.

**35** JUN, C. D., B. M. CHOI, S. U. KIM, S. Y. LEE, H. M. KIM and H. T. CHUNG. 1995. Down-regulation of transforming growth factor-β gene expression by antisense oligodeoxynucleotides increases recombinant interferon-γ-induced nitric oxide synthesis in murine peritoneal macrophages. *Immunology* **85**: 114.

**36** SMYTH, M. J., S. L. STROBL, H. A. YOUNG, J. R. ORTALDO and A. C. OCHOA. 1991. Regulation of lymphokine-activated killer activity and pore-forming protein gene expression in human peripheral blood CD8$^+$ T lymphocytes. Inhibition by transforming growth factor-β. *J. Immunol.* **146**: 3289.

**37** LEE, H. M. and S. RICH. 1993. Differential activation of CD8$^+$ T cells by transforming growth factor-β1. *J. Immunol.* **151**: 668.

**38** MULE, J. J., S. L. SCHWARZ, A. B. ROBERTS, M. B. SPORN and S. A. ROSENBERG. 1988. Transforming growth factor-β inhibits the *in vitro* generation of lymphokine-activated killer cells and cytotoxic T cells. *Cancer Immunol. Immunother.* **26**: 95.

**39** ESPEVIK, T., I. S. FIGARI, G. E. RANGES and M. A. PALLADINO, JR. 1988. Transforming growth factor-β1 (TGF-β1) and recombinant human tumor necrosis factor-α reciprocally regulate the generation of lymphokine-activated killer cell activity. Comparison between natural porcine platelet-derived TGF-β1 and TGF-β2 and recombinant human TGF-β1. *J. Immunol.* **140**: 2312.

**40** ESPEVIK, T., A. WAAGE, A. FAXVAAG and M. R. SHALABY. 1990. Regulation of interleukin-2 and interleukin-6 production from T-cells: involvement of interleukin-1β and transforming growth factor-β. *Cell. Immunol.* **126**: 47.

**41** FARGEAS, C., C. Y. WU, T. NAKAJIMA, D. COX, T. NUTMAN and G. DELESPESSE. 1992. Differential effect of transforming growth factor β on the synthesis of T$_h$1- and T$_h$2-like lymphokines by human T lymphocytes. *Eur. J. Immunol.* **22**: 2173.

**42** LUDVIKSSON, B. R., D. SEEGERS, A. S. RESNICK and W. STROBER. 2000. The effect of TGF-β1 on immune responses of naive versus memory CD4$^+$ T$_h$1/T$_h$2 T cells. *Eur. J. Immunol.* **30**: 2101.

**43** KEHRL, J. H., L. M. WAKEFIELD, A. B. ROBERTS, S. JAKOWLEW, M. ALVAREZ-MON, R. DERYNCK, M. B. SPORN and A. S. FAUCI. 1986. Production of transforming growth factor β by human T lymphocytes and its potential role in the regulation of T cell growth. *J. Exp. Med.* **163**: 1037.

**44** INGE, T. H., K. M. McCOY, B. M. SUSSKIND, S. K. BARRETT, G. ZHAO and H. D. BEAR. 1992. Immunomodulatory effects of transforming growth factor-β on T lymphocytes. Induction of CD8 expression in the CTLL-2 cell line and in normal thymocytes. *J. Immunol.* **148**: 3847.

**45** EBERT, E. C. 1999. Inhibitory effects of transforming growth factor-β (TGF-β) on certain functions of intraepithelial lymphocytes. *Clin. Exp. Immunol.* **115**: 415.

**46** CERWENKA, A., D. BEVEC, O. MAJDIC, W. KNAPP and W. HOLTER. 1994. TGF-β 1 is a potent inducer of human effector T cells. *J. Immunol.* **153**: 4367.

**47** KASID, A., G. I. BELL and E. P. DIRECTOR. 1988. Effects of transforming growth factor-β on human lymphokine-activated killer cell precursors. Autocrine inhibition of cellular proliferation and differentiation to immune killer cells. *J. Immunol.* **141**: 690.

**48** AHUJA, S. S., F. PALIOGIANNI, H. YAMADA, J. E. BALOW and D. T. BOUMPAS. 1993. Effect of transforming growth factor-β on early and late activation events in human T cells. *J. Immunol*. **150**: 3109.

49  PARDOUX, C., C. ASSELIN-PATUREL, J. CHEHIMI, F. GAY, F. MAMI-CHOUAIB and S. CHOUAIB. 1997. Functional interaction between TGF-β and IL-12 in human primary allogeneic cytotoxicity and proliferative response. *J. Immunol*. **158**: 136.

50  BRIGHT, J. J. and S. SRIRAM. 1998. TGF-β inhibits IL-12-induced activation of Jak-STAT pathway in T lymphocytes. *J. Immunol*. **161**: 1772.

51  SUDARSHAN, C., J. GALON, Y. ZHOU and J. J. O'SHEA. 1999. TGF-β does not inhibit IL-12- and IL-2-induced activation of Janus kinases and STATs. *J. Immunol*. **162**: 2974.

52  WELLER, M., D. B. CONSTAM, U. MALIPIERO and A. FONTANA. 1994. Transforming growth factor-β2 induces apoptosis of murine T cell clones without down-regulating bcl-2 mRNA expression. *Eur. J. Immunol*. **24**: 1293.

53  ANDJELIC, S., A. KHANNA, M. SUTHANTHIRAN and J. NIKOLIC-ZUGIC. 1997. Intracellular Ca$^{2+}$ elevation and cyclosporin A synergistically induce TGF-β1-mediated apoptosis in lymphocytes. *J. Immunol*. **158**: 2527.

54  CERWENKA, A., H. KOVAR, O. MAJDIC and W. HOLTER. 1996. Fas- and activation-induced apoptosis are reduced in human T cells preactivated in the presence of TGF-β1. *J. Immunol*. **156**: 459.

55  RICH, S., N. VAN NOOD and H. M. LEE. 1996. Role of $\alpha_5\beta_1$ integrin in TGF-β1-costimulated CD8$^+$ T cell growth and apoptosis. *J. Immunol*. **157**: 2916.

56  ZHANG, X., L. GIANGRECO, H. E. BROOME, C. M. DARGAN and S. L. SWAIN. 1995. Control of CD4 effector fate: transforming growth factor β1 and interleukin 2 synergize to prevent apoptosis and promote effector expansion. *J. Exp. Med*. **182**: 699.

57  SCHIOTT, A., H. O. SJOGREN and M. LINDVALL. 1998. The three isoforms of transforming growth factor-β co-stimulate rat T cells and inhibit lymphocyte apoptosis. *Scand. J. Immunol*. **48**: 371.

58  GENESTIER, L., S. KASIBHATLA, T. BRUNNER and D. R. GREEN. 1999. Transforming growth factor β1 inhibits Fas ligand expression and subsequent activation-induced cell death in T cells via downregulation of c-Myc. *J. Exp. Med*. **189**: 231.

59  CHUNG, E. J., S. H. CHOI, Y. H. SHIM, Y. J. BANG, K. C. HUR and C. W. KIM. 2000. Transforming growth factor-β induces apoptosis in activated murine T cells through the activation of caspase 1-like protease. *Cel.l Immunol*. **204**: 46.

60  SILLETT, H. K., S. M. CRUICKSHANK, J. SOUTHGATE and L. K. TREJDOSIEWICZ. 2001. Transforming growth factor-β promotes "death by neglect" in post-activated human T cells. *Immunology* **102**: 310.

61  ROOK, A. H., J. H. KEHRL, L. M. WAKEFIELD, A. B. ROBERTS, M. B. SPORN, D. B. BURLINGTON, H. C. LANE and A. S. FAUCI. 1986. Effects of transforming growth factor β on the functions of natural killer cells: depressed cytolytic activity and blunting of interferon responsiveness. *J. Immunol*. **136**: 3916.

62  KUPPNER, M. C., M. F. HAMOU, S. BODMER, A. FONTANA and N. DE TRIBOLET. 1988. The glioblastoma-derived T-cell suppressor factor/transforming growth factor β2 inhibits the generation of lymphokine-activated killer (LAK) cells. *Int. J. Cancer* **42**: 562.

63  BROOKS, B., K. CHAPMAN, J. LAWRY, A. MEAGER and R. C. REES. 1990. Suppression of lymphokine-activated killer (LAK) cell induction mediated by interleukin-4 and transforming growth factor-β1: effect of addition of exogenous tumour necrosis factor-α and interferon-γ and measurement of their endogenous production. *Clin. Exp. Immunol*. **82**: 583.

64  MALYGIN, A. M., S. MERI and T. TIMONEN. 1993. Regulation of natural killer cell activity by transforming growth factor-β and prostaglandin E$_2$. *Scand. J. Immunol*. **37**: 71.

65  FONG, L. and E. G. ENGLEMAN. 2000. Dendritic cells in cancer immunotherapy. *Annu. Rev. Immunol*. **18**: 245.

66  BANCHEREAU, J., F. BRIERE, C. CAUX, J. DAVOUST, S. LEBECQUE, Y. J. LIU,

B. Pulendran and K. Palucka. 2000. Immunobiology of dendritic cells. *Annu. Rev. Immunol.* **18**: 767.

**67** Yamaguchi, Y., H. Tsumura, M. Miwa and K. Inaba. 1997. Contrasting effects of TGF-β1 and TNF-α on the development of dendritic cells from progenitors in mouse bone marrow. *Stem Cells* **15**: 144.

**68** Lee, W. C., C. Zhong, S. Qian, Y. Wan, J. Gauldie, Z. Mi, P. D. Robbins, A. W. Thomson and L. Lu. 1998. Phenotype, function and *in vivo* migration and survival of allogeneic dendritic cell progenitors genetically engineered to express TGF-β. *Transplantation* **66**: 1810.

**69** Sato, K., H. Kawasaki, H. Nagayama, M. Enomoto, C. Morimoto, K. Tadokoro, T. Juji and T. A. Takahashi. 2000. TGF-β1 reciprocally controls chemotaxis of human peripheral blood monocyte-derived dendritic cells via chemokine receptors. *J. Immunol.* **164**: 2285.

**70** Won, J., H. Kim, E. J. Park, Y. Hong, S. J. Kim and Y. Yun. 1999. Tumorigenicity of mouse thymoma is suppressed by soluble type II transforming growth factor β receptor therapy. *Cancer Res.* **59**: 1273.

**71** Engel, S., S. Isenmann, M. Stander, J. Rieger, M. Bahr and M. Weller. 1999. Inhibition of experimental rat glioma growth by decorin gene transfer is associated with decreased microglial infiltration. *J. Neuroimmunol.* **99**: 13.

**72** Stander, M., U. Naumann, L. Dumitrescu, M. Heneka, P. Loschmann, E. Gulbins, J. Dichgans and M. Weller. 1998. Decorin gene transfer-mediated suppression of TGF-β synthesis abrogates experimental malignant glioma growth *in vivo*. *Gene Ther.* **5**: 1187.

**73** Stander, M., U. Naumann, W. Wick and M. Weller. 1999. Transforming growth factor-β and p-21: multiple molecular targets of decorin-mediated suppression of neoplastic growth. *Cell Tissue Res.* **296**: 221.

**74** Harthun, N. L., A. M. Weaver, L. H. Brinckerhoff, D. H. Deacon, S. L. Gonias and C. L. Slingluff, Jr.

1998. Activated α₂-macroglobulin reverses the immunosuppressive activity in human breast cancer cell-conditioned medium by selectively neutralizing transforming growth factor-β in the presence of interleukin-2. *J. Immunother.* **21**: 85.

**75** Wojtowicz-Praga, S., U. N. Verma, L. Wakefield, J. M. Esteban, D. Hartmann, A. Mazumder and U. M. Verma. 1996. Modulation of B16 melanoma growth and metastasis by anti-transforming growth factor β antibody and interleukin-2. *J. Immunother. Emphasis Tumor Immunol.* **19**: 169.

**76** Gridley, D. S., S. S. Sura, J. R. Uhm, C. H. Lin and J. D. Kettering. 1993. Effects of anti-transforming growth factor-β antibody and interleukin-2 in tumor-bearing mice. *Cancer Biother.* **8**: 159.

**77** Ohmori, T., J. L. Yang, J. O. Price and C. L. Arteaga. 1998. Blockade of tumor cell transforming growth factor-βs enhances cell cycle progression and sensitizes human breast carcinoma cells to cytotoxic chemotherapy. *Exp. Cell Res.* **245**: 350.

**78** Park, J. A., E. Wang, R. A. Kurt, S. F. Schluter, E. M. Hersh and E. T. Akporiaye. 1997. Expression of an antisense transforming growth factor-β1 transgene reduces tumorigenicity of EMT6 mammary tumor cells. *Cancer Gene Ther.* **4**: 42.

**79** Liau, L. M., H. Fakhrai and K. L. Black. 1998. Prolonged survival of rats with intracranial C6 gliomas by treatment with TGF-β antisense gene. *Neurol. Res.* **20**: 742.

**80** Maggard, M., L. Meng, B. Ke, R. Allen, L. Devgan and D. K. Imagawa. 2001. Antisense TGF-β2 immunotherapy for hepatocellular carcinoma: treatment in a rat tumor model. *Ann. Surg. Oncol* **8**: 32.

**81** Naganuma, H., A. Sasaki, E. Satoh, M. Nagasaka, S. Nakano, S. Isoe and H. Nukui. 1998. Down-regulation of transforming growth factor-β and interleukin-10 secretion from malignant glioma cells by cytokines and anticancer drugs. *J. Neurooncol.* **39**: 227.

82  GLEIZES, P. E., J. S. MUNGER, I. NUNES, J. G. HARPEL, R. MAZZIERI, I. NOGUERA and D. B. RIFKIN. 1997. TGF-β latency: biological significance and mechanisms of activation. *Stem Cells* **15**: 190.

83  KOLI, K., J. SAHARINEN, M. HYYTIAI-NEN, C. CP and J. KESKI-OJA. 2001. Latency, activation and binding proteins of TGF-β. *Microsc. Res. Tech.* **52**: 354.

84  DUBOIS, C. M., F. BLANCHETTE, M. H. LAPRISE, R. LEDUC, F. GRONDIN and N. G. SEIDAH. 2001. Evidence that furin is an authentic transforming growth factor-β1-converting enzyme. *Am. J. Pathol.* **158**: 305.

85  CHU, T. M. and E. KAWINSKI. 1998. Plasmin, substilisin-like endoproteases, tissue plasminogen activator and urokinase plasminogen activator are involved in activation of latent TGF-β1 in human seminal plasma. *Biochem. Biophys. Res. Commun.* **253**: 128.

86  NUNES, I., P. E. GLEIZES, C. N. METZ and D. B. RIFKIN. 1997. Latent transforming growth factor-β binding protein domains involved in activation and transglutaminase-dependent cross-linking of latent transforming growth factor-β. *J. Cell Biol.* **136**: 1151.

87  NUNES, I., R. L. SHAPIRO and D. B. RIFKIN. 1995. Characterization of latent TGF-β activation by murine peritoneal macrophages. *J. Immunol.* **155**: 1450.

88  CRAWFORD, S. E., V. STELLMACH, J. E. MURPHY-ULLRICH, S. M. RIBEIRO, J. LAWLER, R. O. HYNES, G. P. BOIVIN and N. BOUCK. 1998. Thrombospondin-1 is a major activator of TGF-β1 *in vivo*. *Cell* **93**: 1159.

89  RIBEIRO, S. M., M. POCZATEK, S. SCHULTZ-CHERRY, M. VILLAIN and J. E. MURPHY-ULLRICH. 1999. The activation sequence of thrombospondin-1 interacts with the latency-associated peptide to regulate activation of latent transforming growth factor-β. *J. Biol Chem.* **274**: 13586.

90  SASAKI, A., H. NAGANUMA, E. SATOH, T. KAWATAKI, K. AMAGASAKI and H. NUKUI. 2001. Participation of thrombospondin-1 in the activation of latent transforming growth factor-β in malignant glioma cells. *Neurol. Med. Chir (Tokyo)* **41**: 253.

91  HARPEL, J. G., S. SCHULTZ-CHERRY, J. E. MURPHY-ULLRICH and D. B. RIFKIN. 2001. Tamoxifen and estrogen effects on TGF-β formation: role of thrombospondin-1, $\alpha_v\beta_3$ and integrin-associated protein. *Biochem. Biophys. Res. Commun.* **284**: 11.

92  YANG, L., E. E. TREDGET and A. GHAHARY. 2000. Activation of latent transforming growth factor-β1 is induced by mannose 6-phosphate/insulin-like growth factor-II receptor. *Wound Repair Regen.* **8**: 538.

93  DUBOIS, C. M., M. H. LAPRISE, F. BLANCHETTE, L. E. GENTRY and R. LEDUC. 1995. Processing of transforming growth factor β1 precursor by human furin convertase. *J. Biol. Chem.* **270**: 10618.

94  LEITLEIN, J., S. AULWURM, R. WALTEREIT, U. NAUMANN, B. WAGENKNECHT, W. GARTEN, M. WELLER and M. PLATTEN. 2001. Processing of immunosuppressive pro-TGF-β1, 2 by human glioblastoma cells involves cytoplasmic and secreted furin-like proteases. *J. Immunol.* **166**: 7238.

95  ZUJEWSKI, J., A. VAUGHN-COOKE, K. C. FLANDERS, M. A. ECKHAUS, R. A. LUBET and L. M. WAKEFIELD. 2001. Transforming growth factors-β are not good biomarkers of chemopreventive efficacy in a preclinical breast cancer model system. *Breast Cancer Res.* **3**: 66.

96  HASHIMOTO, K., Y. NIO, S. SUMI, T. TOGA, H. OMORI, M. ITAKURA and S. YANO. 2001. Correlation between TGF-β1 and p21 (WAF1/CIP1) expression and prognosis in resectable invasive ductal carcinoma of the pancreas. *Pancreas* **22**: 341.

97  PIERCE, D. F., JR, A. E. GORSKA, A. CHYTIL, K. S. MEISE, D. L. PAGE, R. J. COFFEY, JR and H. L. MOSES. 1995. Mammary tumor suppression by transforming growth factor β1 transgene expression. *Proc. Natl Acad. Sci. USA* **92**: 4254.

98  ASHLEY, D. M., F. M. KONG, D. D. BIGNER and L. P. HALE. 1998. Endogenous expression of transforming growth factor β1 inhibits growth and tumorigenicity and enhances Fas-mediated apopto-

sis in a murine high-grade glioma model. *Cancer Res.* **58**: 302.

**99** MOORE, K. W., R. DE WAAL MALEFYT, R. L. COFFMAN and A. O'GARRA. 2001. Interleukin-10 and the interleukin-10 receptor. *Annu. Rev. Immunol.* **19**: 683.

**100** FIORENTINO, D. F., M. W. BOND and T. R. MOSMANN. 1989. Two types of mouse T helper cell. IV. $T_h2$ clones secrete a factor that inhibits cytokine production by $T_h1$ clones. *J. Exp. Med.* **170**: 2081.

**101** BECKER, J. C., C. CZERNY and E. B. BROCKER. 1994. Maintenance of clonal anergy by endogenously produced IL-10. *Int. Immunol.* **6**: 1605.

**102** ORTEGEL, J. W., E. D. STAREN, L. P. FABER, W. H. WARREN and D. P. BRAUN. 2000. Cytokine biosynthesis by tumor-infiltrating T lymphocytes from human non-small-cell lung carcinoma. *Cancer Immunol. Immunother.* **48**: 627.

**103** COOPER, M. A., T. A. FEHNIGER, S. C. TURNER, K. S. CHEN, B. A. GHAHERI, T. GHAYUR, W. E. CARSON and M. A. CALIGIURI. 2001. Human natural killer cells: a unique innate immunoregulatory role for the CD56(bright) subset. *Blood* **97**: 3146.

**104** LOERCHER, A. E., M. A. NASH, J. J. KAVANAGH, C. D. PLATSOUCAS and R. S. FREEDMAN. 1999. Identification of an IL-10-producing HLA-DR-negative monocyte subset in the malignant ascites of patients with ovarian carcinoma that inhibits cytokine protein expression and proliferation of autologous T cells. *J. Immunol.* **163**: 6251.

**105** HUANG, M., S. SHARMA, J. T. MAO and S. M. DUBINETT. 1996. Non-small cell lung cancer-derived soluble mediators and prostaglandin $E_2$ enhance peripheral blood lymphocyte IL-10 transcription and protein production. *J. Immunol.* **157**: 5512.

**106** SATO, T., P. MCCUE, K. MASUOKA, S. SALWEN, E. C. LATTIME, M. J. MASTRANGELO and D. BERD. 1996. Interleukin 10 production by human melanoma. *Clin. Cancer Res.* **2**: 1383.

**107** HUETTNER, C., S. CZUB, S. KERKAU, W. ROGGENDORF and J. C. TONN. 1997. Interleukin 10 is expressed in human gliomas *in vivo* and increases glioma

cell proliferation and motility *in vitro*. *Anticancer Res.* **17**: 3217.

**108** MORI, N. and D. PRAGER. 1998. Interleukin-10 gene expression and adult T-cell leukemia. *Leuk. Lymph.* **29**: 239.

**109** BARGOU, R. C., M. Y. MAPARA, C. ZUGCK, P. T. DANIEL, M. PAWLITA, H. DOHNER and B. DORKEN. 1993. Characterization of a novel Hodgkin cell line, HD-MyZ, with myelomonocytic features mimicking Hodgkin's disease in severe combined immunodeficient mice. *J. Exp. Med.* **177**: 1257.

**110** VOORZANGER, N., R. TOUITOU, E. GARCIA, H. J. DELECLUSE, F. ROUSSET, I. JOAB, M. C. FAVROT and J. Y. BLAY. 1996. Interleukin (IL)-10 and IL-6 are produced *in vivo* by non-Hodgkin's lymphoma cells and act as cooperative growth factors. *Cancer Res.* **56**: 5499.

**111** MATSUDA, M., F. SALAZAR, M. PETERSSON, G. MASUCCI, J. HANSSON, P. PISA, Q. J. ZHANG, M. G. MASUCCI and R. KIESSLING. 1994. Interleukin 10 pretreatment protects target cells from tumor- and allo-specific cytotoxic T cells and downregulates HLA class I expression. *J. Exp. Med.* **180**: 2371.

**112** SALAZAR-ONFRAY, F., M. PETERSSON, L. FRANKSSON, M. MATSUDA, T. BLANKENSTEIN, K. KARRE and R. KIESSLING. 1995. IL-10 converts mouse lymphoma cells to a CTL-resistant, NK-sensitive phenotype with low but peptide-inducible MHC class I expression. *J. Immunol.* **154**: 6291.

**113** TSURUMA, T., A. YAGIHASHI, K. HIRATA, T. TORIGOE, J. ARAYA, N. WATANABE and N. SATO. 1999. Interleukin-10 reduces natural killer (NK) sensitivity of tumor cells by downregulating NK target structure expression. *Cell. Immunol.* **198**: 103.

**114** ALAS, S., C. EMMANOUILIDES and B. BONAVIDA. 2001. Inhibition of interleukin 10 by rituximab results in down-regulation of *bcl*-2 and sensitization of B-cell non-Hodgkin's lymphoma to apoptosis. *Clin. Cancer Res.* **7**: 709.

**115** BOHLEN, H., M. KESSLER, M. SEXTRO, V. DIEHL and H. TESCH. 2000. Poor clinical outcome of patients with Hodgkin's disease and elevated interleukin-10 serum levels. Clinical significance of interleukin-10 serum levels for Hodgkin's disease. *Ann. Hematol.* **79**: 110.

**116** SARRIS, A. H., K. O. KLICHE, P. PETHAMBARAM, A. PRETI, S. TUCKER, C. JACKOW, O. MESSINA, W. PUGH, F. B. HAGEMEISTER, P. MCLAUGHLIN, M. A. RODRIGUEZ, J. ROMAGUERA, H. FRITSCHE, T. WITZIG, M. DUVIC, M. ANDREEFF and F. CABANILLAS. 1999. Interleukin-10 levels are often elevated in serum of adults with Hodgkin's disease and are associated with inferior failure-free survival. *Ann. Oncol* **10**: 433.

**117** AXDORPH, U., J. SJOBERG, G. GRIMFORS, O. LANDGREN, A. PORWIT-MACDONALD and M. BJORKHOLM. 2000. Biological markers may add to prediction of outcome achieved by the International Prognostic Score in Hodgkin's disease. *Ann. Oncol.* **11**: 1405.

**118** NEMUNAITIS, J., T. FONG, P. SHABE, D. MARTINEAU and D. ANDO. 2001. Comparison of serum interleukin-10 (IL-10) levels between normal volunteers and patients with advanced melanoma. *Cancer Invest.* **19**: 239.

**119** BERGHELLA, A. M., P. PELLEGRINI, T. DEL BEATO, D. ADORNO and C. U. CASCIANI. 1997. IL-10 and sIL-2R serum levels as possible peripheral blood prognostic markers in the passage from adenoma to colorectal cancer. *Cancer Biother. Radiopharm.* **12**: 265.

**120** CHAU, G. Y., C. W. WU, W. Y. LUI, T. J. CHANG, H. L. KAO, L. H. WU, K. L. KING, C. C. LOONG, C. Y. HSIA and C. W. CHI. 2000. Serum interleukin-10 but not interleukin-6 is related to clinical outcome in patients with resectable hepatocellular carcinoma. *Ann. Surg.* **231**: 552.

**121** DE VITA, F., M. ORDITURA, G. GALIZIA, C. ROMANO, E. LIETO, P. IODICE, C. TUCCILLO and G. CATALANO. 2000. Serum interleukin-10 is an independent prognostic factor in advanced solid tumors. *Oncol. Rep.* **7**: 357.

**122** SILVESTRE, J. S., Z. MALLAT, M. DURIEZ, R. TAMARAT, M. F. BUREAU, D. SCHERMAN, N. DUVERGER, D. BRANELLEC, A. TEDGUI and B. I. LEVY. 2000. Antiangiogenic effect of interleukin-10 in ischemia-induced angiogenesis in mice hindlimb. *Circ. Res.* **87**: 448.

**123** HATANAKA, H., Y. ABE, M. NARUKE, T. TOKUNAGA, Y. OSHIKA, T. KAWAKAMI, H. OSADA, J. NAGATA, J. KAMOCHI, T. TSUCHIDA, H. KIJIMA, H. YAMAZAKI, H. INOUE, Y. UEYAMA and M. NAKAMURA. 2001. Significant correlation between interleukin 10 expression and vascularization through angiopoietin/TIE2 networks in non-small cell lung cancer. *Clin. Cancer Res.* **7**: 1287.

**124** DE WAAL MALEFYT, R., J. ABRAMS, B. BENNETT, C. G. FIGDOR and J. E. DE VRIES. 1991. Interleukin 10 (IL-10) inhibits cytokine synthesis by human monocytes: an autoregulatory role of IL-10 produced by monocytes. *J. Exp. Med.* **174**: 1209.

**125** FIORENTINO, D. F., A. ZLOTNIK, T. R. MOSMANN, M. HOWARD and A. O'GARRA. 1991. IL-10 inhibits cytokine production by activated macrophages. *J. Immunol.* **147**: 3815.

**126** BERG, D. J., J. ZHANG, D. M. LAURICELLA and S. A. MOORE. 2001. IL-10 is a central regulator of cyclooxygenase-2 expression and prostaglandin production. *J. Immunol.* **166**: 2674.

**127** GAZZINELLI, R. T., I. P. OSWALD, S. HIENY, S. L. JAMES and A. SHER. 1992. The microbicidal activity of interferon-γ-treated macrophages against *Trypanosoma cruzi* involves an l-arginine-dependent, nitrogen oxide-mediated mechanism inhibitable by interleukin-10 and transforming growth factor-β. *Eur. J. Immunol.* **22**: 2501.

**128** OSWALD, I. P., R. T. GAZZINELLI, A. SHER and S. L. JAMES. 1992. IL-10 synergizes with IL-4 and transforming growth factor-β to inhibit macrophage cytotoxic activity. *J. Immunol.* **148**: 3578.

**129** DE WAAL MALEFYT, R., J. HAANEN, H. SPITS, M. G. RONCAROLO, V. A. TE, C. FIGDOR, K. JOHNSON, R. KASTELEIN, H. YSSEL and J. E. DE VRIES. 1991. Interleukin 10 (IL-10) and viral IL-10 strongly reduce antigen-specific human T cell proliferation by diminishing the antigen-presenting capacity of monocytes via downregulation of class II major histocompatibility complex expression. *J. Exp. Med.* **174**: 915.

**130** KOPPELMAN, B., J. J. NEEFJES, J. E. DE VRIES and R. DE WAAL MALEFYT. 1997.

Interleukin-10 down-regulates MHC class II αβ peptide complexes at the plasma membrane of monocytes by affecting arrival and recycling. *Immunity* **7**: 861.

**131** Ding, L., P. S. Linsley, L. Y. Huang, R. N. Germain and E. M. Shevach. 1993. IL-10 inhibits macrophage costimulatory activity by selectively inhibiting the up-regulation of B7 expression. *J. Immunol.* **151**: 1224.

**132** Willems, F., A. Marchant, J. P. Delville, C. Gerard, A. Delvaux, T. Velu, M. de Boer and M. Goldman. 1994. Interleukin-10 inhibits B7 and intercellular adhesion molecule-1 expression on human monocytes. *Eur. J. Immunol.* **24**: 1007.

**133** Walker, T. M., C. J. Burger and K. D. Elgert. 1994. Tumor growth alters T cell and macrophage production of and responsiveness to granulocyte-macrophage colony-stimulating factor: partial dysregulation through interleukin-10. *Cell Immunol.* **154**: 342.

**134** de Waal Malefyt, R., H. Yssel and J. E. de Vries. 1993. Direct effects of IL-10 on subsets of human CD4+ T cell clones and resting T cells. Specific inhibition of IL-2 production and proliferation. *J. Immunol.* **150**: 4754.

**135** Taga, K. and G. Tosato. 1992. IL-10 inhibits human T cell proliferation and IL-2 production. *J. Immunol.* **148**: 1143.

**136** Barth, R. J., Jr, M. A. Coppola and W. R. Green. 1996. *In vivo* effects of locally secreted IL-10 on the murine antitumor immune response. *Ann. Surg. Oncol.* **3**: 381.

**137** Steinbrink, K., H. Jonuleit, G. Muller, G. Schuler, J. Knop and A. H. Enk. 1999. Interleukin-10-treated human dendritic cells induce a melanoma-antigen-specific anergy in CD8(+) T cells resulting in a failure to lyse tumor cells. *Blood* **93**: 1634.

**138** Steinbrink, K., M. Wolfl, H. Jonuleit, J. Knop and A. H. Enk. 1997. Induction of tolerance by IL-10-treated dendritic cells. *J. Immunol.* **159**: 4772.

**139** Groux, H., M. Bigler, J. E. de Vries and M. G. Roncarolo. 1996. Interleukin-10 induces a long-term antigen-spe-

cific anergic state in human CD4+ T cells. *J. Exp. Med.* **184**: 19.

**140** Chen, M. L., F. H. Wang, P. K. Lee and C. M. Lin. 2001. Interleukin-10-induced T cell unresponsiveness can be reversed by dendritic cell stimulation. *Immunol. Lett.* **75**: 91.

**141** Bejarano, M. T., R. de Waal Malefyt, J. S. Abrams, M. Bigler, R. Bacchetta, J. E. de Vries and M. G. Roncarolo. 1992. Interleukin 10 inhibits allogeneic proliferative and cytotoxic T cell responses generated in primary mixed lymphocyte cultures. *Int. Immunol.* **4**: 1389.

**142** Hsieh, C. L., D. S. Chen and L. H. Hwang. 2000. Tumor-induced immunosuppression: a barrier to immunotherapy of large tumors by cytokine-secreting tumor vaccine. *Hum. Gene Ther.* **11**: 681.

**143** Fitzpatrick, L., A. P. Makrigiannis, M. Kaiser and D. W. Hoskin. 1996. Anti-CD3-activated killer T cells: interferon-γ and interleukin-10 cross-regulate granzyme B expression and the induction of major histocompatibility complex-unrestricted cytotoxicity. *J. Interferon Cytokine Res.* **16**: 537.

**144** Wang, L., E. Goillot and R. I. Tepper. 1994. IL-10 inhibits alloreactive cytotoxic T lymphocyte generation *in vivo*. *Cell. Immunol.* **159**: 152.

**145** Sharma, S., M. Stolina, Y. Lin, B. Gardner, P. W. Miller, M. Kronenberg and S. M. Dubinett. 1999. T cell-derived IL-10 promotes lung cancer growth by suppressing both T cell and APC function. *J. Immunol.* **163**: 5020.

**146** Huang, S., S. E. Ullrich and M. Bar-Eli. 1999. Regulation of tumor growth and metastasis by interleukin-10: the melanoma experience. *J. Interferon Cytokine Res.* **19**: 697.

**147** Zheng, L. M., D. M. Ojcius, F. Garaud, C. Roth, E. Maxwell, Z. Li, H. Rong, J. Chen, X. Y. Wang, J. J. Catino and I. King. 1996. Interleukin-10 inhibits tumor metastasis through an NK cell-dependent mechanism. *J. Exp. Med.* **184**: 579.

**148** Jinquan, T., C. G. Larsen, B. Gesser, K. Matsushima and K. Thestrup-Pedersen. 1993. Human IL-10 is a chemoattractant for CD8$^+$ T lymphocytes and an inhibitor of IL-8-induced CD4$^+$ T lymphocyte migration. *J. Immunol.* **151**: 4545.

149 ROWBOTTOM, A. W., M. A. LEPPER, R. J. GARLAND, C. V. COX and E. G. CORLEY. 1999. Interleukin-10-induced CD8 cell proliferation. *Immunology* **98**: 80.

150 CHEN, W. F. and A. ZLOTNIK. 1991. IL-10: a novel cytotoxic T cell differentiation factor. *J. Immunol.* **147**: 528.

151 MACNEIL, I. A., T. SUDA, K. W. MOORE, T. R. MOSMANN and A. ZLOTNIK. 1990. IL-10, a novel growth cofactor for mature and immature T cells. *J. Immunol.* **145**: 4167.

152 SANTIN, A. D., P. L. HERMONAT, A. RAVAGGI, S. BELLONE, S. PECORELLI, J. J. ROMAN, G. P. PARHAM and M. J. CANNON. 2000. Interleukin-10 increases T$_h$1 cytokine production and cytotoxic potential in human papillomavirus-specific CD8(+) cytotoxic T lymphocytes. *J. Virol.* **74**: 4729.

153 YANG, G., K. E. HELLSTROM, M. T. MIZUNO and L. CHEN. 1995. *In vitro* priming of tumor-reactive cytolytic T lymphocytes by combining IL-10 with B7-CD28 costimulation. *J. Immunol.* **155**: 3897.

154 GROUX, H., F. COTTREZ, M. ROULEAU, S. MAUZE, S. ANTONENKO, S. HURST, T. MCNEIL, M. BIGLER, M. G. RONCAROLO and R. L. COFFMAN. 1999. A transgenic model to analyze the immunoregulatory role of IL-10 secreted by antigen-presenting cells. *J. Immunol.* **162**: 1723.

155 CARSON, W. E., M. J. LINDEMANN, R. BAIOCCHI, M. LINETT, J. C. TAN, C. C. CHOU, S. NARULA and M. A. CALIGIURI. 1995. The functional characterization of interleukin-10 receptor expression on human natural killer cells. *Blood* **85**: 3577.

156 KUNDU, N., T. L. BEATY, M. J. JACKSON and A. M. FULTON. 1996. Antimetastatic and antitumor activities of interleukin 10 in a murine model of breast cancer. *J. Natl Cancer Inst.* **88**: 536.

157 KUNDU, N. and A. M. FULTON. 1997. Interleukin-10 inhibits tumor metastasis, downregulates MHC class I and enhances NK lysis. *Cell Immunol.* **180**: 55.

158 QIN, Z., G. NOFFZ, M. MOHAUPT and T. BLANKENSTEIN. 1997. Interleukin-10 prevents dendritic cell accumulation and vaccination with granulocyte-macrophage colony-stimulating factor gene-modified tumor cells. *J. Immunol.* **159**: 770.

159 ALLAVENA, P., L. PIEMONTI, D. LONGONI, S. BERNASCONI, A. STOPPACCIARO, L. RUCO and A. MANTOVANI. 1998. IL-10 prevents the differentiation of monocytes to dendritic cells but promotes their maturation to macrophages. *Eur. J. Immunol.* **28**: 359.

160 ALLAVENA, P., L. PIEMONTI, D. LONGONI, S. BERNASCONI, A. STOPPACCIARO, L. RUCO and A. MANTOVANI. 1997. IL-10 prevents the generation of dendritic cells from CD14$^+$ blood monocytes, promotes the differentiation to mature macrophages and stimulates endocytosis of FITC–dextran. *Adv. Exp. Med. Biol* **417**: 323.

161 FORTSCH, D., M. ROLLINGHOFF and S. STENGER. 2000. IL-10 converts human dendritic cells into macrophage-like cells with increased antibacterial activity against virulent *Mycobacterium tuberculosis*. *J. Immunol.* **165**: 978.

162 TAKAYAMA, T., H. TAHARA and A. W. THOMSON. 2001. Differential effects of myeloid dendritic cells retrovirally transduced to express mammalian or viral interleukin-10 on cytotoxic T lymphocyte and natural killer cell functions and resistance to tumor growth. *Transplantation* **71**: 1334.

163 CORINTI, S., C. ALBANESI, A. LA SALA, S. PASTORE and G. GIROLOMONI. 2001. Regulatory activity of autocrine IL-10 on dendritic cell functions. *J. Immunol.* **166**: 4312.

164 LUDEWIG, B., D. GRAF, H. R. GELDERBLOM, Y. BECKER, R. A. KROCZEK and G. PAULI. 1995. Spontaneous apoptosis of dendritic cells is efficiently inhibited by TRAP (CD40 ligand) and TNF-α, but strongly enhanced by interleukin-10. *Eur. J. Immunol.* **25**: 1943.

165 ALLEVA, D. G., C. J. BURGER and K. D. ELGERT. 1994. Increased sensitivity of tumor-bearing host macrophages to interleukin-10: a counter-balancing

action to macrophage-mediated suppression. *Oncol. Res.* **6**: 219.

166 HIHARA, J., Y. YAMAGUCHI, K. MINAMI, K. NOMA and T. TOGE. 1999. Down-regulation of IL-10 enhances the efficacy of locoregional immunotherapy using OK-432 against malignant effusion. *Anticancer Res.* **19**: 1077.

167 KIM, B. G., H. G. JOO, I. S. CHUNG, H. Y. CHUNG, H. J. WOO and Y. S. YUN. 2000. Inhibition of interleukin-10 (IL-10) production from MOPC 315 tumor cells by IL-10 antisense oligodeoxynucleotides enhances cell-mediated immune responses. *Cancer Immunol. Immunother.* **49**: 433.

168 MATAR, P., V. R. ROZADOS, A. D. GONZALEZ, D. G. DLUGOVITZKY, R. D. BONFIL and O. G. SCHAROVSKY. 2000. Mechanism of antimetastatic immunopotentiation by low-dose cyclophosphamide. *Eur. J. Cancer* **36**: 1060.

169 SEO, N., Y. TOKURA, M. TAKIGAWA and K. EGAWA. 1999. Depletion of IL-10– and TGF-β-producing regulatory γδ T cells by administering a daunomycin-conjugated specific monoclonal antibody in early tumor lesions augments the activity of CTLs and NK cells. *J. Immunol.* **163**: 242.

170 DI CARLO, E., A. COLETTI, A. MODESTI, M. GIOVARELLI, G. FORNI and P. MUSIANI. 1998. Local release of interleukin-10 by transfected mouse adenocarcinoma cells exhibits pro- and anti-inflammatory activity and results in a delayed tumor rejection. *Eur. Cytokine Netw.* **9**: 61.

171 SUN, H., P. GUTIERREZ, M. J. JACKSON, N. KUNDU and A. M. FULTON. 2000. Essential role of nitric oxide and interferon-γ for tumor immunotherapy with interleukin-10. *J. Immunother.* **23**: 208.

172 BASS, K. K. and M. J. MASTRANGELO. 1998. Immunopotentiation with low-dose cyclophosphamide in the active specific immunotherapy of cancer. *Cancer Immunol. Immunother.* **47**: 1.

173 DRAY, S. and M. B. MOKYR. 1989. Cyclophosphamide and melphalan as immunopotentiating agents in cancer therapy. *Med. Oncol. Tumor Pharmacother.* **6**: 77.

174 MATAR, P., V. R. ROZADOS, S. I. GERVASONI and O. G. SCHAROVSKY. 2001. Down regulation of T-cell-derived IL-10 production by low-dose cyclophosphamide treatment in tumor-bearing rats restores *in vitro* normal lymphoproliferative response. *Int. Immunopharmacol.* **1**: 307.

175 BLOOM, B. R. and B. BENNETT. 1966. Mechanism of a reaction *in vitro* associated with delayed-type hypersensitivity. *Science* **153**: 80.

176 DAVID, J. R. 1966. Delayed hypersensitivity *in vitro*: its mediation by cell-free substances formed by lymphoid cell-antigen interaction. *Proc. Natl Acad. Sci. USA* **56**: 72.

177 BERNHAGEN, J., T. CALANDRA, R. A. MITCHELL, S. B. MARTIN, K. J. TRACEY, W. VOELTER, K. R. MANOGUE, A. CERAMI and R. BUCALA. 1993. MIF is a pituitary-derived cytokine that potentiates lethal endotoxaemia. *Nature* **365**: 756.

178 CALANDRA, T., L. A. SPIEGEL, C. N. METZ and R. BUCALA. 1998. Macrophage migration inhibitory factor is a critical mediator of the activation of immune cells by exotoxins of Gram-positive bacteria. *Proc. Natl Acad. Sci. USA* **95**: 11383.

179 METZ, C. N. and R. BUCALA. 1997. Role of macrophage migration inhibitory factor in the regulation of the immune response. *Adv. Immunol.* **66**: 197.

180 METZ, C. N. and R. BUCALA. 2000. MIF. In: Feldmann, M., Durum, S., Nicola, N., Vilchek, J. and Hirano, T. (eds), *Cytokine Reference*. Academic Press, New York.

181 LEECH, M., C. METZ, L. SANTOS, T. PENG, S. R. HOLDSWORTH, R. BUCALA and E. F. MORAND. 1998. Involvement of macrophage migration inhibitory factor in the evolution of rat adjuvant arthritis. *Arthritis Rheum.* **41**: 910.

182 MIKULOWSKA, A., C. N. METZ, R. BUCALA and R. HOLMDAHL. 1997. Macrophage migration inhibitory factor is involved in the pathogenesis of collagen type II-induced arthritis in mice. *J. Immunol.* **158**: 5514.

183 LEECH, M., C. METZ, L. SANTOS, T. PENG, S. R. HOLDSWORTH, R. BUCALA and

E. F. MORAND. 1998. Involvement of macrophage migration inhibitory factor in the evolution of rat adjuvant arthritis. *Arthritis Rheum.* **41**: 910.

**184** CALANDRA, T., B. ECHTENACHER, D. L. ROY, J. PUGIN, C. N. METZ, L. HULTNER, D. HEUMANN, D. MANNEL, R. BUCALA and M. P. GLAUSER. 2000. Protection from septic shock by neutralization of macrophage migration inhibitory factor. *Nat. Med.* **6**: 164.

**185** LAN, H. Y., M. BACHER, N. YANG, W. MU, D. J. NIKOLIC-PATERSON, C. METZ, A. MEINHARDT, R. BUCALA and R. C. ATKINS. 1997. The pathogenic role of macrophage migration inhibitory factor in Immunologically induced kidney disease in the rat. *J. Exp. Med.* **185**: 1455.

**186** BACHER, M., C. N. METZ, T. CALANDRA, K. MAYER, J. CHESNEY, M. LOHOFF, D. GEMSA, T. DONNELLY and R. BUCALA. 1996. An essential regulatory role for macrophage migration inhibitory factor in T-cell activation. *Proc. Natl Acad. Sci. USA* **93**: 7849.

**187** KITAICHI, N., K. OGASAWARA, K. IWABUCHI, J. NISHIHIRA, K. NAMBA, K. ONOE, J. KONISHI, S. KOTAKE and H. MATSUDA. 2000. Different influence of macrophage migration inhibitory factor (MIF) in signal transduction pathway of various T cell subsets. *Immunobiology* **201**: 356.

**188** MEYER-SIEGLER, K., R. A. FATTOR and P. B. HUDSON. 1998. Expression of macrophage migration inhibitory factor in the human prostate. *Diagn. Mol. Pathol.* **7**: 44.

**189** MEYER-SIEGLER, K. and P. B. HUDSON. 1996. Enhanced expression of macrophage migration inhibitory factor in prostatic adenocarcinoma metastases. *Urology* **48**: 448.

**190** DEL VECCHIO, M. T., S. A. TRIPODI, F. ARCURI, L. PERGOLA, L. HAKO, R. VATTI and M. CINTORINO. 2000. Macrophage migration inhibitory factor in prostatic adenocarcinoma: correlation with tumor grading and combination endocrine treatment-related changes. *Prostate* **45**: 51.

**191** KAMIMURA, A., M. KAMACHI, J. NISHIHIRA, S. OGURA, H. ISOBE, H. DOSAKA-AKITA, A. OGATA, M. SHINDOH, T. OHBUCHI and Y. KAWAKAMI. 2000. Intracellular distribution of macrophage migration inhibitory factor predicts the prognosis of patients with adenocarcinoma of the lung. *Cancer* **89**: 334.

**192** MARKERT, J. M., C. M. FULLER, G. Y. GILLESPIE, J. K. BUBIEN, L. A. MCLEAN, R. L. HONG, K. LEE, S. R. GULLANS, T. B. MAPSTONE and D. J. BENOS. 2001. Differential gene expression profiling in human brain tumors. *Physiol. Genomics* **5**: 21.

**193** MITCHELL, R. A., C. N. METZ, T. PENG and R. BUCALA. 1999. Sustained mitogen-activated protein kinase (MAPK) and cytoplasmic phospholipase A2 activation by macrophage migration inhibitory factor (MIF). Regulatory role in cell proliferation and glucocorticoid action. *J. Biol. Chem.* **274**: 18100.

**194** TAKAHASHI, N., J. NISHIHIRA, Y. SATO, M. KONDO, H. OGAWA, T. OHSHIMA, Y. UNE and S. TODO. 1998. Involvement of macrophage migration inhibitory factor (MIF) in the mechanism of tumor cell growth. *Mol. Med.* **4**: 707.

**195** TAKAHASHI, A., K. IWABUCHI, M. SUZUKI, K. OGASAWARA, J. NISHIHIRA and K. ONOE. 1999. Antisense macrophage migration inhibitory factor (MIF) prevents anti-IgM mediated growth arrest and apoptosis of a murine B cell line by regulating cell cycle progression. *Microbiol. Immunol.* **43**: 61.

**196** TAKAHASHI, N., J. NISHIHIRA, Y. SATO, M. KONDO, H. OGAWA, T. OHSHIMA, Y. UNE and S. TODO. 1998. Involvement of macrophage migration inhibitory factor (MIF) in the mechanism of tumor cell growth. *Mol. Med.* **4**: 707.

**197** HUDSON, J. D., M. A. SHOAIBI, R. MAESTRO, A. CARNERO, G. J. HANNON and D. H. BEACH. 1999. A proinflammatory cytokine inhibits p53 tumor suppressor activity. *J. Exp. Med.* **190**: 1375.

**198** CHESNEY, J., C. METZ, M. BACHER, T. PENG, A. MEINHARDT and R. BUCALA. 1999. An essential role for macrophage migration inhibitory factor (MIF) in angiogenesis and the growth of a murine lymphoma. *Mol. Med.* **5**: 181.

**199** Shimizu, T., R. Abe, H. Nakamura, A. Ohkawara, M. Suzuki and J. Nishihira. 1999. High expression of macrophage migration inhibitory factor in human melanoma cells and its role in tumor cell growth and angiogenesis. *Biochem. Biophys. Res. Commun.* **264**: 751.

**200** Ogawa, H., J. Nishihira, Y. Sato, M. Kondo, N. Takahashi, T. Oshima and S. Todo. 2000. An antibody for macrophage migration inhibitory factor suppresses tumour growth and inhibits tumour-associated angiogenesis. *Cytokine* **12**: 309.

**201** Apte, R. S., D. Sinha, E. Mayhew, G. J. Wistow and J. Y. Niederkorn. 1998. Cutting edge: Role of macrophage migration inhibitory factor in inhibiting NK cell activity and preserving immune privilege. *J. Immunol.* **160**: 5693.

**202** Repp, A. C., E. S. Mayhew, S. Apte and J. Y. Niederkorn. 2000. Human uveal melanoma cells produce macrophage migration-inhibitory factor to prevent lysis by NK cells. *J. Immunol.* **165**: 710.

**203** Abe, R., T. Peng, J. Sailors, R. Bucala and C. N. Metz. 2001. Regulation of the CTL response by macrophage migration inhibitory factor. *J. Immunol.* **166**: 747.

**204** thor Straten, P., P. Guldberg, D. Schrama, M. A. Andersen, U. Moerch, T. Seremet, C. Siedel, R. A. Reisfeld and J. C. Becker. 2001. *In situ* cytokine therapy: redistribution of clonally expanded T cells. *Eur. J. Immunol.* **31**: 250.

**205** Shrikant, P. and M. F. Mescher. 1999. Control of syngeneic tumor growth by activation of CD8⁺ T cells: efficacy is limited by migration away from the site and induction of nonresponsiveness. *J. Immunol.* **162**: 2858.

**206** Hanson, H. L., D. L. Donermeyer, H. Ikeda, J. M. White, V. Shankaran, L. J. Old, H. Shiku, R. D. Schreiber and P. M. Allen. 2000. Eradication of established tumors by CD8⁺ T cell adoptive immunotherapy. *Immunity.* **13**: 265.

**207** Shrikant, P. and M. F. Mescher. 1999. Control of syngeneic tumor growth by activation of CD8⁺ T cells: efficacy is limited by migration away

from the site and induction of nonresponsiveness. *J. Immunol.* **162**: 2858.

**208** Smith, W. L., D. L. DeWitt and R. M. Garavito. 2000. Cyclooxygenases: structural, cellular and molecular biology. *Annu. Rev. Biochem.* **69**: 145.

**209** Eberhart, C. E., R. J. Coffey, A. Radhika, F. M. Giardiello, S. Ferrenbach and R. N. DuBois. 1994. Up-regulation of cyclooxygenase 2 gene expression in human colorectal adenomas and adenocarcinomas. *Gastroenterology* **107**: 1183.

**210** Dimberg, J., A. Samuelsson, A. Hugander and P. Soderkvist. 1999. Differential expression of cyclooxygenase 2 in human colorectal cancer. *Gut* **45**: 730.

**211** Soslow, R. A., A. J. Dannenberg, D. Rush, B. M. Woerner, K. N. Khan, J. Masferrer and A. T. Koki. 2000. COX-2 is expressed in human pulmonary, colonic and mammary tumors. *Cancer* **89**: 2637.

**212** Schrey, M. P. and K. V. Patel. 1995. Prostaglandin E$_2$ production and metabolism in human breast cancer cells and breast fibroblasts. Regulation by inflammatory mediators. *Br. J. Cancer* **72**: 1412.

**213** Lee, D. Y., J. R. Lupton and R. S. Chapkin. 1992. Prostaglandin profile and synthetic capacity of the colon: comparison of tissue sources and subcellular fractions. *Prostaglandins* **43**: 143.

**214** Sitter, T., B. Haslinger, S. Mandl, H. Fricke, E. Held and A. Sellmayer. 1998. High glucose increases prostaglandin E$_2$ synthesis in human peritoneal mesothelial cells: role of hyperosmolarity. *J. Am. Soc. Nephrol.* **9**: 2005.

**215** Hsu, P., M. Shibata and C. W. Leffler. 1993. Prostanoid synthesis in response to high $CO_2$ in newborn pig brain microvascular endothelial cells. *Am. J. Physiol.* **264**: H1485.

**216** Williams, J. A. and E. Shacter. 1997. Regulation of macrophage cytokine production by prostaglandin E$_2$. Distinct roles of cyclooxygenase-1 and -2. *J. Biol. Chem.* **272**: 25693.

**217** Renz, H., J. H. Gong, A. Schmidt, M. Nain and D. Gemsa. 1988. Release of tumor necrosis factor-α from macrophages. Enhancement and suppression are dose-dependently regulated by prostaglandin $E_2$ and cyclic nucleotides. *J. Immunol.* **141**: 2388.

**218** ATTIGA, F. A., P. M. FERNANDEZ, A. T. WEERARATNA, M. J. MANYAK and S. R. PATIERNO. 2000. Inhibitors of prostaglandin synthesis inhibit human prostate tumor cell invasiveness and reduce the release of matrix metalloproteinases. *Cancer Res.* **60**: 4629.

**219** SNYDERMAN, C. H., I. KLAPAN, M. MILANOVICH, D. S. HEO, R. WAGNER, D. SCHWARTZ, J. T. JOHNSON and T. L. WHITESIDE. 1994. Comparison of *in vivo* and *in vitro* prostaglandin $E_2$ production by squamous cell carcinoma of the head and neck. *Otolaryngol. Head. Neck Surg.* **111**: 189.

**220** COHEN, L. A. and R. A. KARMALI. 1984. Endogenous prostaglandin production by established cultures of neoplastic rat mammary epithelial cells. *In Vitro* **20**: 119.

**221** EISENGART, C. A., J. R. MESTRE, H. A. NAAMA, P. J. MACKRELL, D. E. RIVADENEIRA, E. M. MURPHY, P. P. STAPLETON and J. M. DALY. 2000. Prostaglandins regulate melanoma-induced cytokine production in macrophages. *Cell Immunol.* **204**: 143.

**222** YOUNG, M. R., E. WHEELER and M. NEWBY. 1986. Macrophage-mediated suppression of natural killer cell activity in mice bearing Lewis lung carcinoma. *J. Natl Cancer Inst.* **76**: 745.

**223** MILANOVICH, M. R., C. H. SNYDERMAN, R. WAGNER and J. T. JOHNSON. 1995. Prognostic significance of prostaglandin $E_2$ production by mononuclear cells and tumor cells in squamous cell carcinomas of the head and neck. *Laryngoscope* **105**: 61.

**224** SUMITANI, K., R. KAMIJO, T. TOYOSHIMA, Y. NAKANISHI, K. TAKIZAWA, M. HATORI and M. NAGUMO. 2001. Specific inhibition of cyclooxygenase-2 results in inhibition of proliferation of oral cancer cell lines via suppression of prostaglandin $E_2$ production. *J. Oral Pathol. Med.* **30**: 41.

**225** ARVIND, P., E. D. PAPAVASSILIOU, G. J. TSIOULIAS, L. QIAO, C. I. LOVELACE, B. DUCEMAN and B. RIGAS. 1995. Prostaglandin $E_2$ down-regulates the expression of HLA-DR antigen in human colon adenocarcinoma cell lines. *Biochemistry* **34**: 5604.

**226** BEN-EFRAIM, S. and I. L. BONTA. 1994. Modulation of antitumour activity of macrophages by regulation of eicosanoids and cytokine production. *Int. J. Immunopharmacol.* **16**: 397.

**227** SHINOMIYA, S., H. NARABA, A. UENO, I. UTSUNOMIYA, T. MARUYAMA, S. OHUCHIDA, F. USHIKUBI, K. YUKI, S. NARUMIYA, Y. SUGIMOTO, A. ICHIKAWA and S. OH-ISHI. 2001. Regulation of TNFα and interleukin-10 production by prostaglandins I(2) and E(2): studies with prostaglandin receptor-deficient mice and prostaglandin E-receptor subtype-selective synthetic agonists. *Biochem. Pharmacol.* **61**: 1153.

**228** STRASSMANN, G., V. PATIL-KOOTA, F. FINKELMAN, M. FONG and T. KAMBAYASHI. 1994. Evidence for the involvement of interleukin 10 in the differential deactivation of murine peritoneal macrophages by prostaglandin $E_2$. *J. Exp. Med.* **180**: 2365.

**229** PHIPPS, R. P., S. H. STEIN and R. L. ROPER. 1991. A new view of prostaglandin E regulation of the immune response. *Immunol. Today* **12**: 349.

**230** ROPER, R. L. and R. P. PHIPPS. 1994. Prostaglandin $E_2$ regulation of the immune response. *Adv. Prostaglandin Thromboxane Leukot. Res.* **22**: 101.

**231** PLESCIA, O. J., K. GRINWICH and A. M. PLESCIA. 1976. Subversive activity of syngeneic tumor cells as an escape mechanism from immune surveillance and the role of prostaglandins. *Ann. NY Acad. Sci.* **276**: 455.

**232** YOUNG, M. R. and S. HENDERSON. 1982. Enhancement in immunity of tumor bearing mice by immunization against prostaglandin $E_2$. *Immunol. Commun.* **11**: 345.

**233** PARHAR, R. S. and P. K. LALA. 1988. Prostaglandin $E_2$-mediated inactivation of various killer lineage cells by tumor-bearing host macrophages. *J. Leuk. Biol.* **44**: 474.

**234** SNIJDEWINT, F. G., P. KALINSKI, E. A. WIERENGA, J. D. BOS and

M. L. KAPSENBERG. 1993. Prostaglandin $E_2$ differentially modulates cytokine secretion profiles of human T helper lymphocytes. *J. Immunol.* **150**: 5321.

**235** DEMEURE, C. E., L. P. YANG, C. DESJARDINS, P. RAYNAULD and G. DELESPESSE. 1997. Prostaglandin $E_2$ primes naive T cells for the production of anti-inflammatory cytokines. *Eur. J. Immunol.* **27**: 3526.

**236** SUNDER-PLASSMANN, R., H. BREITENEDER, K. ZIMMERMANN, D. STRUNK, O. MAJDIC, W. KNAPP and W. HOLTER. 1996. Single human T cells stimulated in the absence of feeder cells transcribe interleukin-2 and undergo long-term clonal growth in response to defined monoclonal antibodies and cytokine stimulation. *Blood* **87**: 5179.

**237** MESRI, M., J. LIVERSIDGE and J. V. FORRESTER. 1996. Prostaglandin $E_2$ and monoclonal antibody to lymphocyte function-associated antigen-1 differentially inhibit migration of T lymphocytes across microvascular retinal endothelial cells in rat. *Immunology* **88**: 471.

**238** ELLIOTT, L. H. and A. K. LEVAY. 1997. Costimulation with dexamethasone and prostaglandin $E_2$: a novel paradigm for the induction of T-cell anergy. *Cell Immunol.* **180**: 124.

**239** HALE, A. H., D. L. EVANS and L. W. DANIEL. 1982. Effect of prostaglandins on elicitation of anti-viral-cytolytic activity. *Immunol. Lett.* **4**: 171.

**240** WOLF, M. and W. DROEGE. 1982. Inhibition of cytotoxic responses by prostaglandin $E_2$ in the presence of interleukin 2. *Cell Immunol.* **72**: 286.

**241** WALKER, T. M., A. D. YUROCHKO, C. J. BURGER and K. D. ELGERT. 1992. Cytokines and suppressor macrophages cause tumor-bearing host $CD8^+$ T cells to suppress recognition of allogeneic and syngeneic MHC class II molecules. *J. Leuk. Biol.* **52**: 661.

**242** SPECHT, C., S. BEXTEN, E. KOLSCH and H. G. PAUELS. 2001. Prostaglandins, but not tumor-derived IL-10, shut down concomitant tumor-specific CTL responses during murine plasmacytoma progression. *Int. J. Cancer* **91**: 705.

**243** ZIELINSKI, C. C., C. GISINGER, C. BINDER, J. W. MANNHALTER and M. M. EIBL.

1984. Regulation of NK cell activity by prostaglandin $E_2$: the role of T cells. *Cell Immunol.* **87**: 65.

**244** LALA, P. K., R. S. PARHAR and P. SINGH. 1986. Indomethacin therapy abrogates the prostaglandin-mediated suppression of natural killer activity in tumor-bearing mice and prevents tumor metastasis. *Cell Immunol.* **99**: 108.

**245** SCODRAS, J. M., R. S. PARHAR, T. G. KENNEDY and P. K. LALA. 1990. Prostaglandin-mediated inactivation of natural killer cells in the murine decidua. *Cell Immunol.* **127**: 352.

**246** LAUZON, W. and I. LEMAIRE. 1994. Alveolar macrophage inhibition of lung-associated NK activity: involvement of prostaglandins and transforming growth factor-$\beta$ 1. *Exp. Lung Res.* **20**: 331.

**247** BAXEVANIS, C. N., G. J. RECLOS, A. D. GRITZAPIS, G. V. DEDOUSIS, I. MISSITZIS and M. PAPAMICHAIL. 1993. Elevated prostaglandin $E_2$ production by monocytes is responsible for the depressed levels of natural killer and lymphokine-activated killer cell function in patients with breast cancer. *Cancer* **72**: 491.

**248** LI, W. 1992. [Inhibition of growth and metastasis of Lewis lung carcinoma in C57BL mice immunized with $PGE_2$–bovine thyroglobulin conjugate]. *Zhonghua Zhong Liu Za Zhi* **13**: 427.

**249** YOUNG, M. R. and M. DIZER. 1983. Enhancement of immune function and tumor growth inhibition by antibodies against prostaglandin $E_2$. *Immunol. Commun.* **12**: 11.

**250** YOUNG, M. R. and S. KNIES. 1984. Prostaglandin E production by Lewis lung carcinoma: mechanism for tumor establishment *in vivo*. *J. Natl Cancer Inst.* **72**: 919.

**251** MACA, R. D. 1988. Inhibition of the growth of Lewis lung carcinoma by indomethacin in conventional, nude and beige mice. *J. Biol. Resp. Modif.* **7**: 568.

**252** SPECHT, C., S. BEXTEN, E. KOLSCH and H. G. PAUELS. 2001. Prostaglandins, but not tumor-derived IL-10, shut down concomitant tumor-specific CTL responses during murine plasmacytoma progression. *Int. J. Cancer* **91**: 705.

253 STOLINA, M., S. SHARMA, Y. LIN, M. DO-HADWALA, B. GARDNER, J. LUO, L. ZHU, M. KRONENBERG, P. W. MILLER, J. POR-TANOVA, J. C. LEE and S. M. DUBINETT. 2000. Specific inhibition of cyclooxygenase 2 restores antitumor reactivity by altering the balance of IL-10 and IL-12 synthesis. *J. Immunol.* **164**: 361.

254 LONNROTH, C., M. ANDERSSON and K. LUNDHOLM. 2001. Indomethacin and telomerase activity in tumor growth retardation. *Int. J. Oncol.* **18**: 929.

255 WILLIAMS, C. S., M. TSUJII, J. REESE, S. K. DEY and R. N. DUBOIS. 2000. Host cyclooxygenase-2 modulates carcinoma growth. *J. Clin. Invest.* **105**: 1589.

256 CHULADA, P. C., M. B. THOMPSON, J. F. MAHLER, C. M. DOYLE, B. W. GAUL, C. LEE, H. F. TIANO, S. G. MORHAM, O. SMITHIES and R. LANGENBACH. 2000. Genetic disruption of Ptgs-1, as well as Ptgs-2, reduces intestinal tumorigenesis in Min mice. *Cancer Res.* **60**: 4705.

257 KAWAMORI, T., C. V. RAO, K. SEIBERT and B. S. REDDY. 1998. Chemopreventive activity of celecoxib, a specific cyclooxygenase-2 inhibitor, against colon carcinogenesis. *Cancer Res.* **58**: 409.

258 GIARDIELLO, F. M., J. A. OFFERHAUS, A. C. TERSMETTE, L. M. HYLIND, A. J. KRUSH, J. D. BRENSINGER, S. V. BOOKER and S. R. HAMILTON. 1996. Sulindac induced regression of colorectal adenomas in familial adenomatous polyposis: evaluation of predictive factors. *Gut* **38**: 578.

259 NUGENT, K. P., K. C. FARMER, A. D. SPIGELMAN, C. B. WILLIAMS and R. K. PHILLIPS. 1993. Randomized controlled trial of the effect of sulindac on duodenal and rectal polyposis and cell proliferation in patients with familial adenomatous polyposis. *Br. J. Surg.* **80**: 1618.

260 GATELY, S. 2000. The contributions of cyclooxygenase-2 to tumor angiogenesis. *Cancer Metast. Rev.* **19**: 19.

261 HEBY, O. 1981. Role of polyamines in the control of cell proliferation and differentiation. *Differentiation* **19**: 1.

262 DURIE, B. G., S. E. SALMON and D. H. RUSSELL. 1977. Polyamines as markers of response and disease activity in cancer chemotherapy. *Cancer Res.* **37**: 214.

263 UEHARA, N., K. KITA, S. SHIRAKAWA, H. UCHINO and Y. SAEKI. 1980. Elevated polyamine content in erythrocytes of malignant lymphoma patients. *Gann* **71**: 393.

264 HEBY, O. and G. ANDERSSON. 1978. Tumour cell death: the probable cause of increased polyamine levels in physiological fluids. *Acta Pathol. Microbiol. Scand. A* **86**: 17.

265 NISHIOKA, K., K. EZAKI and J. S. HART. 1980. A preliminary study of polyamines in the bone-marrow plasma of adult patients with leukemia. *Clin. Chim. Acta* **107**: 59.

266 ROMANO, M., L. CECCO, M. CERRA, R. MONTUORI and C. DE ROSA. 1980. Polyamines as biological markers of the effectiveness of therapy in acute leukemia. *Tumori* **66**: 677.

267 CHAMAILLARD, L., V. QUEMENER, R. HAVOUIS and J. P. MOULINOUX. 1993. Polyamine deprivation stimulates natural killer cell activity in cancerous mice. *Anticancer Res.* **13**: 1027.

268 REDGATE, E. S., S. BOGGS, A. GRUDZIAK and M. DEUTSCH. 1995. Polyamines in brain tumor therapy. *J. Neurooncol.* **25**: 167.

269 PORTER, C. W. and J. R. SUFRIN. 1986. Interference with polyamine biosynthesis and/or function by analogs of polyamines or methionine as a potential anticancer chemotherapeutic strategy. *Anticancer Res.* **6**: 525.

270 CASERO, R. A. J., B. GO, H. W. THEISS, J. SMITH, S. B. BAYLIN and G. D. LUK. 1987. Cytotoxic response of the relatively difluoromethylornithine-resistant human lung tumor cell line NCI H157 to the polyamine analogue $N^1,N^8$-bis(ethyl)spermidine. *Cancer Res.* **47**: 3964.

271 HERR, H. W., E. L. KLEINERT, P. S. CONTI, J. H. BURCHENAL and W. F. J. WHITMORE. 1984. Effects of α-difluoromethylornithine and methylglyoxal bis(guanylhydrazone) on the growth of experimental renal adenocarcinoma in mice. *Cancer Res.* **44**: 4382.

272 KLEIN, S., J. J. MIRET, I. D. ALGRANATI and E. S. DE LUSTIG. 1985. Effect of α-

difluoromethylornithine in lung metastases before and after surgery of primary adenocarcinoma tumors in mice. *Biol. Cell* **53**: 33.

273 SUNKARA, P. S. and A. L. ROSENBERGER. 1987. Antimetastatic activity of dl-α-difluoromethylornithine, an inhibitor of polyamine biosynthesis, in mice. *Cancer Res.* **47**: 933.

274 MARX, M., C. M. J. TOWNSEND, S. C. BARRANCO, E. J. GLASS and J. C. THOMPSON. 1987. Treatment of hamster pancreatic cancer with α-difluoromethylornithine, an inhibitor of polyamine biosynthesis. *J. Natl Cancer Inst.* **79**: 543.

275 UPP, J. R. J., R. D. BEAUCHAMP, C. M. J. TOWNSEND, S. C. BARRANCO, P. SINGH, S. RAJARAMAN, E. JAMES and J. C. THOMPSON. 1988. Inhibition of human gastric adenocarcinoma xenograft growth in nude mice by α-difluoromethylornithine. *Cancer Res.* **48**: 3265.

276 PRAKASH, N. J., T. L. BOWLIN, G. F. DAVIS, P. S. SUNKARA and A. SJOERDSMA. 1988. Antitumor activity of norspermidine, a structural homologue of the natural polyamine spermidine. *Anticancer Res.* **8**: 563.

277 ANDERSSON, G. and O. HEBY. 1977. Population kinetics of an Ehrlich ascites tumor following treatment with methylglyoxal-bis(guanylhydrazone), a polyamine synthesis inhibitor. *Cancer Lett.* **3**: 59.

278 LUK, G. D., G. GOODWIN, L. J. MARTON and S. B. BAYLIN. 1981. Polyamines are necessary for the survival of human small-cell lung carcinoma in culture. *Proc. Natl Acad. Sci. USA* **78**: 2355.

279 MANNI, A. and C. WRIGHT. 1983. Effect of tamoxifen and α-difluoromethylornithine on clones of nitrosomethylurea-induced rat mammary tumor cells grown in soft agar culture. *Cancer Res.* **43**: 1084.

280 MANNI, A. and C. WRIGHT. 1984. Reversal of the antiproliferative effect of the antiestrogen tamoxifen by polyamines in breast cancer cells. *Endocrinology* **114**: 836.

281 SEIDENFELD, J., A. L. BLOCK, K. A. KOMAR and M. F. NAUJOKAS. 1986. Altered cell cycle phase distributions in cul-

tured human carcinoma cells partially depleted of polyamines by treatment with difluoromethylornithine. *Cancer Res.* **46**: 47.

282 SUNKARA, P. S., C. C. CHANG, N. J. PRAKASH and P. J. LACHMANN. 1985. Effect of inhibition of polyamine biosynthesis by dl-α-difluoromethylornithine on the growth and melanogenesis of B16 melanoma *in vitro* and *in vivo*. *Cancer Res.* **45**: 4067.

283 WALLON, U. M., L. R. SHASSETZ, A. E. CRESS, G. T. BOWDEN and E. W. GERNER. 1994. Polyamine-dependent expression of the matrix metalloproteinase matrilysin in a human colon cancer-derived cell line. *Mol. Carcinogen.* **11**: 138.

284 KUBOTA, S., H. KIYOSAWA, Y. NOMURA, T. YAMADA and Y. SEYAMA. 1997. Ornithine decarboxylase overexpression in mouse 10T1/2 fibroblasts: cellular transformation and invasion. *J. Natl Cancer Inst.* **89**: 567.

285 MCCLOSKEY, D. E., J. YANG, P. M. WOSTER, N. E. DAVIDSON and R. A. J. CASERO. 1996. Polyamine analogue induction of programmed cell death in human lung tumor cells. *Clin. Cancer Res.* **2**: 441.

286 KANEKO, H., H. HIBASAMI, K. MORI, Y. KAWARADA and K. NAKASHIMA. 1998. Apoptosis induction in human breast cancer MRK-nu-1 cells by a polyamine synthesis inhibitor, methylglyoxal bis (cyclopentylamidino-hydrazone) (MGBCP). *Anticancer Res.* **18**: 891.

287 HOLTTA, E., M. AUVINEN and L. C. ANDERSSON. 1993. Polyamines are essential for cell transformation by pp60v-src: delineation of molecular events relevant for the transformed phenotype. *J. Cell Biol.* **122**: 903.

288 TABIB, A. and U. BACHRACH. 1998. Polyamines induce malignant transformation in cultured NIH 3T3 fibroblasts. *Int. J. Biochem. Cell Biol.* **30**: 135.

289 TABIB, A. and U. BACHRACH. 1999. Role of polyamines in mediating malignant transformation and oncogene expression. *Int. J. Biochem. Cell Biol.* **31**: 1289.

290 IWATA, S., Y. SATO, M. ASADA, M. TAKAGI, A. TSUJIMOTO, T. INABA, T. YAMADA, S. SAKAMOTO, J. YATA, T. SHIMOGORI, K. IGARASHI and S. MIZUTANI. 1999. Anti-tumor activity of antizyme which

targets the ornithine decarboxylase (ODC) required for cell growth and transformation. *Oncogene* **18**: 165.

**291** JASNIS, M. A., S. KLEIN, M. MONTE, L. DAVEL, D. L. SACERDOTE and I. D. ALGRANATI. 1994. Polyamines prevent DFMO-mediated inhibition of angiogenesis. *Cancer Lett.* **79**: 39.

**292** TAKIGAWA, M., M. ENOMOTO, Y. NISHIDA, H. O. PAN, A. KINOSHITA and F. SUZUKI. 1990. Tumor angiogenesis and polyamines: α-difluoromethylornithine, an irreversible inhibitor of ornithine decarboxylase, inhibits B16 melanoma-induced angiogenesis *in ovo* and the proliferation of vascular endothelial cells *in vitro*. *Cancer Res.* **50**: 4131.

**293** LUK, G. D. and R. A. J. CASERO. 1987. Polyamines in normal and cancer cells. *Adv. Enz. Reg.* **26**: 91.

**294** KACZMAREK, L., B. KAMINSKA, L. MESSINA, G. SPAMPINATO, A. ARCIDIACONO, L. MALAGUARNERA and A. MESSINA. 1992. Inhibitors of polyamine biosynthesis block tumor necrosis factor-induced activation of macrophages. *Cancer Res.* **52**: 1891.

**295** MESSINA, L., G. SPAMPINATO, A. ARCIDIACONO, L. MALAGUARNERA, M. PAGANO, B. KAMINSKA, L. KACZMAREK and A. MESSINA. 1992. Polyamine involvement in functional activation of human macrophages. *J. Leuk. Biol.* **52**: 585.

**296** SOUTHAN, G. J., C. SZABO and C. THIEMERMANN. 1994. Inhibition of the induction of nitric oxide synthase by spermine is modulated by aldehyde dehydrogenase. *Biochem. Biophys. Res. Commun.* **203**: 1638.

**297** SZABO, C., G. J. SOUTHAN, E. WOOD, C. THIEMERMANN and J. R. VANE. 1994. Inhibition by spermine of the induction of nitric oxide synthase in J774. 2 macrophages: requirement of a serum factor. *Br. J. Pharmacol.* **112**: 355.

**298** HASKO, G., D. G. KUHEL, A. MARTON, Z. H. NEMETH, E. A. DEITCH and C. SZABO. 2000. Spermine differentially regulates the production of interleukin-12 p40 and interleukin-10 and suppresses the release of the T helper 1 cytokine interferon-γ. *Shock* **14**: 144.

**299** LINSALATA, M., L. AMATI, L. CARADONNA, D. CACCAVO, E. JIRILLO and A. DI LEO. 1999. Relationship among red blood cell polyamine content, phagocytic activities and plasma endotoxins in untreated colorectal cancer patients. *Oncol. Rep.* **6**: 1411.

**300** CHAMAILLARD, L., V. CATROS-QUEMENER and J. P. MOULINOUX. 1997. Synergistic activation of macrophage activity by polyamine deprivation and cyclophosphamide. *Anticancer Res.* **17**: 1059.

**301** BOWLIN, T. L., B. J. McKOWN and K. K. SCHROEDER. 1989. Methyl-acetylenicputrescine (MAP), an inhibitor of polyamine biosynthesis, reduces the frequency and cytolytic activity of alloantigen-induced LyT 2.2 positive lymphocytes *in vivo*. *Int. J. Immunopharmacol.* **11**: 259.

**302** BOWLIN, T. L., B. J. McKOWN and P. S. SUNKARA. 1987. Increased ornithine decarboxylase activity and polyamine biosynthesis are required for optimal cytolytic T lymphocyte induction. *Cell Immunol.* **105**: 110.

**303** BOWLIN, T. L., G. F. DAVIS and B. J. McKOWN. 1988. Inhibition of alloantigen-induced cytolytic T lymphocytes *in vitro* with (2R,5R)-6-heptyne-2,5-diamine, an irreversible inhibitor of ornithine decarboxylase. *Cell Immunol.* **111**: 443.

**304** SCHALL, R. P., J. SEKAR, P. M. TANDON and B. M. SUSSKIND. 1991. Difluoromethylornithine (DFMO) arrests murine CTL development in the late, pre-effector stage. *Immunopharmacology* **21**: 129.

**305** CHAMAILLARD, L., V. CATROS-QUEMENER, J. G. DELCROS, J. Y. BANSARD, R. HAVOUIS, D. DESURY, A. COMMEUREC, N. GENETET and J. P. MOULINOUX. 1997. Polyamine deprivation prevents the development of tumour-induced immune suppression. *Br. J. Cancer* **76**: 365.

**306** CHAMAILLARD, L., V. CATROS-QUEMENER, J. G. DELCROS, J. Y. BANSARD, R. HAVOUIS, D. DESURY, A. COMMEUREC, N. GENETET and J. P. MOULINOUX. 1997. Polyamine deprivation prevents the development of tumour-induced immune suppression. *Br. J. Cancer* **76**: 365.

**307** Ho, S. B. and Y. S. Kim. 1991. Carbohydrate antigens on cancer-associated mucin-like molecules. *Semin. Cancer Biol.* **2**: 389.

**308** Ho, J. J. 2000. Mucins in the diagnosis and therapy of pancreatic cancer. *Curr. Pharm. Des.* **6**: 1881.

**309** Agrawal, B., S. J. Gendler and B. M. Longenecker. 1998. The biological role of mucins in cellular interactions and immune regulation: prospects for cancer immunotherapy. *Mol. Med. Today* **4**: 397.

**310** Miles, D. W. and J. Taylor-Papadimitriou. 1999. Therapeutic aspects of polymorphic epithelial mucin in adenocarcinoma. *Pharmacol. Ther.* **82**: 97.

**311** Reddish, M. A., G. D. MacLean, S. Poppema, A. Berg and B. M. Longenecker. 1996. Pre-immunotherapy serum CA27. 29 (MUC-1) mucin level and CD69+ lymphocytes correlate with effects of Theratope sialyl-Tn-KLH cancer vaccine in active specific immunotherapy. *Cancer Immunol. Immunother.* **42**: 303.

**312** MacLean, G. D., M. A. Reddish and B. M. Longenecker. 1997. Prognostic significance of preimmunotherapy serum CA27. 29 (MUC-1) mucin level after active specific immunotherapy of metastatic adenocarcinoma patients. *J. Immunother.* **20**: 70.

**313** Agrawal, B., M. J. Krantz, M. A. Reddish and B. M. Longenecker. 1998. Cancer-associated MUC1 mucin inhibits human T-cell proliferation, which is reversible by IL-2. *Nat. Med.* **4**: 43.

**314** Kim, J. A., M. A. Dayton, W. Aldrich and P. L. Triozzi. 1999. Modulation of CD4 cell cytokine production by colon cancer-associated mucin. *Cancer Immunol. Immunother.* **48**: 525.

**315** Chang, J. F., H. L. Zhao, J. Phillips and G. Greenburg. 2000. The epithelial mucin, MUC1, is expressed on resting T lymphocytes and can function as a negative regulator of T cell activation. *Cell Immunol.* **201**: 83.

**316** Vishwanatha, J. K., Y. Chiang, K. D. Kumble, M. A. Hollingsworth and P. M. Pour. 1993. Enhanced expression of annexin II in human pancreatic carcinoma cells and primary pancreatic cancers. *Carcinogenesis* **14**: 2575.

**317** Schwartz-Albiez, R., K. Koretz, P. Moller and G. Wirl. 1993. Differential expression of annexins I and II in normal and malignant human mammary epithelial cells. *Differentiation* **52**: 229.

**318** Reeves, S. A., C. Chavez-Kappel, R. Davis, M. Rosenblum and M. A. Israel. 1992. Developmental regulation of annexin II (Lipocortin 2) in human brain and expression in high grade glioma. *Cancer Res.* **52**: 6871.

**319** Roseman, B. J., A. Bollen, J. Hsu, K. Lamborn and M. A. Israel. 1994. Annexin II marks astrocytic brain tumors of high histologic grade. *Oncol. Res.* **6**: 561.

**320** Emoto, K., H. Sawada, Y. Yamada, H. Fujimoto, Y. Takahama, M. Ueno, T. Takayama, H. Uchida, K. Kamada, A. Naito, S. Hirao and Y. Nakajima. 2001. Annexin II overexpression is correlated with poor prognosis in human gastric carcinoma. *Anticancer Res.* **21**: 1339.

**321** Aarli, A., J. T. Skeie, E. K. Kristoffersen, A. Bakke and E. Ulvestad. 1997. Inhibition of phytohaemagglutinin-induced lymphoproliferation by soluble annexin II in sera from patients with renal cell carcinoma. *APMIS* **105**: 699.

**322** Aarli, A. and R. Matre. 1998. Suppression of immunoglobulin secretion by soluble annexin II. *Scand. J. Immunol.* **48**: 522.

**323** Reiter, W., P. Stieber, C. Reuter, D. Nagel, U. Lau-Werner and R. Lamerz. 2000. Multivariate analysis of the prognostic value of CEA and CA 19–9 serum levels in colorectal cancer. *Anticancer Res.* **20**: 5195.

**324** Rivoltini, L., G. Cattoretti, F. Arienti, A. Mastroianni and G. Parmiani. 1992. CEA and NCA expressed by colon carcinoma cells affect their interaction with and lysability by activated lymphocytes. *Int. J. Biol. Markers* **7**: 143.

**325** Pellegrini, P., A. M. Berghella, T. Del Beato, D. Maccarone, S. Cencioni, D. Adorno and C. U. Casciani. 1997. The sCEA molecule suppressive role in NK and $T_H1$ cell functions in colorectal cancer. *Cancer Biother. Radiopharm.* **12**: 257.

# 8
# Interleukin-10 in Cancer Immunity
Robert Sabat and Khusru Asadullah

## 8.1
## Introduction

The occurrence and progression of tumors in previously healthy people leads to the question why the malignant cells are not eliminated by the immune system. Two mechanisms have been suggested for this so-called immunological escape of cancers: (1) the loss of tumor antigenicity and (2) the suppression of the immune system.

It has been hypothesized that cytokines, which play an essential role in the intercellular communication network, might contribute to this phenomenon. These are polypeptides with a molecular weight between 7 and 60 kDa that are secreted by a wide variety of stimulated cells, and mediate autocrine, paracrine and, to a lesser extent, even endocrine effects. Cytokines exert their biological effects at concentrations in the picomolar range.

In the early 1990s it became evident that interleukin (IL)-10 represents the most important immunosuppressive cytokine in man. Thus, it has been hypothesized that tumor-associated suppression of the immune system may be mediated by IL-10 [1]. The current status of this hypothesis after 10 years of intense research will be discussed in this chapter.

## 8.2
## IL-10 Protein and IL-10 Receptor (IL-10R)

### 8.2.1
### IL-10 Structure and Expression

IL-10 was first described in 1989 by Moosman et al. [2]. The gene encoding human IL-10 is located on chromosome 1 [3]. Its five exons code for a secreted polypeptide chain of 160 amino acids. The spacial structure of human IL-10 (hIL-10) is well known because four X-ray crystal structures have already been published [4–7]. IL-10 represents a symmetric homodimer formed by the non-covalent intertwining of two identical, oppositely orientated polypeptide chains. This gives rise to the formation

**Tab. 8.1**  Cellular sources of IL-10 *in vitro*

| Cell population | Reference |
|---|---|
| T cells | 2 |
| Monocytes | 42 |
| Macrophages | 43 |
| B cells | 136 |
| NK cells | 137 |
| Eosinophils | 138 |
| Mast cells | 139 |
| Keratinocytes | 140 |

of two structural domains that are oriented in a V-shaped form where each domain is composed of four α helices from one monomer and two α helices from the other. Such a topology was first observed for the interferon (IFN)-γ homodimer [8].

Numerous, different cell populations express IL-10 after activation *in vitro* (Tab. 8.1). With respect to the *in vivo* situation, the immune cells are most likely to be the major producers of this cytokine. Among them, the relevance of an individual cell population for IL-10 production varies depending on the concrete immunological situation. For instance, in the case of tissue-invading pathogens, IL-10 is produced particularly by the resident macrophages and mast cells as a counter-regulation of the initial inflammatory response [9]. In contrast, IL-10 production by regulatory T cells seems to be especially important for the maintenance of peripheral immunological tolerance [10]. Once secreted in the plasma, the half-life of hIL-10 amounts to several hours [11].

### 8.2.2
### IL-10R

IL-10's pleiotropic activities are mediated by a specific cell surface receptor complex. The IL-10R is composed of two different chains, IL-10Rα and IL-10Rβ [12, 13]. Both chains belong to the class II cytokine receptor family (CRF2). Further members of this receptor family are the receptor subunits for IFN-α/β, IFN-γ, IL-20, IL-22 and the membrane tether for coagulation factor VIIa. CRF2 members are usually transmembrane glycoproteins, whose extracellular domains typically consist of about 210 amino acids forming two tandem fibronectin type III domains and have several conserved amino acid positions that are important for the secondary structure. In contrast, their intracellular domains vary in length and do not demonstrate striking sequence homology (reviewed in [14]). Binding of IL-10 to its receptor complex consists of two steps: IL-10 first binds to IL-10Rα. The IL-10/IL-10Rα interaction very probably changes the cytokine conformation allowing the association of the IL-10/IL-10Rα complex with the IL-10Rβ. IL-10Rβ alone is unable to bind IL-10 [13]. The molecular basis of the interaction between human IL-10 and IL-10Rα has been characterized in detail [6, 7, 15]. Recently, an IL-10 epitope becoming available after its conformational change has been proposed to represent the binding site for IL-10Rβ [7, 16]. Activation via the IL-10R complex has been shown to mobilize signaling pathways involving members of the Janus tyrosine kinase (JAK) family and the signal transducers and activators of transcription (STAT) [17]. IL-10 can activate also other signaling pathways such as phosphatidylinositol 3-kinase in macrophages.

IL-10Rα is mainly found on immune cells. Its expression is generally low, varying between 100 and 800 molecules per cell ([18, 19] and R. Sabat, unpublished). As analyzed so far, monocytes and macrophages exhibit the highest IL-10Rα expression (R. Sabat, unpublished). The expression is adjustable, but only a few regulating factors are known so far. In general, the activation of immune cells provokes down-regulation of IL-10Rα expression [20]. In non-immune cells IL-10Rα expression has also been observed [21–23]. Here, cellular activation mostly leads to induction of its expression. In contrast to IL-10Rα, IL-10Rβ is strongly expressed in most cells and tissues, and does not seem to be regulated in its expression levels [24, 25].

### 8.2.3
### IL-10 Homologs

In addition to various mammalian IL-10 homologous molecules (see below), four viral IL-10 homologues are known. They are derived from Epstein–Barr virus (EBV), equine Herpes type 2 virus, poxvirus Orf and cytomegalovirus (CMV) [26–29]. With the exception of CMV IL-10, the similarity of the viral and cellular IL-10s with respect to the amino acid sequence is very high. For instance, the amino acid sequence of the EBV IL-10 (vIL-10) is 84% identical to that of hIL-10. This, apart from marginal differences predominantly in the N-terminal part, results in very similar protein structures [30]. The expression of vIL-10s appears during the lytic phase of virus infection. vIL-10s are suggested to act via the same receptor as cellular IL-10. When compared to hIL-10, however, an about 1000-fold lower efficiency is observed for many effects [31]. This may be explained by a different affinity to IL-10Rα. Unfortunately, most anti-hIL-10 antibodies and ELISA cannot discriminate between hIL-10 and vIL-10.

As well as the viral homologues, novel cellular molecules with homology to IL-10 have been identified. These are combined now in the so-called IL-10 family comprising IL-10, IL-19, IL-20, IL-22, AK155 and the melanoma differentiation associated gene (MDA)-7 ([32–36, reviewed in [37]). Since the identification of these new cytokines is very recent, knowledge of their biology is still limited. It is obvious so far that the sequence homology is not reflected by a shared biological function. IL-20 and IL-22 are suggested to play different roles in inflammatory processes [33, 34]. MDA-7 has been shown to provoke irreversible growth arrest of tumors by induction of apoptosis or differentiation [36]. The biological functions for IL-19 and AK155 have not been described yet [32, 35].

### 8.3
### Biological Activities of IL-10

Numerous IL-10 effects have been demonstrated on a variety of cells *in vitro* (Tab. 8.2). *In vivo*, immune cells, especially monocytes and macrophages, seem to re-

**Tab. 8.2** Effects of IL-10 on immune cells

| Cell population | Suppression | Induction | Reference |
|---|---|---|---|
| Monocytes/ macrophages | TNF-α, IL-1, -8, -12 production; antigen presentation | IL-1RA production; phagocytosis | 42–44, 47–51 |
| DCs | development; antigen presentation | | 39, 40, 141 |
| T cells | IL-2, -4, -5, IFN-γ production; proliferation | | 58, 59, 142, 143 |
| NK cells | | cytotoxic activity; IFN-γ, TNF-α production | 18, 69 |
| B cells | | proliferation; differentiation | 70, 71 |
| Neutrophils | TNF-α, IL-1β, IL-8 production | IL-1RA production | 74, 75 |
| Eosinophils | TNF-α, GM-CSF, IL-8 production | | 77 |
| Mast cells | TNF-α, GM-CSF, NO production | growth; histamine liberation | 78, 79, 144 |

present the major target of IL-10. This is partly due to different levels of IL-10Rα expression among the IL-10-responsive cell populations.

## 8.3.1
### Effects on Myeloid Antigen-Presenting Cells (APC)

Blood monocytes are very sensitive to the presence of IL-10. These cells are not a finally differentiated population. After their 48 h residence in the circulation they emigrate into the stromal tissues where they, depending on the micromilieu, develop into more specialized cell populations, into either macrophages or type 1 dendritic cells (DC1) [38]. IL-10 is able to prevent monocyte differentiation into DC1, which are the most important APCs, especially for primary immune responses [39–41]. During DC1 development the influence of IL-10 on these cells decreases. This is associated with a decrease of cellular IL-10Rα expression (R. Sabat, unpublished). In contrast, IL-10 supports monocyte maturation to macrophages and the sensitivity of macrophages towards IL-10 is comparable to that of monocytes ([40] and R. Sabat, unpublished). The functions of monocytes and macrophages which are regulated by IL-10 can be divided into three groups: (1) production of soluble immunomediators, (2) antigen presentation and (3) phagocytosis. In general, IL-10 inhibits all those activities that favor the inflammatory or specific cellular immune response and enhances those activities that are associated with induction of tolerance in specific immunity as well as with scavenger function. More concretely, IL-10 inhibits the production of pro-inflammatory mediators by monocytes and macrophages, such as endotoxin- and IFN-γ-induced release of IL-1β, IL-6, IL-8, granulocyte colony stimulating factor (CSF), granulocyte macrophage colony stimulating factor (GM-CSF) and tumor necrosis factor (TNF)-α [42, 43]. In addition, it enhances the production of anti-inflammatory mediators like IL-1RA and soluble TNF-α receptors [44–46]. Moreover, IL-10 inhibits the capacity of monocytes and macrophages to present antigen to T cells. This is realized by down-regulation of constitutive and IFN-γ-induced cell surface levels of MHC class II, of co-stimulatory molecules like CD86 and of some adhesion molecules such as CD58 [47–49]. In addition, IL-10 inhibits the monocytic production of IL-12, an essential mediator for the development of specific cellular immune defense [50]. On the other hand, IL-10 favors the phagocytic activity of monocytes and macrophages [51]. This is realized among others by up-regulated expression of specific receptors that mediate the uptake of opsonized and non-opsonized microorganisms. In fact, IL-10-treated monocytes and macrophages show an enhanced expression not only of IgG Fc receptors (CD16, CD32 and CD64) but also of scavenger receptors like CD163 and CD14 [52–55]. Interestingly, IL-10 simultaneously diminishes the killing of ingested microorganisms [56]. The up-regulated expression of scavenger receptors is probably responsible for the observation that IL-10-treated monocytes and macrophages strongly ingest apoptotic cells (W.-D. Döcke and R. Sabat, unpublished). The chemotaxis of monocytes is only weakly impaired by IL-10 [57].

### 8.3.2
### Effects on T Cells

As well as the dominating indirect impact via APCs, IL-10 also exerts a direct effect on T cells (Fig. 8.1). In particular, inhibitory effects have been described on CD4$^+$ T cells. IL-10 inhibits the proliferation as well as the cytokine synthesis of these cells. Concerning the latter, it affects their IL-2 and IFN-γ as well as their IL-4 and IL-5 production as induced by various stimuli [58, 59]. At least in the human system, IL-10 therefore seems to inhibit both the T$_h$1- and T$_h$2-type responses, though the effect on T$_h$1 cells appears to be stronger [60]. The influence of IL-10 on CD4$^+$ T cells is particularly marked on the naive cells. Activated and memory T cells seem to be rather in-

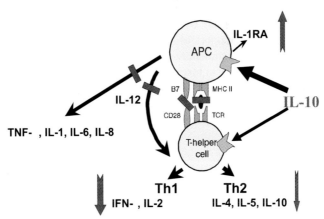

**Fig. 8.1**  Effects of IL-10 on APC–T cell interaction. IL-10 suppresses the expression of pro-inflammatory cytokines and enhances the formation of anti-inflammatory mediators. Moreover, IL-10 inhibits the capacity of monocytes and macrophages to present antigen to T cells. (see color plates page XXV)

sensitive towards this cytokine. This is due to the down-regulation of IL-10Rα upon T cell activation [20]. The interaction between CD28 and IL-10Rα seems to be essential for the influence of IL-10 on these cells [61]. The presence of IL-10 during the activation of CD4$^+$ T cells results in the development of a regulatory phenotype of these cells [62–65]. It is characterized by weak proliferation and a specific cytokine profile after repeated stimulation. Typical for these cells is also their capacity to transfer this phenotype to other T cells with the same antigen specificity. This transfer may not be dependent on soluble mediators, but on cell surface molecules [66]. Whether the influence of IL-10 on CD4$^+$ T cells or on APC *in vivo* is the most important in the generation of such regulatory cells remains to be clarified. *In vitro*, both pathways have been demonstrated. IL-10 does not exert potent direct inhibitory effects on CD8$^+$ T cells. It can even activate CD8$^+$ T cells under certain conditions [67, 68].

### 8.3.3
### Effects on Natural Killer (NK) Cells

The effect of IL-10 on NK cells is mainly stimulatory. IL-10 favors the cytotoxic activity of these cells. It increases the IL-2-induced production of cytokines such as IFN-γ, GM-CSF and TNF-α. Furthermore, it amplifies the IL-2-induced proliferation of the CD56$^{bright}$ NK cell subpopulation [18]. Moreover, IL-10 augments the ability of IL-18 to stimulate NK cells [69].

### 8.3.4
### Effects on other Immune Cells

IL-10 has various, but weak stimulatory effects on B cells. It prevents apoptosis and enhances the proliferation and differentiation towards plasma cells [70, 71]. It also plays a role in Ig switching. In combination with IL-4 it induces IgG4 but inhibits IgE production; in combination with TGF-β, IL-10 induces IgA1 and IgA2 secretion [72, 73].

Very similar to monocytes and macrophages, IL-10 in granulocytes inhibits the production of pro-inflammatory (TNF-α and IL-1β) and induces the production of anti-inflammatory (IL-1RA) mediators. Moreover, it inhibits the release of various chemokines by neutrophils [74, 75]. The synthesis of cyclooxygenase-2 as well as the production of prostaglandin E$_2$ is also inhibited by IL-10 [76]. Another effect of IL-10 is the inhibition of lipopolysaccharide (LPS)-induced synthesis of pro-inflammatory mediators in eosinophils and mast cells [77, 78]. In combination with IL-3 and IL-4, however, IL-10 favors the growth of mast cells [79].

### 8.3.5
### IL-10's Role in the Immune System

Most generally, the immune system can either be divided into the specific and the unspecific or into the humoral and the cellular system. The role of IL-10 particularly concerns the inhibition of the unspecific humoral immunity due to its effects on monocytes, macrophages and also granulocytes. IL-10 exerts inhibitory effects on the specific cellular immunity. By alteration of DC development and of naive $T_h1$ cells, a new immune response is particularly affected. The influence of IL-10 on an established immune response might be associated with the generation of regulatory cells. The overall specific humoral immune responses are only loosely affected by IL-10. It positively influences different functions of B cells, but likewise induces apoptosis of DC2 and inhibits $T_h2$ cells [80]. Finally, it remains to be mentioned that IL-10 enhances the unspecific cellular immunity, especially by modulating NK cells as well as special functions of monocytes and macrophages.

Considering the time course of an immune response, the capacity of IL-10 to interfere appears to be as follows. By inhibiting the inflammation and the establishment of specific cellular immunity, IL-10 regulates the beginning of a new immune response. The ongoing immune reaction is rather insensitive towards IL-10. However, when the immune response slows down the regulatory role of IL-10 becomes important again: IL-10 induces the generation of regulatory T cells and helps the macrophages to 'clean up' the site of reaction. It should be noted that the phagocytosed material is not presented by the macrophages certainly representing a mechanism to prevent the generation of auto-reactive T cells.

## 8.4
## IL-10 Expression in Cancer Patients

Regarding IL-10 in cancer patients, four aspects appear to be especially interesting: (1) the cellular sources of IL-10 (is it produced by tumor or immune cells), (2) the selectivity of IL-10 production (is it only one cytokine among many others produced under these circumstances), (3) the level and the dimension of IL-10 presence (is it locally or systemically distributed, is it temporary or continuously expressed) and (4) the prognostic value of enhanced IL-10 expression.

### 8.4.1
### Cellular Sources of IL-10 in Cancer Patients

The cellular origin of IL-10 found in cancer patients might give hints for its pathophysiological role. Theoretically, IL-10 can be produced by the tumor cells as well as by immune cells that for example infiltrate the tumor. If the first is true it may point to a tumor-favoring role of IL-10. Such tumor-promoting effects could be achieved either in an autocrine (stimulation of malignant cell proliferation) or in a paracrine manner via the suppression of the antitumor immune response. This would support the idea of an IL-10 neutralization as a new therapeutic approach. If IL-10 is produced by immune cells (e.g. tumor-infiltrating cells), at least two different scenarios are possible. One possibility would be that these cells produce IL-10 as part of their antitumor activity, suggesting a tumor suppressive property of IL-10, achieved for instance by direct inhibition of tumor cell growth or the enhancement of the antitumor activity of other immune cells (e.g. NK cells). In this case, a therapeutic application of IL-10 would be reasonable. Another possibility, however, is that IL-10 production by immune cells reflects a normal inflammation-limiting negative feedback response, leading to the very same fatal results as if the tumor produces IL-10 itself. There are a number of scientific groups that have studied the question of IL-10 origin.

Diamantstein's group could demonstrate selective expression of IL-10 mRNA in tissues of primary melanomas and melanoma metastases in comparison to normal skin. Additionally, they showed that some (three of 13) melanoma cell lines strongly expressed IL-10 mRNA and produced biologically active cytokine. In contrast, normal melanocytes, keratinocytes and fibroblasts did not produce detectable IL-10 protein levels [81]. Similar results were reported by Brocker *et al.* This group additionally observed a higher frequency of IL-10 expression in metastases compared to primary tumors [82]. Strieter's group described increased levels of IL-10 protein in tissue homogenates of human bronchogenic carcinomas compared to normal lung tissues. Staining of these tumors illustrated primary localization of IL-10 protein to cancer cells. Additionally, IL-10 protein was present in supernatants of several unstimulated human bronchogenic cell lines [83]. IL-10 protein was also detected in culture supernatants from cell lines of cutaneous carcinomas (basal and squamous cell carcinomas) by ELISA and in the respective primary tumors by immunohistology [84]. Numerous scientific groups have described that cells from B, T and NK cell lymphomas are able to produce biologically active IL-10 [85–90].

The first evidence of other cellular sources of IL-10 production other than tumor cells was found by Kiessling's group. They showed selective expression of IL-10 mRNA in biopsies from epithelial ovarian carcinomas in contrast to normal ovaries and ovarian tumor cell lines. Since these differences could not be explained by the extent of T cell infiltration, they suspected another population of immune cells as the source of IL-10 [91]. Three years afterwards, this group reported similar observations in patients with kidney carcinoma. IL-10 mRNA expression was detected only in tumor samples, not in renal cancer lines, peripheral blood mononuclear cells (PBMC) and non-tumorous kidney tissues from the same patients [92]. An explanation for this might be delivered by results presented by Blay *et al.* This group also detected IL-10 in renal cell carcinoma samples, but not in the culture supernatant of cell lines derived from these tumors. However, these cell lines or their supernatants induced IL-10 production by autologous monocytes and PBMC [93]. Interestingly, very recently a novel subset of monocytes has been identified in peritoneal exudates from patients with ovarian cancer. These monocytes were characterized by production of IL-10 and TGF-β, but not IL-12 and TNF-α. In addition, they expressed CD14, but not HLA-DR, CD86 or CD80 [94].

These examples prove that in tumor patients' tumor cells as well as immune cells may produce IL-10. Whether the IL-10 production by one of these populations dominates may depend on the kind of tumor and the actual state of the immune system.

## 8.4.2
### Selectivity of IL-10 Production

There are only a few studies that quantitatively investigated the expression of IL-10 in malignant tissues in comparison with other cytokines. These few studies suggest that IL-10 may dominate over type 1 (IFN-γ) and Type 2 (IL-4) cytokines [91, 92, 95–98]. Whether IL-10 expression is accompanied by a quantitatively similar inflammatory reaction (TNF-α and IL-1β) cannot be concluded from these studies. It should be mentioned that the systemic deviation of the immune system towards a type 2 phenotype has been postulated in cancer patients [99]. However, to our mind IL-10 is not just a classical type 2 cytokine, and the systemic cytokine phenotype in tumor patients often does not match the classical type 2 phenotype.

### 8.4.3
### IL-10 Presence: Local or Systemic?

The studies described above show good documentation of local IL-10 expression in tumors. Upon tumor progression IL-10 can also be detected in the circulation. As early as 1993 Favrot *et al.* investigated IL-10 serum levels using ELISA which detects both viral and human IL-10 in patients with active non-Hodgkin's lymphoma (NHL) and healthy volunteers. They described the detection of IL-10 in serum from about 50% of these patients but none of the control blood donors. IL-10 was detectable with a similar frequency in all subtypes of NHL and in all clinical stages, as well as in both EBV-seropositive and EBV-seronegative patients [100]. One year later Papa's group demonstrated similar results obtained in patients with aggressive NHL [101]. In the following years these observations were extended to Hodgkin's disease and other lymphoma species, and due to improved sensitivity of ELISA systems it could be shown that lymphoma patients had significantly higher serum levels of IL-10 than healthy volunteers [102–107].

Another study reported by Brocker *et al.* in 1995 shows that IL-10 is detectable especially in serum from progressed melanoma patients [108]. In the following years, elevated levels of serum IL-10 were also observed in patients with other solid tumors compared to healthy subjects. Extensive data are particularly available from patients with lung and gastrointestinal carcinoma [109–114].

### 8.4.4
### Prognostic Value of Enhanced IL-10 Expression

In 1993, Favrot *et al.* reported that IL-10 serum levels in patients with NHL were an independent prognostic factor. In patients with intermediate or high-grade NHL the presence of serum IL-10 correlated with a significantly shorter progression-free and overall survival [100]. The detection of human and viral IL-10 seems to be more relevant than only the human form (reviewed in [103]). A very interesting observation could be demonstrated in patients with chronic lymphocytic leukemia. Even if high IL-10 mRNA expression in leukemic cells from these patients was strongly associated with non-progressive disease [87], high IL-10 serum levels correlated with elevated β$_2$-microglobulin and LDH, and, more importantly, with worse median and 3-year survival [107]. In patients with Hodgkin's disease elevated IL-10 serum levels were also associated with decreased progression-free and overall survival, independently of other established prognostic factors [104–106]. Similar observations could be made in patients with cutaneous T cell lymphoma (mucosis fungoides). Mucosis fungoides progression was associated with significantly higher IL-10 and lower IFN-γ mRNA expression in skin lesions [97].

Elevated IL-10 serum levels have been described as a negative prognostic factor for responsiveness towards treatment, and disease-free and overall survival by patients with melanoma and solid tumors, particularly with lung and gastrointestinal cancer. Moreover, a further significant increase in IL-10 serum levels has been observed in non-responders after chemotherapy [115, 110–113]. Tumor resection resulted in a decrease in IL-10 levels [114].

## 8.5
### Effects of IL-10 in Cancer Models

Several experimental investigations has been performed to analyze the role of IL-10 on tumor development. The data from *in vitro, ex vivo* and animal experiments are complex, pointing to opposite directions regarding the influence of IL-10 on the cancer: depending on the experimental model, IL-10 seems to favor or inhibit the existence and progression of tumors.

### 8.5.1
#### Tumor-Promoting Effects of IL-10

IL-10 is able to directly stimulate the growth of certain tumor cells. Klein *et al.* have shown that IL-10 is an IL-6-unrelated growth factor for myeloma cells. By inducing the expression of co-receptors for oncostatin M on myeloma cells IL-10 provoked an autocrine growth loop [116, 117]. IL-10 is also an autocrine growth factor for other B cell lymphomas [86, 88, 90]. The role of IL-10 in B chronic lymphocytic leukemia (B-CLL) is discussed. Some investigators reported that IL-10 enhanced the survival of B-CLL cells by inhibiting the process of apoptotic cell death, whereas others described that IL-10 decreased Bcl-2 protein levels and induced apoptosis [85, 118]. Moreover, IL-10 also acts as an autocrine growth factor for melanoma cells by enhancing proliferation and prolonged the survival of these cells [119].

IL-10 can convert tumor cells to a cytotoxic T cell lysis (CTL)-resistant phenotype. In 1994, Kiessling *et al.* reported an about 50% reduction of MHC class I expression in human melanoma cells after IL-10 treatment. This pretreatment resulted in a dose-dependent and up to 100% inhibition of autologous CTL-mediated, tumor-specific lysis [120]. Three years later the same group demonstrated that this was mediated by reduced expression of the so-called transporter associated with antigen processing (TAP)-1 and -2 which results in reduced translocation of peptides to the endoplasmic reticulum, and therefore in diminished MHC class I peptide loading and cell surface levels [121]. However, the down-regulation of MHC class I expression results in higher sensitivity of these cells towards NK cell activity that also can fight tumors ([122] and see below).

IL-10 can inhibit the antitumor immune reactions. One would expect a negative impact on the function of monocytes, macrophages, CD4⁺ T cells and on the generation of DCs (see above). In line with this, Strieter's group reported that PBMC cultured with supernatants from human bronchogenic cell lines only in the presence of anti-IL-10 antibodies increased their TNF-α and IL-6 production [83]. As mentioned above, cutaneous carcinoma produces IL-10. T cells lines established from tumor-infiltrating lymphocytes proliferated in the presence of autologous tumor cells dependent on the addition of anti-IL-10 antibodies [84]. Similar results were reported for the newly identified subset of monocytes from malignant ascites of patients with ovarian carcinoma. These monocytes inhibited the proliferation of autologous T cells in response to phytohemagglutinin. Moreover, this inhibition could be reversed by addition of anti-IL-10 and anti-TGF-β antibodies [94]. The consequence of IL-10 presence and thereby inhibition of the antitumor immune reaction might be the uncontrolled development of cancers. This has been demonstrated in transgenic mice expressing IL-10 under the control of the IL-2 promoter. These animals are unable to limit the growth of immunogenic tumors. However, administration of anti-IL-10 antibodies restored the anticancer response [123]. Not surprisingly, these mice show defects not only in T cells but also in APC. The latter have suppressed capacity to produce IL-12 production and to induce a T cell reaction [124].

These examples show that IL-10 is able to favor tumor growth both directly by affecting the tumor cells and indirectly by affecting the immune cells.

## 8.5.2
### Tumor-Inhibiting Effects of IL-10

IL-10 can directly exert a negative effect on tumor cells. For instance, it inhibits the spontaneous proliferation of acute myelogenous leukemia blast cells. This is an irreversible inhibitory effect as inhibition could also be demonstrated when the cytokine was present only at the beginning of culture. However, independently on the effect on proliferation, IL-10 reduces IL-1α/β, TNF-α, GM-CSF and IL-6 secretion by these cells [125]. Similar effects are seen on chronic myelomonocytic leukemia cells. IL-10 dose-dependently inhibits the growth of these cells. This is due to a decrease of GM-CSF mRNA and protein [126]. Another direct negative effect of IL-10 on tumor survival has been described by Fulton's group. They observed that IL-10 gene transfer in murine mammalian tumor cells was associated with increased expression of the inducible isoform of NO synthase (iNOS). The activity of this enzyme was elevated as well. This can result in elevated levels of NO in transfected tumor cells [127]. NO is known to have potent antitumor activity.

IL-10 can inhibit the generation of new vessels within the tumor both directly by acting on the tumor cells and indirectly by influencing infiltrating immune cells. IL-10 induced the tissue inhibitor of metalloproteinase (TIMP)-2 in primary human prostate cancer cells. Simultaneously, it reduced the secretion of matrix metalloproteinase (MMP)-2 and -9 from these cells. The consequence was the inhibition of microvessel formation [128]. Interestingly, TGF-β induced the expression of MMP-2 and this induction was prevented by IL-10. When primary human prostate cancer cells either expressing TGF-β or IL-10 were implanted in SCID mice, TGF-β promoted tumor growth, angiogenesis and metastasis. In contrast, IL-10 reduced growth rates, angiogenesis and metastasis. More importantly, none of the mice bearing TGF-β-expressing tumor cells survived compared to 80% of those expressing IL-10 [129]. IL-10 can inhibit the angiogenesis also by inhibiting tumor-resident macrophages. Bar-Eli *et al.* reported that the transplantation of human melanoma cells that had been transfected with the murine IL-10 cDNA into nude mice resulted in fewer lung metastases and significant inhibition of tumor growth. The authors suggested that this was due to inhibition of angiogenesis by IL-10. They referred to the fact that IL-10 down-regulated the production of vascular endothelial growth factor in the tumor-associated macrophages. Other factors involved in neovascularization such as IL-1β, TNF-α and IL-6 were also inhibited [130, 131].

Different groups described the positive effect of IL-10 on NK cell activity resulting in an indirect negative effect on cancer growth. NK cell activity is especially important in cases of diminished MHC class I expression by the tumor cells. Low MHC class I expression can be the normal feature of this cell type, but might also be induced by immune mediators like IL-10. Velu *et al.* demonstrated a loss of tumorigenicity of melanoma cells injected into syngeneic mice after previous retroviral transfection of these cells with IL-10 cDNA. Host T cells and NK cells might be involved in the observed tumor eradication because IL-10-producing tumor cells grew in nude mice and in CD8+ T or NK cell-depleted mice [132]. Similar observations have been reported by Fulton's group. They described that injection of the murine mammary tumor cell line 410.4 in syngeneic mice resulted in progressive growth and death from pulmonary metastases. In contrast, transfection of IL-10 cDNA in these cell lines resulted in complete inhibition of growth and metastatic disease. Interestingly, the antimetastatic activity of IL-10 is expressed in T cell-deficient mice but is lost when NK cell activity is suppressed. These authors also point out the importance of IL-10-mediated reduction of MHC class I expression by tumor cells [133].

## 8.6
## Conclusions

Various tumors are associated with locally, and upon tumor progression also systemically, elevated IL-10 levels. IL-10 was found to be produced by both the tumor cells as well as immune cells. Elevated IL-10 serum levels are associated with a poor prognosis. Several experimental investigations pointed to opposite directions regarding the influence of IL-10 on the cancer – either to favor or to inhibit the existence and progression of tumors. In summary, it remains difficult to give a clear postulate concerning the role of IL-10 in tumor development as it induces numerous and contrary effects. Whether it will act as an inhibitor or stimulator of the tumor may depend on different factors such as the species of tumor and the stage of disease. Three questions appear to be especially important in context of the species of tumor:

1. Does IL-10 directly modulate the proliferation of the tumor cells?
2. Is the neovascularization essential for the progression of the tumor?

3.  How immunogenic are the tumor cells? What is the most relevant mechanism
    for protection against the tumor – the NK-cell mediated lysis or the specific im-
    munity (DC1, CD4$^+$ and CD8$^+$ T cells)?

Thus it is understandable that IL-10 enhances the growth of some tumors like certain lymphomas (IL-10 enhances the proliferation of these cells, no relevance of neovascularization, immune protection particularly given through specific immunity),
while inhibiting other tumor species (important role of neovascularization, protection given by NK cells).

In addition, at least two further aspects are likely to be relevant for the final effect of
IL-10:

1.  The concentration of the cytokine.
2.  The time and duration of its presence.

The IL-10 concentration does not only seem to be relevant for the quantity but also
for quality of the effects. Based on our recent *in vivo* and *in vitro* observations we
speculate that low concentrations of IL-10 are efficient for negative effects on immune cells, whereas higher concentrations are needed for stimulatory effects. As discussed before, negative regulatory effects of IL-10 are only seen when applied early
in an immune response. Overall, we think that for the majority of tumors IL-10 contributes to tumor escape from an immune response, especially in the beginning of
the disease.

Whatever the role of IL-10 on tumors might be, the question arises whether the
modulation of IL-10 levels will result in therapeutic effects. A decrease of IL-10
serum levels can be safely achieved by anti-IL-10 antibodies [135]. Reduction of IL-10
levels might only be useful in tumors where IL-10 acts as an autocrine growth factor.
For most of the patients submitted to the hospital it may not work as they are already
in a late stage of disease with reduced antitumor immunity. Additionally, regulatory
T cells might already be generated. On the other hand, depletion of IL-10 could increase the inflammatory activity of monocytes and macrophages, resulting in further
dysregulation of the immune system (massive inflammation does inhibit specific
immunity).

The opposite treatment – application of IL-10 – has also been performed in healthy
volunteers and numerous, different patients [11, 60]. Application of IL-10 may be
useful in some tumors, especially at progressed stages. Specific immunity is already
inhibited, thus negative effects should not be expected. In contrast, IL-10 could increase NK cell-mediated tumor lysis and inhibit angiogenesis. Importantly, proliferative effects on the tumor need to be excluded before IL-10 application.

Ongoing trials will show whether theory will fit with nature.

## References

1 SPITS H, DE WAAL MALEFYT R. Functional characterization of human IL-10. *Int Arch Allergy Immunol* 1992; **99**: 8–15.

2 FIORENTINO DF, BOND MW, MOSMANN TR. Two types of mouse T helper cell. IV. T$_h$2 clones secrete a factor that inhibits cytokine production by T$_h$1 clones. *J Exp Med* 1989; **170**: 2081–95.

3 KIM JM, BRANNAN CI, COPELAND NG, JENKINS NA, KHAN TA, MOORE KW. Structure of the mouse IL-10 gene and chromosomal localization of the mouse and human genes. *J Immunol* 1992; **148**: 3618–23.

4 ZDANOV A, SCHALK-HIHI C, GUSTCHINA A, TSANG M, WEATHERBEE J, WLODAWER A. Crystal structure of interleukin-10 reveals the functional dimer with an unexpected topological similarity to interferon γ. *Structure* 1995; **3**: 591–601.

5 WALTER MR, NAGABHUSHAN TL. Crystal structure of interleukin 10 reveals an interferon γ-like fold. *Biochemistry* 1995; **34**: 12118–25.

6 ZDANOV A, SCHALK-HIHI C, WLODAWER A. Crystal structure of human interleukin-10 at 1.6 A resolution and a model of a complex with its soluble receptor. *Protein Sci* 1996; **5**: 1955–62.

7 JOSEPHSON K, LOGSDON NJ, WALTER MR. Crystal structure of the IL-10/IL-10R1 complex reveals a shared receptor binding site. *Immunity* 2001; **15**: 35–46.

8 EALICK SE, COOK WJ, VIJAY-KUMAR S, *et al.* Three-dimensional structure of recombinant human interferon-γ. *Science* 1991; **252**: 698–702.

9 AJUEBOR MN, DAS AM, VIRAG L, FLOWER RJ, SZABO C, PERRETTI M. Role of resident peritoneal macrophages and mast cells in chemokine production and neutrophil migration in acute inflammation: evidence for an inhibitory loop involving endogenous IL-10. *J Immunol* 1999; **162**: 1685–91.

10 ASSEMAN C, MAUZE S, LEACH MW, COFFMAN RL, POWRIE F. An essential role for interleukin 10 in the function of regulatory T cells that inhibit intestinal inflammation. *J Exp Med* 1999; **190**: 995–1004.

11 HUHN RD, RADWANSKI E, O'CONNELL SM, *et al.* Pharmacokinetics and immunomodulatory properties of intravenously administered recombinant human interleukin-10 in healthy volunteers. *Blood* 1996; **87**: 699–705.

12 HO AS, LIU Y, KHAN TA, HSU DH, BAZAN JF, MOORE KW. A RECEPTOR FOR INTERLEUKIN 10 IS RELATED TO INTERFERON RECEPTORS. *Proc Natl Acad Sci USA* 1993; **90**: 11267–71.

13 KOTENKO SV, KRAUSE CD, IZOTOVA LS, POLLACK BP, WU W, PESTKA S. IDENTIFICATION AND FUNCTIONAL CHARACTERIZATION OF A SECOND CHAIN OF THE INTERLEUKIN-10 RECEPTOR COMPLEX. *EMBO J* 1997; **16**: 5894–903.

14 KOTENKO SV, PESTKA S. JAK–STAT SIGNAL TRANSDUCTION PATHWAY THROUGH THE EYES OF CYTOKINE CLASS II RECEPTOR COMPLEXES. *Oncogene* 2000; **19**: 2557–65.

15 REINEKE U, SABAT R, VOLK HD, SCHNEIDER-MERGENER J. MAPPING OF THE INTERLEUKIN-10/INTERLEUKIN-10 RECEPTOR COMBINING SITE. *Protein Sci* 1998; **7**: 951–60.

16 REINEKE U, SCHNEIDER-MERGENER J, GLASER RW, *et al.* Evidence for conformationally different states of interleukin-10: binding of a neutralizing antibody enhances accessibility of a hidden epitope. *J Mol Recognit* 1999; **12**: 242–8.

17 FINBLOOM DS, WINESTOCK KD. IL-10 INDUCES THE TYROSINE PHOSPHORYLATION OF TYK2 AND JAKI AND THE DIFFERENTIAL ASSEMBLY OF STAT1 α AND STAT3 COMPLEXES IN HUMAN T CELLS AND MONOCYTES. *J Immunol* 1995; **155**: 1079–90.

18 CARSON WE, LINDEMANN MJ, BAIOCCHI R, *et al.* The functional characterization of interleukin-10 receptor expression on human natural killer cells. *Blood* 1995; **85**: 3577–85.

19 JURLANDER J, LAI CF, TAN J, *et al.* Characterization of interleukin-10 receptor expression on B-cell chronic lymphocy-

tic leukemia cells. *Blood* 1997; **89**: 4146–52.

20 LIU Y, WEI SH, HO AS, DE WAAL MALE-FYT R, MOORE KW. Expression cloning and characterization of a human IL-10 receptor. *J Immunol* 1994; **152**: 1821–9.

21 WEBER-NORDT RM, MERAZ MA, SCHREIBER RD. Lipopolysaccharide-dependent induction of IL-10 receptor expression on murine fibroblasts. *J Immunol* 1994; **153**: 3734–44.

22 ROTH I, FISHER SJ. IL-10 is an autocrine inhibitor of human placental cytotrophoblast MMP-9 production and invasion. *Dev Biol* 1999; **205**: 194–204.

23 DENNING TL, CAMPBELL NA, SONG F, *et al.* Expression of IL-10 receptors on epithelial cells from the murine small and large intestine. *Int Immunol* 2000; **12**: 133–9.

24 LUTFALLA G, GARDINER K, UZE G. A new member of the cytokine receptor gene family maps on chromosome 21 at less than 35 kb from IFNAR. *Genomics* 1993; **16**: 366–73.

25 GIBBS VC, PENNICA D. CRF2–4: isolation of cDNA clones encoding the human and mouse proteins. *Gene* 1997; **186**: 97–101.

26 HSU DH, DE WAAL MALEFYT R, FIOREN-TINO DF, *et al.* Expression of interleukin-10 activity by Epstein–Barr virus protein BCRF1. *Science* 1990; **250**: 830–2.

27 RODE HJ, JANSSEN W, ROSEN-WOLFF A, *et al.* The genome of equine herpesvirus type 2 harbors an interleukin 10 (IL10)-like gene. *Virus Genes* 1993; **7**: 111–6.

28 FLEMING SB, MCCAUGHAN CA, AN-DREWS AE, NASH AD, MERCER AA. A homolog of interleukin-10 is encoded by the poxvirus orf virus. *J Virol* 1997; **71**: 4857–61.

29 KOTENKO SV, SACCANI S, IZOTOVA LS, MIROCHNITCHENKO OV, PESTKA S. Human cytomegalovirus harbors its own unique IL-10 homolog (cmvIL-10). *Proc Natl Acad Sci USA* 2000; **97**: 1695–700.

30 ZDANOV A, SCHALK-HIHI C, MENON S, MOORE KW, WLODAWER A. Crystal structure of Epstein–Barr virus protein BCRF1, a homolog of cellular interleukin-10. *J Mol Biol* 1997; **268**: 460–7.

31 LIU Y, DE WAAL MALEFYT R, BRIERE F, *et al.* The EBV IL-10 homologue is a selective agonist with impaired binding to the IL-10 receptor. *J Immunol* 1997; **158**: 604–13.

32 GALLAGHER G, DICKENSHEETS H, ESK-DALE J, *et al.* Cloning, expression and initial characterization of interleukin-19 (IL-19), a novel homologue of human interleukin-10 (IL-10). *Genes Immun* 2000; **1**: 442–50.

33 BLUMBERG H, CONKLIN D, XU WF, *et al.* Interleukin 20: discovery, receptor identification, and role in epidermal function. *Cell* 2001; **104**: 9–19.

34 DUMOUTIER L, LOUAHED J, RENAULD JC. Cloning and characterization of IL-10–related T cell-derived inducible factor (IL-TIF), a novel cytokine structurally related to IL-10 and inducible by IL-9. *J Immunol* 2000; **164**: 1814–9.

35 KNAPPE A, HOR S, WITTMANN S, FICK-ENSCHER H. Induction of a novel cellular homolog of interleukin-10, AK155, by transformation of T lymphocytes with herpesvirus saimiri. *J Virol* 2000; **74**: 3881–7.

36 JIANG H, LIN JJ, SU ZZ, GOLDSTEIN NI, FISHER PB. Subtraction hybridization identifies a novel melanoma differentiation associated gene, *mda-7*, modulated during human melanoma differentiation, growth and progression. *Oncogene* 1995; **11**: 2477–86.

37 VOLK H, KHUSRU A, GALLAGHER G, SA-BAT R, GRUTZ G. IL-10 and its homologs: important immune mediators and emerging immunotherapeutic targets. *Trends Immunol* 2001; **22**: 414–7.

38 RANDOLPH GJ, BEAULIEU S, LEBECQUE S, STEINMAN RM, MULLER WA. Differentiation of monocytes into dendritic cells in a model of transendothelial trafficking. *Science* 1998; **282**: 480–3.

39 BUELENS C, VERHASSELT V, DE GROOTE D, THIELEMANS K, GOLDMAN M, WILL-EMS F. Interleukin-10 prevents the generation of dendritic cells from human peripheral blood mononuclear cells cultured with interleukin-4 and granulocyte/macrophage-colony-stimulating factor. *Eur J Immunol* 1997; **27**: 756–62.

40 ALLAVENA P, PIEMONTI L, LONGONI D, *et al.* IL-10 prevents the differentiation

of monocytes to dendritic cells but promotes their maturation to macrophages. *Eur J Immunol* 1998; **28**: 359–69.

41 BANCHEREAU J, STEINMAN RM. Dendritic cells and the control of immunity. *Nature* 1998; **392**: 245–52.

42 DE WAAL MALEFYT R, ABRAMS J, BENNETT B, FIGDOR CG, DE VRIES JE. Interleukin 10 (IL-10) inhibits cytokine synthesis by human monocytes: an autoregulatory role of IL-10 produced by monocytes. *J Exp Med* 1991; **174**: 1209–20.

43 FIORENTINO DF, ZLOTNIK A, MOSMANN TR, HOWARD M, O'GARRA A. IL-10 inhibits cytokine production by activated macrophages. *J Immunol* 1991; **147**: 3815–22.

44 JENKINS JK, MALYAK M, AREND WP. The effects of interleukin-10 on interleukin-1 receptor antagonist and interleukin-1 β production in human monocytes and neutrophils. *Lymphokine Cytokine Res* 1994; **13**: 47–54.

45 JOYCE DA, GIBBONS DP, GREEN P, STEER JH, FELDMANN M, BRENNAN FM. Two inhibitors of pro-inflammatory cytokine release, interleukin-10 and interleukin-4, have contrasting effects on release of soluble p75 tumor necrosis factor receptor by cultured human monocytes. *Eur J Immunol* 1994; **24**: 2699–705.

46 HART PH, HUNT EK, BONDER CS, WATSON CJ, FINLAY-JONES JJ. Regulation of surface and soluble TNF receptor expression on human monocytes and synovial fluid macrophages by IL-4 and IL-10. *J Immunol* 1996; **157**: 3672–80.

47 DE WAAL MALEFYT R, HAANEN J, SPITS H, *et al.* Interleukin 10 (IL-10) and viral IL-10 strongly reduce antigen-specific human T cell proliferation by diminishing the antigen-presenting capacity of monocytes via downregulation of class II major histocompatibility complex expression. *J Exp Med* 1991; **174**: 915–24.

48 CREERY WD, DIAZ-MITOMA F, FILION L, KUMAR A. Differential modulation of B7–1 and B7–2 isoform expression on human monocytes by cytokines which influence the development of T helper cell phenotype. *Eur J Immunol* 1996; **26**: 1273–7.

49 WILLEMS F, MARCHANT A, DELVILLE JP, *et al.* Interleukin-10 inhibits B7 and intercellular adhesion molecule-1 expression on human monocytes. *Eur J Immunol* 1994; **24**: 1007–9.

50 D'ANDREA A, ASTE-AMEZAGA M, VALIANTE NM, MA X, KUBIN M, TRINCHIERI G. Interleukin 10 (IL-10) inhibits human lymphocyte interferon γ-production by suppressing natural killer cell stimulatory factor/IL-12 synthesis in accessory cells. *J Exp Med* 1993; **178**: 1041–8.

51 BUCHWALD UK, GEERDES-FENGE HF, VOCKLER J, ZIEGE S, LODE H. Interleukin-10: effects on phagocytosis and adhesion molecule expression of granulocytes and monocytes in a comparison with prednisolone. *Eur J Med Res* 1999; **4**: 85–94.

52 TE VELDE AA, DE WAAL MALEFIJT R, HUIJBENS RJ, DE VRIES JE, FIGDOR CG. IL-10 stimulates monocyte Fc γ R surface expression and cytotoxic activity. Distinct regulation of antibody-dependent cellular cytotoxicity by IFN-γ, IL-4, and IL-10. *J Immunol* 1992; **149**: 4048–52.

53 SPITTLER A, SCHILLER C, WILLHEIM M, TEMPFER C, WINKLER S, BOLTZ-NITULESCU G. IL-10 augments CD23 expression on U937 cells and down-regulates IL-4-driven CD23 expression on cultured human blood monocytes: effects of IL-10 and other cytokines on cell phenotype and phagocytosis. *Immunology* 1995; **85**: 311–7.

54 CALZADA-WACK JC, FRANKENBERGER M, ZIEGLER-HEITBROCK HW. Interleukin-10 drives human monocytes to CD16 positive macrophages. *J Inflamm* 1996; **46**: 78–85.

55 RITTER M, BUECHLER C, LANGMANN T, ORSO E, KLUCKEN J, SCHMITZ G. The scavenger receptor CD163: regulation, promoter structure and genomic organization. *Pathobiology* 1999; **67**: 257–61.

56 ROILIDES E, ANASTASIOU-KATSIARDANI A, DIMITRIADOU-GEORGIADOU A, *et al.* Suppressive effects of interleukin-10 on human mononuclear phagocyte function against *Candida albicans* and *Staphylococcus aureus*. *J Infect Dis* 1998; **178**: 1734–42.

57 VICIOSO MA, GARAUD JJ, REGLIER-POU-PET H, LEBEAUT A, GOUGEROT-POCI-DALO MA, CHOLLET-MARTIN S. Moderate inhibitory effect of interleukin-10 on human neutrophil and monocyte chemotaxis *in vitro*. *Eur Cytokine Netw* 1998; **9**: 247–53.

58 DEL PRETE G, DE CARLI M, ALMERI-GOGNA F, GIUDIZI MG, BIAGIOTTI R, ROMAGNANI S. Human IL-10 is produced by both type 1 helper (T$_h$1) and type 2 helper (T$_h$2) T cell clones and inhibits their antigen-specific proliferation and cytokine production. *J Immunol* 1993; **150**: 353–60.

59 GROUX H, BIGLER M, DE VRIES JE, RON-CAROLO MG. Interleukin-10 induces a long-term antigen-specific anergic state in human CD4$^+$ T cells. *J Exp Med* 1996; **184**: 19–29.

60 ASADULLAH K, STERRY W, STEPHANEK K, *et al.* IL-10 is a key cytokine in psoriasis. Proof of principle by IL-10 therapy: a new therapeutic approach. *J Clin Invest* 1998; **101**: 783–94.

61 JOSS A, AKDIS M, FAITH A, BLASER K, AKDIS CA. IL-10 directly acts on T cells by specifically altering the CD28 co-stimulation pathway. *Eur J Immunol* 2000; **30**: 1683–90.

62 GROUX H, O'GARRA A, BIGLER M, *et al.* A CD4$^+$ T-cell subset inhibits antigen-specific T-cell responses and prevents colitis. *Nature* 1997; **389**: 737–42.

63 ZELLER JC, PANOSKALTSIS-MORTARI A, MURPHY WJ, RUSCETTI FW, NARULA S, RONCAROLO MG, BLAZAR BR. Induction of CD4$^+$ T cell alloantigen-specific hyporesponsiveness by IL-10 and TGF-β. *J Immunol* 1999; **163**: 3684–91.

64 LEVINGS MK, SANGREGORIO R, GAL-BIATI F, SQUADRONE S, DE WAAL MALE-FYT R, RONCAROLO MG. IFN-α and IL-10 induce the differentiation of human type 1 T regulatory cells. *J Immunol* 2001; **166**: 5530–9.

65 LEVINGS MK, SANGREGORIO R, RON-CAROLO MG. Human CD25(+)CD4(+) T regulatory cells suppress naive and memory T cell proliferation and can be expanded *in vitro* without loss of function. *J Exp Med* 2001; **193**: 1295–302.

66 JONULEIT H, SCHMITT E, SCHULER G, KNOP J, ENK AH. Induction of interleu-kin 10-producing, nonproliferating CD4(+) T cells with regulatory properties by repetitive stimulation with allogeneic immature human dendritic cells. *J Exp Med* 2000; **192**: 1213–22.

67 GROUX H, BIGLER M, DE VRIES JE, RON-CAROLO MG. Inhibitory and stimulatory effects of IL-10 on human CD8$^+$ T cells. *J Immunol* 1998; **160**: 3188–93.

68 SANTIN AD, HERMONAT PL, RAVAGGI A, *et al.* Interleukin-10 increases T$_h$1 cytokine production and cytotoxic potential in human papillomavirus-specific CD8(+) cytotoxic T lymphocytes. *J Virol* 2000; **74**: 4729–37.

69 CAI G, KASTELEIN RA, HUNTER CA. IL-10 enhances NK cell proliferation, cytotoxicity and production of IFN-γ when combined with IL-18. *Eur J Immunol* 1999; **29**: 2658–65.

70 LEVY Y, BROUET JC. Interleukin-10 prevents spontaneous death of germinal center B cells by induction of the bcl-2 protein. *J Clin Invest* 1994; **93**: 424–8.

71 ROUSSET F, PEYROL S, GARCIA E, *et al.* Long-term cultured CD40-activated B lymphocytes differentiate into plasma cells in response to IL-10 but not IL-4. *Int Immunol* 1995; **7**: 1243–53.

72 JEANNIN P, LECOANET S, DELNESTE Y, GAUCHAT JF, BONNEFOY JY. IgE versus IgG4 production can be differentially regulated by IL-10. *J Immunol* 1998; **160**: 3555–61.

73 DEFRANCE T, VANBERVLIET B, BRIERE F, DURAND I, ROUSSET F, BANCHEREAU J. Interleukin 10 and transforming growth factor β cooperate to induce anti-CD40-activated naive human B cells to secrete immunoglobulin A. *J Exp Med* 1992; **175**: 671–82.

74 CASSATELLA MA, MEDA L, BONORA S, CESKA M, CONSTANTIN G. Interleukin 10 (IL-10) inhibits the release of proinflammatory cytokines from human polymorphonuclear leukocytes. Evidence for an autocrine role of tumor necrosis factor and IL-1 β in mediating the production of IL-8 triggered by lipopolysaccharide. *J Exp Med* 1993; **178**: 2207–11.

75 KASAMA T, STRIETER RM, LUKACS NW, BURDICK MD, KUNKEL SL. Regulation of neutrophil-derived chemokine ex-

pression by IL-10. *J Immunol* 1994; **152**: 3559–69.

**76** NIIRO H, OTSUKA T, IZUHARA K, *et al.* Regulation by interleukin-10 and interleukin-4 of cyclooxygenase-2 expression in human neutrophils. *Blood* 1997; **89**: 1621–8.

**77** TAKANASKI S, NONAKA R, XING Z, O'BYRNE P, DOLOVICH J, JORDANA M. Interleukin 10 inhibits lipopolysaccharide-induced survival and cytokine production by human peripheral blood eosinophils. *J Exp Med* 1994; **180**: 711–5.

**78** AROCK M, ZUANY-AMORIM C, SINGER M, BENHAMOU M, PRETOLANI M. Interleukin-10 inhibits cytokine generation from mast cells. *Eur J Immunol* 1996; **26**: 166–70.

**79** LIN TJ, BEFUS AD. Differential regulation of mast cell function by IL-10 and stem cell factor. *J Immunol* 1997; **159**: 4015–23.

**80** RISSOAN MC, SOUMELIS V, KADOWAKI N, *et al.* Reciprocal control of T helper cell and dendritic cell differentiation. *Science* 1999; **283**: 1183–6.

**81** KRUGER-KRASAGAKES S, KRASAGAKIS K, GARBE C, *et al.* Expression of interleukin 10 in human melanoma. *Br J Cancer* 1994; **70**: 1182–5.

**82** DUMMER W, BASTIAN BC, ERNST N, SCHANZLE C, SCHWAAF A, BROCKER EB. Interleukin-10 production in malignant melanoma: preferential detection of IL-10-secreting tumor cells in metastatic lesions. *Int J Cancer* 1996; **66**: 607–10.

**83** SMITH DR, KUNKEL SL, BURDICK MD, *et al.* Production of interleukin-10 by human bronchogenic carcinoma. *Am J Pathol* 1994; **145**: 18–25.

**84** KIM J, MODLIN RL, MOY RL, *et al.* IL-10 production in cutaneous basal and squamous cell carcinomas. A mechanism for evading the local T cell immune response. *J Immunol* 1995; **155**: 2240–7.

**85** KITABAYASHI A, HIROKAWA M, MIURA AB. The role of interleukin-10 (IL-10) in chronic B-lymphocytic leukemia: IL-10 prevents leukemic cells from apoptotic cell death. *Int J Hematol* 1995; **62**: 99–106.

**86** MASOOD R, ZHANG Y, BOND MW, *et al.* Interleukin-10 is an autocrine growth factor for acquired immunodeficiency syndrome-related B-cell lymphoma. *Blood* 1995; **85**: 3423–30.

**87** SJOBERG J, AGUILAR-SANTELISES M, SJOGREN AM, *et al.* Interleukin-10 mRNA expression in B-cell chronic lymphocytic leukaemia inversely correlates with progression of disease. *Br J Haematol* 1996; **92**: 393–400.

**88** BEATTY PR, KRAMS SM, MARTINEZ OM. Involvement of IL-10 in the autonomous growth of EBV-transformed B cell lines. *J Immunol* 1997; **158**: 4045–51.

**89** BOULLAND ML, MEIGNIN V, LEROY-VIARD K, *et al.* Human interleukin-10 expression in T/natural killer-cell lymphomas: association with anaplastic large cell lymphomas and nasal natural killer-cell lymphomas. *Am J Pathol* 1998; **153**: 1229–37.

**90** JONES KD, AOKI Y, CHANG Y, MOORE PS, YARCHOAN R, TOSATO G. Involvement of interleukin-10 (IL-10) and viral IL-6 in the spontaneous growth of Kaposi's sarcoma herpesvirus-associated infected primary effusion lymphoma cells. *Blood* 1999; **94**: 2871–9.

**91** PISA P, HALAPI E, PISA EK, *et al.* Selective expression of interleukin 10, interferon γ, and granulocyte-macrophage colony-stimulating factor in ovarian cancer biopsies. *Proc Natl Acad Sci USA* 1992; **89**: 7708–12.

**92** NAKAGOMI H, PISA P, PISA EK, *et al.* Lack of interleukin-2 (IL-2) expression and selective expression of IL-10 mRNA in human renal cell carcinoma. *Int J Cancer* 1995; **63**: 366–71.

**93** MENETRIER-CAUX C, BAIN C, FAVROT MC, DUC A, BLAY JY. Renal cell carcinoma induces interleukin 10 and prostaglandin E2 production by monocytes. *Br J Cancer* 1999; **79**: 119–30.

**94** LOERCHER AE, NASH MA, KAVANAGH JJ, PLATSOUCAS CD, FREEDMAN RS. Identification of an IL-10–producing HLA-DR-negative monocyte subset in the malignant ascites of patients with ovarian carcinoma that inhibits cytokine protein expression and proliferation of autologous T cells. *J Immunol* 1999; **163**: 6251–60.

**95** YAMAMURA M, MODLIN RL, OHMEN JD, MOY RL. Local expression of antiinflammatory cytokines in cancer. *J Clin Invest* 1993; **91**: 1005–10.

**96** FILGUEIRA L, ZUBER M, MERLO A, *et al.* Cytokine gene transcription in renal cell carcinoma. *Br J Surg* 1993; **80**: 1322–5.

**97** ASADULLAH K, DOCKE WD, HAEUSSLER A, STERRY W, VOLK HD. Progression of mycosis fungoides is associated with increasing cutaneous expression of interleukin-10 mRNA. *J Invest Dermatol* 1996; **107**: 833–7.

**98** ASADULLAH K, GELLRICH S, HAEUSSLER-QUADE A, *et al.* Cytokine expression in primary cutaneous germinal center cell lymphomas. *Exp Dermatol* 2000; **9**: 71–6.

**99** FILELLA X, ALCOVER J, ZARCO MA, BEARDO P, MOLINA R, BALLESTA AM. Analysis of type T1 and T2 cytokines in patients with prostate cancer. *Prostate* 2000; **44**: 271–4.

**100** BLAY JY, BURDIN N, ROUSSET F, *et al.* Serum interleukin-10 in non-Hodgkin's lymphoma: a prognostic factor. *Blood* 1993; **82**: 2169–74.

**101** STASI R, ZINZANI L, GALIENI P, *et al.* Detection of soluble interleukin-2 receptor and interleukin-10 in the serum of patients with aggressive non-Hodgkin's lymphoma. Identification of a subset at high risk of treatment failure. *Cancer* 1994; **74**: 1792–800.

**102** CORTES JE, TALPAZ M, CABANILLAS F, SEYMOUR JF, KURZROCK R. Serum levels of interleukin-10 in patients with diffuse large cell lymphoma: lack of correlation with prognosis. *Blood* 1995; **85**: 2516–20.

**103** CORTES J, KURZROCK R. Interleukin-10 in non-Hodgkin's lymphoma. *Leuk Lymph.* 1997; **26**: 251–9.

**104** SARRIS AH, KLICHE KO, PETHAMBARAM P, *et al.* Interleukin-10 levels are often elevated in serum of adults with Hodgkin's disease and are associated with inferior failure-free survival. *Ann Oncol* 1999; **10**: 433–40.

**105** BOHLEN H, KESSLER M, SEXTRO M, DIEHL V, TESCH H. Poor clinical outcome of patients with Hodgkin's disease and elevated interleukin-10 serum levels. Clinical significance of interleu-kin-10 serum levels for Hodgkin's disease. *Ann Hematol* 2000; **79**: 110–3.

**106** VASSILAKOPOULOS TP, NADALI G, ANGELOPOULOU MK, *et al.* Serum interleukin-10 levels are an independent prognostic factor for patients with Hodgkin's lymphoma. *Haematologica* 2001; **86**: 274–81.

**107** FAYAD L, KEATING MJ, REUBEN JM, *et al.* Interleukin-6 and interleukin-10 levels in chronic lymphocytic leukemia: correlation with phenotypic characteristics and outcome. *Blood* 2001; **97**: 256–63.

**108** DUMMER W, BECKER JC, SCHWAAF A, LEVERKUS M, MOLL T, BROCKER EB. Elevated serum levels of interleukin-10 in patients with metastatic malignant melanoma. *Melanoma Res* 1995; **5**: 67–8.

**109** FORTIS C, FOPPOLI M, GIANOTTI L, *et al.* Increased interleukin-10 serum levels in patients with solid tumors. *Cancer Lett* 1996; **104**: 1–5.

**110** WOJCIECHOWSKA-LACKA A, MATECKA-NOWAK M, ADAMIAK E, LACKI JK, CERKASKA-GLUSZAK B. Serum levels of interleukin-10 and interleukin-6 in patients with lung cancer. *Neoplasma* 1996; **43**: 155–8.

**111** DE VITA F, ORDITURA M, GALIZIA G, *et al.* Serum interleukin-10 levels in patients with advanced gastrointestinal malignancies. *Cancer* 1999; **86**: 1936–43.

**112** DE VITA F, ORDITURA M, GALIZIA G, *et al.* Serum interleukin-10 levels as a prognostic factor in advanced non-small cell lung cancer patients. *Chest* 2000; **117**: 365–73.

**113** DE VITA F, ORDITURA M, GALIZIA G, *et al.* Serum interleukin-10 is an independent prognostic factor in advanced solid tumors. *Oncol Rep* 2000; **7**: 357–61.

**114** CHAU GY, WU CW, LUI WY, *et al.* Serum interleukin-10 but not interleukin-6 is related to clinical outcome in patients with resectable hepatocellular carcinoma. *Ann Surg* 2000; **231**: 552–8.

**115** NEMUNAITIS J, FONG T, SHABE P, MARTINEAU D, ANDO D. Comparison of serum interleukin-10 (IL-10) levels between normal volunteers and patients with advanced melanoma. *Cancer Invest* 2001; **19**: 239–47.

116 LU ZY, ZHANG XG, RODRIGUEZ C, *et al.* Interleukin-10 is a proliferation factor but not a differentiation factor for human myeloma cells. *Blood* 1995; **85**: 2521–7.

117 GU ZJ, COSTES V, LU ZY, *et al.* Interleukin-10 is a growth factor for human myeloma cells by induction of an oncostatin M autocrine loop. *Blood* 1996; **88**: 3972–86.

118 FLUCKIGER AC, DURAND I, BANCHEREAU J. Interleukin 10 induces apoptotic cell death of B-chronic lymphocytic leukemia cells. *J Exp Med* 1994; **179**: 91–9.

119 YUE FY, DUMMER R, GEERTSEN R, HOFBAUER G, LAINE E, MANOLIO S, BURG G. Interleukin-10 is a growth factor for human melanoma cells and down-regulates HLA class-I, HLA class-II and ICAM-1 molecules. *Int J Cancer* 1997; **71**: 630–7.

120 MATSUDA M, SALAZAR F, PETERSSON M, *et al.* Interleukin 10 pretreatment protects target cells from tumor- and allospecific cytotoxic T cells and downregulates HLA class I expression. *J Exp Med* 1994; **180**: 2371–6.

121 SALAZAR-ONFRAY F, CHARO J, PETERSSON M, *et al.* Down-regulation of the expression and function of the transporter associated with antigen processing in murine tumor cell lines expressing IL-10. *J Immunol* 1997; **159**: 3195–202.

122 SALAZAR-ONFRAY F, PETERSSON M, FRANKSSON L, *et al.* IL-10 converts mouse lymphoma cells to a CTL-resistant, NK-sensitive phenotype with low but peptide-inducible MHC class I expression. *J Immunol* 1995; **154**: 6291–8.

123 HAGENBAUGH A, SHARMA S, DUBINETT SM, *et al.* Altered immune responses in interleukin 10 transgenic mice. *J Exp Med* 1997; **185**: 2101–10.

124 SHARMA S, STOLINA M, LIN Y, *et al.* T cell-derived IL-10 promotes lung cancer growth by suppressing both T cell and APC function. *J Immunol* 1999; **163**: 5020–8.

125 BRUSERUD O, TORE GJERTSEN B, TERJE BRUSTUGUN O, *et al.* Effects of interleukin 10 on blast cells derived from patients with acute myelogenous leukemia. *Leukemia* 1995; **9**: 1910–20.

126 GEISSLER K, OHLER L, FODINGER M, *et al.* Interleukin 10 inhibits growth and granulocyte/macrophage colony-stimulating factor production in chronic myelomonocytic leukemia cells. *J Exp Med* 1996; **184**: 1377–84.

127 KUNDU N, DORSEY R, JACKSON MJ, *et al.* Interleukin-10 gene transfer inhibits murine mammary tumors and elevates nitric oxide. *Int J Cancer* 1998; **76**: 713–9.

128 STEARNS ME, RHIM J, WANG M. Interleukin 10 (IL-10) inhibition of primary human prostate cell-induced angiogenesis: IL-10 stimulation of tissue inhibitor of metalloproteinase-1 and inhibition of matrix metalloproteinase (MMP)-2/MMP-9 secretion. *Clin Cancer Res* 1999; **5**: 189–96.

129 STEARNS ME, GARCIA FU, FUDGE K, RHIM J, WANG M. Role of interleukin 10 and transforming growth factor β1 in the angiogenesis and metastasis of human prostate primary tumor lines from orthotopic implants in severe combined immunodeficiency mice. *Clin Cancer Res* 1999; **5**: 711–20.

130 HUANG S, XIE K, BUCANA CD, ULLRICH SE, BAR-ELI M. Interleukin 10 suppresses tumor growth and metastasis of human melanoma cells: potential inhibition of angiogenesis. *Clin Cancer Res* 1996; **2**: 1969–79.

131 HUANG S, ULLRICH SE, BAR-ELI M. Regulation of tumor growth and metastasis by interleukin-10: the melanoma experience. *J Interferon Cytokine Res* 1999; **19**: 697–703.

132 GERARD CM, BRUYNS C, DELVAUX A, *et al.* Loss of tumorigenicity and increased immunogenicity induced by interleukin-10 gene transfer in B16 melanoma cells. *Hum Gene Ther* 1996; **7**: 23–31.

133 KUNDU N, FULTON AM. Interleukin-10 inhibits tumor metastasis, downregulates MHC class I, and enhances NK lysis. *Cell Immunol* 1997; **180**: 55–61.

134 LLORENTE L, RICHAUD-PATIN Y, GARCIA-PADILLA C, *et al.* Clinical and biologic effects of anti-interleukin-10 monoclonal antibody administration in systemic lupus erythematosus. *Arthritis Rheum* 2000; **43**: 1790–800.

**135** MOORE KW, DE WAAL MALEFYT R, COFF-
MAN RL, O'GARRA A. Interleukin-10
and the interleukin-10 receptor. Annu
Rev Immunol 2001; **19**:683–765.

**136** O'GARRA A, STAPLETON G, DHAR V, *et al.*
Production of cytokines by mouse B
cells: B lymphomas and normal B cells
produce interleukin 10. *Int Immunol*
1990; **2**: 821–32.

**137** MEHROTRA PT, DONNELLY RP, WONG S,
*et al.* Production of IL-10 by human natural killer cells stimulated with IL-2
and/or IL-12. *J Immunol* 1998; **160**:
2637–44.

**138** NAKAJIMA H, GLEICH GJ, KITA H. Constitutive production of IL-4 and IL-10
and stimulated production of IL-8 by
normal peripheral blood eosinophils.
*J Immunol* 1996; **156**: 4859–66.

**139** MARIETTA EV, CHEN Y, WEIS JH. Modulation of expression of the anti-inflammatory cytokines interleukin-13 and in-
terleukin-10 by interleukin-3. *Eur J Immunol* 1996; **26**: 49–56.

**140** RIVAS JM, ULLRICH SE. Systemic suppression of delayed-type hypersensitivity by supernatants from UV-irradiated
keratinocytes. An essential role for kera-
tinocyte-derived IL-10. *J Immunol* 1992;
**149**: 3865–71.

**141** MACATONIA SE, DOHERTY TM, KNIGHT
SC, O'GARRA A. DIFFERENTIAL EFFECT
OF IL-10 ON DENDRITIC CELL-INDUCED
T CELL PROLIFERATION AND IFN-γ PRO-
DUCTION. *J Immunol* 1993; **150**: 3755–
65.

**142** DE WAAL MALEFYT R, YSSEL H, DE
VRIES JE. Direct effects of IL-10 on subsets of human CD4$^+$ T cell clones and
resting T cells. Specific inhibition of IL-
2 production and proliferation. *J Immunol* 1993; **150**: 4754–65.

**143** TAGA K, MOSTOWSKI H, TOSATO G. Human interleukin-10 can directly inhibit
T-cell growth. *Blood* 1993; **81**: 2964–71.

**144** THOMPSON-SNIPES L, DHAR V, BOND
MW, MOSMANN TR, MOORE KW, RE-
NNICK DM. Interleukin 10: a novel stimulatory factor for mast cells and their
progenitors. *J Exp Med* 1991; **173**: 507–
10.

**Part 3**
**Strategies for Cancer Immunology**

# 9

# Dendritic Cells and Cancer: Prospects for Cancer Vaccination

DEREK N. J. HART, DAVID JACKSON and FRANK NESTLE

## 9.1
## Introduction

Effective therapeutic cancer vaccination is an old dream, now rekindled by modern advances in cell biology and immunology. Several key facts have inspired the current optimism for clinical immunotherapy trials. First, the realization that, by definition, every malignant cell must express at least one gene product in an abnormal fashion means that theoretically there is at least one tumor-associated antigen (TAA) (it may be an autoantigen) available as a target. Secondly, we now know that any cellular protein (membrane, cytoplasmic or nuclear) may be presented as a peptide, in the context of major histocompatibility complex (MHC) molecules, for recognition by the T lymphocyte receptor complex. Thirdly, whilst it is clear that the immune response has failed the cancer patient, it is also true that it has not suffered irreversible meltdown, i.e. deletion of tumor-reactive T lymphocytes. Finally, it is now recognized that dendritic cells (DCs) are the key cellular elements for initiating and directing immune responses. As DC biology appears to be abnormal in cancer patients, the simplest hypothesis of the day is to use activated DCs to present relevant TAAs to the patient's immune system and thus generate an effective therapeutic response. This chapter will review the physiology of DC biology in the cancer patient, DC preparations and clinical trial results, whilst predicting areas requiring attention in order to optimize DC cancer vaccination for future patient benefit.

## 9.2
## DC Properties

DCs originate from $CD34^+$ hematopoietic stem cells, circulate in peripheral blood and are found in virtually all tissues of the body. In peripheral blood, DCs are a morphologically heterogeneous cell population, including DCs with membrane processes ("myeloid DC") and DCs with plasmacytoid morphology ("plasmacytoid monocytes", "plasmacytoid T lymphocyte", "lymphoid DCs") [1, 2]. In the skin, DCs are present as epidermal Langerhans cells (LCs) with their characteristic Birbeck granules [3] and dermal DCs [4, 5], which have a subtly different morphology and phenotype. In secondary lymphoid tissues they are present as interdigitating DCs with prominent membrane processes in the T cell area and as "plasmacytoid monocytes" around high endothelial venules (HEVs) [6]. Monocytes may also differentiate directly into DC-like cells in sites of inflammation [7]. Whilst there is some uncertainty about the identity of the different DC populations and their differentiation, it is clear that a variety of growth factors and cytokines drive DC development [8]. Furthermore, chemokines direct their migration [9] and other soluble compounds influence their function.

Blood DCs are commonly defined as lineage negative (Lin⁻), MHC class II positive (MHC-II⁺) cells, lacking the CD14 (monocyte), CD3 (T cell), CD19 (B cell) and CD56 [natural killer (NK) cell] lineage markers, but expressing MHC class II molecules at high density, on their surface. They express various adhesion molecules including CD11a (LFA-1), CD58 (LFA-3), CD54 (ICAM-1), CD50 (ICAM-3), CD102 (ICAM-2) and CD62L (L-selectin) [1, 10]. Co-stimulatory molecules such as CD80, CD86 and CD40 are expressed at low levels on steady-state DCs [11]. Subsets of DCs express Fcγ receptor (CD16, CD32 and CD64), complement receptors CD11c (CR4), CD11b (CR3) and CD88 (CR5a), and lectin receptors [12, 13]. Blood DCs express high levels of the skin homing molecule, cutaneous leukocyte antigen (CLA) [14] and L-selectin [1,6]. Certain subsets of DC precursors circulating in the blood can express CD2, CD14 and CD34 initially, but expression of these antigens is lost with their differentiation into DCs [7, 15–17].

The human DC population is currently subdivided into two broad subsets based on the reciprocal expression of the CD11c and CD123 [interleukin (IL)-3 receptor] markers. Myeloid CD11c⁺ DCs express myeloid markers (CD33 and CD13), whilst the "lymphoid" CD123⁺ DCs lack myeloid markers and express more CD4 [1, 18, 19]. Alternatively, the DC population can be subdivided into two subsets based on the expression of immunoglobulin-like transcript (ILT) molecules. The ILT3⁺/1⁺ subset corresponds in the main to the CD11c⁺ DCs, whilst the ILT3⁺/ILT1⁺ subset corresponds predominantly to the CD123⁺ DCs [6], but further subtleties in these DC subpopulations, particularly in CD11c⁺ DCs are emerging ([20] and MacDonald *et al.*, submitted.

Surveillance DCs possess the unique ability to capture, process and present antigen as peptide–MHC complexes to naive T cells and to deliver the co-stimulatory signals necessary for T cell activation. DCs take up antigen in peripheral non-lymphoid tissues such as skin or mucosa by pinocytosis, through the CD206 (macrophage mannose receptor), and potentially through other lectin-like antigen uptake receptors such as CD205 [21, 22], perhaps CD209 (DC-SIGN receptor) [23] and CD207 (Langerin) [24]. Other molecular candidates for antigen uptake "receptors" such as the Toll-like receptors (TLRs) are now being investigated as receptors for DNA and other microorganism-derived molecules [25].

Natural sources of antigen for DC presentation can include viral or bacterial proteins [26, 27], apoptotic/necrotic cells [28] or exosomes [29]. DCs process antigen via the so-called classical pathways: the endogenous antigens via the proteasome into the MHC class I compartment and exogenous antigens via endocytic lysosomes into the

MHC class II compartment [30]. DCs also use alternative pathways of antigen processing and can route exogenous antigen into the MHC class I pathway, through a mechanism known as cross-priming [31]. They may utilize molecules such as heat shock proteins (e. g. hsp96) to deliver antigenic chaperoned peptides through CD91 into MHC class I compartments [32, 33]. An alternative use of the term cross-priming refers to the possibility that other cells, e. g. macrophages or DCs themselves, may transfer antigen, perhaps in a modified form, to DCs.

In addition to encountering antigen, DCs are thought to require an antigen-independent "danger" signal to induce a characteristic process of terminal differentiation often referred to as "maturation". These include signals from cytokines, bacteria [34, 35]s viruses [36], apoptotic or necrotic cells [28, 37, 38]. Depending on the differentiation/activating stimulus, DCs may respond with a variety of important changes. Examples include increased expression of MHC class II molecules and the co-stimulatory CD80 and CD86 molecules [11]; generation of a new chemokine receptor repertoire, especially CCR7 [39, 40]; and the induction of molecules like CD40 and the tumor necrosis factor (TNF)-related activation-induced cytokine receptor (TRANCE-R) essential for DC survival and stimulation [41, 42]. The down-regulation of E-cadherin on LCs may reduce their adhesion to other epithelial cells [43]. DC migration requires key intracellular signaling events (e. g. relB expression) and these processes are initiated at the site of antigen exposure [44]. Functional differentiation/maturation coincidences with the down-regulation of antigen-uptake and -processing capabilities, and up-regulation of antigen-presenting function [45].

Upon receiving appropriate signals, the surveillance, DCs migrate from the tissues into the afferent lymphatics. Key mediators, i. e. the so-called "danger" signals mentioned above, initiate these events, but there also appears to be a substantial basal rate of DC trafficking. The differentiating/activated DCs migrate into the T cell-rich paracortex of the draining lymph nodes, guided by chemokines MIP-3P and SLC [46, 47]. Again, recent data suggests that a complex set of DC subpopulations is present in lymph node/tonsil, including a population of less-activated DCs, which might play a role in peripheral tolerance [48].

Within the secondary lymphoid tissues, two key events occur with regard to an exogenous antigen-driven immune response. Firstly, activated $CD4^+$ T lymphocytes can further mature DC through CD40–CD40 ligand (CD40L) interactions and this provides a survival signal to the DCs [41]. Secondly, mature DCs secrete chemokines such as DC-CKI, MDC, IL-8 and RANTES that attract naive and memory T and B lymphocytes, respectively [49–51]. Mature DCs also secret cytokines including IL-7 [52] and IL-12 [53], which contribute to their antigen-presenting function. IL-7 can induce CD4 and CD8 T and B lymphocyte proliferation and B lymphocyte differentiation [54]. IL-12 biases T helper responses toward a $T_h1$ effector immune response [55]. In secondary lymphoid tissues, a stimulatory cytokine/chemokine milieu produced by mature DCs, combined with the presentation of peptide/MHC complexes and expression of co-stimulatory molecules, contributes to generation of potent antigen specific immune responses [56].

The role of the "lymphoid" $CD123^+$ DC in these processes is unclear. These cells appear to migrate from the blood via the HEVs into the T cell areas in secondary lymphoid tissue. They produce interferon (IFN)-α in these locations and are thought to contribute to the innate immune response [6]. Recent data suggesting that they can be recruited to inflammatory sites [57] and can present antigen for primary T lymphocyte responses (Vuckovic *et al.*, in preparation) suggests an even more complex set of cellular interactions than formally thought is possible within responding secondary lymphoid tissues.

Preliminary evidence also exists for the ability of DCs to interact directly with NK cells and activate them [58]. DCs and NK cells might interact at a peripheral site (e.g. tumor site), where they can be recruited through chemokines. Their activity may result in tumor lysis, releasing apoptotic or necrotic bodies that will be taken up, transported and presented by DCs to T lymphocytes. Cross-talk between DCs and NK cells may serve as another mechanism through which DCs can elicit and enhance an effector immune responses, and link the innate and adaptive immune responses.

## 9.3
## DC in Human Cancer

If the DCs are to mount a protective response to an early cancer, the DCs must sense "danger", react appropriately and present relevant TAAs to the immune system. This has now been studied in several human cancers. Immunohistological analysis of renal cell carcinoma suggested that DCs were present in normal numbers in the malignant tissue and no evidence of increased activation was found [59]. Similar findings were made in prostate cancer [60], and by us [61] and others [62] in breast cancer. Bladder cancers likewise had normal numbers of DC1a⁻ DCs present, consistent with their superficial epithelial location [63]. It proved possible to isolate the DCs from renal cell carcinoma and basal cell carcinoma [64], and these cells appeared to have low stimulatory capacity. Notably, the DCs present in draining lymph nodes likewise had apparently reduced allostimulatory capacity [65].

These findings may be integrated with a more extensive body of literature using S100 staining to identify DC in human tumors, notably head and neck as well as gastrointestinal tumors [66, 67]. In these studies, a correlation between S100 staining and positive prognosis has been a common finding. A correlation between S100 staining and the subset of activated DCs identified by the CMRF-44 mAb [68] suggests that a good prognosis relates to the number of DC which are activated in the tumor environment – exactly as predicted.

Reduced blood DC counts in cancer patients have been described [69]; however, this finding may vary with the stage of disease as our studies suggest (Ho *et al.*, in preparation). DC counts are preserved in patients with stage I and II breast cancer. Likewise, blood DC counts in patients with multiple myeloma appear to be relatively preserved but systemic defects in the ability of the DC to up-regulate co-stimulator molecules were noted [70]. A subset of Lin⁻ HLA-DR⁻ cells present in the blood of cancer patients identified as immature myeloid cells has also been suggested to inhibit blood DC function [71].

Abnormalities in monocyte function have been described in cancer. Consistent with this, some investigators [72–75] have reported difficulties in generating [76] monocyte-derived DCs (Mo-DCs) in cancer patients, whereas others have not [73]. Cancers may also influence DC production at an even earlier level and vascular endothelial growth factor (VEGF) has been suggested to suppress DC production in the bone marrow [77].

Thus, the data to date suggests that cancers fail to activate DCs sufficiently and, furthermore, that they liberate a variety of mediators, which compromise DC function. Thus, there appears to be a clear defect in the immune response to cancer, which is an opportunity to be tested for remedial action.

## 9.4
## Blood DC Counts and DC Mobilization

The ability to count DCs in the blood and to monitor them in the tissues is fundamental to studying DC biology in cancer. It is also a pre-requisite to plan DC mobilization and therapeutic procedures. Fortunately, modern flow cytometry techniques allow this relatively rare cell to be tracked in the blood [78, 79]. Most laboratories prepare human blood DC using a mixture of monoclonal antibodies (mAbs) to lineage antigens (the choice is critical) and then a variety of immunoselection procedures to remove these cells prior to further analysis or use them in functional assays. How the cells are prepared and just what subsets of blood DCs are present is being redefined at present as a result of recent studies ([20] and MacDonald et al., submitted). Whilst it is still convenient to describe a $CD11c^+$ $(CD123^{lo})$ myeloid subset and $CD11c^-$ $CD123^{hi}$ lymphoid subset, it is clear that other (perhaps even functionally distinct) myeloid subsets can be defined (MacDonald et al., submitted). Laboratories, used to counting rare cell populations, are now starting to analyze blood DCs in whole blood or in peripheral blood mononuclear cell (PBMC) populations.

Blood DCs represent (depending on the phenotypic definition) 0.5–1.5% of PBMCs. A range of 0.15–0.70% or $3–17 \times 10^6$ DC/l was obtained using the mAb CMRF-44 [79]. Studies on patients undergoing surgery showed an acute rise in absolute blood DC counts, which peaked before monocytes [80]. Interestingly, blood DC counts are not increased in patients with chronic myelomonocytic leukemia [81].

Blood DC counts have been studied following hematopoietic stem cell mobilization for autologous and allogeneic stem cell transplants [79]. In normals, granulocyte colony stimulating cell (G-CSF) mobilization appears to increase $CD123^+$ DC counts selectively over the CD11c population [82]. This effect is less obvious in cyclophosphamide/G-CSF mobilized patients with multiple myeloma and low-grade non-Hodgkin's lymphoma (NHL) (Vuckovic et al., submitted) and patients who have received chronic myelosuppressive chemotherapy, patients may have lower numbers of circulating DCs. Flt-3 ligand (Flt-3L) and Flt-3L/G-CSF have now been used to mobilize blood DCs. Myeloid DCs counts increase approximately 40-fold with a 10-fold increase in the lymphoid subset in normal individuals [83] and increases are reported in cancer patients [84, 85]. Nonetheless, DCs may mobilize less effectively with Flt-3L [85] and Flt-3L/G-CSF (D Ashley personal communication) in cancer patients.

Further studies in cancer patients are clearly necessary to establish what DC populations are available to be harvested for immunotherapy. Studies in multiple myeloma and low-grade NHL suggest sufficient numbers of blood DCs for immunotherapy may be available without mobilization (Vuckovic *et al.*, submitted).

## 9.5
## DC Preparations for Immunotherapy

In vivo targeting of DCs for immunotherapy has yet to be explored, but there have been attempts to mobilize DCs into tumors or the skin for vaccination purposes using granulocyte macrophage colony stimulating factor (GM-CSF)/IL-4 [86] or GM-CSF/TNF-$\alpha$ [87]. Flt-3L proved efficacious in generating anticancer responses in mice, perhaps as a result of NK activation, but does not seem to achieve a clinical effect on its own apart from DC mobilization. Thus, most investigators take the approach of removing DCs from the patient and loading them with TAAs, whilst activating them in the test tube. The down side to this, of course, is that the complexity of normal DC function may be compromised in this process. In broad terms, at least three types of DCs preparations are being tested for immunotherapy as described below.

The availability of CD34$^+$ mobilized and immunoselected stem cells has encouraged a few groups to differentiate DCs from these for therapeutic purposes [88–90]. Whilst some cell expansion occurs and a range of different growth factor/cytokine cocktails have been reported to produce reasonable yields of DCs, it seems a biologically difficult process to control and the end result may be something akin to Mo-DCs preparations. Others have used different protocols and carefully characterized two potential DCs populations – CD1a$^{hi}$ and CD1a$^{lo}$ [91].

The majority of attention has focused on Mo-DCs using multiple myeloma variations of the original protocol described by Sallusto and Lanzavecchia [45, 92, 93]. GM-CSF and IL-4 are used routinely in varying concentrations to develop a so-called "immature" Mo-DCs after 5–7 days *in vitro* culture. These have been exposed to antigen and then injected using the argument that a natural maturation process would take place *in vivo*. Another argument to justify this approach is that the cells might retain normal migratory capacity and indeed a small proportion do [94, 95]. GM-CSF/IL-4-generated Mo-DCs are not stable. Upon cytokine removal the re-adhere, convert to macrophages and lose allostimulatory function. Adding macrophage colony stimulating factor (M-CSF) hastens CD14 re-expression and the proportion of adherent spindle-shaped macrophages *in vitro* [96]. Immature Mo-DCs are also sensitive to the effects of IL–10 [97]. The clinical imperative has bypassed some basic studies. Recent data [98] would suggest that the differentiated Mo-DC is an effective antigen-presenting cell (APC) but suggests caution in the use of the undifferentiated Mo-DC: in two patients tested, reduced specific immune responses were documented [99]. A semimature variant of Mo-DCs with higher expression of co-stimulatory molecules is obtained in the presence of fetal calf serum. An alternative approach has been to further mature these cells using monocyte-derived conditioning medium or TNF-α [100]. Other differentiating or "maturing" agents include a cocktail of TNF-α, IL-1β, IL-6 and prostaglandin E$_2$ [101], and calcium ionophores [102]. These more-differentiated Mo-DCs have greater stimulatory activity in cellular assays *in vitro* and also appear to be active *in vivo*, but comparative migration data with blood DCs is not available. At a practical level how the preparations are made is absolutely critical, e.g. the use of PBMCs or CD14-selected monocytes, the presence of serum, etc. The prolonged culture period and numerous components involved make the good manufacturing practice (GMP) quality requirements a serious exercise. Several commercial companies are now providing this facility.

The third possible cell preparation is to use one or more of the natural blood DC population(s) circulating in a patient [103–105]. These might be postulated to be in the most appropriate stage of the DC "life cycle" for use (Fig. 9.1). Blood DCs were used for the first clinical DC therapeutic trial, which used low-grade NHL patients [106].

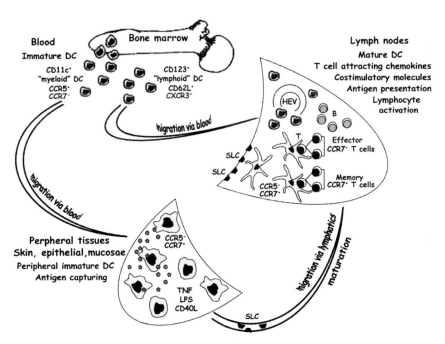

**Fig. 9.1** The DC Life Cycle. Hematopoietic stem cells in bone marrow produce DCs into the blood stream. Blood myeloid DCs and lymphoid DCs use adhesion molecules and chemokine receptors (CD62L, CXCR3 and CCR5) to traffic to peripheral tissues (CD11c$^+$ myeloid) or directly to lymph nodes (DC123$^+$ lymphoid) via HEVs. In peripheral tissues immature myeloid DCs which encounter antigens and accompany microbial products (TNF and lipopolysaccharide) and signals from activated T cells (CD40L) start to differentiate. These DCs move toward lymphatics using chemokine receptors (CCR7), whose ligand SLC, is found both in lymphatic endothelium and in secondary lymphoid tissue. In the lymph node mature DCs produce chemokines, which attract naive and activated T cells. Complex interactions with the local microenvironment (perhaps including lymphoid DCs) increase co-stimulatory molecules, optimize antigen presentation, and induce further lymphocyte activation and the production of effector and memory T lymphocytes. DCs also contribute to B lymphocyte activation and antibody production. (see color plates page XXVI)

Blood DCs may be obtained as part of a mononuclear cell preparation and then isolated via a range of techniques. Gradient techniques have been developed commercially [107]. Given the potential for other cell populations to contribute confounding regulatory influences, a relatively pure DC population seems advisable in the longer term. Attempts to use mAb-based selection of DC have therefore been initiated in at least two or three laboratories. Using the CMRF-44 [108] or CMRF-56 mAb it appears that reasonable numbers of relatively pure DCs can be obtained (Lopez *et al.*, submitted). Of course, this method of selection allows for DC subset selection, and this might allow both stimulatory and regulatory DC preparations to be obtained. Despite the similarities, there are notable differences between Mo-DCs and myeloid CD11c$^+$ DCs. Differences include expression of presumed regulatory Ig family molecules (Clark *et al.*, in preparation) and cell surface lectins, e.g. CD205, CD206 and CD209 [20]. Functional data [109] suggests that myeloid blood CD11c$^+$ are capable of inducing a greater percentage of effector T lymphocytes *in vitro* and that these DC preparations should be assessed independently.

Whilst there are established methods for purifying stem cells using CD34 or CD133 reagents for antibody-based cell selection, this, plus the mobilization, are significant preliminary steps before the *in vitro* culture and generation of DCs. One of the attractive features of Mo-DCs to investigators is that venesection may provide enough cells [101]; however, there is an increasing trend to use apheresis procedures to obtain larger number of mononuclear cells for the *in vitro* cultures [76]. Apheresis will certainly be essential if blood DCs are to be used but recent data suggests that they "mobilize" during the procedure [110] and that sufficient numbers will be available even without mobilization in cancer patients (Vuckovic *et al.*, submitted). Quality control of these preparations will become a big issue as raised elsewhere [111].

## 9.6
## Loading DC with Antigens

Having chosen the DC preparation for immunotherapy, the next challenge is to optimize the conditions for antigen loading. The state of Mo-DC maturation, the media, and the presence and type of serum/protein additives all make a difference [76, 101]. However, perhaps one of the more important variables is the time of incubation – this not only influences antigen loading, but may also determine the type of immune responses initiated. These variables are also important for blood DC preparations [104].

The choice of methodology for providing the antigen is critical. The field began with irradiated tumor cells or tumor cell lysates or partial peptide preparations. These were appropriate to initiate investigations, but they are difficult to standardize and may contain critical DC-activating or -modulating capacity, e.g. heat shock proteins, that needs better defining. Now the cell biology revolution has given us the opportunity to consider many different potential forms of TAAs.

TAA peptides, which bind class I and class II, are now readily predicted and validated. They are easy to manufacture and produce under GMP conditions. They can be linked to include multiple (including helper and cytotoxic) epitopes and different structures investigated [112] to optimize delivery. Mouse models validate the role of DCs in delivering effective antitumor responses (reviewed in [66]). Comparative data in a mouse model suggests DC peptide administration is more effective than naked DNA vaccination [113].

An alternative, which bypasses the need to consider HLA-restricting elements, is to use recombinant proteins – these can of course be engineered if necessary to remove any potentially harmful epitopes. Cost is a consideration, but the quantities required may be relatively small. Engineering targeting components as described for the GM-CSF prostatic acid phosphatase fusion protein may be very effective [107].

New strategies have also seen a revival of the whole-cell vaccine approach in the form of pulsing DC with apoptotic bodies. Necrotic material from tumors may be relevant as it is likely that DC have sophisticated mechanisms to distinguish necrosis from apoptosis, theoretically, with different outcomes. DC/tumor cell hybrids are also being explored. The injection of DC/tumors hybrids in mice generated cure of advanced metastatic disease [114]. Tumor fusions have now been generated with human cells and hybrids produced in the presence of polyethylene glycol (PEG) yielded measurable specific responses against breast cancer cells [115, 116]. Moreover, striking clinical responses were reported with the use of electroporated hybrid preparations [117]. Further detailed studies on the quality of the cells injected and the nature of the immune response generated are eagerly anticipated. A number of clinical trials using both allogeneic and autologous DC are currently underway in various centers and the initial results should emerge soon (P. Walden, personal communication).

Recombinant viruses DNA or RNA constructs may be used to deliver polytopes (multiple peptide epitopes) or recombinant protein to DCs. This technique has been very effective in mouse models. It is also capable of eliciting human cytotoxic T lymphocyte (CTL)-specific responses *in vitro* [118–120]. Electroporated RNA may be superior to DNA plasmid expression of RNA [121]. Clinical trials in patients with prostate cancer using this technique are underway. Retrovirus vectors have been used to deliver both class I and II epitopes [122]. Adeno [123] and canarypox [124] viruses known to replicate poorly in humans have also been used.

Much excitement has been engendered by the use of RNA to deliver specific TAAs and also total tumor RNA [118, 125]. Now alternatives are being considered including delivering the antigens via DC surface antigen receptors [21] and by targeting proteins using intracellular locations signals such as HIV tat [126].

## 9.7
### Dose Delivery and Vaccination Schedule

Dose-finding studies in DC vaccination has been difficult in the past because of questionable endpoints. An endpoint such as induction of an immune response is not necessarily correlated with clinical response. A potential but unsatisfactory way is to titrate DC numbers injected against T cell response to a strong test immunogen by measuring HLA/peptide tetramer (which bind specific T cell receptors) responses or possibly delayed-type hypersensitivity (DTH) reactions *in vivo*. Empirical dosing of DCs and schedules suggest a minimal cell number is required, currently accepted as approximately $10^6$, but 10-fold less may suffice. The few dose-escalation studies have not shown a clear cell dose effect [127], although there are suggestions that this is a relevant variable [72].

The issue is further complicated by the choice of the DC injection site. One million DCs injected into a lymph node will produce a different outcome to the same number of DCs injected intradermally (i.d.) or intravenously (i.v.). Currently available migration studies [94, 128] predict that about 1% of Mo-DCs injected into the skin will reach a draining lymph node. Rapid migration of CD34$^+$ DCs into lymph nodes occurred following intralymphatic injection but DC administered i.v. located in lung and liver and ultimately the spleen but not lymph nodes [129]. The consensus from animal data is that of the conventional parenteral administrations; delivery via the skin [i.d. rather than subcutaneous (s.c.)] is preferable to i.v. administration [130, 131]. The clinical data accrued to date now needs a formal comparison to direct the next generation of trials. Migration is likely to differ accordingly to the type of DC preparation, as they have different chemokine receptors and adhesion-mediating properties. Intranodal injection under ultrasound guidance was used in the first melanoma vaccination study [132]. A recent paper [133] compared T lymphocyte and antibody responses to blood DCs loaded with recombinant mouse prostatic and phosphatase injected i.v., i.d. or into cannulated lymphatics. Only the latter two routes resulted in T lymphocyte IFN-γ production (T proliferation occurred in each) and the i.v. route resulted in more antibody responses.

Injection schedules to date are derived from experiences in animal models and human vaccination studies in infectious diseases. Weekly injections with monthly boosting or monthly injection schedules are currently being performed. Again, data optimizing these is urgently required given suggestions that frequent administration may be counter-productive [131]. Given DC are critical for priming responses, it may be that alternative vehicles for revaccinating may be possible, improving the feasibility of the procedure.

The cautionary data suggesting that DCs in certain forms may in certain circumstances have a negative influence on anti-tumor responses [99, 134] will need to be heeded.

## 9.8
### Phase I/II Clinical Trials

A summary is provided in Tab. 9.1. The initial clinical trials involving four patients in relapsed low-grade NHL fortunately produced encouraging results without side effects [106]. The most encouraging feature was the first demonstration that patients could be immunized to generate T lymphocyte responses to the idiotype protein antigen. The excellent results in low-grade NHL patients with minimal residual disease (MRD) using GM-GSF and keyhole limpet hemocyanin (KLH)-conjugated idiotype indicate the potential in this disease [135]. Longer-term follow-up has shown a

**Tab. 9.1** Reports on the use of DC for cancer immunotherapy

| Type of cancer | Antigen | Center | DC type | Route of immuni- zation | Number of individuals immunized | Response reported | Reference |
|---|---|---|---|---|---|---|---|
| NHL | idiotype | Standford | Im Mo | i.v. > s.c. | 4 | 1 CR, 1 PR; antigen-specific lymphocyte proliferation | 106 |
| Multiple myeloma | idiotype protein | Cardiff | Im Mo | i.v. | 1 | antigen-specific lymphocyte prolif- eration response, antibodies | 137 |
| Multiple myeloma | idiotype protein + KLH | Stanford | blood | i.v. | 12 | 11/12 KLH, 2/12 idiotype-specific lymphocyte proliferation (CR) | 139 |
| Multiple myeloma (follow-up) | idiotype protein + KLH | Stanford | blood | i.v. | 26 | 24/26 KLH, 4/26 idiotype-specific lymphocyte proliferation (CR) | 140 |
| Multiple myeloma | idiotype protein + KLH | Cardiff | Im Mo | i.v. | 6 | Increase CTL proliferation in 3/6; antibodies; idiotype proliferation; IFN-$\gamma$ ELISA | 174 |
| Chronic myeloid leukemia | leukemic DC (Ph1$^+$) | Ninomaru | Ma Mo | i.v. | 1 | Ph1-specific CTL | 161 |
| Melanoma | Mart-1, gp100 peptides | Bethesda | Im Mo | i.v. | 10 | increased CTL 1/5, 1 PR; metastasis regression | 76 |
| Melanoma | Melan-A, gp100 | Freiburg | CD34$^+$ | i.v. | 14 | peptide DTH, met regression, vitiligo | 89 |
| Melanoma | Melan-A, tyrosinase, MAGE3 + influenza MP | Dallas | CD34$^+$ | i.d. | 18 | antigen-specific ELISPOT 16/18; met regression; delayed progression | 91 |
| Melanoma | lysate/pep- tide mix + KLH | Zürich | Im Mo | i.n. | 16 | DTH to peptide and KLH, 2 CR, 3 PR, met regres- sion | 132 |
| Melanoma | MAGE A1/ A3 peptide | Brussels | Im Mo | i.v. > s.c. | 24 | increase in peptide- specific CTL 14/24 | 142 |
| Melanoma | tyrosinase, gp100 peptides | Los Angeles | Im Mo | i.v. | 16 | 1 CR, 2 SD, 5/16 IFN-$\gamma$ ELISA response | 143 |
| Melanoma | Melan-A or MAGE-1 tyrosinase | Mainz | Im Mo versus Ma Mo | i.n. | 11 | 3 PR, 2 SD of 8 evaluable 5/7 CTL Ma Mo; 1/7 CTL Im Mo | 144 |

**Tab. 9.1** (continued)

| Type of cancer | Antigen | Center | DC type | Route of immuni-zation | Number of individuals immunized | Response reported | Reference |
|---|---|---|---|---|---|---|---|
| Melanoma | MAGE-3A1, HLA-A1 peptide | Erlangen | Ma Mo | s.c., i.d. > i.v. | 11 | Peptide-specific CTL 6/11, metastasis regression 6/11 | 176 |
| Melanoma | MAGE-3A1, HLA-A2 peptide | Erlangen | Ma Mo | s.c., i.d. > i.v. | 8 | peptide-specific CTL 8/8 | 177 |
| Melanoma | tumor/allo peripheral blood mononuclear cell hybrid | Berlin | Activated peripheral blood mononuclear cells | s.c. | 16 | 1 CR, 1 PR, 5 SD | 178 |
| Breast/ovarian | Her2/neu, MUC-1 peptides | Tübingen | Ma Mo | s.c. | 10 | 5/10 CTL | 159 |
| Breast | tumor lysate | Osaka | Mo | i.n. | 1 | metastasis regression | 160 |
| Prostate | fusion protein GM-CSF + PAP | Seattle | blood | i.v. | 31 | lymphocyte proliferation to GM-CSF and PAP | 72 |
| Prostate | PSMA P1 and P2 peptides | Seattle | Im Mo | i.v. | 51 | 7 PR, peptide-specific CTL | 148 |
| Prostate | PMSA P1 and P2 peptides | Seattle | Im Mo | i.v. | 37 | 1 CR, 10 PR | 149 |
| Prostate (follow-up) | PMSA P1 and P2 peptides | Seattle | Im Mo | i.v. | 37 | DTH and cytokine production relates to clinical response | 151 |
| Prostate | fusion protein GM-CSF + PAP | Rochester | blood | i.v. | 13 | Peptide-specific lymphocyte proliferation to T antibody PAP in 20/31 (delayed disease pro-gression) | 157 |
| Renal cell carcinoma | tumor/allo DC hybrid | Göttingen | Ma Mo | i.v. | 17 | 4 CR, metastasis regression, 1 mass reduction >0% | 117 |
| Renal cell carcinoma | cell lysate + KLH | Innsbruck | Ma Mo | i.v. | 4 | 1 PR; KLH IFN-γ responses | 145 |

**Tab. 9.1**  (continued)

| Type of cancer | Antigen | Center | DC type | Route of immuni-zation | Number of individuals immunized | Response reported | Reference |
|---|---|---|---|---|---|---|---|
| Renal cell carcinoma | cell lysate + KLH | Innsbruck | Ma Mo | i.v. | 12 | renal cell carcinoma, normal kidney and KLH proliferation | 146 |
| Metastatic CEA expressing | CAP-1 peptide/ RNA | Durham | Im Mo | i.v. | 17 | CEA-specific CTL equal response in peptide and RNA cohorts | 118 |
| Metastatic CEA expressing | CAP-1 peptide | Durham | Im Mo | i.v. | 21 | 1 SD | 158 |
| Pancreas | tumor lysate + KLH | Dusseldorf | Ma Mo | s.c. | 1 | vaccine DTH, lymphocyte prolif-eration, decreased marker; metastasis regression | 179 |
| Gastro-intestinal | MAGE peptide | Kyushu | Im Mo | i.v. | 12 | peptide-specific CTL 4/8; reduced tumor marker 7/12 | 180 |
| Glioma | Acid-eluted peptide | Los Angeles | Im Mo | s.c. | 7 | CTL infiltrate in tumor; prolonged survival | 163 |
| Glioma | tumor/auto DC fusion | Tokyo | Ma Mo | i.d. | 8 | 2 PR | 164 |
| Solid tumors (pediatric) | tumor lysate + KLH | Ann Arbor | Im Mo | i.d. | 8 | tumor regression | 162 |

CAE: carcinoembrionic antigen; CAP: peptide fragment of CAE; Ph1: Philadelphia chromosome; i.n.: intranodal; Im: Immature; Ma: mature; Mo: Mo-DC; SD: stable disease.

variable outcome, but it is now recognized that on going vaccination may be necessary to maintain immunity.

Multiple myeloma has also attracted attention. Again there is data to suggest patients can mount T-mediated anti-idiotype responses [136]. *In vitro* studies confirm the ability of autologous Mo-DCs to generate such responses [137, 138] and the one clinical study suggested that DCs generated anti-idiotype responses after autologous stem cell transplantation [139]. Multiple myeloma patients may be more immuno-suppressed and idiotype may be a weak TAA, but as all these studies have employed the i.v. route of immunization this may account for the relatively low frequency of anti-idiotype responses (four of 26 versus 24 of 26 KLH control in [140]). Interestingly, three-quarters of responders in the later study were in complete disease remission. Another study performed in the post-transplant setting [107] remains to be fully reported; however, it too suggests responses may occur in the MRD setting after autologous stem cell transplant for multiple myeloma. A remarkable nine out of 18 clinical responses [five complete responses (CRs) and four partial responses (PRs)] were seen in this context (F. H. Valone, personal communication)

It is perhaps in melanoma that greatest interest was aroused and there are a plethora of trials in progress. Few have been formally reported, but the follow-up from the first description of the use of Mo-DCs and melanoma peptides/tumor lysates [132] shows two CRs and three PRs in 21 patients with metastatic disease, indicating an ongoing control of disease in the proportion of patients who responded with a mean survival of over 47 months in responder patients. This protocol induced peptide-specific T cell responses in 10 out of 10 HLA-A2 patients. A second trial [141] used Mo-DCs matured in monocyte-conditioned medium s.c. and i.d. induced specific CTL expansion in eight out of 11 HLA/A1 patients, but notably these responses declined after further i.v. injections. Regression of metastases occurred in six out of 11 patients. Notably, the same group has reported poor clinical results (no regressions in eight evaluable patients) in a third study involving HLA-A2 individuals, but using the same MAGE-3 antigen. Curiously, the later patient group had active melanoma peptide-specific IFN-γ effector CD8$^+$ T cells (confirmatory cytotoxic studies were not performed) present and received DCs by the possibly more optimal s.c. protocol.

However, a fourth published study [76] using immature Mo-DCs administered i.d. produced poor cytotoxic responses and had only one partial clinical response in seven patients evaluated. A protocol which used CD34$^+$-derived DCs administered s.c. enhanced immunity in at least one assay (ELISPOT or proliferation) in 16 of 18 patients – DTH responses were independent of blood assay results [91]. During a 10-week evaluation, four patients with multiple lesions experience regression at one or more disease sites and three with limited disease cleared evidence of the disease. In broad terms, immunological responses predicted for disease response. Another trial made use of CD34$^+$-derived DCs but gave them i.v. – the monitoring of immunological responses was limited, but these patients had a lesser clinical response, again suggesting that perhaps the i.v. route is less effective [89].

A consensus (including unpublished studies) is emerging despite the different approaches that in advanced melanoma some 20–30% of patients have a significant clinical response. The use of immature Mo-DCs may be associated with a lesser outcome [89, 142] in melanoma unless their preparation and antigen loading involves activation, as may have occurred in the first trial. Immunological tests may predict for the group with some clinical response [143]. A formal comparison of immature versus mature Mo-DCs used different DCs preparations and antigens in the same patients [144]; it was not possible to allocate the positive clinical outcomes to a particular preparation although, as commented earlier, differences in T cell responses were seen.

Other most encouraging results have been obtained in renal cell carcinoma [145–147]. The use of allogeneic tumor cell–DC hybrids was pioneered in this area [117] – the excellent results are being investigated further. Again, it is perhaps relevant that this is a disease in which immune responses are known to occur, e.g. following IL-2/LAK therapy.

There has been a large cohort of prostate cancer patients studied by two groups [72, 148–157], perhaps in part because prostate organ-specific antigens [e.g. prostate-specific membrane antigen (PSMA) and prostatic acid phosphatase (PAP)] can also be considered as TAAs. Mo-DCs used in conjunction with PSMA peptides have been used in a phase II trial, which described one CR and 10 PRs amongst 37 patients with presumed local recurrence [149]. There was a strong association between clinical responders and pre-existing immune competence [151]. A protocol which uses blood DCs and the novel DC-activating GM-CSF–PAP compound has been show to generate T cell responses to PAP [157] and decreases in PSA levels as a tumor marker stimulated a phase III study of patients with progressive metastatic disease.

Other cancers are also being addressed. Immune responses have resulted following DC vaccination with carcinoembryonic antigen as RNA [118] or peptide [158]. Peptide-pulsed DCs have now been reported to produce cytotoxic responses in breast and ovarian cancer patients [159], and a single case report describes a clinical response in breast cancer [160]. A single chronic myeloid leukemia patient produced CTLs after DC vaccination [161]. DC vaccination with tumor lysates showed some benefits in children with fibrosacroma [162].

Results in renal cell carcinoma appear to be promising, but perhaps more unexpected have been the responses noted in patients with brain tumors [161, 163, 165]. However, as gliomas break the classic blood–brain barrier, the ability to deliver effector T lymphocytes to this site is probably unimpaired.

What lessons have been learnt! As stated earlier, extensive immunological monitoring to establish the surrogate markers is now mandatory. It appears that the immunosuppressed patient with advanced cancer is not a good candidate for immunotherapy. Other cautious conclusions may be drawn: immature Mo-DCs (lacking activation) should not be used, the i.v. route may be less favorable and follow-up vaccination may be essential (and an ethical obligation) in responding patients.

## 9.9
### Phase III Clinical Trials

A phase III study in prostate cancer has been completed in patients with hormone-refractory progressive metastatic prostatic cancer and is about to undergo its first analysis [107]. A second phase III trial in hormone-sensitive patients is being initiated. Further phase II studies are being explored prior to a phase III study on multiple myeloma [107].

A phase III study performed by the Dermato-Oncology Working Group in melanoma [111] will compare Mo-DC vaccination with melanoma peptides with conventional treatment with dacarbazine. Other phase II studies are establishing protocols which will encourage phase III studies. It is hoped that clinicians and scientists alike will encourage and support these cooperative studies.

## 9.10
## Side Effects

Fortunately, adverse events have been limited. Minor discomfort at injection sites is reported formally, together with minor febrile reactions hypotension (with infusions) and myalgia. No definite treatment-related hematological hepatic or renal toxicity has resulted. The greatest concern has been the possibility of life-threatening or debilitating autoimmune reactions, which would undo the benefits of the beneficial antitumor response. One view is that this problem has been minimal because relatively weak immune responses have been generated. The alternative view is that where patients have been at risk, the natural tolerance or regulating mechanisms have prevented such detrimental self-reactivity. In the case of melanoma, vaccination against melanoma differentiation antigens might lead to destruction of melanocyte-containing tissue compartments such as the brain or the eye. To date, no serious autoimmune-related events have been reported, although an allergic reaction to exogenous protein has [165]. A few patients present with antinuclear antibodies or antithyroid antibodies without evolving further. Interestingly, the use of melanoma tumor lysates as antigens will induce widespread vitiligo in 43% of patients with metastasizing melanoma (Nestle *et al.*, submitted). These data demonstrate the power of immune activation against self-antigens using DCs pulsed with tumor lysates and emphasize that careful selection of target antigens will continue to be a major issue.

Given the animal model predictions, the paucity of autoimmune problems is most intriguing. As most TAAs generate low-affinity CTL responses, it is argued that this may be protective [125]. An interesting experiment attempting to generate a deliberate autoantigen response *in vitro* suggested that tolerance was preserved in the RNA-loading system used [120].

## 9.11
## Monitoring Immune Responses

There is an urgent need to identify credible surrogate markers of an immune response which will correlate with clinical responses. Until these techniques are identified or validated, the encouraging results to date can only be progressed via careful trial design, notably by selecting homogenous patient groups to study and documenting their clinical response by well-accepted clinical monitoring using current radiological or laboratory (tumor marker) methods. If and when surrogate immunological markers are validated these may be used to test the multiplicity of variables discussed, which have yet to be optimized. These can be incorporated into phase III trials. At present, it is essential that DC vaccination studies are carried out in association with laboratory facilities that can provide a full range of immunological laboratory studies

It is assumed but not yet proven (given the limited phase I/II clinical data showing a correlation) that DC vaccination should be optimized to produce maximal TAA-specific CTL responses. DC vaccination may be able to boost the frequency of an existing CTL precursor pool, but maintaining this as a memory response appears to be difficult [141, 142]. Again, it is hoped that the crucial high-affinity responses [166] will be developed by DC vaccination. Chromium-release assays using tumor cell targets is a laudable goal; however, this is clearly not widely achievable. Nonetheless, the ability to isolate tumor RNA and amplifying it allows autologous tumor target substitutes to be created from patients' Epstein–Barr virus-transformed B cells or other cell sources [118, 120]. The ELISPOT technique is now being widely applied and with observer-independent counting methodology now available this is providing useful information regarding IFN-γ-producing CD8 T lymphocyte responses; providing that sensitization *in vitro* is done first, flow cytometry detection of cytokine-producing cells may also be as sensitive. This technique can also be combined with specific T cell receptor analysis. Analysis of specific T cell receptors for HLA class I-restricted peptides is now possible using biotinylated soluble HLA-A2 (i.e. locus allele specific) TAA peptide-loaded tetramers and these detected by flow cytometry. Alternative technology uses different recombinant soluble (Fc/HLA-A2) dimers loaded with TAA peptide. Data in melanoma, chronic myeloid leukemia and bowel cancer suggests that the pre-existing TAA-specific T cell frequency is of the order of 0.1–2.0% [167, 168] and this can be expanded. However, it is very clear that TAA-specific T lymphocytes do not necessarily have antitumor activity. Thus, the limited correlation to date suggests cytotoxic assays will not. The functional contribution of the tetramer-positive cells may even be a negative one. Most studies necessarily sample the blood, but it is a valid point that direct tumor sampling may be required as effective CTLs may traffic from the blood to the tumor site.

There is good evidence that $CD4^+$ helper T lymphocyte responses driven by DCs contribute to CTL development. $CD4^+$ TAA-specific responses have also be shown to contribute to antitumor responses, not only as direct cytotoxic (class II-restricted) effectors), but also indirectly via recruitment and activation of other cells types. Classically, this is considered to be measured as part of the DTH response. An increase in the DTH response has been documented after DC vaccination and there may be some correlation with clinical outcome [91, 132]. DCs are also capable of activating NK responses [58] and Flt-3L effects have been shown to be at least in part due to a direct NK-activating effect [169].

## 9.12
## Tumor Escape

Cancers evolve other methods of immune evasion apart from avoiding DC initiation and presentation of the immune response. In patients who disease has progressed through conventional therapy there has been extensive opportunity for selective pressure to evolve tumor variants. The malignant cells may produce a host of factors which directly compromise immune cell function, e.g. transforming growth factor-β, VEGF and even products such as PSA, which has only recently been shown to have immunosuppressive qualities [170]. More importantly in terms of CTL effectors, defects in tumor antigen-processing and antigen display may influence the TAA tumors display – whether this merits individualizing therapy at this juncture is a mute point. However, loss of MHC antigens in advanced disease may reflect a hopeless situation and some would argue that rational trial design would exclude such cases rather than waste resources in uninformative cases.

There is clear consensus that the best results will be obtained in patients with minimal residual disease. This not only minimizes the risk of tumor escape, but may provide an optimal immune environment for DC initiation of an effective immune response. Like chemotherapy protocols, the aim must be tumor eradication and not just control. Careful study design is required for this population and integrating DC immunotherapy into an overall treatment program involving other modalities (with a functional immune system) is a problem. Common diseases susceptible to immunotherapy without standard curative protocols, such as multiple myeloma and low-grade NHL, should be investigated early [103].

## 9.13
### New Developments in DC Immunotherapy

Phase III studies of DC in multiple myeloma, prostate cancer and melanoma are underway. The preliminary data in multiple myeloma and prostate cancer are encouraging. Thus, we can anticipate more phase III studies. Given the low toxicity of DC immunotherapy, these are likely to be initiated in earlier disease. However, a major limitation remains the paucity of well-recognized TAAs apart from melanoma, whereby the TAAs (Mart-1/Melan-A. gp100, Tyrosinase) are virtually standard. Additionally, antigens, e.g. MAGE-1 and -3, have been key additions to the repertoire and novel antigens, e.g. the recently described embryonic TAA [171], are likely.

One can anticipate a rapid standardization of DC preparations as a result of commercial input and the new appropriate regulatory environment monitoring biological therapies. Key questions remain as how to load DCs with antigen effectively. This may involve modifying antigen (protein, peptide, DNA or RNA) targeting DC membrane receptors such as the Toll receptor, DEC-205 and Langerin or targeting DC intracellular pathways, e.g. with HIV tat [93].

Activating/differentiating DCs in an optimal fashion will also require careful experimentation. CD40L is already in use, CpG [172] likewise – other more potent compounds are likely to energy. These will need to be assessed to ensure they do not compromise DC migration.

Finally, to improve on DCs as the specialist APC, additional IL-12 or IL-2 may encourage T lymphocyte expansion. Genetic manipulation of DCs to enhance T lymphocyte recruitment has been suggested [173]. Equally, passive TAA-specific T lymphocytes generated *in vitro* for infusion [174] might be boosted *in vivo* by DC vaccinations.

Although HLA-matched allogeneic DCs may themselves be effective, it is possible that allografting an immune system in its entirety may be extended from hematological malignancies to other cancers. Thus, allogeneic stem cell transplants are effective in renal cell carcinoma and DC vaccination may be used to boost the anticancer response once immune reconstitution has been achieved. The allogeneic transplant procedure itself, may be facilitated by further DC engineering.

Finally, one might anticipate a shift from *ex vivo* DC loading to *in vivo* DC targeting of patients as part of their primary consolidation therapy.

## 9.14
## Conclusion

There is a strong basic scientific argument to support the argument for DC immunotherapy. Early trials using non-optimized systems have produced encouraging results. Equally, systems that are not optimized on the basis of basic scientific data have not. Phase III data is needed to justify ongoing clinical evaluation and trials are underway. Further gains may be possible if the treatment is applied in the context of minimal residual disease. The apparent low toxicity including autoimmune phenomenon justifies earlier application in the trial context.

### References

1 ROBINSON SP, PATTERSON S, ENGLISH N, DAVIES D, KNIGHT SC, REID CD. *Eur J Immunol* 1999; **29**: 2769–2778.

2 HART DNJ. *Pathology* 2001; **33**: 478–491.

3 KATZ SI, TAMAKI K, SACHS DH. *Nature* 1979; **282**: 324–326.

4 NELSON DJ, HOLT PG. *J Immunol* 1995; **155**: 3517–3524.

5 McLELLAN AD, HEISER A, SORG RV, FEARNLEY DB, HART DN. *J Invest Dermatol* 1998; **111**: 841–849.

6 CELLA M, JARROSSAY D, FACCHIETTI F, ALEBARDI O, NAKAJIMA H, LANZAVECCHIA A, COLONNA M. *Nat Med* 1999; **8**: 919–929.

7 RANDOLPH GJ, BEAULIEU S, LEBECQUE S, STEINMAN RM, MULLER WA. *Science* 1998; **282**: 479–482.

8 VUCKOVIC S, FLORIN THJ, KHALIL D, ZHANG MF, PATEL K, HAMILTON I, HART DNJ. *Am J Gastroenterol* 2001; **96**: 2946–2956.

9 SALLUSTO F, LANZAVECCHIA A. *Immunol Rev* 2000; **177**: 134–140.

10 HART DNJ. *Blood* 1997; **90**: 3245–3287.

11 McLELLAN AD, SORG RV, WILLIAMS LA, HART DNJ. *Eur J Immunol* 1996; **26**: 1204–1210.

12 HART DN, CLARK GJ, DEKKER JW, FEARNLEY DB, KATO M, HOCK BD, McLELLAN AD, NEIL T, SORG RV, SORG U, SUMMERS KL, VUCKOVIC S. *Adv Exp Med Biol* 1997; **417**: 439–442.

13 EL SHERBINI H, HOCK B, FEARNLEY D, McLELLAN A, VUCKOVIC S, HART DN. *Cell Immunol* 2000; **200**: 36–44.

14 STRUNK D, EGGER C, LEITNER G, HANAU D, STINGL G. *J Exp Med* 1997; **185**: 1131–1136.

15 TAKAMIZAWA M, RIVAS A, FAGNONI F, BENIKE C, KOSEK J, HYAKAWA H, ENGELMAN EG. *J Immunol* 1997; **158**: 2134–2142.

16 CRAWFORD K, GABUZDA D, VP, XU J, CLEMENT C, REINHERZ E, ALPER C. *J Immunol* 1999; **163**: 5920–5928.

17 FERRERO E, BONDANZA A, LEONE BE, MANICI S, POGGI A, ZOCCHI MR. *J Immunol* 1998; **160**: 2675–2683.

18 GROUARD G, RISSOAN M-C, FILGUEIRA L, DURAND I, BANCHEREAU J, LIU Y-J. *J Exp Med* 1997; **185**: 1101–1111.

19 OLWEUS J, BITMANSOUR A, WARNKE R, THOMPSON PA, CARBALLIDO J, PICKER LJ, LUND-JOHANSEN F. *Proc Natl Acad Sci USA* 1997; **94**: 12551–12556.

20 HART DNJ, CLARK GJ, MACDONALD K, KATO M, VUCKOVIC S, LOPEZ JA, WYKES M. IN: *Leucocyte Typing VII*. Oxford: Oxford University Press 2002: 283–294.

21 MAHNKE K, GUO M, LEE S, SEPULVEDA H, SWAIN SL, NUSSENZWEIG M, STEINMAN RM. *J Cell Biol* 2000; **151**: 673–684.

22 KATO M, MACDONALD K, MUNSTER D, VUCKOVIC S, CLARK G, HART DNJ. IN: *Leucocyte Typing VII*. Oxford: Oxford University Press 2002: 298–300.

23 GEIJTENBEEK TB, KWON DS, TORENSMA R, VAN VLIET SJ, VAN DUIJNHOVEN GC, MIDDEL J, CORNELISSEN IL, NOTTET HS, KEWALRAMANI VN, LITTMAN DR, FIGDOR CG, VAN KOOYK Y. *Cell* 2000; **100**: 587–597.

24 VALLADEAU J, RAVEL O, DEZUTTER-DAMBUYANT C, MOORE K, KLEIJMEER M, LIU Y, DUVERT-FRANCES V, VINCENT C, SCHMITT D, DAVOUST J, CAUX C, LEBECQUE S, SAELAND S. *Immunity* 2000; **12**: 71–81.

25 HEMMI H, TAKEUCHI O, KAWAI T, KAISHO T, SATO S, SANJO H, MATSUMOTO M, HOSHINO K, WAGNER H, TAKEDA K, AKIRA S. *Nature* 2000; **408**: 740–745.

26 MILONE MC, FITZGERALD-BOCARSLY P. *J Immunol* 1998; **161**: 2391–2399.

27 KADOWAKI N, ANTONENKO S, LIU YJ. *J Immunol* 2001; **166**: 2291–2295.

28 ALBERT ML, SAUTER B, BHARDWAJ N. *Nature* 1998; **392**: 86–89.

29 WOLFERS J, LOZIER A, RAPOSO G, REGNAULT A, THERY C, MASURIER C, FLAMENT C, POUZIEUX S, FAURE F, TURSZ T, ANGEVIN E, AMIGORENA S, ZITVOGEL L. *Nat Med* 2001; **7**: 297–303.

30 LANZAVECCHIA A. *Curr Opin Immunol* 1996; **8**: 348–354.

31 NORBURY CC, CHAMBERS BJ, PRESCOTT AR, LJUNGGREN H-G, WATTS C. *Eur J Immunol* 1997; **27**: 280–288.

32 ARNOLD-SCHILD D, HANAU D, SPEHNER D, SCHMID C, RAMMENSEE HG, DE LA SALLE H, SCHILD H. *J Immunol* 1999; **162**: 3757–3760.

33 BASU S, BINDER RJ, RAMALINGAM T, SRIVASTAVA PK. *Immunity* 2001; **14**: 303–313.

34 ROAKE JA, RAO AS, MORRIS PJ, LARSEN CP, HANKINS DF, AUSTYN JM. *J Exp Med* 1995; **181**: 2237–2247.

35 SPARWASSER T, KOCH ES, VABULAS RM, HEEG K, LIPFORD GB, ELLWART JW, WAGNER H. *Eur J Immunol* 1998; **28**: 2045–2054.

36 BHARDWAJ N. *J Exp Med* 1997; **186**: 795–799.

37 SAUTER B, ALBERT ML, FRANCISCO L, LARSSON M, SOMERSAN S, BHARDWAJ N. *J Exp Med* 2000; **191**: 423–434.

38 GALLUCCI S, LOLKEMA M, MATZINGER P. *Nat Med* 1999; **5**: 1249–1255.

39 SALLUSTO F, LANZAVECCHIA A, MACKAY CR. *Immunol Today* 1998; **19**: 568–574.

40 FORSTER R, SCHUBEL A, BREITFELD D, KREMMER E, RENNER-MULLER I, WOLF E, LIPP M. *Cell* 1999; **99**: 23–33.

41 MCLELLAN A, HELDMANN M, TERBECK G, WEIH F, LINDEN C, BROCKER EB, LEVERKUS M, KAMPGEN E. *Eur J Immunol* 2000; **30**: 2612–2619.

42 WONG BR, JOSIEN R, LEE SY, SAUTER B, LI HL, STEINMAN RM, CHOI Y. *J Exp Med* 1997; **186**: 2075–2080.

43 RIEDL E, STOCKL J, MAJDIC O, SCHEINECKER C, KNAPP W, STROBL H. *Blood* 2000; **96**: 4276–4284.

44 CLARK GJ, GUNNINGHAM SP, TROY AJ, VUCKOVIC S, HART DN. *Immunology* 1999; **98**: 189–196.

45 SALLUSTO F, LANZAVECCHIA A. *J Exp Med* 1994; **179**: 1109–1118.

46 DIEU M-C, VANBERVLIET B, VICARI A, BRIDON J-M, OLDHAM E, AIT-YAHIA S, BRIERE F, ZLOTNIK A, LEBECQUE S, CAUX C. *J Exp Med* 1998; **188**: 373–386.

47 CHAN VWF, KOTHAKOTA S, ROHAN MC, PANGANIBAN-LUSTAN L, GARDNER JP, WACHOWICZ MS, WINTER JA, WILLIAMS LT. *Blood* 1999; **93**: 3610–3616.

48 SUMMERS KL, HOCK BD, MCKENZIE JL, HART DN. *Am J Pathol* 2001; **159**: 285–295.

49 ADEMA GJ, HARTGERS F, VERSTRATEN R, DE VRIES E, MARLAND G, MENON S, FOSTER J, XU Y, NOOYEN P, MCCLANAHAN T, BACON KB, FIGDOR CG. *Nature* 1997; **387**: 713–715.

**50** Tang HLl, Cyster JG. *Science* 1999; **284**: 819–822.

**51** Luther SA, Gulbranson-Judge A, Acha-Orbea H, MacLennan IC. *J Exp Med* 1997; **185**: 551–562.

**52** Sorg RV, McLellan AD, Hock BD, Fearnley DB, Hart DN. *Immunobiology* 1998; **198**: 514–526.

**53** Cella M, Scheidegger D, Palmer-Lehmann K, Lane P, Lanzavecchia A, Alber G. *J Exp Med* 1996; **184**: 747–752.

**54** Armitage RJ, Namen AE, Sassenfeld HM, Grabstein KH. *J Immunol* 1990; **144**: 938–941.

**55** Heufler C, Koch F, Stanzl U, Topar G, Wysocka M, Trinchieri G, Enk A, Steinman RM, Romani N, Schuler G. *Eur J Immunol* 1996; **26**: 659–668.

**56** Steinman RM. *Annu Rev Immunol* 1991; **9**: 271–296.

**57** Jahnsen FL, Lund-Johansen F, Dunne JF, Farkas L, Haye R, Brandtzaeg P. *J Immunol* 2000; **165**: 4062–4068.

**58** Fernandez NC, Lozier A, Flament C, Ricciardi-Castagnoli P, Bellet D, Suter M, Perricaudet M, Tursz T, Maraskovsky E, Zitvogel L. *Nat Med* 1999; **5**:405–411.

**59** Troy AJ, Summers KL, Davidson PJ, Atkinson CA, Hart DN. *Clin Cancer Res* 1998; **4**: 585–593.

**60** Troy A, Davidson P, Atkinson C, Hart D. *J Urol* 1998; **160**: 214–219.

**61** Coventry BJ. *Anticancer Res* 1999; **19**: 3183–3187.

**62** Bell D, Chomarat P, Broyles D, Netto G, Harb G, Lebecque S, Valladeau J, Davoust J, Palucka K, Banchereau J. *J Exp Med* 1999; **190**: 1417–1425.

**63** Troy AJ, Davidson PJ, Atkinson CH, Hart DN. *J Urol* 1999; **161**: 1962–1967.

**64** Nestle FO, Burg G, Fah J, Wrone-Smith T, Nickoloff BJ. *Am J Pathol* 1997; **150**: 641–651.

**65** Almand B, Resser JR, Lindman B, Nadaf S, Clark JI, Kwon ED, Carbone DP, Gabrilovich DI. *Clin Cancer Res* 2000; **6**: 1755–1766.

**66** Troy AJ, Hart DNJ. *J Hematother* 1997; **6**: 523–533.

**67** Lotze MT, Jaffe R. In: *Dendritic Cells: Biology and Clinical Applications.* New York: Academic Press 2001: 425–437.

**68** Troy AC, Hart DNJ. *Urologic Oncology* 1998; **4**: 17–23.

**69** Savary CA, Grazziutti ML, Melichar B, Przepiorka D, Freedman RS, Cowart RE, Cohen DM, Anaissie EJ, Woodside DG, McIntyre BW, Pierson DL, Pellis NR, Rex JH. *Cancer Immunol Immunother* 1998; **45**: 234–240.

**70** Brown RD, Pope B, Murray A, Esdale W, Sze DM, Gibson J, Ho PJ, Hart D, Joshua D. *Blood* 2001; **98**: 2992–2998.

**71** Almand B, Clark JI, Nikitina E, van Beynen J, English NR, Knight SC, Carbone DP, Gabrilovich DI. *J Immunol* 2001; **166**: 678–689.

**72** Small EJ, Fratesi P, Reese DM, Strang G, Laus R, Peshwa MV, Valone FH. *J Clin Oncol* 2000; **18**: 3894–3903.

**73** Salgaller ML, Thurnher M, Bartsch G, Boynton AL, Murphy GP. *Cancer* 1999; **86**: 2674–2683.

**74** Kiertscher SM, Luo J, Dubinett SM, Roth MD. *J Immunol* 2000; **164**: 1269–1276.

**75** Remmel E, Terracciano L, Noppen C, Zajac P, Heberer M, Spagnoli GC, Padovan E. *Hum Immunol* 2001; **62**: 39–49.

**76** Panelli MC, Wunderlich J, Jeffries J, Wang E, Mixon A, Rosenberg SA, Marincola FM. *J Immunother* 2000; **23**: 487–498.

**77** Gabrilovich DI, Chen HL, Girgis KR, Cunningham HT, Meny GM, Nadaf S, Kavanaugh D, Carbone DP. *Nat Med* 1996; **2**: 1096.

**78** Ho CS, Munster D, Pyke CM, Hart DN, Lopez JA. *Blood* 2002; **99**: 2897–2904.

**79** Fearnley DB, Whyte LF, Carnoutsos SA, Cook AH, Hart DN. *Blood* 1999; **93**: 728–736.

**80** Ho CS, Lopez JA, Vuckovic S, Pyke CM, Hockey RL, Hart DN. *Blood* 2001; **98**: 140–145.

**81** Vuckovic S, Fearnley DB, Gunningham SP, Spearing RL, Patton WN, Hart DN. *Br J Haematol* 1999; **105**: 974–985.

**82** ARPINATI M, GREEN CL, HEIMFELD S, HEUSER JE, ANASETTI C. *Blood* 2000; **95**: 2484–2490.

**83** MARASKOVSKY E, DARO E, ROUX E, TEEPE M, MALISZEWSKI CR, HOEK J, CARON D, LEBSACK ME, MCKENNA HJ. *Blood* 2000; **96**: 878–884.

**84** FONG L, HOU Y, RIVAS A, BENIKE C, YUEN A, FISHER GA, DAVIS MM, ENGLEMAN EG. *Proc Natl Acad Sci USA* 2001; **98**: 8809–8814.

**85** MORSE MA, NAIR S, FERNANDEZ-CASAL M, DENG Y, ST PETER M, WILLIAMS R, HOBEIKA A, MOSCA P, CLAY T, CUMMING RI, FISHER E, CLAVIEN P, PROIA AD, NIEDZWIECKI D, CARON D, LYERLY HK. *J Clin Oncol* 2000; **18**: 3883–3893.

**86** ROTH MD, GITLITZ BJ, KIERTSCHER SM, PARK AN, MENDENHALL M, MOLDAWER N, FIGLIN RA. *Cancer Res* 2000; **60**: 1934–1941.

**87** JANIK JE, MILLER LL, KOPP WC, TAUB DD, DAWSON H, STEVENS D, KOSTBOTH P, CURTI BD, CONLON KC, DUNN BK, DONEGAN SE, ULLRICH R, ALVORD WG, GAUSE BL, LONGO DL. *Clin Immunol* 1999; **93**: 209–221.

**88** BERNHARD H, DISIS ML, HEIMFELD S, HAND S, GRALOW JR, CHEEVER MA. *Cancer Res* 1995; **55**: 1099–1104.

**89** MACKENSEN A, HERBST B, CHEN JL, KOHLER G, NOPPEN C, HERR W, SPAGNOLI GC, CERUNDOLO V, LINDEMANN A. *Int J Cancer* 2000; **86**: 385–392.

**90** MONJI T, PETERSONS JT, VUCKOVIC S, SAUND NK, HART DNJ, AUDITORE-HARGREAVES K, RISDON G. *Immunol Cell Biol* 2001; in press.

**91** BANCHEREAU J, PALUCKA AK, DHODAPKAR M, BURKEHOLDER S, TAQUET N, ROLLAND A, TAQUET S, COQUERY S, WITTKOWSKI KM, BHARDWAJ N, PINEIRO L, STEINMAN R, FAY J. *Cancer Res* 2001; **61**: 6451–6458.

**92** VUCKOVIC S, FEARNLEY DB, MANNERING SI, DEKKER J, WHYTE LF, HART DN. *Exp Hematol* 1998; **26**: 1255–1264.

**93** VUCKOVIC S, CLARK GJ, HART DNJ. *Current Pharmaceutical Design* 2002; **8**: 125–133.

**94** THOMAS R, CHAMBERS M, BOYTAR R, BARKER K, CAVANAGH LL, MACFADYEN S, SMITHERS M, JENKINS M, ANDERSEN J. *Melanoma Res* 1999; **9**: 474–481.

**95** BARRATT-BOYES SM, WATKINS SC, FINN OJ. *J Immunol* 1997; **158**: 4543–4547.

**96** PALUCKA KA, TAQUET N, SANCHEZ-CHAPUIS F, GLUCKMAN JC. *J Immunol* 1998; **160**: 4587–4595.

**97** STEINBRINK K, WOLFL M, JONULEIT H, KNOP J, ENK A. *J Immunol* 1997; **159**: 4772–4780.

**98** DHODAPKAR MV, KRASOVSKY J, STEINMAN RM, BHARDWAJ N. *J Clin Invest* 2000; **105**: R9–R14.

**99** DHODAPKAR MV, STEINMAN RM, KRASOVSKY J, MUNZ M, BHARDWAJ N. *J. Exp Med* 2001; **193**: 233–238.

**100** ROMANI N, REIDER D, HEUER M, EBNER S, KAMPGEN E, EIBL B, NIEDERWIESER D, SCHULER G. *J Immunol Methods* 1996; **196**: 137–151.

**101** JONULEIT H, KUHN U, MULLER G, STEINBRINK K, PARAGNIK L, SCHMITT E, KNOP J, ENK AH. *Eur J Immunol* 1997; **27**: 3135–3142.

**102** CZERNIECKI BJ, CARTER C, RIVOLTINI L, KOSKI GK, KIM HI, WENG DE, ROROS JG, HIJAZI YM, XU S, ROSENBERG SA, COHEN PA. *J Immunol* 1997; **159**: 3823–3837.

**103** HART DN, HILL GR. *Immunol Cell Biol* 1999; **77**: 451–459.

**104** MANNERING SI, MCKENZIE JL, HART DN. *J Immunol Methods* 1998; **219**: 69–83.

**105** HART DNJ. *Pathology* 2001; **33**: 478–491.

**106** HSU FJ, BENIKE C, FAGNONI F, LILES TM, CZERWINSKI D, TAIDI B, ENGELMAN EG, LEVY R. *Nat Med* 1996; **2**: 52–58.

**107** VALONE FH, SMALL E, MACKENZIE M, BURCH P, LACY M, PESHWA MV, LAUS R. *Cancer J* 2001; **7**(suppl 2): S53–61.

**108** FEARNLEY DB, MCLELLAN AD, MANNERING SI, HOCK BD, HART DNJ. *Blood* 1997; **89**: 3708–3716.

**109** OSUGI Y, VUCKOVIC S, HART DNJ. *Blood*; in press.

**110** LOPEZ JA, CROSBIE GV, KELLY C, MCGEE A, WILLIAMS K, SCHUYLER R, RODWELL R, WRIGHT SJ, TAYLOR KM, HART DN. *J Immunol Methods*; in press.

111 NESTLE FO, BANCHEREAU J, HART D. *Nat Med* 2001; **7**: 761–765.

112 ZENG W, GHOSH S, MACRIS M, PAGNON J, JACKSON DC. *Vaccine* 2001; **19**: 3843–3852.

113 BELLONE M, CANTARELLA D, CASTIGLIONI P, CROSTI MC, RONCHETTI A, MORO M, GARANCINI MP, CASORATI G, DELLABONA P. *J Immunol* 2000; **165**: 2651–2656.

114 GONG J, CHEN D, KASHIWABA M, KUFE D. *Nat Med* 1997; **3**: 558–561.

115 GONG J, AVIGAN D, CHEN D, WU Z, KOIDO S, KASHIWABA M, KUFE D. *Proc Natl Acad Sci USA* 2000; **97**: 2715–2718.

116 GONG J, NIKRUI N, CHEN D, KOIDO S, WU Z, TANAKA Y, CANNISTRA S, AVIGAN D, KUFE D. *J Immunol* 2000; **165**: 1705–1711.

117 KUGLER A, STUHLER G, WALDEN P, ZOLLER G, ZOBYWALSKI A, BROSSART P, TREFZER U, ULLRICH S, MULLER CA, BECKER V, GROSS AJ, HEMMERLEIN B, KANZ L, MULLER GA, RINGERT RH. *Nat Med* 2000; **6**: 332–336.

118 NAIR SK, HULL S, COLEMAN D, GILBOA E, LYERLY HK, MORSE MA. *Int J Cancer* 1999; **82**: 121–124.

119 NAIR SK, HEISER A, BOCZKOWSKI D, MAJUMDAR A, NAOE M, LEBKOWSKI JS, VIEWEG J, GILBOA E. *Nat Med* 2000; **6**: 1011–1017.

120 HEISER A, MAURICE MA, YANCEY DR, WU NZ, DAHM P, PRUITT SK, BOCZKOWSKI D, NAIR SK, BALLO MS, GILBOA E, VIEWEG J. *J Immunol* 2001; **166**: 2953–2960.

121 VAN TENDELOO VF, PONSAERTS P, LARDON F, NIJS G, LENJOU M, VAN BROECKHOVEN C, VAN BOCKSTAELE DR, BERNEMAN ZN. *Blood* 2001; **98**: 49–56.

122 LAPOINTE R, ROYAL RE, REEVES ME, ALTOMARE I, ROBBINS PF, HWU P. *J Immunol* 2001; **167**: 4758–4764.

123 WAN Y, BRAMSON J, CARTER R, GRAHAM F, GAULDIE J. *Hum Gene Ther* 1997; **8**: 1355–1363.

124 ENGELMAYER J, LARSSON M, LEE A, LEE M, COX WI, STEINMAN RM, BHARDWAJ N. *J Virol* 2001; **75**: 2142–2153.

125 GILBOA E. *Nat Immunol* 2001; **2**: 789–792.

126 FAWELL S, SEERY J, DAIKH Y, MOORE C, CHEN LL, PEPINSKY B, BARSOUM J. *Proc Natl Acad Sci USA* 1994; **91**: 664–668.

127 FONG L, ENGLEMAN EG. *Annu Rev Immunol* 2000; **18**: 245–273.

128 MORSE MA, COLEMAN RE, AKABANI G, NIEHAUS N, COLEMAN D, LYERLY HK. *Cancer Res* 1999; **59**: 56–58.

129 MACKENSEN A, KRAUSE T, BLUM U, UHRMEISTER P, MERTELSMANN R, LINDEMANN A. *Cancer Immunol Immunother* 1999; **48**: 118–122.

130 EGGERT A, SCHREURS M, BOERMAN O, OYEN W, BOER A, PUNT C, FIGDOR C, ADEMA G. *Cancer Res* 1999; **59**: 3340–3345.

131 SERODY JS, COLLINS EJ, TISCH RM, KUHNS JJ, FRELINGER JA. *J Immunol* 2000; **164**: 4961–4967.

132 NESTLE FO, ALIJAGIC S, GILLIET M, SUN Y, GRABBE S, DUMMER R, BURG G, SCHADENDORF D. *Nat Med* 1998; **4**: 328–332.

133 FONG L, BROCKSTEDT D, BENIKE C, WU L, ENGLEMAN EG. *J Immunol* 2001; **166**: 4254–4259.

134 STEINBRINK K, JONULEIT H, MULLER G, SCHULER G, KNOP J, ENK AH. *Blood* 1999; **93**: 1634–1642.

135 BENDANDI M, GOCKE CD, KOBRIN CB, BENKO FA, STERNAS LA, PENNINGTON R, WATSON TM, REYNOLDS CW, GAUSE BL, DUFFEY PL, JAFFE ES, CREEKMORE SP, LONGO DL, KWAK LW. *Nat Med* 1999; **5**: 1171–1177.

136 OSTERBORG A, YI Q, HENRIKSSON L, FAGERBERG J, BERGENBRANT S, JEDDI-TEHRANI M, RUDEN V, LEFVERT AK, HOLM G, MELLSTEDT H. *Blood* 1998; **91**: 2549.

137 WEN YJ, LING M, BAILEY-WOOD R, LIM SH. *Clin Cancer Res* 1998; **4**: 957.

138 DABADGHAO S, BERGENBRANT S, ANTON D, HE W, HOLM G, YI Q. *Br J Haematol* 1998; **100**: 647–654.

139 REICHARDT VL, OKADA CY, LISO A, BENIKE CJ, STOCKERL-GOLDSTEIN KE, ENGLEMAN EG, BLUME KG, LEVY R. *Blood* 1999; **93**: 2411–2419.

140 LISO A, STOCKERL-GOLDSTEIN KE, AUFFERMANN-GRETZINGER S, BENIKE CJ, REICHARDT V, VAN BECKHOVEN A, RAJAPAKSA R, ENGLEMAN EG, BLUME KG,

LEVY R. *Biol Blood Marrow Transplant* 2000; **6**: 621–627.

141 THURNER B, HAENDLE I, RODER C, DIECKMANN D, KEIKAVOUSSI P, JONULEIT H, BENDER A, MACZEK C, SCHREINER D, VON DEN DRIESCH P, BROCKER EB, STEINMAN RM, ENK A, KAMPGEN E, SCHULER G. *J Exp Med* 1999; **190**: 1669–1678.

142 TOUNGOUZ M, LIBIN M, BULTE F, FAID L, LEHMANN F, DURIAU D, LAPORTE M, GANGJI D, BRUYNS C, LAMBERMONT M, GOLDMAN M, VELU T. *J Leuk Biol* 2001; **69**: 937–943.

143 LAU R, WANG F, JEFFERY G, MARTY V, KUNIYOSHI J, BADE E, RYBACK ME, WEBER J. *J Immunother* 2001; **24**: 66–78.

144 JONULEIT H, GIESECKE-TUETTENBERG A, TUTING T, THURNER-SCHULER B, STUGE TB, PARAGNIK L, KANDEMIR A, LEE PP, SCHULER G, KNOP J, ENK AH. *Int J Cancer* 2001; **93**: 243–251.

145 RIESER C, RAMONER R, HOLTL L, ROGATSCH H, PAPESH C, STENZL A, BARTSCH G, THURNHER M. *Urol Int* 2000; **63**: 151–159.

146 HOLTL L, RIESER C, PAPESH C, RAMONER R, HEROLD M, KLOCKER H, RADMAYR C, STENZL A, BARTSCH G, THURNHER M. *J Urol* 1999; **161**: 777–782.

147 THURNHER M, RIESER C, HOLTL L, PAPESH C, RAMONER R, BARTSCH G. *Urol Int* 1998; **61**: 67–71.

148 MURPHY G, TJOA B, RAGDE H, KENNY G, BOYNTON A. *Prostate* 1996; **29**: 371–380.

149 MURPHY GP, TJOA BA, SIMMONS SJ, RAGDE H, ROGERS M, ELGAMAL A, KENNY GM, TROYCHAK MJ, SALGALLER ML, BOYNTON AL. *Prostate* 1999; **39**: 54–59.

150 MURPHY GP, TJOA BA, SIMMONS SJ, JARISCH J, BOWES VA, RAGDE H, ROGERS M, ELGANAL A, KENNY GM, COBB OE, IRETON RC, TROYCHAK MJ, SALGALLER ML, BOYNTON AL. *Prostate* 1999; **38**: 73–78.

151 LODGE PA, JONES LA, BADER RA, MURPHY GP, SALGALLER ML. *Cancer Res* 2000; **60**: 829–833.

152 MURPHY GP, SNOW P, SIMMONS SJ, TJOA BA, ROGERS MK, BRANDT J, HEALY CG, BOLTON WE, RODBOLD D. *Prostate* 2000; **42**: 67–72.

153 TJOA BA, MURPHY GP. *Immunol Lett* 2000; **74**: 87–93.

154 TJOA BA, SIMMONS SJ, BOWES VA, RAGDE H, ROGERS M, ELGAMAL A, KENNY GM, COBB OE, IRETON RC, TROYCHAK MJ, SALGALLER ML, BOYNTON AL, MURPHY GP. *Prostate* 1998; **36**: 39–44.

155 TJOA BA, SIMMONS SJ, ELGAMAL A, ROGERS M, RAGDE H, KENNY GM, TROYCHAK MJ, BOYNTON AL, MURPHY GP. *Prostate* 1999; **40**: 125–129.

156 SALGALLER ML, LODGE PA, MCLEAN JG, TJOA BA, LOFTUS DJ, RAGDE H, KENNY GM, ROGERS M, BOYNTON AL, MURPHY GP. *Prostate* 1998; **35**: 144–151.

157 BURCH PA, BREEN JK, BUCKNER JC, GASTINEAU DA, KAUR JA, LAUS RL, PADLEY DJ, PESHWA MV, PITOT HC, RICHARDSON RL, SMITS BJ, SOPAPAN P, STRANG G, VALONE FH, VUK-PAVLOVIC S. *Clin Cancer Res* 2000; **6**: 2175–2182.

158 MORSE M, DENG Y, COLEMAN D, HULL S, KITRELL-FISHER E, NAIR S, SCHLOM J, RYBACK M, LYERLY H. *Clin Cancer Res* 1999; **5**: 1331–1338.

159 BROSSART P, WIRTHS S, STUHLER G, REICHARDT VL, KANZ L, BRUGGER W. *Blood* 2000; **96**: 3102–3108.

160 KOBAYASHI T, SHINOHARA H, TOYODA M, IWAMOTO S, TANIGAWA N. *Surg Today* 2001; **31**: 513–516.

161 FUJII S, SHIMIZU K, FUJIMOTO K, KIYOKAWA T, SHIMOMURA T, KINOSHITA M, KAWANO F. *Jpn J Cancer Res* 1999; **90**: 1117–1129.

162 GEIGER J, HUTCHINSON R, HOHENKIRK L, MCKENNA E, CHANG A, MULE J. *Lancet* 2000; **356**: 1163–1165.

163 YU JS, WHEELER CJ, ZELTZER PM, YING H, FINGER DN, LEE PK, YONG WH, INCARDONA F, THOMPSON RC, RIEDINGER MS, ZHANG W, PRINS RM, BLACK KL. *Cancer Res* 2001; **61**: 842–847.

164 KIKUCHI T, AKASAKI Y, IRIE M, HOMMA S, ABE T, OHNO T. *Cancer Immunol Immunother* 2001; **50**: 337–344.

165 MACKENSEN A, DRAGER R, SCHLESIER M, MERTELSMANN R, LINDEMANN A. *Cancer Immunol Immunother* 2000; **49**: 152–156.

**166** ZEH HJ, PERRY-LALLEY D, DUDLEY ME, ROSENBERG SA, YANG JC. *J Immunol* 1999; **162**: 989–994.

**167** LEE PP, YEE C, SAVAGE PA, FONG L, BROCKSTEDT D, WEBER JS, JOHNSON D, SWETTER S, THOMPSON J, GREENBERG PD, ROEDERER M, DAVIS MM. *Nat Med* 1999; **5**: 677–685.

**168** MOLLDREM JJ, LEE PP, WANG C, FELIO K, KANTARJIAN HM, CHAMPLIN RE, DAVIS MM. *Nat Med* 2000; **6**: 1018–1023.

**169** LYNCH DH, ANDREASEN A, MARASKOVSKY E, WHITMORE J, MILLER RE, SCHUH JCL. *Nat Med* 1997; **3**: 625–630.

**170** KENNEDY-SMITH AG, MCKENZIE JL, OWEN MC, DAVIDSON PJT, VUCKOVIC S, HART DNJ. *J Urol*; in press.

**171** MONK M, HOLDING C. *Oncogene* 2001; **20**: 8085–8091.

**172** HARTMANN G, WEINER GJ, KRIEG AM. *Proc Natl Acad Sci USA* 1999; **96**: 9305–9310.

**173** CAO X, ZHANG W, HE L, XIE Z, MA S, TAO Q, YU Y, HAMADA H, WANG J. *J Immunol* 1998; **161**: 6238–6244.

**174** SANTIN AD, HERMONAT PL, RAVAGGI A, BELLONE S, COWAN C, COKE C, PECORELLI S, CANNON MJ, PARHAM GP. *Gynecol Obstet Invest* 2000; **49**: 194–203.

**175** LIM SH, BAILEY-WOOD R. *Int J Cancer* 1999; **83**: 215–222.

**176** THURNER B, RODER C, DIECKMANN D, HEUER M, KRUSE M, GLASER A, KEIKAVOUSSI P, KAMPGEN E, BENDER A, SCHULER G. *J Immunol Methods* 1999; **223**: 1–15.

**177** SCHULER-THURNER B, DIECKMANN D, KEIKAVOUSSI P, BENDER A, MACZEK C, JONULEIT H, RODER C, HAENDLE I, LEISGANG W, DUNBAR R, CERUNDOLO V, VON DEN DRIESCH P, KNOP J, BROCKER EB, ENK A, KAMPGEN E, SCHULER G. *J Immunol* 2000; **165**: 3492–3496.

**178** TREFZER U, WEINGART G, CHEN Y, HERBERTH G, ADRIAN K, WINTER H, AUDRING H, GUO Y, STERRY W, WALDEN P. *Int J Cancer* 2000; **85**: 618–626.

**179** SCHOTT M, FELDKAMP J, LETTMANN M, SIMON D, SCHERBAUM WA, SEISSLER J. *Clin Endocrinol (Oxford)* 2001; **55**: 271–277.

**180** SADANAGA N, NAGASHIMA H, MASHINO K, TAHARA K, YAMAGUCHI H, OHTA M, FUJIE T, TANAKA F, INOUE H, TAKESAKO K, AKIYOSHI T, MORI M. *Clin Cancer Res* 2001; **7**: 2277–2284.

# 10

# The Immune System in Cancer: If It Isn't Broken, Can We Fix It?

Dragan Terremovic and Richard G. Vile

## 10.1
## Commitment and the Modern Immune System

The importance of immune effector cells in protecting against the emergence of tumors within immunocompetent hosts has been a point of controversy for many years. In the 1970s, Burnet proposed that lymphocytes patrol the body and react to, and remove, tumor cells that have escaped normal controls of growth and differentiation, giving rise to the concept of "cancer immunosurveillance" [1]. However, this attractive (and comforting) theory became less credible with the observation that athymic nude mice, lacking functional T cells, develop tumors at the same rate as their immunocompetent wild-type counterparts. To understand these competing views better, it is important to realize that immune recognition of tumors is only one of the roles that the modern immune system has evolved to fulfill. Probably higher on its list of priorities comes its ability to recognize and respond to invading pathogens. However, along with this need for vigorous reactivity against non-self antigens, comes an equally important need to ignore self antigens (see Appendix). Hence, the modern immune system is constantly pulled in opposite directions with stringent twin requirements of aggressive responses against infectious foreign pathogens whilst maintaining a complete lack of response to self antigens to avoid autoimmunity.

Within the confines of these two extremes is the need to deal with the threat posed by the uncontrolled growth and dissemination of cancer cells. In order to understand how the immune system should evolve to be able to meet all of the demands that are asked of it, let us consider the two extreme models (Fig. 10.1). In one model (Fig. 10.1A), immune recognition of tumors might have become finely tuned to recognize all emerging tumor cells and the molecular mutations associated with them. A second option, erring on the side of preventing autoimmune disease, would be an immune system that has no capacity to respond to emerging tumor cells at all (Fig. 10.1B). In reality, the most likely situation, which offers maximal benefit to the species, falls between these two extremes of immunological hypersensitivity and immunological ignorance (Fig. 10.1).

| | Model A | Model B |
|---|---|---|
| | Hypersensitivity to tumor-associated mutations | Unresponsiveness to tumor associated mutations |
| Level of self/ near-self recognition | Exquisite | Zero |
| Time of cancer onset | Late life/not at all | Early life |
| Incidence of cancers | Low | High |
| Risk of death by cancer | Low | **High** |
| Risk of death autoimmune disease | **High** | Low |
| Risk to species | High | High |

**Fig. 10.1**  Two models for antitumor immunity. The level of sensitivity with which the immune system can evolve to respond to tumor-associated mutations is shaped by competing influences. The two extreme models are (A) that the immune system has evolved to treat tumors as it would a foreign pathogen and be hyper-responsive to even small mutations in cellular oncoproteins or (B) that it is completely unresponsive to tumors, which are essentially self, to avoid the consequences of autoimmunity. The bottom line shows that the immune system cannot afford to adopt either of these two extremes. Therefore, it has evolved a broad, rather than exquisite, recognition of tumor-associated mutations as a compromise that ensures the balance between disease control and disease promotion. In general terms, this delays cancer occurrence and makes it a disease of later life.

## 10.2
## Evolutionary Tuning

The immune system has in place very sophisticated mechanisms to avoid recognizing self antigens, through thymic T cell deletion and the generation of immunological tolerance (see Box 10.1). The question then arises as to how good can it ever be at recognizing the altered self antigens that arise from tumorigenic mutations (see below)?

If the immune system did no immunoediting [1, 2], the number of oncogenic mutations that would be tolerated within tumor cells might be much greater than the repertoire that is currently observed (Fig. 10.2). This would allow cellular transformation to occur much more quickly and cancer would become a disease of early life. If individuals routinely died of cancer before reproductive efficiency was maximal, the evolution of enhanced immune mechanisms that recognize tumor-associated mutations would provide an enormous selective advantage (Figs. 10.1 and 10.2).

Therefore, we would expect some degree of "immunoediting" of tumors to occur; in other words, the immune system would attack and destroy cells expressing mutant proteins whose structures are sufficiently different from wild-type that they are no longer recognized as self. Is there any evidence for this? Recently, Shankaran *et al.* provided elegant proof that the growth of spontaneously arising tumors in immunocompetent mice is indeed edited by the immune system [2]. These authors used mice in which specific subsets of immune cells were genetically deleted. They showed that both transplantable and spontaneously arising tumors grow more rapidly in animals deficient in certain immune effector pathways than in animals where the immune system is intact, indicating that highly immunogenic tumor-associated mutations arise in the absence of a functional immune system. These animal studies are consistent with observations that the oncogenic mutations seen in clinically apparent human cancer cells are often very subtle, e.g. single amino acid changes in oncoproteins such as Ras and Myc. This probably represents selection of those mutations that do not *per se* give rise to immunogenic epitopes (see Appendix). A prediction of this hypothesis is that there might be a much broader range of mutations in cellular proto-oncogenes/tumor-suppressor genes that can promote uncontrolled cellular proliferation but that are never actually seen in human cancer cells because they are immunoedited out (Fig. 10.2C and D) [2]. This theory can now be tested by analyzing the spontaneous tumors that arise in immunodeficient mice. Are the apparently tight restraints that are placed oncogenic mutations that arise in immunocompetent animals relieved in tumors growing in immunodeficient animals? Experiments along these lines should help to establish whether the immune system is a prime driver of selection of tumor genotype.

In summary, neither immune hypersensitivity nor immune ignorance to tumors (Fig. 10.1) is likely to be the most beneficial situation to have evolved within the context of the other competing commitments that the immune system has to keep. However, immunoediting [2] of gross mutations in transforming oncoproteins would provide a 'third way' – one that provides a delaying tactic so that most individuals can pass their genes on to their progeny before dying of cancer. There is also

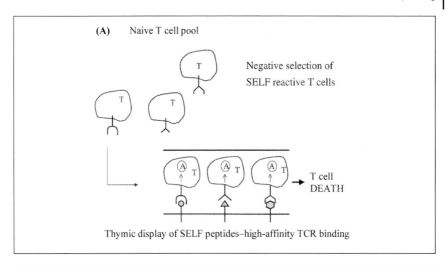

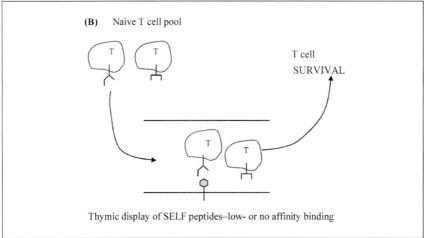

**Box 10.1** Thymic selection of T cells and the generation of tolerance to self. The immune system has evolved to ignore self antigens to prevent the onset of autoimmune disease through the generation of tolerance. (A) Negative selection of T cells with TCRs that recognize self antigens eradicates T cells with autoimmune capability. Naive T cells express TCRs which can recognize peptides in the context of MHC molecules presented by thymic DCs [91, 92]. Any T cell with a TCR that binds to an MHC molecule expressing an epitope derived from a *self* antigen in the thymus is induced to die by apoptosis. Thus, tolerance to *self* peptides is established by negative selection of autoreactive T cells in the thymus (central tolerance). Other less well-defined mechanisms may also exist to establish tolerance to *self* antigens in the peripheral circulation, possibly by a population of DCs which continually display *self* antigens to T cells in the lymph nodes in a tolerogenic rather activating environment [6, 61]. (B) Any other T cells are not negatively selected in the thymus, either because they recognize self antigens that do not have access to the thymus, or that are not expressed until after generation of the T cell repertoire in the thymus, or because they have TCR which recognize *non-self* epitopes. Alternatively, they have a TCR that binds only weakly to a self peptide displayed in the thymus, allowing the T cell to escape thymic selection. Those T cells that do not recognize any self antigens pass to the periphery to seek non-self antigens.

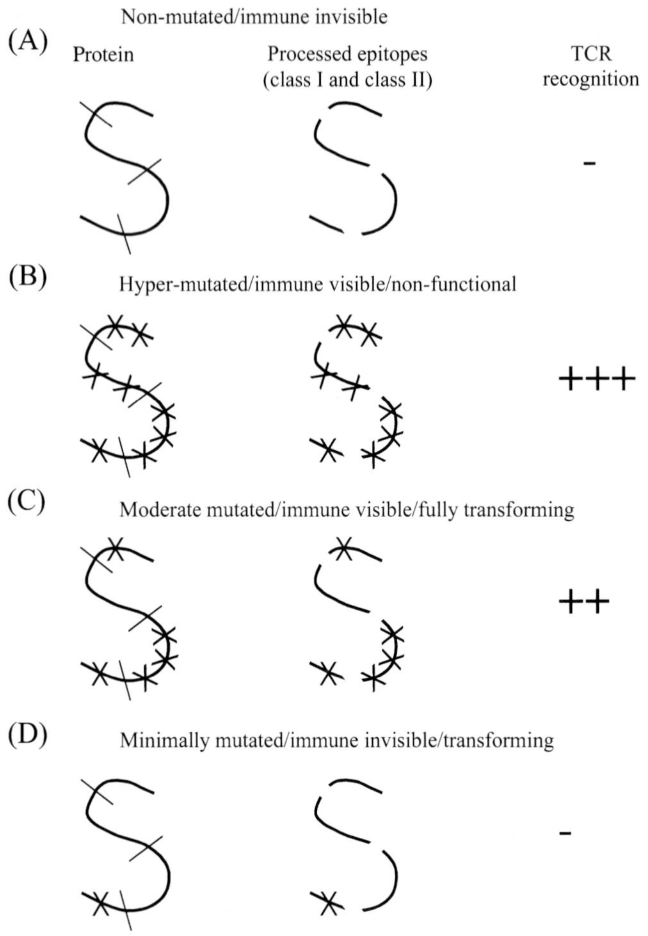

**Fig. 10.2** How immune selection might determine the range of mutations that are clinically observed in oncoproteins. (A) A wild-type protein involved in control of cell growth/differentiation is a self antigen that is invisible to the immune system because there are no T cells with TCR specificity to any of the antigenic epitopes derived from it. (B) Hyper-mutation of this protein would lead to loss of function, so the protein would be non-transforming and highly immunogenic. (C) A smaller number of defined mutations might make the protein optimally onco-genic. These mutations would generate a significant number of foreign epitopes that would be recognized by circulating T cells. Therefore, cells containing these proteins would be rejected by the immune system. (D) A protein containing a minimal number of mutations might be less transforming but would generate epitopes that were so weakly recognized (if at all) by peripheral T cells that the protein would be oncogenic but in-visible to the immune system. Cells carrying such mutations would sur-vive immune-selection and contribute to cancer etiology. This model might explain in part why many transforming mutations in human cancers are very subtle.

backup help from the many checkpoints that must be overcome purely at the level of cell growth and differentiation control to generate a malignant cell [3]. Simultaneously, autoimmune disease is also largely avoided by not having a trigger-happy immune system perpetually able to recognize small variants of self antigens. So, if the sensitivity of the immune system is set at a level that is optimal for propagation of the species, might we be able to give it a boost by tipping the balance towards recognition of tumor antigens? To find out whether this is possible, we need to understand the nature of tumor antigens and immune responses to them.

## 10.3
## Tumor Antigens and Responses to Them

At best, tumor-associated antigens (TAAs) are overtly foreign, e. g. many cervical cancer cells express the papillomavirus oncoproteins E6 and E7. However, much more commonly they are either immunologically 'near-self' or 'self'. Self antigens are not altered in any way with respect to the same protein expressed in normal cells. Other proteins in a cancer cell are mutated versions of the corresponding normal protein. These mutations are most often directly responsible for cellular transformation and/ or metastasis. Epitopes derived from the mutated parts of these antigens will have a different structure from those epitopes derived from the normal cellular counterparts. The differences are usually at only one or a few amino acid positions and so these antigens are termed near-self (Fig. 10.2D). As near-self epitopes diverge in structure (sequence) from the corresponding self epitopes, so the chances of T cells with T cell receptors (TCRs) reactive to them increases – the dividing line between where near-self becomes foreign determines the ability of the immune system to recognize and destroy tumor cells (Fig. 10.3). In addition, some non-mutated self proteins can be expressed on tumor cells but not expressed on other adult tissues. Thus, some melanoma-associated antigens are only expressed normally during early development, but are switched off at later times (except in a very few restricted tissues). These antigens, when expression is reactivated within tumor cells, can therefore serve as target antigens since they are effectively now tumor specific. Finally, tumor cells can also express self antigens which are expressed at higher levels than they are normally expressed on other tissue types. Since density of expression can act as a signal for T cell recognition of antigens, especially for T cells with low-affinity TCR recognition of antigen, self antigens can also be effectively near-self if they are over-expressed on the tumor cells (Fig. 10.2) [4, 5].

## 10.4
## Antigen Presentation – A Resume

So, at least in theory, tumors are likely to express at least some epitopes that could form the basis of immune recognition. However, antigen expression alone is not enough. For antigens to be recognized, and reacted to, by the immune system, they

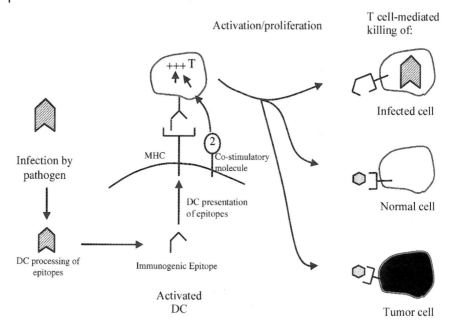

**Fig. 10.3**  Generation of autoreactive and tumor-reactive responses. If a pathogenic infection is associated with a protein that resembles a self antigen, presentation of that antigen by activated DCs could activate a T cell that has high affinity for the pathogenic epitope but retains some affinity for the self-derived epitope. Activation and prolifera-tion of this T cell would induce recognition of cells infected by the pathogen but also now normal cells expressing the self peptide on its own MHC molecules. In addition, if the *self* peptide is actually a tumor-associated peptide, these T cells will also recognize tumor cells.

have to be presented by dendritic cells (DCs) or other professional antigen-present-ing cells (APCs) in the appropriate context. For optimal immune activation against an antigen it has to be taken up by an APC within the context of a highly immunosti-mulatory (cytokine-rich) environment. This environment both recruits APCs to the site of antigen release and, critically, activates them. Activation of APCs means that they not only process and present the epitopes from the antigen, but they also ex-press high levels of co-stimulatory molecules (see Appendix), such as adhesion mole-cules and those of the B7 family. A T cell will only be fully activated to respond to an epitope if it receives signals from binding the epitope/MHC molecule and additional co-stimulatory signals provided by binding to these co-stimulatory molecules on the surface of the activated APCs (see also Fig. 10.4A). Simultaneously, within the target cells (in our case tumor cells) cellular antigens are continually processed within the cell and presented as small peptides (8–13 amino acids) in the context of major histo-compatibility complex (MHC) class I molecules. In this way, the immune system can continually sample the antigenic content of cells through TCR recognition. As already described, T cells with TCRs which can bind self epitopes bound to MHC class I molecules have been negatively selected and so will not be present to bind these epitopes. However, any T cells which can bind an epitope through presentation by an activated APC will now recognize any cell that displays these epitopes on their surface class I molecules. This then illustrates the critical link between the uptake of antigen by APC in a fully co-stimulatory environment, and the subsequent effector phase of target cell recognition and killing by fully activated T cells.

In the case of tumor antigens, therefore, the antigen displayed by the tumor cell in the context of MHC class I needs to be recognized by peripheral T cells bearing TCRs with the acuity to bind the epitopes derived from the mutated regions of these proteins, whilst distinguishing these from epitopes derived from wild-type versions of the proteins (Fig. 10.3). One type of tumor antigen that stands a high chance of doing this is one that contains novel epitopes created by fusion of self proteins, such as the Bcr–Abl junction fragment [5]. However, as we discussed above, many onco-genic mutations are very subtle (e.g. point mutations in oncoproteins such as Ras). There are likely to be only a few T cells with TCRs which have the fine structure to distinguish a *self* from a *near-self* epitope (Fig. 10.3B), unless the changes in the *near-self* epitope are very significant. Any such T cells would be critically valuable in clear-ing tumor cells, but not related, normal cells (Fig. 10.3C). In addition, a small num-ber of peripheral T cells might retain the ability to recognize unaltered self epitopes, There are three reasons why this might occur: (1) a self antigen might resemble a foreign antigen – a phenomenon known as molecular mimicry (see Appendix), (2) T cells carrying low-affinity TCR for an antigen might have been overlooked by the pro-cess of thymic deletion as described in Box 10.1 and Fig. 10.3 or (3) there might be a lack of central tolerance to the antigen because it is inaccessible to thymic APCs dur-ing the formation of the T cell repertoire [6]. Therefore, the T cell armory available for the war on cancer is probably populated by T cells carrying, at best, TCRs that can only weakly recognize subdominant epitopes (see Appendix) of self proteins and/or weakly immunogenic epitopes of TAAs derived from mutated self proteins (Fig. 10.3). The existence of such T cells is tolerated (Box 10.1) because even if they be-come inadvertently activated to recognize self antigens, that recognition might not lead to catastrophic autoimmune disease. An example of this is vitiligo, the skin de-pigmentation that occurs in some patients undergoing treatment with melanoma vaccines, when an effective immune response is generated not only against the mela-noma cells, but also against melanocytes [7].

It is this army of "second-rate" T cells that we must collaborate with in devising anti-tumor immunization strategies (Fig. 10.3). The next question, then, is how we ma-nipulate these intrinsically weak responses to make them resemble responses to truly foreign antigens.

## 10.5
### Playing to Strengths

In the immune responses against pathogenic infection, the immune system is work-ing against a set of clearly defined, outstandingly foreign antigens. These antigens are usually associated with overtly inflammatory, pathological situations – such as

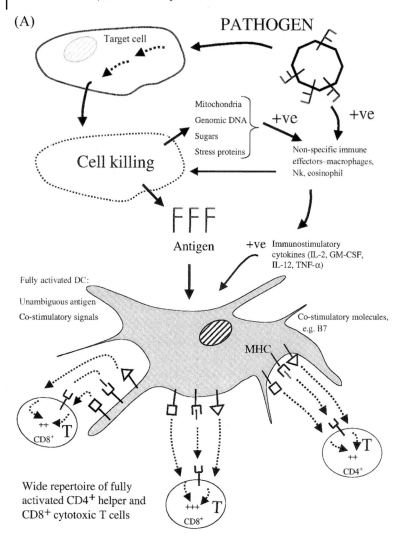

**Fig. 10.4** Lessons for tumor immunotherapy from normal immune function. (A) What the immune system does well. An invading pathogen activates non-specific immune effectors such as natural killer cells, macrophages and eosinophils. This releases cellular contents and foreign antigens into a highly immunostimulatory environment that recruits and activates APCs such as DCs. Uptake, processing and presentation of the tumor antigens in this environment occurs in the presence of full co-stimulation (adhesion molecules and those of the B7 family). This presentation activates a large pool of T cells with receptors (TCRs) that can recognize foreign epi-topes from the pathogen's proteins. (B) What the immune system does poorly. In the case of tumor growth, there is normally no invading pathogen and little or no physiologically abnormal cell death. Any antigen that is released is either self or near-self. Therefore, even if these antigens are ingested by APCs they are presented in an immunosuppressive environment lacking co-stimulation. Very few T cells have TCRs that can recognize tumor-associated epitopes and any T cells bearing these TCRs are likely to be rendered anergic by presentation of the epitopes in the absence of full APC activation.

(B)

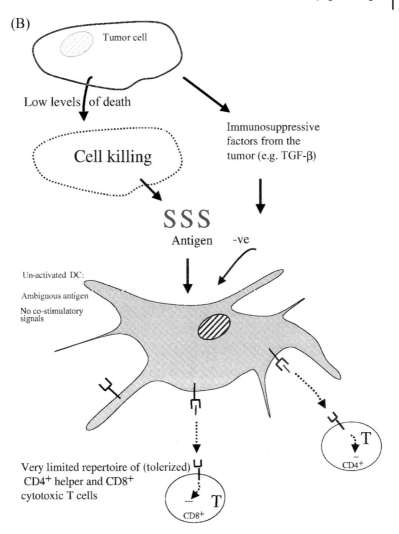

Tumor cell

Low levels of death

Cell killing

Immunosuppressive factors from the tumor (e.g. TGF-β)

S S S
Antigen    -ve

Un-activated DC:

Ambiguous antigen

No co-stimulatory signals

Very limited repertoire of (tolerized) CD4+ helper and CD8+ cytotoxic T cells

T
CD4+

T
CD8+

cell death of infected cells and cytokine-rich environments created by reactivity against the antigens (Fig. 10.4A). There is also likely to be a large number of naive T cells with TCR specificities that can bind epitopes from the immunogens when presented by APCs (Fig. 10.3). The APCs will also have been activated by the inflammatory milieu. This will provide high levels of co-stimulatory molecules in association with which the antigenic epitopes will be presented to the T cells – resulting in a vigorous and potent clearative response (Fig. 10.4A).

In the case of tumor cell recognition (Fig. 10.4B), however, the repertoire of antigenic targets is far less clearly defined and is much more subversive [8]. Until the tumor develops a necrotic core, which occurs when its growth has outstripped its blood supply, there is minimal cell death occurring and few tumor antigens are released, so the immune system has no particular reason to react to tumor growth [9]. There is often no reason for APCs to be attracted to the tumor; indeed, tumors often se-crete factors, such as transforming growth factor (TGF)-β or interleukin (IL)-10, that actively inhibit such migration [10] (Fig. 10.4B). Moreover, as discussed above, any antigen that is released from the tumor cells will be of a very different nature from those presented by invading pathogens. This means that the repertoire of T cells with any chance of recognizing TAAs is small (Figs 10.3 and 10.4B). Indeed, any antigen that is presented by host APCs in the absence of adequate levels of activation of the APC might even be worse than no antigen at all, because the presentation of antigen in the absence of co-stimulation will tolerize the host to the antigen [6, 11, 12]. Reactive T cells die on encountering antigen in the absence of a co-stimulatory signal [13] – a fail-safe mechanism whose primary function is to block autoimmunity (Fig. 10.4B) [14]. Finally, even if T cells can be activated against tumor antigens, T cells might not be able to kill the tumor cell because many tumors lose expression of MHC molecules, making recognition of the cells by activated T cells very difficult. So what hope do we have of turning this at best, feeble, and at worst, tolerizing, envir-onment into one that resembles infection? We know that there are situations in which the immune system mounts a vigorous attack on self antigens; when this oc-curs, autoimmune disease is the result. So can autoimmunity teach us anything about how to boost an antitumor response?

## 10.6
### Exploiting Weaknesses: Autoimmunity

The simplest model for the development of most autoimmune disease is the initia-tion of autoreactivity to a single self antigen (Fig. 10.5A) [15]. This may later spread to reactivity against several antigens as a result of epitope spreading. This is the si-tuation where a strong immune reactivity is generated against a potently immuno-genic antigen (i. e. one to which TCR reactivity is strong) through transfer of the anti-gen into APC, their full activation and presentation of epitopes derived from the anti-gen to reactive T cells. At the same time as this occurs, other poorly immunogenic antigens (i. e. ones to which weak TCR reactivity might exist) will also be transferred into the APC, processed and presented to the T cell repertoire in the context of full co-stimulation. Any T cells which can then bind epitopes from these other antigens will also be activated. In this way, an immune reactivity to a weakly immunogenic antigen can also be generated through the process of generating a response to a strongly immunogenic antigen. This process of epitope spreading is probably criti-cally important in the generation of autoimmune reactivity to autoantigens – and can be exploited to generate responses against weak tumor antigens. Most tissues can be subjected to immune attack against an antigen expressed exclusively in that organ (e. g. neurons in multiple sclerosis [16] or β cells in type 1 diabetes) [15]. The pathology is usually mediated by T cells [17], but autoantibodies can also be responsi-ble through the provision of CD4$^+$ T cell help (see Appendix) (Fig. 10.5A) [18]. Sus-ceptibility to autoimmune disease is determined by genetic and environmental factors that determine "the overall reactivity and quality of cells of the immune system" [15]. Genetic linkages to autoimmune diseases [19] that affect genes involved in general immunoreactivity [20] include genes encoding cytokines, molecules involved in cell proliferation and inhibitors of apoptosis, as well as genes involved specifically in antigen presentation and recognition [15, 21, 22]. For example, there is a strong genetic contribution to the development of rheumatoid arthritis at various HLA-DR alleles (especially HLA-DRB1*0401 and *0404 in Europeans [15, 21, 22]). These data suggest that such individuals may be able to present epitopes from self-derived antigens more effectively than other members of the population. If so, it may be that cancer patients of particular haplotypes may be more capable of presenting self, or near-self, epitopes derived from oncogenic mutations that arise in particular cancer types. Such correlative studies are only in their infancy, but may provide the cancer immunotherapy field with a rich resource in diagnostic information for the design of cancer vaccine strategies on a patient-by-patient basis.

It has also been anecdotally reported that infections (usually with unknown agents) are associated with the onset of many autoimmune diseases and the nature of the response to infections can skew immune responses in directions that can promote autoimmune development (Fig. 10.5A) [23]. In animal models of autoimmune disease, the injection of adjuvants (see Appendix) is usually necessary [24] – and sometimes sufficient [25, 26] – to induce the pathology. This is directly reminiscent of one of the few truly successful immunotherapy treatments for cancer; thus, treatment of bladder cancer can be effective by treatment with BCG which is believed to work by acting as a powerful adjuvant to stimulate both non-specific and specific antitumor immune effector cells to clear the tumor cell population. Thus, adjuvants can either improve immune responses to unrelated self antigens (Fig. 10.5A) [27], promote cross-reaction with autoantigens through molecular mimicry (see Appendix) (Fig. 10.3) [28] or act to inhibit T cell death following activation and killing [29, 30].

These characteristics of autoimmune disease offer significant encouragement for the development of tumor immunotherapies [31–35]. If self antigens exist in most tissues that can be the targets of T and B cell immune reactivity, cancers of most histological types could potentially be targeted by immune responses if the appropriate target antigens could be identified. The other side of the coin is clearly that there is a concomitant danger of developing autoimmunity against the tissue from which the tumor derives (see below). It might also be possible to exploit an understanding of the genetic determinants of autoimmunity to tip the balance towards antitumor immune reactivity (Fig. 10.3). In particular, genes affecting T cell recognition of peptides (e. g. specific MHC haplotypes) are often central to the development of autoimmune disease [15, 20, 22]. Finally, the mechanisms that promote the unintentional turning of the immune system against self targets also means that it might be possible to copy these mechanisms to enhance the immunogenicity of self or near-self tumor antigens [23]. So, it might be possible to use the initiating agents for autoimmune disease [24–27, 30] as adjuvants in immunotherapy. In addition, mimicry of tumor antigens by other closely related antigens [36] from naturally occurring microorganisms might, if they can be found, yield tumor antigen-specific vaccination strategies. In addition, if the presumed infectious agent that initiates, for example, mul-

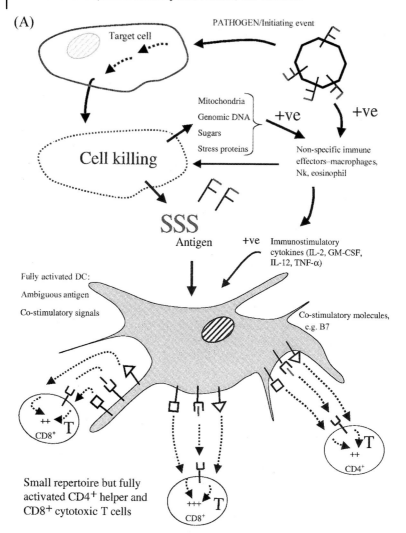

**Fig. 10.5** How the immune system could be manipulated for effective antitumor immunotherapy. (A) What the immune system should not do: In autoimmune disease, it is believed that some initiating factor, e.g. viral or bacterial infection, serves as an adjuvant to initiate cell death of the target tissue. Antigen release occurs in the context of full immune activation. Molecular mimicry of a self antigen by a pathogenic antigen or direct activation of a potentially self-reactive T cell leads to activation of an autoimmune response from a small repertoire of such T cells. (B) What we would like the immune system to do. Effective immunotherapy strategies for cancer will combine elements from Figs 10.4 (A) and 10.5 (A) (e.g. identification of foreign pathogens or autoimmune initiating agents along with gene transfer) to stimulate tumor cell killing and promote the creation of a highly immunostimulatory environment associated with release of tumor antigens. Although the antigens released will be predominantly self or near-self, they will be presented in a stimulatory fashion to a small pool of potentially reactive T cells that might have the ability to initiate and maintain antitumor immune responses.

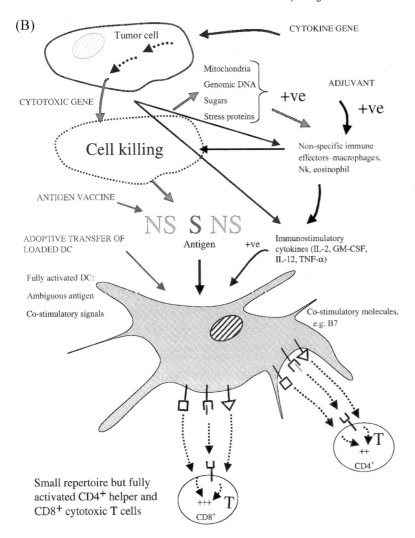

(B)

tiple sclerosis could be identified, perhaps it could be used in a modified form or context as an adjuvant for tumor vaccination (although clearly whatever the context, or form, of the agent is that promotes multiple sclerosis would have to be nullified). Many autoimmune diseases also proceed through a series of cycles of relapse and remission, perhaps stimulated by periodic trauma or episodes of inflammation. Might immunotherapies directed against predominantly self or near-self tumor antigens be most effective if given as repeated vaccinations to overcome the natural waning of T cell responses [37]? We should, therefore, be able to learn a great deal about how to induce tumor immunity by understanding how the immune system is duped during autoimmune disease initiation and progression.

**10.7**
**Combining the Best of Both Worlds**

It is already clear from both *in vitro* and *in vivo* tumor model systems [31–35, 38, 39], as well as from clinical experience of autoimmune disease, that the immune system can be re-educated to recognize self/near-self antigens to the point of mounting clearative immune responses against them. In fact, a surprisingly wide variety of different approaches (Fig. 10.6) have proved effective in animal models of tumor rejection [4, 5, 12, 40–56]. The literature of tumor immunotherapy in (transplantable) rodent models (i.e. immunocompetent mice injected with tumor cells derived from syngeneic mice) is so full of different success stories that it would seem that curing cancer in mice is little more than a case of choose your gene and use it! Yet immunotherapy in human oncology remains only very much at the periphery of clinical utility [57]. This discrepancy highlights the deficiencies of the animal models of tumorigenesis that have been used in the past and, in reality, such systems may more faithfully represent models of parasitic infections than growth of human tumors. This is because many of the tumor cell lines used to establish tumors in animal models have been passaged for many years in tissue culture and may have lost many of the characteristics that define true tumors which develop over time in the presence of an intact host immune system [58]. Nonetheless, despite criticisms of the models used, it is now possible to rationalize the apparently highly diverse range of successful approaches into a few common principles. Most successful immunotherapies for cancer culminate in a common pathway that starts by *tumor cell killing* (Figs 10.5B and 10.6).

Tumor cell killing can be achieved in many ways – directly by cytotoxic gene expression or indirectly through activation of both specific (T cells) or non-specific [59] (natural killer, eosinophils, macrophages) immune mechanisms through expression of co-stimulatory molecules, adjuvants, cytokines, immunogens and so on (Figs 10.5B and 10.6). However, not all tumor cell death is equal [9, 37, 60–63]. In general, it is not only important to kill tumor cells, but to make sure that they 'suffer' as they die, i.e. that they show biochemical markers of a 'stressful death' [60]. This labels them as 'pathologically abnormal' to the immune system (Fig. 10.4A) – distinguishing them from cells that are undergoing 'normal' cell death, such as occurs during development [9, 37, 64]. In particular, cells dying a stressful death express heat shock proteins [48, 60, 62, 65] and cause the unhindered [60, 66] release of intracellular molecules that are natural activators of DCs [61, 63, 67, 68] (Fig. 10.5B). By contrast, 'normal' cell death is likely to lead both to induction of tolerance to cellular antigens at the level of DC function [6] and to the neat packaging and removal of all of these materials by phagocytes before they can signal immunological danger (see Appendix) [37, 60, 66, 69–71].

There is also a fine balance between the mechanisms of cell death and the levels of that death. Even if cells die a stress-free death by apoptosis, if the levels of apoptosis are too high for phagocytes to clear up the debris, autoimmune pathology results [72, 73]. It might be possible to exploit the reactions to this form of cell death for antitumor vaccination [74, 75]: if a good source of tumor antigen is available, then

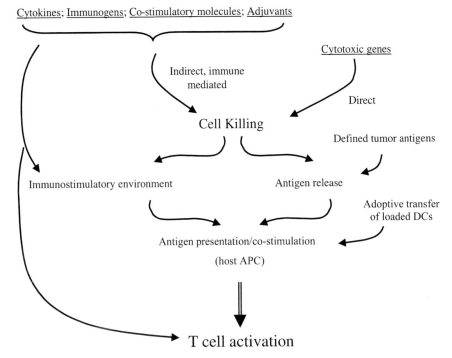

Cytokines; Immunogens; Co-stimulatory molecules; Adjuvants

Cytotoxic genes

Indirect, immune mediated

Direct

Cell Killing

Defined tumor antigens

Immunostimulatory environment

Antigen release

Adoptive transfer of loaded DCs

Antigen presentation/co-stimulation

(host APC)

T cell activation

**Fig. 10.6** Multiple different strategies lead to successful vaccination in tumor models by convergence into a common mechanistic pathway. A wide variety of different approaches have proved effective in animal models of tumor rejection [40], including transfer of genes encoding multiple cytokines [41, 42], co-stimulatory molecules [43, 44], foreign immunogens [45], allogeneic MHC molecules [46, 47], cytotoxic genes [48], heat shock proteins [49], etc. Vaccinations have been achieved with defined tumor antigens [4, 5], antigen-loaded DCs [12, 50–53] and auto-logous/allogeneic cell vaccines [88, 90]. In addition, there is a much older history of the use of adjuvants based on various bacterial and other materials [54–56]. It is, however, now possible to rationalize the apparently highly diverse range of successful approaches into a few common principles. A synthesis of the literature indicates that most successful immunotherapies for cancer culminate in a common pathway which starts by tumor cell killing leading to antigen release, uptake by APCs and presentation in a fully activated environment.

most of the above steps can be bypassed by simply loading activated DCs with tumor antigen *ex vivo* and using adoptive transfer of these cells to the patient, although caution must always be retained in case the antitumor therapy becomes so successful in breaking tolerance to tumor antigens that it is accompanied by the induction of auto-immunity to the related normal tissues [76]. Clinical trials using DCs loaded with tumor antigens have already shown considerable promise, confirming that these cells, their antigenic load and their state of activation lie firmly on the key pathways to effective tumor vaccination (see, e.g. [50, 77]).

The outstanding significance of tumor cell killing is that it leads to *antigen release* and the mechanism of cell killing is important because it needs to lead to antigen release within an environment that is highly immunostimulatory. Regardless of whether the fuel that lights this immunostimulatory fire is cytokines, adjuvant or the release of stressful markers of death (Fig. 10.5B), the important result is that APCs are recruited to the site of tumor antigen release. The APCs can then take up the released antigens, process them and present them, and, because of the immunostimulatory environment, will mature and express the full complement of co-stimulatory molecules [12, 78–81]. In this way, previously immunologically silent antigens are now 'visible' in the context of the complete repertoire of fully activated antigen-presentation pathways.

Once antigen has been provided in the context of co-stimulatory cross-presentation by host APCs [78–81], the success of the next phase of this generic tumor vaccination protocol (Fig. 10.5B) depends upon whether any T cells exist that can respond to epitopes from TAAs. As discussed above, we know that such T cells exist [5, 82] and how they might have escaped thymic selection (see Appendix) (Box 10.1). The next challenge, assuming that the full range of tumor-associated antigens is now displayed on mature APCs [78–81], is presenting the associated epitopes to the T cell repertoire in the lymph nodes to where activated APC traffick following acquisition of antigen and subsequent maturation (Fig. 10.5B). This is precisely what is likely to occur when the triggers for autoimmune diseases lead to presentation of self antigen to host T cells (Fig. 10.5A). It is not so surprising, then, and is even encouraging, that some effective tumor vaccines show signs of autoimmune side effects, in both model and clinical systems. The best-documented example of this is the induction of vitiligo in both animals and in human patients following immunotherapeutic treatments for malignant melanoma. In these cases, activation of immune responses against melanoma-associated antigens have also led to the induction of reactivity against similar, or the same, antigens expressed on normal melanocytes [14, 39, 50, 83–86].

Clearly, however, there are serious risks associated with inducing autoimmunity against self or near-self tumor antigens [76]. Immunostimulatory tumor cell killing will release not only the relevant tumor antigens, but also a flood of cellular antigens. All are equally likely to be taken up by suitably activated APCs to be presented in the context of a full co-stimulatory phenotype. If we postulate that some low-affinity T cells will exist that recognize tumor antigen-associated epitopes, it is probable that similar cells also exist to recognize cellular antigen-associated epitopes with no relevance to the tumor. How can we ensure that the immune system sifts out those antigens to which we do not want it to react (those with cellular autoimmune potential) but does develop immunity to those that we do (tumor associated autoimmunity)? This problem is not specific to induction of antitumor immunity (Fig. 10.5B); it is also relevant to normal infection, when the death of infected cells liberates both foreign and normal cellular antigens (Fig. 10.4A) [6]. Recently it has been suggested that a population of immature DCs [87] continually induces peripheral (as opposed to central or thymic) tolerance to self antigens, by ingesting antigens in apoptotic bodies released by normal turnover of tissues [6, 61] and subsequently presenting them to T cells in the lymph nodes. Since these antigens are taken up in a tolerogenic manner by the DCs (i.e. the absence of co-stimulatory molecules) any T cells with reactive TCR are induced to die. During infection, antigens released from the infected tissue will be released in the immunostimulatory environment created by the infection (Fig. 10.5A). Now, DCs which pick up the pathogenic antigens will be able to prime T cell responses against them whilst tolerance has previously been established for all other cellular antigens which are co-released. This does not bode well for the development of cancer vaccines because the antigens involved are predominantly self and will have been sampled previously – indeed this may be one mechanism by which immune unresponsiveness (tolerance) to tumor antigens develop since the tumor site is usually a site of immunosuppression and the DCs picking up antigens from there will not be activated. However, once again, the fact that autoimmune disease can develop despite such processes gives hope that inducing reactivity to self or near-self tumor antigens will, at least in some circumstances, be viable [35].

The greatest challenge, then, lies in developing antitumor vaccination strategies that combine efficacy (breaking tolerance to TAAs) with safety (preventing widespread autoimmunity). These considerations argue strongly that the safest form of antitumor vaccination would come from protocols using one, or a few, defined, tumor-specific antigens for which the potential for presentation of specific epitopes of that antigen is known in the context of the specific MHC haplotype of each patient. In general, the present view on the most efficacious approach is the converse – the relative paucity of known tumor antigens means that vaccines based on whole-cell preparations should provide a broader portfolio of antigens relevant to the tumor [88]. However, the whole-cell vaccine approach also increases the risk of liberating non-TAAs to which potentially self reactivity will be detrimental. If we have a clearer understanding of exactly which cellular antigens can form the basis of autoimmune reactions then we may be able to design the cell vaccine approach more precisely to exclude the possibility of generating deleterious autoimmune reactivity whilst inducing beneficial antitumor reactivity. This is also a concern when the tumor antigens are themselves not exclusively restricted to the tumor, but are also expressed on other, normal cells. In some situations, such as the development of vitiligo whilst undergoing immune therapies for malignant melanoma [50, 83], the trade-off between autoimmune destruction of normal tissue and continued development of malignant disease might be an acceptable bargain. However, in others, such as the prospect of autoimmune destruction of the colon or brain during immune-mediated treatment for colorectal cancer or glioma, this might not be the case [32, 34].

## 10.8
## The Way Forward

So, in many cancer patients the immune system is probably functioning as well as it can within the confines of its responsibilities to protect against infectious disease while avoiding autoimmune disease. We now need to learn how to manipulate antitumor immunity within these confines and push it in the direction of, but not too far towards, the generation of autoimmune-like reactivity.

Key advances in the coming years will come from the ability to profile each type of tumor to determine the range of antigens that are expressed. Eventually it will be possible to match these expression profiles with those antigens known to be truly self, and against which no residual T cell reactivity can exist within a specific patient's MHC haplotype. In contrast, other antigens will match with those for which some T cells are likely to exist with at least some capacity to recognize self or near-self-derived epitopes. To get to this stage, deeper understanding of the mechanisms of central and peripheral tolerance will be required [6]; greater numbers of immunologically relevant tumor-specific antigens will have to be described [4, 5]; the epitopes of these antigens will need to be mapped and their relationship to different MHC haplotypes determined. In this way, it might genuinely be possible to match tumor expression and patient MHC haplotype profiles to predict which antigen-based vaccine strategies stand a reasonable chance of success. Simultaneously, it will be necessary to develop effective ways to associate the expression of these antigens with immunologically dangerous/pathological situations that resemble the situations to which the immune system reacts extremely aggressively (Fig. 10.4). One particularly good way to do this might simply be to place those antigens in appropriately activated DCs for adoptive transfer to the patient [51, 52]. In addition, study of autoimmune initiating mechanisms will help immunotherapists understand the activities and therapeutic value of novel adjuvants, both in the context of molecular mimicry with tumor antigens and in their ability to initiate epitope spreading [36]. Advances in the treatment of autoimmune disease will also provide safety nets for cancer immunotherapists who may, at some point, want to dampen down effective tumor vaccination protocols that threaten to become too aggressive in the patient. Improved vaccination schedules may also be devised based on the observed waxing/waning patterns of progression of autoimmune disease. Finally it should eventually become possible to exploit analogous, but opposite, approaches to those used in autoimmune therapy to enhance antitumor immune reactivity – such as [38] and [14] or [89] and [41].

In much the same way that not everybody develops autoimmune disease, so the success of immunotherapy for different cancers will depend heavily on several factors: (1) the histological type of the tumor and the range of antigens that it expresses, (2) the individual tumor profile within that histological type and (3) the genetic constitution of the individual patient. Perhaps there are certain combinations of tumors and hosts for which there will never be a good match between immunizing antigens and potentially reactive T cells. So it will be important to manage the expectations of the clinical oncology community and raise the possibility that universally effective immune therapies might not be an achievable goal.

Up to a certain point, the similarities between what those agents that trigger autoimmune disease can achieve, and what tumor immunologists would like to achieve, coincide very closely. The existence of autoimmune disease provides hope that immunotherapy can be successful. Perhaps if these two fields of immunology combined forces, e. g. through creation of interdisciplinary meetings and scientific collaborations, we could not only learn how to induce potent antitumor immune responses, but also how to prevent autoimmune disease by mimicking those mechanisms that tumors recruit to avoid triggering what are effectively autoimmune responses. However, before any of us can hope to appreciate the interests of others, we will all have to start by understanding our self.

## Acknowledgments

I thank Toni Higgins for expert secretarial assistance. R. V. is supported by the Mayo Foundation and some of the ideas for this review came from support from NIH grant RO1 CA85931.

## Appendix: Glossary

*Adjuvants.* Materials (often derived from microorganisms) which stimulate the innate immune system. This stimulates the production of inflammatory cytokines, and leads to recruitment and activation of APCs by inducing expression of MHC class II molecules as well as co-stimulatory proteins.

*Antigen/epitope.* Any protein expressed in a cell. Antigens are continually proteolytically processed within the cell and presented as small fragments (8–13 amino acids) – known as *epitopes* – in the context of MHC class I or II molecules to T cells. Any T cells which express a TCR with a high enough affinity for any of the epitope/MHC complexes will recognize cells expressing the parent antigen from which the epitope was derived.

*CD4 T cell help.* Generation of an effective immune response to an antigen requires presentation of epitopes of the antigen to both CD8$^+$ T cells and CD4$^+$ T cells. CD4 T cell activation leads to the secretion of helper cytokines which activate other immune cells (including the CD8 T cells) important in generating a potent immune response to the antigen.

*Central tolerance.* APCs in the thymus display epitopes of self proteins in the context of MHC molecules to naive T cells. Any T cells which express a TCR with a high enough binding affinity for any self/MHC complex is induced to die by apoptosis This *thymic deletion* of potentially self-reactive T cells helps to induce immunological tolerance whereby antigen-specific cells can co-exist with antigen expressing cells in the periphery (see Box 10.1).

*Co-stimulatory molecules.* A naive T cell will only be fully activated when binding an epitope/MHC molecule on the surface of an APC if it also receives additional activating signals. These are provided by binding of co-stimulatory molecules – such as B7 and OX-40L – on the surface of the APC to receptors on the T cell surface.

*FOREIGN* antigens. Cells infected by invading pathogens express proteins from the pathogen. Processing of these *foreign* antigens usually yields epitopes which are distinct from *self* epitopes.

*Immunological danger signals.* Antigens must be presented in the appropriate context of a highly immunostimulatory environment (the key component of which are proinflammatory cytokines) to recruit APC and, critically, to activate them to express high levels of co-stimulatory molecules. Molecules that initiate the creation of this immunostimulatory environment may be referred to as danger signals [37, 60, 66, 69–71].

*Molecular mimicry.* Processed epitopes of different proteins may resemble each other in amino acid sequence sufficiently that, when bound to the same MHC molecule, a single TCR will recognize either complex and become activated. The activated T cells will then recognize cells expressing either of the two proteins (see Fig. 10.3).

*NEAR-SELF tumor antigens.* Some cellular proteins in a cancer cell will be mutated. Epitopes derived from the mutated parts of these antigens will have a different structure from those epitopes derived from the normal cellular counterparts and so there are likely to be only a few T cells with TCR which have the fine structure to distinguish a *self* from a *near-self* epitope.

*SELF antigens.* Normal (unmutated) cellular antigens. Generally no, or very few, T cells exist that recognize them.

*Subdominant epitopes.* Following vaccination with a given antigen, the majority of the T cell response (at least initially) will be directed against only one, or a few, dominant epitopes derived from that antigen. The remaining minority of the reactive T cells will recognize other subdominant epitopes. The nature of an epitope as dominant or subdominant will be determined by a variety of factors, including the affinity with which the epitope binds to MHC molecules and its interactions with other components of the antigen-presenting pathway.

*Tumor antigen.* Any cellular antigen that is expressed exclusively or predominantly by tumor cells. Epitopes from tumor antigens have the potential to stimulate tumor-specific immune reactivity, provided T cells with appropriate TCR exist to recognize them.

# References

1  BURNET FM. The concept of immunological surveillance. *Prog Exp Tumor Res* 1970; **13**: 1–27.

2  SHANKARAN V, IKEDA H, BRUCE AT, WHITE JM, SWANSON PE, OLD LJ, SCHREIBER RD. IFN-γ and lymphocytes prevent primary tumour development and shape tumour immunogenicity. *Nature* 2001; **410**: 1107–1111.

3  VOGELSTEIN B, KINZLER KW. The multi-step nature of cancer. *Trends Genet* 1993; **9**: 138–141.

4  BOON T, VAN DER BRUGGEN P. Human tumor antigens recognized by T lymphocytes. *J Exp Med* 1996; **183**: 725–729.

5  ROSENBERG SA. Progress in human tumour immunology and immunotherapy. *Nature* 2001; **411**: 380–384.

6  STEINMAN RM, TURLEY S, MELLMAN I, INABA K. The induction of tolerance by dendritic cells that have captured apoptotic cells [Comment]. *J Exp Med* 2000; **191**: 411–416.

7  BARNHILL RL. Malignant melanoma – pathology and prognostic factors. *Curr Opin Oncol* 1993; **5**: 364–376.

8  SPEISER DE, MIRANDA R, ZAKARIAN A, BACHMANN MF, MCKALL-FAIENZA K, ODERMATT B, HANAHAN D, ZINKERNAGEL R, OHASHI PS. Self antigens expressed by solid tumors do not efficiently stimulate naive or activated T cells: implications for immunotherapy. *J Exp Med* 1997; **186**: 645–653.

9  MELCHER AA, GOUGH MJ, TODRYK S, VILE RG. Apoptosis or necrosis for tumour immunotherapy – what's in a name? *J Mol Med* 1999; **77**: 824–833.

10  GORELIK L, FLAVELL RA. Immune-mediated eradication of tumors through the blockade of transforming growth factor-β signaling in T cells. *Nat Med* 2001; **7**: 1118–1122.

11  ANDERSON CC, MATZINGER P. Immunity or tolerance: opposite outcomes of microchimerism from skin grafts. *Nat Med* 2001; **7**: 80–87.

12  BANCHEREAU J, STEINMAN RM. Dendritic cells and the control of immunity. *Nature* 1998; **392**: 245–252.

13  ALLISON JP, KRUMMEL MF. The Yin and Yan of T cell costimulation. *Science* 1995; **270**: 932–933.

14  VAN ELSAS A, HURWITZ AA, ALLISON JP. Combination immunotherapy of B16 melanoma using anti-cytotoxic T lymphocyte-associated antigen 4 (CTLA-4) and granulocyte/macrophage colony-stimulating factor (GM-CSF)-producing vaccines induces rejection of subcutaneous and metastatic tumors accompanied by autoimmune depigmentation. *J Exp Med* 1999; **190**: 355–366.

15  MARRACK P, KAPPLER J, KOTZIN BL. Autoimmune disease: why and where it occurs. *Nat Med* 2001; **7**: 899–905.

16  STEINMAN L. Multiple sclerosis: a coordinated immunological attack against myelin in the central nervous system. *Cell* 1996; **85**: 299–302.

17  WONG FS, VISINTIN I, WEN L, FLAVELL RA, JANEWAY CA JR. CD8 T cell clones from young nonobese diabetic (NOD) islets can transfer rapid onset of diabetes in NOD mice in the absence of CD4 cells. *J Exp Med* 1996; **183**: 67–76.

18  KOTZIN BL. Systemic lupus erythematosus. *Cell* 1996; **85**: 303–306.

19  BELL JI, LATHROP GM. Multiple loci for multiple sclerosis. *Nat Genet* 1996; **13**: 377–378.

20  POLTORAK A, SMIRNOVA I, HE X, LIU MY, VAN HUFFEL C, MCNALLY O, BIRDWELL D, ALEJOS E, SILVA M, DU X, THOMPSON P, CHAN EK, LEDESMA J, ROE B, CLIFTON S, VOGEL SN, BEUTLER B. Genetic and physical mapping of the Lps locus: identification of the Toll-4 receptor as a candidate gene in the critical region. *Blood Cells Mol Dis* 1998; **24**: 340–355.

21  SEKO Y, TAKAHASHI N, AZUMA M, YAGITA H, OKUMURA K, YAZAKI Y. Expression of costimulatory molecule CD40 in murine heart with acute myocarditis and reduction of inflammation by treatment with anti-CD40L/B7–1 monoclonal antibodies. *Circ Res* 1998; **83**: 463–469.

22  QUAYLE AJ, WILSON KB, LI SG, KJELDSEN-KRAGH J, OFTUNG F, SHINNICK T,

Sioud M, Forre O, Capra JD, Natvig JB. Peptide recognition, T cell receptor usage and HLA restriction elements of human heat-shock protein (hsp) 60 and mycobacterial 65-kDa hsp-reactive T cell clones from rheumatoid synovial fluid. *Eur J Immunol* 1992; **22**: 1315–1322.

23 Lucey DR, Clerici M, Shearer GM. Type 1 and type 2 cytokine dysregulation in human infectious, neoplastic, and inflammatory diseases. *Clin Microbiol Rev* 1996; **9**: 532–562.

24 Segal BM, Klinman DM, Shevach EM. Microbial products induce autoimmune disease by an IL-12-dependent pathway. *J Immunol* 1997; **158**: 5087–5090.

25 Brackertz D, Mitchell GF, Mackay IR. Antigen-induced arthritis in mice. I. Induction of arthritis in various strains of mice. *Arthritis Rheum* 1977; **20**: 841–850.

26 Esquivel PS, Rose NR, Kong YC. Induction of autoimmunity in good and poor responder mice with mouse thyroglobulin and lipopolysaccharide. *J Exp Med* 1977; **145**: 1250–1263.

27 Chiller JM, Skidmore BJ, Morrison DC, Weigle WO. Relationship of the structure of bacterial lipopolysaccharides to its function in mitogenesis and adjuvanticity. *Proc Natl Acad Sci USA* 1973; **70**: 2129–2133.

28 Dell A, Antone SM, Gauntt CJ, Crossley CA, Clark WA, Bunningham MW. Autoimmune determinants of rheumatic carditis: localisation of epitopes in human cardiac myosin. *Eur Heart J* 1991; **12**: 158–162.

29 Kearney ER, Pape KA, Loh DY, Jenkins MK. Visualization of peptide-specific T cell immunity and peripheral tolerance induction *in vivo*. *Immunity* 1994; **1**: 327–339.

30 Vella AT, Mitchell T, Groth B, Linsley PS, Green JM, Thompson CB, Kappler JW, Marrack P. CD28 engagement and proinflammatory cytokines contribute to T cell expansion and long-term survival *in vivo*. *J Immunol* 1997; **158**: 4714–4720.

31 Bowne WB, Srinivasan R, Wolchok JD, Hawkins WG, Blachere NE, Dyall R, Lewis JJ, Houghton AN.

Coupling and uncoupling of tumor immunity and autoimmunity. *J Exp Med* 1999; **190**: 1717–1722.

32 Houghton AN. Cancer antigens: immune recognition of self and altered self. *J Exp Med* 1994; **180**: 1–4.

33 Golumbek P, Levitsky H, Jaffee E, Pardoll DM. The antitumor immune response as a problem of self–nonself discrimination: implications for immunotherapy. *Immunol Res* 1993; **12**: 183–192.

34 Pardoll DM. Inducing autoimmune disease to treat cancer. *Proc Natl Acad Sci USA* 1999; **96**: 5340–5342.

35 Parmiani G. Tumor immunity as autoimmunity: tumor antigens include normal self proteins which stimulate anergic peripheral T cells. *Immunol Today* 1993; **14**: 536–538.

36 Naftzger C, Takechi Y, Kohda H, Hara I, Vijayasaradhi S, Houghton AN. Immune response to a differentiation antigen induced by altered antigen: a study of tumor rejection and autoimmunity. *Proc Natl Acad Sci USA* 1996; **93**: 14809–14814.

37 Matzinger P. An innate sense of danger. *Semin Immunol* 1998; **10**: 399–415.

38 Harlan DM, Hengartner H, Huang ML, Kang YH, Abe R, Moreadith RW, Pircher H, Gray GS, Ohashi PS, Freeman GJ, Nadler LM, June CH, Aichele P. Mice expressing both B7-1 and viral glycoprotein on pancreatic β cells along with glycoprotein-specific transgenic T cells develop diabetes due to a breakdown of T-lymphocyte unresponsiveness. *Proc Natl Acad Sci USA* 1994; **91**: 3137–3141.

39 Overwijk WW, Lee DS, Surman DR, Irvine KR, Touloukian CE, Chan C, Carroll MW, Moss B, Rosenberg SA, Restifo NP. Vaccination with a recombinant vaccinia virus encoding a self antigen induced autoimmune vitiligo and tumor cell destruction in mice: requirement for CD4[+] T lymphocytes. *Proc Natl Acad Sci USA* 1999; **96**: 2982–2987.

40 Vile RG, Castleden SC, Upton C, Chong HC. Gene therapy for cancer using a combination of cytotoxic and

immunomodulatory genes. In: Boiron M, Marty M, eds. *Eurocancer 96.* Paris: John Libbey 1996.

**41** PARDOLL DM. Paracrine cytokine adjuvants in cancer immunotherapy. *Annu Rev Immunol* 1995; **13**: 399–415.

**42** COLOMBO MP, FORNI G. Immunotherapy: cytokine gene transfer strategies. *Cancer Metastasis Rev* 1996; **15**: 317–328.

**43** HELLSTROM KE, HELLSTROM I, CHEN L. Can co-stimulated tumor immunity be therapeutically efficacious? *Immunol Rev* 1995; **145**: 123–145.

**44** HUANG AYC, BRUCE AT, PARDOLL DM, LEVITSKY HI. Does B7–1 expression confer antigen-presenting cell capacity to tumors *in vivo*? *J Exp Med* 1996; **183**: 769–776.

**45** SCHIRRMACHER V, HAAS C, BONIFER R, AHLERT T, GERHARDS R, ERTEL C. Human tumor cell modification by virus infection: an efficient and safe way to produce cancer vaccine with pleiotropic immune stimulatory properties when using Newcastle disease virus. *Gene Ther* 1999; **6**: 63–73.

**46** NABEL GJ, CHANG A, NABEL EG, PLAUTZ G, FOX BA, HUANG L, SHU S. Clinical protocol: immunotherapy of malignancy by *in vivo* gene transfer into tumors. *Hum Gene Ther* 1992; **3**: 399–410.

**47** FABRE JW. The allogeneic response and tumor immunity. *Nat Med* 2001; **7**: 649–652.

**48** MELCHER AA, TODRYK S, HARDWICK N, FORD M, JACOBSON M, VILE RG. Tumor immunogenicity is determined by the mechanism of cell death via induction of heat shock protein expression. *Nat Med* 1998; **4**: 581–587.

**49** SRIVASTAVA PK, MENORET A, BASU S, BINDER RJ, McQUADE KL. Heat shock proteins come of age: primitive functions acquire new roles in an adaptive world. *Immunity* 1998; **8**: 657–665.

**50** BANCHEREAU J, PALUCKA AK, DHODAPKAR M, BURKEHOLDER S, TAQUET N, ROLLAND A, TAQUET S, COQUERY S, WITTKOWSKI KM, BHARDWAJ N, PINEIRO L, STEINMAN R, FAY J. Immune and clinical responses in patients with metastatic melanoma to CD34+ progenitor-derived dendritic cell vaccine. *Cancer Res* 2001; **61**: 6451–6458.

**51** NESTLE FO, BANCHEREAU J, HART D. Dendritic cells: on the move from the bench to the bedside. *Nat Med* 2001; **7**: 761–765.

**52** MELERO I, VILE RG, COLOMBO MP. Feeding dendritic cells with tumor antigens: self-service buffet or a la carte? *Gene Ther* 2000; **7**: 1167–1170.

**53** ALBERT ML, SAUTER B, BHARDWAJ N. Dendritic cells acquire antigen from apoptotic cells and induce class I-restricted CTLs. *Nature* 1998; **392**: 86–89.

**54** DALGLEISH A. The case for therapeutic vaccines. *Melanoma Res* 1996; **6**: 5–10.

**55** HOCK H, DORSCH M, KUNZENDORF U, UBERLA K, QIN Z, DIAMANSTEIN T, BLANKENSTEIN T. Vaccinations with tumor cells genetically engineered to produce different cytokines: effectivity not superior to a classical adjuvant. *Cancer Res* 1993; **53**: 714–716.

**56** SINGH M, O'HAGAN D. Advances in vaccine adjuvants. *Nat Biotechnol* 1999; **17**: 1075–1081.

**57** FORNI G, LOLLINI PL, MUSIANI P, COLOMBO MP. Immunoprevention of cancer: is the time ripe? *Cancer Res* 2000; **60**: 2571–2575.

**58** WILSON JM. Perspective series: molecular medicine in genetically engineered animals. *J Clin Invest* 1996; **97**: 1138–1141.

**59** DI CARLO E, FORNI G, LOLLINI P, COLOMBO MP, MODESTI A, MUSIANI P. The intriguing role of polymorphonuclear neutrophils in antitumor reactions. *Blood* 2001; **97**: 339–345.

**60** GOUGH MJ, MELCHER AA, AHMED A, CRITTENDEN MR, RIDDLE DS, LINARDAKIS E, RUCHATZ AN, VILE RG. Macrophages orchestrate the immune response to tumor cell death. *Cancer Res* 2001; **61**: 7240–7247.

**61** SAUTER B, ALBERT ML, FRANCISCO L, LARSSON M, SOMERSAN S, BHARDWAJ N. Consequences of cell death: exposure to necrotic tumor cells, but not primary tissue cells or apoptotic cells, induces the maturation of immunostimulatory dendritic cells. *J Exp Med* 2000; **191**: 423–434.

62 Basu S, Binder RJ, Suto R, Anderson KM, Srivastava PK. Necrotic but not apoptotic cell death releases heat shock proteins, which deliver a partial maturation signal to dendritic cells and activate the NF-κB pathway. *Int Immunol* 2000; **12**: 1539–1546.

63 Gallucci S, Lolkema M, Matzinger P. Natural adjuvants: endogenous activators of dendritic cells. *Nat Med* 1999; **5**: 1249–1255.

64 Fuchs EJ, Matzinger P. Is cancer dangerous to the immune system? *Semin Immunol* 1996; **8**: 271–280.

65 Todryk S, Melcher AA, Hardwick N, Linardakis E, Bateman A, Colombo MP, Stoppacciaro A, Vile RG. Heat shock protein 70 induced during tumor cell killing induces T$_h$1 cytokines and targets immature dendritic cell precursors to enhance antigen uptake. *J Immunol* 1999; **163**: 1398–1408.

66 Savill J, Fadok V. Corpse clearance defines the meaning of cell death. *Nature* 2000; **407**: 784–788.

67 Ishii KJ, Suzuki K, Coban C, Takeshita F, Itoh Y, Matoba H, Kohn LD, Klinman DM. Genomic DNA released by dying cells induces the maturation of APCs. *J Immunol* 2001; **167**: 2602–2607.

68 Vabulas RM, Pircher H, Lipford GB, Hacker H, Wagner H. CpG-DNA activates in vivo T cell epitope presenting dendritic cells to trigger protective antiviral cytotoxic T cell responses. *J Immunol* 2000; **164**: 2372–2378.

69 Piacentini M. Apoptosis and autoimmunity: two sides to the coin. *Cell Death Differ* 1999; **6**: 1–2.

70 Ren Y, Savill J. Apoptosis: the importance of being eaten. *Cell Growth Differ* 1998; **5**: 563–568.

71 Matzinger P. Tolerance, danger and the extended family. *Annu Rev Immunol* 1994; **12**: 991–1045.

72 Kalled SL, Cutler AH, Burkly LC. Apoptosis and altered dendritic cell homeostasis in lupus nephritis are limited by anti-CD154 treatment. *J Immunol* 2001; **167**: 1740–1747.

73 Seery JP, Cattell V, Watt FM. Cutting edge: amelioration of kidney disease in a transgenic mouse model of lupus nephritis by administration of the caspase

inhibitor carbobenzoxy-valyl-alanyl-aspartyl-(β-O-methyl)-fluoromethylketone. *J Immunol* 2001; **167**: 2452–2455.

74 Kurts C, Miller JFAP, Subramaniam RM, Carbone FR, Heath WR. Major histocompatibility complex class I-restricted cross-presentation is biased towards high dose antigens and those released during cellular destruction. *J Exp Med* 1998; **188**: 409–414.

75 Ronchetti A, Rovere P, Iezzi G, Galati G, Heltai S, Pia Protti M, Paola Garancini M, Manfredi AA, Rugarli C, Bellone M. Immunogenicity of apoptotic cells in vivo: role of antigen load, antigen-presenting cells, and cytokines. *J Immunol* 1999; **163**: 130–136.

76 Ludewig B, Ochsenbein AF, Odermatt B, Paulin D, Hengartner H, Zinkernagel RM. Immunotherapy with dendritic cells directed against tumor antigens shared with normal host cells results in severe autoimmune disease. *J Exp Med* 2000; **191**: 795–804.

77 Kugler A, Stuhler G, Walden P, Zoller G, Zobywalski A, Brossart P, Trefzer U, Ullrich S, Muller CA, Becker V, Gross AJ, Hemmerlein B, Kanz L, Muller GA, Ringert RH. Regression of human metastatic renal cell carcinoma after vaccination with tumor cell–dendritic cell hybrids. *Nat Med* 2000; **6**: 332–336.

78 Huang AYC, Golumbek P, Ahmadzadeh M, Jaffee E, Pardoll D, Levitsky H. Role of bone marrow derived cells in presenting MHC class I-restricted tumor antigens. *Science* 1994; **264**: 961–965.

79 Huang AYC, Bruce AT, Pardoll DM, Levitsky HI. In vivo cross-priming of MHC class I-restricted antigens requires a TAP transporter. *Immunity* 1996; **4**: 349–355.

80 Levitsky HI, Lazenby A, Hayashi RJ, Pardoll D. In vivo priming of two distinct antitumor effector populations: the role of MHC class I expression. *J Exp Med* 1994; **179**: 1215–1224.

81 Cayeux S, Richter G, Becker C, Pezzutto A, Dorken B, Blankenstein T. Direct and indirect T cell priming by dendritic cell vaccines. *Eur J Immunol* 1999; **29**: 255–234.

**82** BOON T, CEROTTINI JC, VAN DEN EYNDE B, VAN DER BRUGGEN P, VAN PEL A. Tumor antigens recognized by T lymphocytes. *Annu Rev Immunol* 1994; **12**: 337–365.

**83** YEE C, THOMPSON JA, ROCHE P, BYRD DR, LEE PP, PIEPKORN M, KENYON K, DAVIS MM, RIDDELL SR, GREENBERG PD. Melanocyte destruction after antigen-specific immunotherapy of melanoma: direct evidence of T cell-mediated vitiligo. *J Exp Med* 2000; **192**: 1637–1644.

**84** COLELLA TA, BULLOCK TN, RUSSELL LB, MULLINS DW, OVERWIJK WW, LUCKEY CJ, PIERCE RA, RESTIFO NP, ENGELHARD VH. Self-tolerance to the murine homologue of a tyrosinase-derived melanoma antigen: implications for tumor immunotherapy. *J Exp Med* 2000; **191**: 1221–1232.

**85** OSANTO S, SCHIPHORST PP, WEIJL NI, DIJKSTRA N, VAN WEES A, BROUWENSTEIN N, VAESSEN N, VAN KRIEKEN JH, HERMANS J, CLETON FJ, SCHRIER PI. Vaccination of melanoma patients with an allogeneic, genetically modified interleukin 2-producing melanoma cell line. *Hum Gene Ther* 2000; **11**: 739–750.

**86** STEITZ J, BRUCK J, STEINBRINK K, ENK A, KNOP J, TUTING T. Genetic immunization of mice with human tyrosinase-related protein 2: implications for the immunotherapy of melanoma. *Int J Cancer* 2000; **86**: 89–94.

**87** HUANG FP, PLATT N, WYKES M, MAJOR JR, POWELL TJ, JENKINS CD, MACPHERSON GG. A discrete subpopulation of dendritic cells transports apoptotic intestinal epithelial cells to T cell areas of mesenteric lymph nodes. *J Exp Med* 2000; **191**: 435–443.

**88** JAFFEE EM, HRUBAN RH, BIEDRZYCKI B, LAHERU D, SCHEPERS K, SAUTER PR, GOEMANN M, COLEMAN J, GROCHOW L, DONEHOWER RC, LILLEMOE KD, O'REILLY S, ABRAMS RA, PARDOLL DM, CAMERON JL, YEO CJ. Novel allogeneic granulocyte-macrophage colony-stimulating factor-secreting tumor vaccines for pancreatic cancer: a phase I trial of safety and immune activation. *J Clin Oncol* 2001; **19**: 145–156.

**89** PRUD'HOMME GJ. Gene therapy of autoimmune diseases with vectors encoding regulatory cytokines or inflammatory cytokine inhibitors. *J Gene Med* 2000; **2**: 222–232.

**90** SIMONS JW, JAFFEE EM, WEBER CE, LEVITSKY HI, NELSON WG, CARDUCCI MA, LAZENBY AJ, COHEN LK, FINN CC, CLIFT SM, HAUDA KM, BECK LA, LEIFERMAN KM, OWENS AH, PIANTADOSI S, DRANOFF G, MULLIGAN RC, PARDOLL DM, MARSHAL FF. Bioactivity of autologous irradiated renal cell carcinoma vaccines generated by *ex vivo* granulocyte-macrophage colony-stimulating factor gene transfer. *Cancer Res* 1997; **57**: 1537–1546.

**91** MATZINGER P, GUERDER S. Does T cell tolerance require a dedicated antigen presenting cell? *Nature* 1989; **338**: 74–76.

**92** ZAL TA, VOLKMANN A, STOCKINGER B. Mechanisms of tolerance induction in major histocompatibility complex class II-restricted T cells specific for a blood borne self-antigen. *J Exp Med* 1994; **180**: 2089–2099.

## 11
# Hybrid Cell Vaccination for Cancer Immune Therapy
PETER WALDEN, GERNOT STUHLER and UWE TREFZER

### 11.1
### Introduction

Cases of spontaneous regressions of tumors reported for a variety of cancers have long been interpreted as the result of tumor-specific immune reactions [1]. Burnet had forged these observations from clinical cases together with the results of pathological studies and a number of animal model experiments into the concept of immune surveillance of cancer, and thereby summed up about a century of tumor immunology [2–4]. Regression zones occasionally observed in melanoma lesions are frequently referred to as illustrations of cellular immune reactions against the tumor and correlated with a better prognosis [5, 6]. Such clinical observation together with an increasing number of reports that demonstrate greatly expanded frequencies of tumor-specific T cells in cancer patients [7–28] are indicative of active antitumor immune responses. For several tumor-associated antigens (TAAs), expanded frequencies of specific T cells have even been demonstrated in healthy individuals [29]. However, regression areas in melanoma are often seen together with simultaneous tumor progression at the border zones of the same tumor and, at later stages of the disease, increasing immune dysfunctions are described in many patients which gradually eliminate effective specific antitumor immune responses. All these observations suggest an ongoing struggle of the tumor and the immune system, with tumor progression being the result of a shift in favor of the tumor and tumor regression a shift in favor of the immune system. Vaccination for cancer immune therapy thus seems to aim at a specific modulation of the quality and quantity of this balance, and, maybe, induction of new antitumor cytotoxic cellular immune responses. Currently, vaccination in cancer is primarily a therapeutic intervention in contrast to the situation in the case of infectious diseases. Preventive vaccination against cancer is not yet possible in humans, but might be attempted in future in specific high-risk situations.

Prerequisite of an active role of adaptive immune responses against cancer is a specific antigenicity of the tumor cells. The development of specific vaccination strategies for cancer immune therapy depends on TAAs, but also on the identification of the effector mechanism used by the immune system. Burnet *et al.* had suggested already some 30 years ago that T lymphocytes are the solely most important effector cells in these immune responses [3]. Although the critical role of MHC class I-restricted CD8$^+$ T cells in tumor rejects had been demonstrated in animal models and in cancer patients previously [30–32], the specific function and dominant role of these cells could be proven only after the first tumor-associated T cell epitopes and the corresponding antigens had been identified [33, 34]. In parallel developments, great progress has been made in the understanding of the differentiation and physiology of effector T cells, and of the cellular and molecular requirements of the induction and activation of these cells. This knowledge has been used for a rational development and thorough evaluation of new vaccination therapies, although many aspects of the T cell biology in antitumor immune responses still await elucidation.

The development of vaccination strategies for cancer immune therapy has to design vaccines that combine relevant TAAs with a means to induce efficient T cell responses. Hybrid cell vaccination (HCV) as one of these vaccination strategies uses the patient's tumor cells as antigen, and renders them immunogenic and into potent T cell stimulators by fusion with antigen-presenting cells (APCs) such as dendritic cells (DCs) [35]. In this chapter we will discuss the immunological basis and the results of the initial preclinical and clinical studies of this therapeutic approach.

## 11.2
## Immunological Basis of the HCV Approach to Cancer Immune Therapy

### 11.2.1
### Tumor Antigenicity

After several reports of clear but indirect evidence for TAAs recognized by cytotoxic T cells in cancer patients [31, 32, 36] and the demonstration of a tumor-associated T cell epitope in a mouse tumor model [33], the first human TAA was identified by Thierry Boon *et al.* and published in 1991 [34]. Since that time about 250 tumor-associated T cell epitopes derived from about 60 different proteins have been reported [37, 38]. The vast majority of the antigens were identified for melanoma and are MHC class I-restricted. Some of the antigen originally found for melanoma have later also been demonstrated in other tumors. According to the source and expression pattern TAAs can be classified as follows:

*Differentiation antigens*: proteins expressed by all cells of the tumor histotype lineage (e. g. tyrosinase, gp100, MART/Melan) [39–45].
*Embryonic antigens*: epitopes derived from antigens normally expressed in embryonic cells (e. g. CEA, AFP) [46, 47].
*Tumor-testis antigens*: epitopes of proteins expressed by the tumor cells and cells of the testes (e. g. MAGE, BAGE, GAGE) [34, 48–50].
*Over-expressed cellular proteins*: the presentation of peptides due to over-expression of a protein (e. g. HER-2/neu) [46, 51–54].
*Antigens resulting from mutations*: antigens induced by mutations in the tumor cells (e. g. cdk4, MUM, idiotypes) [55–57].

*Viral antigens*: antigens derived from oncogenic viruses (e. g. human papilloma virus) [58–60].

Of these categories, the first four are public antigens, which are not restricted to the tumors cells. Embryonic antigens and antigens of the tumor-testis group are relatively tumor-specific as they are either not expressed in normal adult tissue (embryonic antigens) or, besides the tumor, only in the immune-privileged organ testis (tumor-testis antigens). However, differentiation antigens which often dominate antitumor immune responses are expressed also by normal adult tissue. Thus, expectedly, autoimmune reactions against normal melanocytes are seen in some melanoma patients [61]. These autoimmune responses were shown to be mediated by the same T cell clones that are found among the tumor-infiltrating lymphocytes of the melanoma lesion [62–65]. Sometimes such autoimmune responses occur in the context of a vaccination therapy. Cytotoxic T cells with specificity for differentiation antigens should, according to conventional knowledge, not exist. They should have been eliminated in the course of the establishment of self-tolerance. To explain their existence in cancer patients and even in healthy individuals [28, 29] it has been proposed that their antigen receptors might be of low avidity and the T cells thus of too low efficiency to eliminate the tumor cells.

T cell epitopes resulting from tumor-specific mutations are private to the tumor and, therefore, ideal targets for immune therapy. Studies in mouse tumor models suggest that these tumor-specific mutations might be most important for antitumor immune responses [33, 66]. However, only very few such mutated epitopes have been identified for human cancer. Viral antigens play a role only in those cases in which oncogenic viruses are involved in tumorigenesis. They may, however, be interesting target structures for the development of preventive cancer vaccines in these cases.

The majority of the tumor-associated T cell epitopes have been identified using tumor-specific T cells as indicator cells. Serological responses to cancer, however, have long been described and exploited in cancer diagnostic. The very systematic approach to identifying serological antitumor specificity SEREX (see Chapter 2) has yielded a large number of antigens recognized by antibodies of the serum of cancer patients. Although there are a few cases in which a serologically identified antigen also harbors epitopes for MHC class I-restricted T cells [19, 67], for the majority of these antigens, no MHC class I-restricted T cell epitopes have so far been found.

The identification of these TAAs and T cell epitopes and their use to study the tumor-specific immune responses in cancer patients have confirmed that CD8[+] cytotoxic T cells are the most important effector cells in antitumor immunity. After most of the initial work to elucidate the function of these cells in cancer immunity was done in melanoma, increasing evidence is now being presented that demonstrates tumor-specific CD8[+] T cell responses in other tumors [27, 46, 47, 51–60]. In contrast to the large number of MHC class I-restricted epitopes, only a few MHC class II-restricted T cell epitopes have been identified to date [38, 68, 69]. Many of the cited studies have shown that the tumor cells display a complex antigenicity and that the immune responses directed against the tumor cells are of correspondingly complex specificity [70]. This complexity is further emphasized by the heterogeneity of the tumor cells with regard to antigen expression. Differences in the expression of TAAs have been described for melanoma within single lesions, between different lesions of the same patient as well as in the same patient at different times in the course of the disease.

## 11.2.2
### T–T Cell Collaboration in the Induction of Cellular Cytotoxic Immune Responses

The dependence of the induction, activation and expansion of MHC class I-restricted, CD8[+] T cells on T cell help has long been suggested by the crucial role of interleukin (IL)-2 as growth factor for these cells [36, 71–75] and the finding that activated MHC class II-restricted CD4[+] T cells are the main source for this cytokine [76]. Raulet and Bevan [77], and later Juretić *et al.* [78] have studied the immunogenetics of the induction of cytotoxic T cells in further detail, and found that these responses are MHC class I- as well as MHC class II-restricted, again suggesting a crucial role of CD4[+] T cells in the induction of CD8[+] T cell responses. Initially T cell help was seen as paracrine delivery of IL-2 by the helper T cell to the cytotoxic precursor cell [75]. It was believed that the efficacy of paracrine IL-2 was dependent on the microenvironment in which induction of the cytotoxic T cell takes place and a relatively close proximity of the two cells.

More detailed studies by Mitchison *et al.* [79, 80] and by our group [81] on the mode of interaction of helper and cytotoxic precursor T cells have yielded evidence for the direct involvement of the stimulator or APC in this interaction. Effective interaction of the two T cell types requires that the APC expresses MHC class I as well as MHC class II molecules and T cell epitopes for both T cell types [79–83]. Thus, it is the APC that organizes the interaction of the helper and effector compartment of cellular immunity. In analogy to the epitope linkage requirement for induction of T cell-dependent B cells, there is an epitope linkage requirement for the T–T cell collaboration in the induction of cellular cytolytic T cell responses with the APC linking the two epitopes [79, 81]. However, a number of studies have shown that the antigens for the two interacting T cells need not to be related on the molecular level [81, 82]. Thus, there is a 2-fold MHC restriction and potentially 2-fold antigen specificity that controls the induction of cytotoxic T cell responses in contrast to T–B cell collaboration for induction of secondary antibody responses, which is controlled solely by MHC class II molecules, and where the T and B cell epitopes need to be linked in a single antigen molecule [84]. This complex mode of antigenic and co-stimulatory control of the induction of cytolytic effector T cell responses provides additional protection against potential autoimmune reactions, but also poses restrictions on the induction of cellular immunity where it is needed, as in the case of cancer or viral infections.

Recognition of cognate peptides together with their specific MHC class I and II molecules on the surface of the APC by the two T cell types induces a complex array of molecular interaction between the cells. Both T cells communicate with the APC and with each other via cell surface molecules and soluble factors. Some of these molecules are constitutively expressed; others are induced or modulated in their expression. They may be a result of the maturation of the participating cells as CD28, B7 and 4–1BB [85–88], or they may be activation-induced such as the cytokines IL-2 and interferon (IFN)-γ and their receptors or CD40 and CD40 ligand [75, 89–97]. The expression of cytokines, IL-2 as growth and differentiation factor for cytotoxic T lymphocytes (CTLs) provided by the helper T cell [71–73, 75, 76, 90], and IFN-γ, a major differentiation factor of CTLs which can be produced by both T cells types [74, 91, 98, 99], is strictly activation-dependent. Moreover, also the capacity to respond to the cytokines, i. e. the expression of high-affinity cytokine receptors is induced by the activation of the T cell via its antigen receptor [89, 90, 100–102]. Recent reports suggest that additional constitutional or activation-induced factors regulate the interaction of the APC and the precursor cytotoxic T cell, although their exact molecular nature or mode of action has not been clarified [103]. It thus appears that the molecular and cellular mechanisms of the induction and activation of cytotoxic effector T cells have not yet been completely uncovered. Still, new players are discovered and are added to the list or are implicated by indirect evidence. The factors so-far identified provide signals of very different nature acting as co-stimulating factors that affect survival, growth, differentiation, and mode and extent of the molecular and cellular responses of the T cells. All these signals are essential for the development of cellular immunity. The activation of some of these receptors without simultaneous activation of certain other receptors often results in anergy or activation-induced cell death rather than activation and maturation [92]. An example of such adverse signaling is the activation of T cells without involvement of CD28, which among many other effects results in a block of signaling via the IL-2 receptor. IL-12, on the other hand, is a cytokine that can block cell death and anergy, and might be critical for sustained expansion and functional capacity of the activated T cell [25]. It thus appears critical not only to address the T cell receptors of the interacting T cells, but also to arrange the cellular and molecular components required for induction of cytotoxic T cells such that cytotoxic precursor cells and helper T cells are attracted and activated in a coordinated way involving all the essential co-stimulating factors and receptors [104, 105].

Although several MHC class II-expressing cells can serve as APCs in these three cell interactions, the DC is clearly the most potent cell for antigen harvesting, processing and presentation, for organizing the regulatory cell clusters, and for co-stimulation [97, 106–108]. The cellular interactions involved are dynamic in nature with the cells responding pair-wise to be modulated and responsive to productive interaction with the third partner. A recent series of publications have reported that DCs, upon antigen-dependent interaction with helper T cells, become charged to provide crucial co-stimulating signals to the CD8[+] T cell [93, 95, 96]. The exact nature of the molecular factors and interactions that regulate these events still awaits elucidation. In contrast to the multiple regulatory interactions required for the induction of cytotoxic T cells, the execution of the effector functions, i. e. the cytolysis of the target cells, is only dependent on MHC/peptide complexes and cell adhesion. In addition to the requirement for specific APCs, it seems that the environment where the interacting cells meet, the lymphoid organs, is also important. The impact of the specific architecture of the lymphoid organs on the efficiency of the interactions and of the induction of effector T cell is largely unexplored. However, non-lymphoid tissue appears to be a far less potent promoter of immune responses [109].

**11.3**
**Vaccination Strategies for Cancer Immune Therapy**

Both the concept of therapeutic vaccination for immune therapy in general as well as that of tumor vaccination have a long history dating back to the 19th century. A systematic exploration of vaccination approaches to cancer therapy is, however, a relatively recent development based on the rapidly expanding knowledge of tumor antigenicity and the regulatory requirements of the induction of tumor-specific immune responses. A number of different strategies have been developed during the past 20 or so years, each reflecting the current understanding of tumor immunology. Earlier attempts have focused on the induction of antibody responses against tumor cell surface antigens using the tumor cells themselves or tumor lysates. This work has been extended to the development of diagnostic tools, and of therapeutic agents such as immunotoxins and immunocytokines, which are discussed elsewhere in this volume (see Chapter 17).

With increasing appreciation of the importance of MHC class I-restricted CD8$^+$ T cells in antitumor immunity, tumor cells have also been employed to stimulate specific antitumor cytotoxic T cell responses [110]. A number of modifications were introduced to enhance the immunogenicity of the tumor cells: allogenic tumor cells [111, 112], allogenic, MHC class I-matched tumor cells [113, 114] or tumor cell lysates [115], haptenized tumor cells [116–119] or gene technologically altered tumor cells that were transfected with genes coding for allogenic MHC class II molecules to activate helper T cells [120], granulocyte-macrophage colony-stimulating factor (GM-CSF) to enhance antigen presentation and DC function [121–124], IFN-γ to support the differentiation of tumor-specific cytotoxic T cells [125–127], or factors such as B7 to enhance co-stimulation of the cytotoxic T cells [120, 128].

Following the discovery of the first TAAs and T cell epitopes, these antigens and synthetic peptides were used as vaccines [129, 130]. In the earliest studies, neat peptides or peptides in incomplete Freund's adjuvant (IFA) were injected into patients to induce antitumor T cell responses [131–134]. The initial clinical trials with these protocols have yielded some cases of clinical responses, but overall the response rates were low. These experiences together with the emergence of new concepts and technologies for the generation of vaccines have led to the design of new types of vaccines. Peptides with epitopes for tumor-specific cytotoxic T cells were combined with helper T cell epitopes and IFA [135], the genes coding for the entire TAAs were engineered into plasmid vectors or into virus DNA and used for naked DNA [135, 137] or virus vaccination [138, 139], thus making use of the strong immunogenicity of the virus, in most cases adenovirus. With the development of techniques for large-scale production of DCs and the discovery that DCs are uniquely capable of taking up and processing peptides, protein antigens or polynucleic acids, this cell is being extensively explored as an antigen carrier and adjuvant for the induction of antitumor T cell responses (see Chapter 9). DCs have been loaded with synthetic peptides [140–144], antigen-coding DNA or RNA [145–147], tumor lysates [143], exosomes or apoptotic bodies from tumor cells [148] or heat shock proteins extracted from tumor cells (see Chapter 12), or have been fused to the tumor cells [149–159], all to generate a potent immune stimulator cell. All these different approaches to cancer vaccination therapy are being tested in clinical trials – some of which are discussed in different chapters of this volume. The initial observations reported from these trials include a number of clinical responses of varying degree in late-stage cancer. A thorough evaluation of these attempts, however, will have to await the conclusion of these trials. There is, however, an increasing appreciation of the antigenic complexity of tumor cells and the need to address with the tumor vaccines as many specificities, i.e. tumor-associated T cell epitopes, and as many T cells as possible to induce a strong antitumor immune response and to minimize the selection for specific antigen-loss variants of the tumor cells. Antigen loss as effect of antigen-specific immune selection induced by antigen-specific vaccination might in fact be among the most serious side effects of vaccination therapy. In addition to this, all these trials have shown that vaccination therapy is remarkably well tolerated by the patients. Some cases of autoimmune reactions seen (usually restricted vitiligo) have been reported from different trials, but, so far, no case of vaccination-associated autoimmune disease has been seen [160]. Other adverse effects are very limited and signs of vaccine-induced immune responses.

## 11.4
## HCV

### 11.4.1
### Conceptual Basis

The HCV approach to cancer immune therapy attempts to render antigenic tumor cells immunogenic by fusing them with potent APCs, activated B cells or DCs [35, 158, 161–163]. Using the tumor cell itself as source and carrier of the tumor antigens should ensure the broadest possible representation of the tumor's antigenicity in the vaccine, including tumor-specific mutations. Two different designs of the hybrid cells have been tested. The one relies on the co-stimulatory capacity of the activated B cell or DC alone and uses autologous fusion cell combinations [162], whereas the other fuses autologous tumor cells with allogeneic APCs to recruit and activate helper T cells to support the induction of tumor-specific cytotoxic T cells [161]. While the majority of tumor cells express MHC class I molecules, constitutive expression of MHC class II expression is limited to a few cell types of the immune system (see Chapter 9). Accordingly, the probability for a tumor cell to simultaneously express both MHC class I and II in conjunction with suitable tumor antigens that can address the helper and precursor cytotoxic T cells of the patients at the same time is low. The use of allogeneic MHC class II molecules for the induction of T cell help eliminates the need for MHC class II-restricted TAAs for the activation of CD4$^+$ helper T cells and the reliably induced strong T cell responses against allogeneic MHC class II molecules does not require prior priming of these T cells. Moreover, recent reports suggest that the immune stimulatory function of DCs in cancer patients might be impaired and that allogeneic DCs prepared from the peripheral blood of healthy individuals might thus have the additional advantage of being an unrestricted source of competent immune stimulatory cells [164, 165].

In summary, the HCV approach was designed:

- To utilize a large variety of usually unidentified TAAs.
- To provide co-stimulating signals.
- To recruit and activate T cell help for the induction of tumor specific cytotoxic T cells.

Classical hybridoma technology aims at long-term lines that are selected on the basis of, primarily, their resistance to cytostatic drugs and, subsequently, according to the specific functionality desired. Usually, both fusion partners cells are of the same tissue origin and are controlled by very similar genetic programs. One of the fusion partners is a tumor cell selected for good growth properties. The hybrid cells needed for cancer immune therapy are very different [35]. First, the fusion partners are usually heterogeneous, i.e. they are of very different tissue origin controlled by different genetic programs, and, second, the tumor cell has in most cases not been adapted for stable growth in culture. On the other hand, long-term survival and growth of the hybrid cell is not required for the vaccination effect. Just the opposite – it must be ensured that the hybrid cells cannot survive and proliferate after injection into the patient. The vaccines are irradiated prior to inoculation to prevent tumor spreading in the vaccinee.

Since usually the hybrid cells cannot be expanded, the fusion technology must be designed to yield high fusion efficiencies independent of the specific types of cells used for hybridization. Electrofusion is one of the options for this purpose as it has a relatively high efficiency of hybrid cell generation and is relatively independent of the cell types that shall be fused [166, 167]. As the exact fusion conditions are defined by the setting of the electrical parameter of the power suppliers and pulsers, this technique is well reproducible.

## 11.4.2
### HCV in Preclinical Studies

The HCV concept has been tested successfully in a number of different animal tumor models including intradermal thymoma [161], liver cell and other carcinomas [149, 154, 156, 159, 162, 168], brain tumors such as neuroblastoma [152, 155], melanoma [169], and hematological cancers [170]. The fusion partners in the earlier works were B lymphoma cells; in the recent reports, DCs. Therapeutic vaccinations as well as primary immunizations with the hybrid cells were tested in the very first experiments [161, 162]. In all cases eradication of established tumors and induction of specific long-lasting antitumor immunity was induced by a single injection of the vaccine. The thymoma [161] study provided evidence of the need for cell hybridization, i.e. only the fused tumor and APCs induced tumor rejection and antitumor immunity, but not the parental cells mock-fused to themselves, or mixtures of these mock-fused cells. It could also be demonstrated that helper T cells specific for the allogeneic MHC are involved in the induction of the immune response. The eradication of the tumor, on the other hand, was shown to depend solely on tumor-specific, self-MHC-restricted CD8$^+$ cytotoxic T cells. Moreover, the initial liver cell carcinoma study [162] showed that the co-stimulatory molecule B7–1 is required for effective induction of tumor rejection *in vivo*. The reported efficiencies in all the animal model experiments were very similar, and no difference was seen between B cells and DCs as fusion partners. The inferior APC capacity of B cells might be overcome by the vigor of the T cell responses against the allogeneic MHC molecules [161]. These initial observations were extended in the subsequent studies that yielded further evidence for the need to hybridize the tumor and DC, and the involvement of both CD4$^+$ and CD8$^+$ T cells in the induction of the antitumor immune response [149]. This work, done with an adenocarcinoma model, also demonstrated that HCV can prime naive T cells [149]. More recently, the same group has demonstrated antitumor immunity in MUC1 transgenic mice from vaccination with allogeneic DCs fused with carcinoma cells [156]. In a lymphoma as well as in a melanoma model where protective immunity, reduced tumor incidence and prolonged survival was seen in hybrid cell treated animals, it was demonstrated that hybrids express MHC class I and II antigens and co-stimulatory molecules, as well as DC-specific and tumor-derived surface markers. In these experiments it was shown that a fusion rate of 20 % in the vaccine is sufficient for the vaccination effect and, most interestingly, adoptive transfer of T cells led to tumor regression in recipient mice. The results of HCV attempts in brain tumor models [155] which have provided evidence for tumor rejection without detectable side effects are particularly interesting as patients with brain tumors or brain metastases are often excluded from clinical studies because of fear of serious adverse effects such as inflammation and edema which could seriously harm the vaccinee and which would require immune-suppressive treatment.

In addition to the animal model experiment, the efficacy of tumor/DC hybrids for induction of tumor-specific CD8$^+$ T cell responses has also been analyzed in *in vitro* test systems using human tumor cells and peripheral blood cells as sources for precursor effector cells [157, 158, 170]. As well as demonstrating the efficacy of hybrid cells as inducers of primary and recall tumor-specific cytotoxic T cell responses, these *in vitro* test systems are also well suited to analyzing and validating hybrid cell vaccines for new types of tumors, demonstrating the existence of specific TAAs and establishing tumor-specific T cell lines.

## 11.4.3
### Clinical Experience with HCV

The two initial clinical cancer immune therapy trials to test the HCV strategy were performed with patients suffering from malignant melanoma [171, 172] or renal cell carcinoma [151, 173]. The main objective of these initial clinical trials was to test the toxicity, feasibility and antitumor activity of this treatment. The patients were therefore mostly stage IV patients. The vaccines were prepared by fusion of autologous tumor cells with allogeneic activated B cells and given intracutaneously or intradermally. A tumor response was seen in three out of thirteen patients with renal cell carcinoma. In patients with metastatic melanoma, two out of 16 patients showed objective tumor responses, while in five other patients, stable disease was induced after previous progression. Interestingly, stable disease was maintained under repeated booster injections for more than 2 years in some of the patients. Some of these patients remained in stable disease with periodic HCVs for more than 2 years. Antitumor immune responses were seen only in patients who still had the capacity to mount delayed-type hypersensitivity responses to at least one of a set of common recall antigens. As evidenced by histological analyses of tumor lesions that became inflamed after vaccinations, the vaccination induced or mediated T cell relocation into tumor nodules [171].

The first study with HCV using allogeneic DCs and autologous tumor cells was completed with 17 patients with metastatic renal cell carcinoma [151]. HLA-A2-restricted cytotoxic T cells reactive with the Muc1 TAA were shown to be induced and it could be demonstrated that $CD8^+$ T lymphocytes were recruited into tumor challenge sites. Again, side effects were minor. There were four complete and two partial responses, and one patient had a mixed response, indicating that this approach might be safe and effective in patients with renal cell carcinoma.

A very interesting report was recently published of a first HCV trial with eight patients with glioma [153]. Two of these patients experienced partial responses. No serious adverse effects were observed in any of the patients, whereas most of the patients showed signs of changes in their immune status as evidenced by increased lymphocyte counts and enhanced IFN levels in the peripheral blood. Three of the four clinical HCV trials which have yielded cases of objective clinical responses, i. e. complete responses or reduction of the tumor mass by 50 %, have used hybrids of autologous tumor cells with allogeneic APCs, activated B cells or DCs. These initial observations might indicate that the T cell response against the allogeneic MHC molecules indeed provides additional co-stimulatory support for the tumor-specific T cell responses.

So far, renal cell carcinoma patients seem to benefit more often than melanoma patients from a HCV therapy [151, 171–173]. The number of patients treated in the glioma trial is too low to support any conclusions in this direction [153]. Both tumors, renal cell carcinoma and melanoma, are considered to be relatively immunogenic tumors whereby the known melanoma-associated antigens by far outnumber the antigens associated with renal cell carcinoma [38]. The difference in clinical responses seen in the HCV trials might reflect a difference in antigenicity, but more likely is related to the biology of these tumors, with malignant melanoma being considered more aggressive, or to the treatments received by the patients before the vaccination therapy. Whereas the majority of the melanoma patients in the clinical vaccination trials had received chemotherapy before, this was the case only for a few exceptional patients with renal cell carcinoma. In addition to the general immune suppression often associated with chemotherapy, a recent report demonstrated that chemotherapy can selectively eliminate tumor-specific T cells from the circulation of the patients [26]. Chemotherapy is certainly incompatible with specific vaccination therapy and these two regiments are not combined. However, so far there is no information available as to the extent to which the cellular immune response capacity of patients can recover after chemotherapy, i. e. if a complete or at least sufficient recovery is possible; there is also information lacking regarding the kinetics of this process.

The side effects seen in the trials were mild and all signs of vaccination-induced immune responses. They included erythema at the sites of inoculation, some cases of fever and others of strong but temporal perspiration. In some of the malignant melanoma patients a locally restricted vitiligo occurred after vaccination which again is indicative of the activity of cytotoxic T cells with specificity for public melanoma associated antigens. No other signs of vaccination-induced autoimmune reactivity were observed. Such low toxicity is, as discussed before, common to all vaccination therapy trials reported so far.

## 11.5
## Conclusion and Prospects

HCV has proven to be a feasible strategy for the treatment of cancer patients and well-suited for individualized therapy, and the responses achieved so far in advanced-stage cancer patients are encouraging. The hallmark of this approach is the use of the patients own tumor cells, which is the broadest possible representation of the antigen spectrum of the tumor and which also includes, besides shared TAAs, the specific mutations private to the specific tumor cell clones of the patient. Other vaccination strategies with this potential to address a broad spectrum of TAAs and to induce a broad repertoire of tumor-specific T cells use heat shock proteins (gp96 or HSP70; discussed in Chapter 12) or DCs pulsed with tumor lysates [174, 175], peptides eluted from tumor cells [176, 177], or amplified total mRNA obtained from tumor cell lines or micro-dissected tumor material [175, 178–180]. The latter three strategies make use of the unique capacity of DCs to take up antigenic material and to process it for presentation to T cells. The preparation of heat shock proteins, peptides or lysates from tumor cells will require large tumor masses which in many cases might be difficult to obtain from the patients. The HCV approach is burdened by the same problem. It could be possible to use established tumor cell lines for the preparation of the vaccines. However, such cultured cell lines might not express the same antigens as the tumor in the patients. In fact, preliminary observations from the initial HCV trials with melanoma patients indicate that autologous tumor cell lines represent a different antigenicity than the original tumor and are less efficient in the vaccine preparations [171]. Amplified mRNA of tumor cells might become a promising solution for these problems if it becomes possible to ensure that the amplified mRNA represents a sufficiently broad spectrum of the tumor antigens and that these complex mixtures of RNA can be introduced into the DCs efficiently. The best type and optimal maturation state of the APCs will depend on the vaccination strategy and the mode of antigen transfer. The generation of hybrid cell vaccines will certainly require mature DCs as most potent APCs and T cell stimulators [144]. For those approaches that require active antigen processing, immature DCs might be the better choice.

The repeated observation that patients who do not experience complete responses can be treated with hybrid cell vaccines for prolonged times and stay in a stable disease state throughout opens the option of vaccination therapy as a maintenance therapy. Since such therapies are well tolerated by the patients, this appears to be an attractive option; however, it requires that tumor material for vaccine production is available for long periods.

While the clinical responses observed in the initial trials are promising, cure is a rare exception and the question is how to improve the vaccination therapies in order to improve the response rates and, in future, offer vaccination therapy as a standard therapy for the treatment of various cancer. Late-stage cancers are certainly not targets for cancer immune therapy. The tumor burden is often very high, the patients often already suffer from disease-related immune suppression and the tumor cells might already be highly diversified. The selection of an immune-escape variant of the tumor is a possible adverse effect of specific immune intervention. It is conceivable to combine HCV with other treatment modalities that can help to reduce the tumor burden and to provide relief from some of the immune-suppressive activities of the tumors. It might be necessary to include in the treatment cytokines that can stabilize the tumor-specific T cell responses, and aid their long-term expansion and functional integrity.

## References

1 BURNET FM. Immunological aspects of malignant disease. *Lancet* 1967; **1**: 1171–4.

2 BURNET FM. The concept of immunological surveillance. *Prog Exp Tumor Res* 1970; **13**: 1–27.

3 BURNET FM. Immunological surveillance in neoplasia. *Transplant Rev* 1971; **7**: 3–25.

4 BURNET FM. Implications of immunological surveillance for cancer therapy. *Isr J Med Sci* 1971; **7**: 9–16.

5 BLESSING K, McLAREN KM. Histological regression in primary cutaneous melanoma: recognition, prevalence and significance. *Histopathology* 1992; **20**: 315–22.

6 BARNHILL RL, FINE JA, ROUSH GC, BERWICK M. Predicting five-year outcome for patients with cutaneous melanoma in a population-based study. *Cancer* 1996; **78**: 427–32.

7 VALMORI D, DUTOIT V, RUBIO-GODOY V, CHAMBAZ C, LIENARD D, GUILLAUME P, ROMERO P, CEROTTINI JC, RIMOLDI D. Frequent cytolytic T-cell responses to peptide MAGE-A10(254–262) in melanoma. *Cancer Res* 2001; **61**: 509–12.

8 SCHEIBENBOGEN C, ROMERO P, RIVOLTINI L, HERR W, SCHMITTEL A, CEROT-

TINI JC, WOELFEL T, EGGERMONT AM, KEILHOLZ U. Quantitation of antigen-reactive T cells in peripheral blood by IFN-γ-ELISPOT assay and chromium-release assay: a four-centre comparative trial. *J Immunol Methods* 2000; **244**: 81–9.

9 ROMERO P, PITTET MJ, VALMORI D, SPEISER DE, CERUNDOLO V, LIENARD D, LEJEUNE F, CEROTTINI JC. Immune monitoring in cancer immunotherapy. *Ernst Schering Res Found Workshop* 2000; **30**: 75–97.

10 VALMORI D, DUTOIT V, LIENARD D, LEJEUNE F, SPEISER D, RIMOLDI D, CERUNDOLO V, DIETRICH PY, CEROTTINI JC, ROMERO P. Tetramer-guided analysis of TCR β-chain usage reveals a large repertoire of melan-A-specific CD8$^+$ T cells in melanoma patients. *J Immunol* 2000; **165**: 533–8.

11 VALMORI D, PITTET MJ, VONARBOURG C, RIMOLDI D, LIENARD D, SPEISER D, DUNBAR R, CERUNDOLO V, CEROTTINI JC, ROMERO P. Analysis of the cytolytic T lymphocyte response of melanoma patients to the naturally HLA-A*0201-associated tyrosinase peptide 368–376. *Cancer Res* 1999; **59**: 4050–5.

12 D'SOUZA S, RIMOLDI D, LIENARD D, LEJEUNE F, CEROTTINI JC, ROMERO P.

Circulating Melan-A/Mart-1 specific cytolytic T lymphocyte precursors in HLA-A2$^+$ melanoma patients have a memory phenotype. *Int J Cancer* 1998; **78**: 699–706.

13 ROMERO P, DUNBAR PR, VALMORI D, PITTET M, OGG GS, RIMOLDI D, CHEN JL, LIENARD D, CEROTTINI JC, CERUNDOLO V. *Ex vivo* staining of metastatic lymph nodes by class I major histocompatibility complex tetramers reveals high numbers of antigen-experienced tumor-specific cytolytic T lymphocytes. *J Exp Med* 1998; **188**: 1641–50.

14 ROMERO P, GERVOIS N, SCHNEIDER J, ESCOBAR P, VALMORI D, PANNETIER C, STEINLE A, WOLFEL T, LIENARD D, BRICHARD V, VAN PEL A, JOTEREAU F, CEROTTINI JC. Cytolytic T lymphocyte recognition of the immunodominant HLA-A*0201-restricted Melan-A/MART-1 antigenic peptide in melanoma. *J Immunol* 1997; **159**: 2366–74.

15 VALMORI D, LIENARD D, WAANDERS G, RIMOLDI D, CEROTTINI JC, ROMERO P. Analysis of MAGE-3-specific cytolytic T lymphocytes in human leukocyte antigen-A2 melanoma patients. *Cancer Res* 1997; **57**: 735–41.

16 ZAROUR H, DE SMET C, LEHMANN F, MARCHAND M, LETHE B, ROMERO P, BOON T, RENAULD JC. The majority of autologous cytolytic T-lymphocyte clones derived from peripheral blood lymphocytes of a melanoma patient recognize an antigenic peptide derived from gene Pmel17/gp100. *J Invest Dermatol* 1996; **107**: 63–7.

17 ROMERO P. Cytolytic T lymphocyte responses of cancer patients to tumor-associated antigens. *Springer Semin Immunopathol* 1996; **18**: 185–98.

18 GNJATIC S, NAGATA Y, JAGER E, STOCKERT E, SHANKARA S, ROBERTS BL, MAZZARA GP, LEE SY, DUNBAR PR, DUPONT B, CERUNDOLO V, RITTER G, CHEN YT, KNUTH A, OLD LJ. Strategy for monitoring T cell responses to NY-ESO-1 in patients with any HLA class I allele. *Proc Natl Acad Sci USA* 2000; **97**: 10917–22.

19 JAGER E, NAGATA Y, GNJATIC S, WADA H, STOCKERT E, KARBACH J, DUNBAR PR, LEE SY, JUNGBLUTH A, JAGER D,

ARAND M, RITTER G, CERUNDOLO V, DUPONT B, CHEN YT, OLD LJ, KNUTH A. Monitoring CD8 T cell responses to NY-ESO-1: correlation of humoral and cellular immune responses. *Proc Natl Acad Sci USA* 2000; **97**: 4760–5.

20 ROMERO P, DUNBAR PR, VALMORI D, PITTET M, OGG GS, RIMOLDI D, CHEN JL, LIENARD D, CEROTTINI JC, CERUNDOLO V. *Ex vivo* staining of metastatic lymph nodes by class I major histocompatibility complex tetramers reveals high numbers of antigen-experienced tumor-specific cytolytic T lymphocytes. *J Exp Med* 1998; **188**: 1641–50.

21 OGG GS, ROD DUNBAR P, ROMERO P, CHEN JL, CERUNDOLO V. High frequency of skin-homing melanocyte-specific cytotoxic T lymphocytes in autoimmune vitiligo. *J Exp Med* 1998; **188**: 1203–8.

22 ANICHINI A, MOLLA A, MORTARINI R, TRAGNI G, BERSANI I, DI NICOLA M, GIANNI AM, PILOTTI S, DUNBAR R, CERUNDOLO V, PARMIANI G. An expanded peripheral T cell population to a cytotoxic T lymphocyte (CTL)-defined, melanocyte-specific antigen in metastatic melanoma patients impacts on generation of peptide-specific CTLs but does not overcome tumor escape from immune surveillance in metastatic lesions. *J Exp Med* 1999; **190**: 651–67.

23 VALMORI D, PITTET MJ, VONARBOURG C, RIMOLDI D, LIENARD D, SPEISER D, DUNBAR R, CERUNDOLO V, CEROTTINI JC, ROMERO P. Analysis of the cytolytic T lymphocyte response of melanoma patients to the naturally HLA-A*0201-associated tyrosinase peptide 368–376. *Cancer Res* 1999; **59**: 4050–5.

24 SCHULER-THURNER B, DIECKMANN D, KEIKAVOUSSI P, BENDER A, MACZEK C, JONULEIT H, RODER C, HAENDLE I, LEISGANG W, DUNBAR R, CERUNDOLO V, VON DEN DRIESCH P, KNOP J, BROCKER EB, ENK A, KAMPGEN E, SCHULER G. Mage-3 and influenza-matrix peptide-specific cytotoxic T cells are inducible in terminal stage HLA-A2.1$^+$ melanoma patients by mature monocyte-derived dendritic cells. *J Immunol* 2000; **165**: 3492–6.

25  MORTARINI R, BORRI A, TRAGNI G, BERSANI I, VEGETTI C, BAJETTA E, PILOTTI S, CERUNDOLO V, ANICHINI A. Peripheral burst of tumor-specific cytotoxic T lymphocytes and infiltration of metastatic lesions by memory CD8⁺ T cells in melanoma patients receiving interleukin 12. *Cancer Res* 2000; **60**: 3559–68.

26  LEE PP, YEE C, SAVAGE PA, FONG L, BROCKSTEDT D, WEBER JS, JOHNSON D, SWETTER S, THOMPSON J, GREENBERG PD, ROEDERER M, DAVIS MM. Characterization of circulating T cells specific for tumor-associated antigens in melanoma patients. *Nat Med* 1999; **5**: 677–85.

27  MOLLDREM JJ, LEE PP, WANG C, FELIO K, KANTARJIAN HM, CHAMPLIN RE, DAVIS MM. Evidence that specific T lymphocytes may participate in the elimination of chronic myelogenous leukemia. *Nat Med* 2000; **6**: 1018–23.

28  VALMORI D, DUTOIT V, LIENARD D, RIMOLDI D, PITTET MJ, CHAMPAGNE P, ELLEFSEN K, SAHIN U, SPEISER D, LEJEUNE F, CEROTTINI JC, ROMERO P. Naturally occurring human lymphocyte antigen-A2 restricted CD8⁺ T-cell response to the cancer testis antigen NY-ESO-1 in melanoma patients. *Cancer Res* 2000; **60**: 4499–506.

29  PITTET MJ, VALMORI D, DUNBAR PR, SPEISER DE, LIENARD D, LEJEUNE F, FLEISCHHAUER K, CERUNDOLO V, CEROTTINI JC, ROMERO P. High frequencies of naive Melan-A/MART-1-specific CD8⁺ T cells in a large proportion of human histocompatibility leukocyte antigen (HLA)-A2 individuals. *J Exp Med* 1999; **190**: 705–15.

30  LAMOUSE-SMITH E, CLEMENTS VK, OSTRAND-ROSENBERG S. Beta 2M⁻/⁻ knockout mice contain low levels of CD8⁺ cytotoxic T lymphocyte that mediate specific tumor rejection. *J Immunol* 1993; **151**: 6283–90.

31  DARROW TL, SLINGLUFF CL JR, SEIGLER HF. The role of HLA class I antigens in recognition of melanoma cells by tumor-specific cytotoxic T lymphocytes. Evidence for shared tumor antigens. *J Immunol* 1989; **142**: 3329–35.

32  CROWLEY NJ, DARROW TL, QUINN-ALLEN MA, SEIGLER HF. MHC-restricted recognition of autologous melanoma by tumor-specific cytotoxic T cells. Evidence for restriction by a dominant HLA-A allele. *J Immunol* 1991; **146**: 1692–9.

33  VAN PEL A, WARNIER G, VAN DEN EYNDE B, LETHE B, LURQUIN C, BOON T. Tum⁻ antigens, TSTA, and T cell immune surveillance. *Ann NY Acad Sci* 1991; **636**: 43–51.

34  VAN DER BRUGGEN P, TRAVERSARI C, CHOMEZ P, LURQUIN C, DE PLAEN E, VAN DEN EYNDE B, KNUTH A, BOON T. A gene encoding an antigen recognized by cytolytic T lymphocytes on a human melanoma. *Science* 1991; **254**: 643–7.

35  WALDEN P. Hybrid cell vaccination for cancer immunotherapy. *Adv Exp Med Biol* 2000; **465**: 347–54.

36  DE VRIES JE, SPITS H. Cloned human cytotoxic T lymphocyte (CTL) lines reactive with autologous melanoma cells. I. In vitro generation, isolation, and analysis to phenotype and specificity. *J Immunol* 1984; **132**: 510–9.

37  VAN DEN EYNDE BJ, BOON T. Tumor antigens recognized by T lymphocytes. *Int J Clin Lab Res* 1997; **27**: 81–6.

38  RENKVIST N, CASTELLI C, ROBBINS PF, PARMIANI G. A listing of human tumor antigens recognized by T cells. *Cancer Immunol Immunother* 2001; **50**: 3–15.

39  BRICHARD V, VAN PEL A, WOLFEL T, WOLFEL C, DE PLAEN E, LETHE B, COULIE P, BOON T. The tyrosinase gene codes for an antigen recognized by autologous cytolytic T lymphocytes on HLA-A2 melanomas. *J Exp Med* 1993; **178**: 489–95.

40  KAWAKAMI Y, ELIYAHU S, DELGADO CH, ROBBINS PF, SAKAGUCHI K, APPELLA E, YANNELLI JR, ADEMA GJ, MIKI T, ROSENBERG SA. Identification of a human melanoma antigen recognized by tumor-infiltrating lymphocytes associated with *in vivo* tumor rejection. *Proc Natl Acad Sci USA* 1994; **91**: 6458–62.

41  KAWAKAMI Y, ELIYAHU S, SAKAGUCHI K, ROBBINS PF, RIVOLTINI L, YANNELLI JR, APPELLA E, ROSENBERG SA. Identification of the immunodominant peptides of the MART-1 human melanoma antigen recognized by the majority of HLA-A2-restricted tumor infiltrating lymphocytes. *J Exp Med* 1994; **180**: 347–52.

**42** BAKKER AB, SCHREURS MW, DE BOER AJ, KAWAKAMI Y, ROSENBERG SA, ADEMA GJ, FIGDOR CG. Melanocyte lineage-specific antigen gp100 is recognized by melanoma-derived tumor-infiltrating lymphocytes. *J Exp Med* 1994; **179**: 1005–9.

**43** WOLFEL T, VAN PEL A, BRICHARD V, SCHNEIDER J, SELIGER B, MEYER ZUM BUSCHENFELDE KH, BOON T. Two tyrosinase nonapeptides recognized on HLA-A2 melanomas by autologous cytolytic T lymphocytes. *Eur J Immunol* 1994; **24**: 759–64.

**44** VALMORI D, GERVOIS N, RIMOLDI D, FONTENEAU JF, BONELO A, LIENARD D, RIVOLTINI L, JOTEREAU F, CEROTTINI JC, ROMERO P. Diversity of the fine specificity displayed by HLA-A*0201-restricted CTL specific for the immunodominant Melan-A/MART-1 antigenic peptide. *J Immunol* 1998; **161**: 6956–62.

**45** SKIPPER JC, KITTLESEN DJ, HENDRICKSON RC, DEACON DD, HARTHUN NL, WAGNER SN, HUNT DF, ENGELHARD VH, SLINGLUFF CL JR. Shared epitopes for HLA-A3-restricted melanoma-reactive human CTL include a naturally processed epitope from Pmel-17/gp100. *J Immunol* 1996; **157**: 5027–33.

**46** KAWASHIMA I, TSAI V, SOUTHWOOD S, TAKESAKO K, SETTE A, CELIS E. Identification of HLA-A3-restricted cytotoxic T lymphocyte epitopes from carcinoembryonic antigen and HER-2/neu by primary *in vitro* immunization with peptide-pulsed dendritic cells. *Cancer Res* 1999; **59**: 431–5.

**47** TSANG KY, ZAREMBA S, NIERODA CA, ZHU MZ, HAMILTON JM, SCHLOM J. Generation of human cytotoxic T cells specific for human carcinoembryonic antigen epitopes from patients immunized with recombinant vaccinia–CEA vaccine. *J Natl Cancer Inst* 1995; **87**: 982–90.

**48** ROMERO P, PANNETIER C, HERMAN J, JONGENEEL CV, CEROTTINI JC, COULIE PG. Multiple specificities in the repertoire of a melanoma patient's cytolytic T lymphocytes directed against tumor antigen MAGE-1.A1. *J Exp Med* 1995; **182**: 1019–28.

**49** BOEL P, WILDMANN C, SENSI ML, BRASSEUR R, RENAULD JC, COULIE P,

BOON T, VAN DER BRUGGEN P. BAGE: a new gene encoding an antigen recognized on human melanomas by cytolytic T lymphocytes. *Immunity* 1995; **2**: 167–75.

**50** TANZARELLA S, RUSSO V, LIONELLO I, DALERBA P, RIGATTI D, BORDIGNON C, TRAVERSARI C. Identification of a promiscuous T-cell epitope encoded by multiple members of the MAGE family. *Cancer Res* 1999; **59**: 2668–74.

**51** FISK B, BLEVINS TL, WHARTON JT, IOANNIDES CG. Identification of an immunodominant peptide of HER-2/neu protooncogene recognized by ovarian tumor-specific cytotoxic T lymphocyte lines. *J Exp Med* 1995; **181**: 2109–17.

**52** PEOPLES GE, GOEDEGEBUURE PS, SMITH R, LINEHAN DC, YOSHINO I, EBERLEIN TJ. Breast and ovarian cancer-specific cytotoxic T lymphocytes recognize the same HER2/neu-derived peptide. *Proc Natl Acad Sci USA* 1995; **92**: 432–6.

**53** KONO K, RONGCUN Y, CHARO J, ICHIHARA F, CELIS E, SETTE A, APPELLA E, SEKIKAWA T, MATSUMOTO Y, KIESSLING R. Identification of HER2/neu-derived peptide epitopes recognized by gastric cancer-specific cytotoxic T lymphocytes. *Int J Cancer* 1998; **78**: 202–8.

**54** RONGCUN Y, SALAZAR-ONFRAY F, CHARO J, MALMBERG KJ, EVRIN K, MAES H, KONO K, HISING C, PETERSSON M, LARSSON O, LAN L, APPELLA E, SETTE A, CELIS E, KIESSLING R. Identification of new HER2/neu-derived peptide epitopes that can elicit specific CTL against autologous and allogeneic carcinomas and melanomas. *J Immunol* 1999; **163**: 1037–44.

**55** COULIE PG, LEHMANN F, LETHE B, HERMAN J, LURQUIN C, ANDRAWISS M, BOON T. A mutated intron sequence codes for an antigenic peptide recognized by cytolytic T lymphocytes on a human melanoma. *Proc Natl Acad Sci USA* 1995; **92**: 7976–80.

**56** WOLFEL T, HAUER M, SCHNEIDER J, SERRANO M, WOLFEL C, KLEHMANN-HIEB E, DE PLAEN E, HANKELN T, MEYER ZUM BUSCHENFELDE KH, BEACH D. A p16INK4a-insensitive CDK4 mutant targeted by cytolytic T lymphocytes in a human melanoma. *Science* 1995; **269**: 1281–4.

57 ROBBINS PF, EL-GAMIL M, LI YF, KAWA-KAMI Y, LOFTUS D, APPELLA E, ROSEN-BERG SA. A mutated β-catenin gene encodes a melanoma-specific antigen recognized by tumor infiltrating lymphocytes. *J Exp Med* 1996; **183**: 1185–92.

58 FELTKAMP MC, SMITS HL, VIER-BOOM MP, MINNAAR RP, DE JONGH BM, DRIJFHOUT JW, TER SCHEGGET J, ME-LIEF CJ, KAST WM. Vaccination with cytotoxic T lymphocyte epitope-containing peptide protects against a tumor induced by human papillomavirus type 16-transformed cells. *Eur J Immunol* 1993; **23**: 2242–9.

59 RESSING ME, SETTE A, BRANDT RM, RUPPERT J, WENTWORTH PA, HART-MAN M, OSEROFF C, GREY HM, MELIEF CJ, KAST WM. Human CTL epitopes encoded by human papillomavirus type 16 E6 and E7 identified through *in vivo* and *in vitro* immunogenicity studies of HLA-A*0201-binding peptides. *J Immunol* 1995; **54**: 5934–43.

60 ELLIS JR, KEATING PJ, BAIRD J, HOUN-SELL EF, RENOUF DV, ROWE M, HOP-KINS D, DUGGAN-KEEN MF, BARTHOLO-MEW JS, YOUNG LS, STERN PL. The association of an HPV16 oncogene variant with HLA-B7 has implications for vaccine design in cervical cancer. *Nat Med* 1995; **1**: 464–70.

61 ROSENBERG SA, WHITE DE. Vitiligo in patients with melanoma: normal tissue antigens can be targets for cancer immunotherapy. *J Immunother Emphasis Tumor Immunol* 1996; **19**: 81–4.

62 KAWAKAMI Y, ELIYAHU S, JENNINGS C, SAKAGUCHI K, KANG X, SOUTHWOOD S, ROBBINS PF, SETTE A, APPELLA E, ROSEN-BERG SA. Recognition of multiple epitopes in the human melanoma antigen gp100 by tumor-infiltrating T lymphocytes associated with *in vivo* tumor regression. *J Immunol* 1995; **154**: 3961–8.

63 KAWAKAMI Y, ROBBINS PF, WANG X, TUPESIS JP, PARKHURST MR, KANG X, SAKAGUCHI K, APPELLA E, ROSEN-BERG SA. Identification of new melanoma epitopes on melanosomal proteins recognized by tumor infiltrating T lymphocytes restricted by HLA-A1,

-A2, and -A3 alleles. *J Immunol* 1998; **161**: 6985–92.

64 PANELLI MC, BETTINOTTI MP, LALLY K, OHNMACHT GA, LI Y, ROBBINS P, RIKER A, ROSENBERG SA, MARIN-COLA FM. A tumor-infiltrating lymphocyte from a melanoma metastasis with decreased expression of melanoma differentiation antigens recognizes MAGE-12. *J Immunol* 2000; **164**: 4382–92.

65 BECKER JC, GULDBERG P, ZEUTHEN J, BROCKER EB, STRATEN PT. Accumulation of identical T cells in melanoma and vitiligo-like leukoderma. *J Invest Dermatol* 1999; **113**: 1033–8.

66 DUDLEY ME, ROOPENIAN DC. Loss of a unique tumor antigen by cytotoxic T lymphocyte immunoselection from a 3-methylcholanthrene-induced mouse sarcoma reveals secondary unique and shared antigens. *J Exp Med* 1996; **184**: 441–7.

67 JAGER E, CHEN YT, DRIJFHOUT JW, KAR-BACH J, RINGHOFFER M, JAGER D, ARAND M, WADA H, NOGUCHI Y, STOCK-ERT E, OLD LJ, KNUTH A. Simultaneous humoral and cellular immune response against cancer-testis antigen NY-ESO-1: definition of human histocompatibility leukocyte antigen (HLA)-A2-binding peptide epitopes. *J Exp Med* 1998; **187**: 265–70.

68 CHAUX P, VANTOMME V, STROOBANT V, THIELEMANS K, CORTHALS J, LUITEN R, EGGERMONT AM, BOON T, VAN DER BRUGGEN P. Identification of MAGE-3 epitopes presented by HLA-DR molecules to CD4+ T lymphocytes. *J Exp Med* 1999; **189**: 767–78.

69 JAGER E, JAGER D, KARBACH J, CHEN YT, RITTER G, NAGATA Y, GNJATIC S, STOCK-ERT E, ARAND M, OLD LJ, KNUTH A. Identification of NY-ESO-1 epitopes presented by human histocompatibility antigen (HLA)-DRB4*0101–0103 and recognized by CD4+ T lymphocytes of patients with NY-ESO-1-expressing melanoma. *J Exp Med* 2000; **191**: 625–30.

70 DIETRICH PY, WALKER PR, QUIQUE-REZ AL, PERRIN G, DUTOIT V, LIENARD D, GUILLAUME P, CEROTTINI JC, ROMERO P, VALMORI D. Melanoma patients respond to a cytotoxic T lymphocyte-defined self-

peptide with diverse and nonoverlapping T-cell receptor repertoires. *Cancer Res* 2001; **61**: 2047–54.

**71** KASAKURA S, LOWENSTEIN L. A factor stimulating DNA synthesis derived from the medium of leukocyte cultures. *Nature* 1965; **208**: 794–5.

**72** MORGAN DA, RUSCETTI FW, GALLO R. Selective *in vitro* growth of T lymphocytes from normal human bone marrows. *Science* 1976; **193**: 1007–8.

**73** GILLIS S, UNION NA, BAKER PE, SMITH KA. The *in vitro* generation and sustained culture of nude mouse cytolytic T-lymphocytes. *J Exp Med* 1979; **149**: 1460–76.

**74** RAULET DH. Expression and function of interleukin-2 receptors on immature thymocytes. *Nature* 1985; **314**: 101–3.

**75** KROEMER G, ANDREU JL, GONZALO JA, GUTIERREZ-RAMOS JC, MARTINEZ C. Interleukin-2, autotolerance, and autoimmunity. *Adv Immunol* 1991; **50**: 147–235.

**76** MOSMANN TR, CHERWINSKI H, BOND MW, GIEDLIN MA, COFFMAN RL. Two types of murine helper T cell clone. I. Definition according to profiles of lymphokine activities and secreted proteins. *J Immunol* 1986; **136**: 2348–57.

**77** RAULET DH, BEVAN MJ. Helper T cells for cytotoxic T lymphocytes need not be I region restricted. *J Exp Med* 1982; **155**: 1766–84.

**78** JURETIC A, MALENICA B, JURETIC E, KLEIN J, NAGY ZA. Helper effects required during *in vivo* priming for a cytolytic response to the H-Y antigen in nonresponder mice. *J Immunol* 1985; **134**: 1408–14.

**79** MITCHISON NA, O'MALLEY C. Three-cell-type clusters of T cells with antigen-presenting cells best explain the epitope linkage and noncognate requirements of the *in vivo* cytolytic response. *Eur J Immunol* 1987; **17**: 1579–83.

**80** MITCHISON NA. An exact comparison between the efficiency of two- and three-cell-type clusters in mediating helper activity. *Eur J Immunol* 1990; **20**: 699–702.

**81** STUHLER G, WALDEN P. Collaboration of helper and cytotoxic T lymphocytes. *Eur J Immunol* 1993; **23**: 2279–86.

**82** BORGES E, WIESMULLER KH, JUNG G, WALDEN P. Efficacy of synthetic vaccines in the induction of cytotoxic T lymphocytes. Comparison of the costimulating support provided by helper T cells and lipoamino acid. *J Immunol Methods* 1994; **173**: 253–63.

**83** BAXEVANIS CN, VOUTSAS IF, TSITSILONIS OE, GRITZAPIS AD, SOTIRIADOU R, PAPAMICHAIL M. Tumor-specific CD4$^+$ T lymphocytes from cancer patients are required for optimal induction of cytotoxic T cells against the autologous tumor. *J Immunol* 2000; **164**: 3902–12.

**84** MITCHISON NA, RAJEWSKY K, TAYLOR RB. In: Sterzle J, Riha I, eds. *Developmental aspects of antibody formation and structure.* New York: Academic Press 1970: 547.

**85** MUELLER DL, JENKINS MK, SCHWARTZ RH. An accessory cell-derived costimulatory signal acts independently of protein kinase C activation to allow T cell proliferation and prevent the induction of unresponsiveness. *J Immunol* 1989; **142**: 2617–28.

**86** MUELLER DL, JENKINS MK, SCHWARTZ RH. Clonal expansion versus functional clonal inactivation: a costimulatory signalling pathway determines the outcome of T cell antigen receptor occupancy. *Annu Rev Immunol* 1989; **7**: 445–80.

**87** LINSLEY PS, CLARK EA, LEDBETTER JA. T-cell antigen CD28 mediates adhesion with B cells by interacting with activation antigen B7/BB-1. *Proc Natl Acad Sci USA* 1990; **87**: 5031–5.

**88** CHEN L, ASHE S, BRADY WA, HELLSTROM I, HELLSTROM KE, LEDBETTER JA, McGOWAN P, LINSLEY PS. Costimulation of antitumor immunity by the B7 counterreceptor for the T lymphocyte molecules CD28 and CTLA-4. *Cell* 1992; **71**: 1093–102.

**89** CANTRELL DA, SMITH KA. Transient expression of interleukin 2 receptors. Consequences for T cell growth. *J Exp Med* 1983; **158**: 1895–911.

**90** RAULET DH, BEVAN MJ. A differentiation factor required for the expression of cytotoxic T-cell function. *Nature* 1982; **296**: 754–7.

**91** KLEIN JR, RAULET DH, PASTERNACK MS, BEVAN MJ. Cytotoxic T lymphocytes produce immune interferon in response to antigen or mitogen. *J Exp Med* 1982; **155**: 1198–203.

92 FILGUEIRA L, ZUBER M, JURETIC A, LUSCHER U, CAETANO V, HARDER F, GAROTTA G, HEBERER M, SPAGNOLI GC. Differential effects of interleukin-2 and CD3 triggering on cytokine gene transcription and secretion in cultured tumor infiltrating lymphocytes. *Cell Immunol* 1993; **150**: 205–18.

93 BENNETT SR, CARBONE FR, KARAMALIS F, FLAVELL RA, MILLER JF, HEATH WR. Help for cytotoxic-T-cell responses is mediated by CD40 signalling. *Nature* 1998; **393**: 478–80.

94 REID CD. The biology and clinical applications of dendritic cells. *Transfus Med* 1998; **8**: 77–86.

95 RIDGE JP, DI ROSA F, MATZINGER P. A conditioned dendritic cell can be a temporal bridge between a CD4$^+$ T-helper and a T-killer cell. *Nature* 1998; **393**: 474–8.

96 SCHOENBERGER SP, TOES RE, VAN DER VOORT EI, OFFRINGA R, MELIEF CJ. T-cell help for cytotoxic T lymphocytes is mediated by CD40–CD40L interactions. *Nature* 1998; **393**: 480–3.

97 LANZAVECCHIA A. Licence to kill. *Nature* 1998; **393**: 413–4.

98 SIEGEL JP. Effects of interferon-γ on the activation of human T lymphocytes. *Cell Immunol* 1988; **111**: 461–72.

99 TUTTLE TM, MCCRADY CW, INGE TH, SALOUR M, BEAR HD. γ-Interferon plays a key role in T-cell-induced tumor regression. *Cancer Res* 1993; **53**: 833–9.

100 TALMADGE JE. Therapeutic potential of cytokines: a comparison of preclinical and clinical studies. *Prog Exp Tumor Res* 1988; **32**: 154–73.

101 TAKESHITA T, ASAO H, OHTANI K, ISHII N, KUMAKI S, TANAKA N, MUNAKATA H, NAKAMURA M, SUGAMURA K. Cloning of the gamma chain of the human IL-2 receptor. *Science* 1992; **257**: 379–82.

102 SMITH KA. Lowest dose interleukin-2 immunotherapy. *Blood* 1993; **81**: 1414–23.

103 STUHLER G, SCHLOSSMAN SF. Antigen organization regulates cluster formation and induction of cytotoxic T lymphocytes by helper T cell subsets. *Proc Natl Acad Sci USA* 1997; **94**: 622–7.

104 STUHLER G, ZOBYWALSKI A, GRUNEBACH F, BROSSART P, REICHARDT VL, BARTH H, STEVANOVIC S, BRUGGER W, KANZ L, SCHLOSSMAN SF. Immune regulatory loops determine productive interactions within human T lymphocyte-dendritic cell clusters. *Proc Natl Acad Sci USA* 1999; **96**: 1532–5.

105 PAWELEC G, REES RC, KIESSLING R, MADRIGAL A, DODI A, BAXEVANIS C, GAMBACORTI-PASSERINI C, MASUCCI G, ZEUTHEN J. Cells and cytokines in immunotherapy and gene therapy of cancer. *Crit Rev Oncogenes* 1999; **10**: 83–127.

106 BANCHEREAU J, STEINMAN RM. Dendritic cells and the control of immunity. *Nature* 1998; **392**: 245–52.

107 SHORTMAN K, CAUX C. Dendritic cell development: multiple pathways to nature's adjuvants. *Stem Cells* 1997; **15**: 409–19.

108 PORGADOR A, GILBOA E. Bone marrow-generated dendritic cells pulsed with a class I-restricted peptide are potent inducers of cytotoxic T lymphocytes. *J Exp Med* 1995; **182**: 255–60.

109 URBAN JL, SCHREIBER H. Host–tumor interactions in immunosurveillance against cancer. *Prog Exp Tumor Res* 1988; **32**: 17–68.

110 BERD D, MAGUIRE HC JR, MCCUE P, MASTRANGELO MJ. Treatment of metastatic melanoma with an autologous tumor-cell vaccine: clinical and immunologic results in 64 patients. *J Clin Oncol* 1990; **8**: 1858–67.

111 MORTON DL, FOSHAG LJ, HOON DS, NIZZE JA, FAMATIGA E, WANEK LA, CHANG C, DAVTYAN DG, GUPTA RK, ELASHOFF R, IRIE RF. Prolongation of survival in metastatic melanoma after active specific immunotherapy with a new polyvalent melanoma vaccine. *Ann Surg* 1992; **216**: 463–82.

112 MORTON DL, BARTH A. Vaccine therapy for malignant melanoma. *CA Cancer J Clin* 1996; **46**: 225–44.

113 CROWLEY NJ, SLINGLUFF CL JR, DARROW TL, SEIGLER HF. Generation of human autologous melanoma-specific cytotoxic T-cells using HLA-A2-matched allo-

geneic melanomas. *Cancer Res* 1990; **50**: 492–8.

114 CROWLEY NJ, DARROW TL, SEIGLER HF. Generation of autologous tumor-specific cytotoxic T-cells using HLA-A region matched allogeneic melanoma. *Curr Surg* 1989; **46**: 393–6.

115 MITCHELL MS. Perspective on allogeneic melanoma lysates in active specific immunotherapy. *Semin Oncol* 1998; **25**: 623–35.

116 FUJIWARA H, AOKI H, YOSHIOKA T, TOMITA S, IKEGAMI R, HAMAOKA T. Establishment of a tumor-specific immunotherapy model utilizing TNP-reactive helper T cell activity and its application to the autochthonous tumor system. *J Immunol* 1984; **133**: 509–14.

117 BERD D, KAIRYS J, DUNTON C, MASTRANGELO MJ, SATO T, MAGUIRE HC JR. Autologous, hapten-modified vaccine as a treatment for human cancers. *Semin Oncol* 1998; **25**: 646–53.

118 BERD D, MAGUIRE HC JR, SCHUCHTER LM, HAMILTON R, HAUCK WW, SATO T, MASTRANGELO MJ. Autologous hapten-modified melanoma vaccine as postsurgical adjuvant treatment after resection of nodal metastases. *J Clin Oncol* 1997; **15**: 2359–70.

119 BERD D, MURPHY G, MAGUIRE HC JR, MASTRANGELO MJ. Immunization with haptenized, autologous tumor cells induces inflammation of human melanoma metastases. *Cancer Res* 1991; **51**: 2731–4.

120 BASKAR S, NABAVI N, GLIMCHER LH, OSTRAND-ROSENBERG S. Tumor cells expressing major histocompatibility complex class II and B7 activation molecules stimulate potent tumor-specific immunity. *J Immunother* 1993; **14**: 209–15.

121 DRANOFF G, JAFFEE E, LAZENBY A, GOLUMBEK P, LEVITSKY H, BROSE K, JACKSON V, HAMADA H, PARDOLL D, MULLIGAN RC. Vaccination with irradiated tumor cells engineered to secrete murine granulocyte-macrophage colony-stimulating factor stimulates potent, specific, and long-lasting anti-tumor immunity. *Proc Natl Acad Sci USA* 1993; **90**: 3539–43.

122 DRANOFF G, SOIFFER R, LYNCH T, MIHM M, JUNG K, KOLESAR K, LIEBSTER L, LAM P, DUDA R, MENTZER S, SINGER S, TANABE K, JOHNSON R, SOBER A, BHAN A, CLIFT S, COHEN L, PARRY G, ROKOVICH J, RICHARDS L, DRAYER J, BERNS A, MULLIGAN RC. A phase I study of vaccination with autologous, irradiated melanoma cells engineered to secrete human granulocyte-macrophage colony stimulating factor. *Hum Gene Ther* 1997; **8**: 111–23.

123 SOIFFER R, LYNCH T, MIHM M, JUNG K, RHUDA C, SCHMOLLINGER JC, HODI FS, LIEBSTER L, LAM P, MENTZER S, SINGER S, TANABE KK, COSIMI AB, DUDA R, SOBER A, BHAN A, DALEY J, NEUBERG D, PARRY G, ROKOVICH J, RICHARDS L, DRAYER J, BERNS A, CLIFT S, DRANOFF G, COHEN LK, MULLIGAN RC. Vaccination with irradiated autologous melanoma cells engineered to secrete human granulocyte-macrophage colony-stimulating factor generates potent antitumor immunity in patients with metastatic melanoma. *Proc Natl Acad Sci USA* 1998; **95**: 13141–6.

124 MACH N, GILLESSEN S, WILSON SB, SHEEHAN C, MIHM M, DRANOFF G. Differences in dendritic cells stimulated *in vivo* by tumors engineered to secrete granulocyte-macrophage colony-stimulating factor or Flt3-ligand. *Cancer Res* 2000; **60**: 3239–46.

125 ABDEL-WAHAB Z, WELTZ C, HESTER D, PICKETT N, VERVAERT C, BARBER JR, JOLLY D, SEIGLER HF. A Phase I clinical trial of immunotherapy with interferon-gamma gene-modified autologous melanoma cells: monitoring the humoral immune response. *Cancer* 1997; **80**: 401–12.

126 NEMUNAITIS J, BOHART C, FONG T, MEYER W, EDELMAN G, PAULSON RS, ORR D, JAIN V, O'BRIEN J, KUHN J, KOWAL KJ, BURKEHOLDER S, BRUCE J, OGNOSKIE N, WYNNE D, MARTINEAU D, ANDO D. Phase I trial of retroviral vector-mediated interferon (IFN)-gamma gene transfer into autologous tumor cells in patients with metastatic melanoma. *Cancer Gene Ther* 1998; **5**: 292–300.

127 DRANOFF G, JAFFEE E, LAZENBY A, GOLUMBEK P, LEVITSKY H, BROSE K, JACK-

son V, Hamada H, Pardoll D, Mulligan RC. Vaccination with irradiated tumor cells engineered to secrete murine granulocyte-macrophage colony-stimulating factor stimulates potent, specific, and long-lasting anti-tumor immunity. *Proc Natl Acad Sci USA* 1993; **90**: 3539–43.

128  Baskar S, Ostrand-Rosenberg S, Nabavi N, Nadler LM, Freeman GJ, Glimcher LH. Constitutive expression of B7 restores immunogenicity of tumor cells expressing truncated major histocompatibility complex class II molecules. *Proc Natl Acad Sci USA* 1993; **90**: 5687–90.

129  Pardoll DM. Cancer vaccines. *Nat Med* 1998; **4**: 525–31.

130  Chen JL, Dunbar PR, Gileadi U, Jager E, Gnjatic S, Nagata Y, Stockert E, Panicali DL, Chen YT, Knuth A, Old LJ, Cerundolo V. Identification of NY-ESO-1 peptide analogues capable of improved stimulation of tumor-reactive CTL. *J Immunol* 2000; **165**: 948–55.

131  Salgaller ML, Marincola FM, Cormier JN, Rosenberg SA. Immunization against epitopes in the human melanoma antigen gp100 following patient immunization with synthetic peptides. *Cancer Res* 1996; **56**: 4749–57.

132  Cormier JN, Salgaller ML, Prevette T, Barracchini KC, Rivoltini L, Restifo NP, Rosenberg SA, Marincola FM. Enhancement of cellular immunity in melanoma patients immunized with a peptide from MART-1/Melan A. *Cancer J Sci Am* 1997; **3**: 37–44.

133  Rosenberg SA, Yang JC, Schwartzentruber DJ, Hwu P, Marincola FM, Topalian SL, Restifo NP, Dudley ME, Schwarz SL, Spiess PJ, Wunderlich JR, Parkhurst MR, Kawakami Y, Seipp CA, Einhorn JH, White DE. Immunologic and therapeutic evaluation of a synthetic peptide vaccine for the treatment of patients with metastatic melanoma. *Nat Med* 1998; **4**: 321–7.

134  Marchand M, van Baren N, Weynants P, Brichard V, Dreno B, Tessier MH, Rankin E, Parmiani G, Arienti F, Humblet Y, Bourlond A,

Vanwijck R, Lienard D, Beauduin M, Dietrich PY, Russo V, Kerger J, Masucci G, Jager E, De Greve J, Atzpodien J, Brasseur F, Coulie PG, van der Bruggen P, Boon T. Tumor regressions observed in patients with metastatic melanoma treated with an antigenic peptide encoded by gene MAGE-3 and presented by HLA-A1. *Int J Cancer* 1999; **80**: 219–30.

135  Valmori D, Romero JF, Men Y, Maryanski JL, Romero P, Corradin G. Induction of a cytotoxic T cell response by co-injection of a T helper peptide and a cytotoxic T lymphocyte peptide in incomplete Freund's adjuvant (IFA): further enhancement by pre-injection of IFA alone. *Eur J Immunol* 1994; **24**: 1458–62.

136  Corr M, Lee DJ, Carson DA, Tighe H. Gene vaccination with naked plasmid DNA: mechanism of CTL priming. *J Exp Med* 1996; **184**: 1555–60.

137  Corr M, Tighe H, Lee D, Dudler J, Trieu M, Brinson DC, Carson DA. Costimulation provided by DNA immunization enhances antitumor immunity. *J Immunol* 1997; **159**: 4999–5004.

138  Rosenberg SA, Zhai Y, Yang JC, Schwartzentruber DJ, Hwu P, Marincola FM, Topalian SL, Restifo NP, Seipp CA, Einhorn JH, Roberts B, White DE. Immunizing patients with metastatic melanoma using recombinant adenoviruses encoding MART-1 or gp100 melanoma antigens. *J Natl Cancer Inst* 1998; **90**: 1894–900.

139  Brossart P, Goldrath AW, Butz EA, Martin S, Bevan MJ. Virus-mediated delivery of antigenic epitopes into dendritic cells as a means to induce CTL. *J Immunol* 1997; **158**: 3270–6.

140  Mukherji B, Chakraborty NG, Yamasaki S, Okino T, Yamase H, Sporn JR, Kurtzman SK, Ergin MT, Ozols J, Meehan J, Mauri F. Induction of antigen-specific cytolytic T cells *in situ* in human melanoma by immunization with synthetic peptide-pulsed autologous antigen presenting cells. *Proc Natl Acad Sci USA* 1995; **92**: 8078–82.

141  Celluzzi CM, Mayordomo JI, Storkus WJ, Lotze MT, Falo LD Jr. Peptide-pulsed dendritic cells induce anti-

gen-specific CTL-mediated protective tumor immunity. *J Exp Med* 1996; **183**: 283–7.

142 HU X, CHAKRABORTY NG, SPORN JR, KURTZMAN SH, ERGIN MT, MUKHERJI B. Enhancement of cytolytic T lymphocyte precursor frequency in melanoma patients following immunization with the MAGE-1 peptide loaded antigen presenting cell-based vaccine. *Cancer Res* 1996; **56**: 2479–83.

143 NESTLE FO, ALIJAGIC S, GILLIET M, SUN Y, GRABBE S, DUMMER R, BURG G and SCHADENDORF D. Vaccination of melanoma patients with peptide- or tumor lysate-pulsed dendritic cells. *Nat Med* 1998; **4**: 328–32.

144 SALIO M, SHEPHERD D, DUNBAR PR, PALMOWSKI M, MURPHY K, WU L, CERUNDOLO V. Mature dendritic cells prime functionally superior melan-A-specific CD8$^+$ lymphocytes as compared with nonprofessional APC. *J Immunol* 2001; **167**: 1188–97.

145 CONDON C, WATKINS SC, CELLUZZI CM, THOMPSON K, FALO LD JR. DNA-based immunization by *in vivo* transfection of dendritic cells. *Nat Med* 1996; **2**: 1122–8.

146 KOIDO S, KASHIWABA M, CHEN D, GENDLER S, KUFE D, GONG J. Induction of antitumor immunity by vaccination of dendritic cells transfected with MUC1 RNA. *J Immunol* 2000; **165**: 5713–9.

147 VAN TENDELOO VF, PONSAERTS P, LARDON F, NIJS G, LENJOU M, VAN BROECKHOVEN C, VAN BOCKSTAELE DR, BERNEMAN ZN. Highly efficient gene delivery by mRNA electroporation in human hematopoietic cells: superiority to lipofection and passive pulsing of mRNA and to electroporation of plasmid cDNA for tumor antigen loading of dendritic cells. *Blood* 2001; **98**: 49–56.

148 CELLUZZI CM, FALO LD JR. Physical interaction between dendritic cells and tumor cells results in an immunogen that induces protective and therapeutic tumor rejection. *J Immunol* 1998; **160**: 3081–5.

149 GONG J, CHEN D, KASHIWABA M, KUFE D. Induction of antitumor activity by immunization with fusions of den-

dritic and carcinoma cells. *Nat Med* 1997; **3**: 558–61.

150 WANG J, SAFFOLD S, CAO X, KRAUSS J, CHEN W. Eliciting T cell immunity against poorly immunogenic tumors by immunization with dendritic cell-tumor fusion vaccines. *J Immunol* 1998; **161**: 5516–24.

151 KUGLER A, STUHLER G, WALDEN P, ZOLLER G, ZOBYWALSKI A, BROSSART P, TREFZER U, ULLRICH S, MULLER CA, BECKER V, GROSS AJ, HEMMERLEIN B, KANZ L, MULLER GA, RINGERT RH. Regression of human metastatic renal cell carcinoma after vaccination with tumor cell-dendritic cell hybrids. *Nat Med* 2000; **6**: 332–6.

152 ORENTAS RJ, SCHAUER D, BIN Q, JOHNSON BD. Electrofusion of a weakly immunogenic neuroblastoma with dendritic cells produces a tumor vaccine. *Cell Immunol* 2001; **213**: 4–13.

153 KIKUCHI T, AKASAKI Y, IRIE M, HOMMA S, ABE T, OHNO T. Results of a phase I clinical trial of vaccination of glioma patients with fusions of dendritic and glioma cells. *Cancer Immunol Immunother* 2001; **50**: 337–44.

154 HOMMA S, TODA G, GONG J, KUFE D, OHNO T. Preventive antitumor activity against hepatocellular carcinoma (HCC) induced by immunization with fusions of dendritic cells and HCC cells in mice. *J Gastroenterol* 2001; **36**: 764–71.

155 AKASAKI Y, KIKUCHI T, HOMMA S, ABE T, KOFE D, OHNO T. Antitumor effect of immunizations with fusions of dendritic and glioma cells in a mouse brain tumor model. *J Immunother* 2001; **24**: 106–13.

156 GONG J, APOSTOLOPOULOS V, CHEN D, CHEN H, KOIDO S, GENDLER SJ, MCKENZIE IF, KUFE D. Selection and characterization of MUC1-specific CD8$^+$ T cells from MUC1 transgenic mice immunized with dendritic-carcinoma fusion cells. *Immunology* 2000; **101**: 316–24.

157 GONG J, NIKRUI N, CHEN D, KOIDO S, WU Z, TANAKA Y, CANNISTRA S, AVIGAN D, KUFE D. Fusions of human ovarian carcinoma cells with autologous or allogeneic dendritic cells in-

duce antitumor immunity. *J Immunol* 2000; **165**: 1705–11.

158 GONG J, AVIGAN D, CHEN D, WU Z, KOIDO S, KASHIWABA M, KUFE D. Activation of antitumor cytotoxic T lymphocytes by fusions of human dendritic cells and breast carcinoma cells. *Proc Natl Acad Sci USA* 2000; **97**: 2715–8.

159 GONG J, CHEN D, KASHIWABA M, LI Y, CHEN L, TAKEUCHI H, QU H, ROWSE GJ, GENDLER SJ, KUFE D. Reversal of tolerance to human MUC1 antigen in MUC1 transgenic mice immunized with fusions of dendritic and carcinoma cells. *Proc Natl Acad Sci USA* 1998; **95**: 6279–83.

160 YEE C, THOMPSON JA, ROCHE P, BYRD DR, LEE PP, PIEPKORN M, KENYON K, DAVIS MM, RIDDELL SR, GREENBERG PD. Melanocyte destruction after antigen-specific immunotherapy of melanoma: direct evidence of t cell-mediated vitiligo. *J Exp Med* 2000; **192**: 1637–44.

161 STUHLER G and WALDEN P. Recruitment of helper T cells for induction of tumor rejection by cytolytic T lymphocytes. *Cancer Immunol Immunother* 1994; **39**: 342–5.

162 GUO Y, WU M, CHEN H, WANG X, LIU G, LI G, MA J, SY MS. Effective tumor vaccine generated by fusion of hepatoma cells with activated B cells. *Science* 1994; **263**: 518–20.

163 STUHLER G, TREFZER U, WALDEN P. Hybrid cell vaccination in cancer immunotherapy. Recruitment and activation of T cell help for induction of anti tumour cytotoxic T cells. *Adv Exp Med Biol* 1998; **451**: 277–82.

164 SATTHAPORN S, EREMIN O. Dendritic cells (I): biological functions. *J R Coll Surg Edinb* 2001; **46**: 9–19.

165 SATTHAPORN S, EREMIN O. Dendritic cells (II): role and therapeutic implications in cancer. *J R Coll Surg Edinb* 2001; **46**: 159–67.

166 SCOTT-TAYLOR TH, PETTENGELL R, CLARKE I, STUHLER G, LA BARTHE MC, WALDEN P, DALGLEISH AG. Human tumor and dendritic cell hybrids generated by electrofusion: potential for cancer vaccines. *Biochim Biophys Acta* 2000; **1500**:2 65–79.

167 TREFZER U, WEINGART G, STERRY W, WALDEN P. Hybrid cell vaccination in patients with metastatic melanoma. *Methods Mol Med*. 2000; **35**: 469–75.

168 TANAKA Y, KOIDO S, CHEN D, GENDLER SJ, KUFE D, GONG J. Vaccination with allogeneic dendritic cells fused to carcinoma cells induces antitumor immunity in MUC1 transgenic mice. *Clin Immunol* 2001; **101**:192–200.

169 SOUBERBIELLE BE, WESTBY M, GANZ S, KAYAGA J, MENDES R, MORROW WJ, DALGLEISH AG. Comparison of four strategies for tumour vaccination in the B16-F10 melanoma model. *Gene Ther* 1998; **5**: 1447–54.

170 DUNNION DJ, CYWINSKI AL, TUCKER VC, MURRAY AK, RICKINSON AB, COULIE P, BROWNING MJ. Human antigen-presenting cell/tumor cell hybrids stimulate strong allogeneic responses and present tumor-associated antigens to cytotoxic T cells *in vitro*. *Immunology* 1999; **98**: 541–50.

171 TREFZER U, WEINGART G, CHEN Y, HERBERTH G, ADRIAN K, WINTER H, AUDRING H, GUO Y, STERRY W, WALDEN P. Hybrid cell vaccination for cancer immune therapy: first clinical trial with metastatic melanoma. *Int J Cancer* 2000; **85**: 618–26.

172 TREFZER U, HERBERTH G, STERRY W, WALDEN P. The hybrid cell vaccination approach to cancer immunotherapy. *Ernst Schering Res Found Workshop* 2000; **30**: 154–66.

173 KUGLER A, SESEKE F, THELEN P, KALLERHOFF M, MULLER GA, STUHLER G, MULLER C, RINGERT RH. Autologous and allogenic hybrid cell vaccine in patients with metastatic renal cell carcinoma. *Br J Urol* 1998; **82**: 487–93.

174 GILBOA E, NAIR SK, LYERLY HK. Immunotherapy of cancer with dendritic-cell-based vaccines. *Cancer Immunol Immunother* 1998; **46**: 82–7.

175 ASHLEY DM, FAIOLA B, NAIR S, HALE LP, BIGNER DD, GILBOA E. Bone marrow-generated dendritic cells pulsed with tumor extracts or tumor RNA induce antitumor immunity against central nervous system tumors. *J Exp Med* 1997; **186**: 1177–82.

**176** PORGADOR A, GILBOA E. Bone marrow-generated dendritic cells pulsed with a class I-restricted peptide are potent inducers of cytotoxic T lymphocytes. *J Exp Med* 1995; **182**: 255–60.

**177** NAIR SK, BOCZKOWSKI D, SNYDER D, GILBOA E. Antigen-presenting cells pulsed with unfractionated tumor-derived peptides are potent tumor vaccines. *Eur J Immunol* 1997; **27**: 589–97.

**178** BOCZKOWSKI D, NAIR SK, SNYDER D, GILBOA E. Dendritic cells pulsed with RNA are potent antigen-presenting cells *in vitro* and *in vivo*. *J Exp Med* 1996; **184**: 465–72.

**179** BOCZKOWSKI D, NAIR SK, NAM JH, LYERLY HK, GILBOA E. Induction of tumor immunity and cytotoxic T lymphocyte responses using dendritic cells transfected with messenger RNA amplified from tumor cells. *Cancer Res* 2000; **60**: 1028–34.

**180** HEISER A, MAURICE MA, YANCEY DR, WU NZ, DAHM P, PRUITT SK, BOCZKOWSKI D, NAIR SK, BALLO MS, GILBOA E, VIEWEG J. Induction of polyclonal prostate cancer-specific CTL using dendritic cells transfected with amplified tumor RNA. *J Immunol* 2001; **166**: 2953–60.

# 12

# Principles and Strategies Employing Heat Shock Proteins for Immunotherapy of Cancers

ZIHAI LI

## 12.1
### The Thesis

Fueled by the idea of immunosurveillance [1] and the dream that tumors can be dealt with by vaccinations, tumor immunologists have contributed significantly to the development of immunology, such as in the discovery of major histocompatibility complex (MHC) molecules, certain cell types like natural killer (NK) cells and cytokines, including tumor necrosis factor (TNF), and the development of monoclonal antibody technologies [2]. The immunological properties of heat shock proteins (HSPs) began to emerge in the 1980s when it was found that HSPs purified from tumor cells can immunize animals against tumor challenge, despite the fact that there are no tumor-specific structural changes of HSPs themselves [3]!

HSPs are a family of extremely conserved (from single-celled organisms to *Homo sapiens*) "housekeeping" molecules that have everything to do with protein folding and unfolding in the cell [4, 5]. They are subclassified customarily according to their molecular weight (kDa), such as the family of HSP90, HSP70, HSP60, and low and high molecular weight HSPs. There are multiple members in each family. For example, the HSP90 family encompasses cytosolic HSP90$\alpha$, HSP90$\beta$ and the endoplasmic reticular counterpart of HSP90, gp96 or grp94 [6]. On the one hand, HSPs are detergent-like molecules inside of the cell to prevent millions of millions of proteins and their intermediates from sticking to one another [7]. On the other hand, the roles of HSPs in the prevention of protein denaturation and apoptosis explain why they are often induced by heat (hence the name HSP), or other conditions that lead to protein unfolding or misfolding [8].

Over the last two decades, several immunological principles of HSPs have been uncovered (Fig. 12.1). It is now clear that HSPs play broader roles in both innate and adaptive immunity [3, 9].

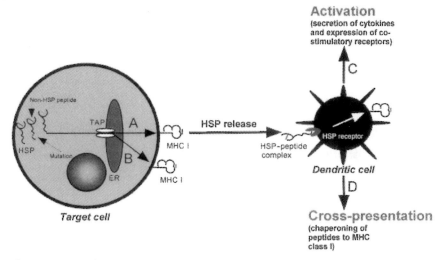

**Fig. 12.1** Immunological principles of HSPs. At least four immunological principles of HSP in tumor immunity have been described. (A) HSPs are rarely tumor-specific antigens due to altered structure or mutations. (B) HSPs are carriers for intracellular antigenic peptides. (C) HSPs activate DCs by binding directly to HSP receptor(s) on DCs. (D) HSP chaperoned peptides can be cross-presented to MHC molecules on DCs for cross-priming of T cells.

### 12.1.1
### HSPs *per se* are rarely Tumor Antigens

HSPs are well-conserved molecules in evolution with limited polymorphism. Although HSP expression can be down-regulated and up-regulated in relation to cancers, no cancer specific "hotspots" of mutations have been described. In only one published example, mutation of HSP70 occurred in renal cell carcinoma and the mutated HSP70 molecule served as the target for tumor-specific cytotoxic T lymphocytes (CTLs) [10]. This is an exception rather than a rule.

### 12.1.2
### HSPs are Molecular Chaperones for Antigenic Peptides

This concept was proposed to explain the dilemma that immunization with structurally normal HSPs purified from tumor cells, but not from normal cells, confers tumor specific immunity [11, 12]. The principle has since been confirmed structurally and immunologically in the HSP70 and HSP90 family. The resolution of the HSP–peptide complex is largely achieved by studying if HSPs can associate with immunologically defined peptides [3]. For example, gp96 purified from vesicular stomatitis virus (VSV)-infected cells, but not uninfected cells, was associated with an 8mer VSV-derived peptide as revealed by both structural and immunological assays [13]. Similarly, it was shown that highly purified gp96 from cells expressing β-galactosidase, minor histocompatibility antigens [14], ovalbumin [15, 16] and murine leukemia Rl male symbol antigens [17] associated with respective peptides derived from these proteins. Furthermore, it was found in patients with hepatitis virus B-associated hepatocellular carcinomas that a virus-specific peptide is associated with gp96 [18]. The peptide-binding property of gp96 has also been supported by a number of biophysical and structural assays [19–23]. By protease mapping and cross-linking approaches, the minimal peptide-binding site of gp96 was mapped to amino acid residues 624–630 in a highly conserved region [21]. In case of HSP70, the peptides can be dissociated with ATP [24]. As expected, treatment of HSP70–peptide complex with ATP leads to loss of immunogenicity [25]. Studies have also shown that HSP70 purified from human melanoma can activate T cells to recognize melanoma differentiation antigens such as MART-1, gp100 and TRP-2 in a MHC-restricted manner [26]. Moreover, HSP70 isolated from an allogeneic melanoma cell line can pulse gp100-negative target cells for specific recognition by anti-gp100 CTL clones, indicating that peptide binding by HSP70 is not restricted by MHC haplotypes. Structurally, the peptide-binding pocket of DnaK, a prokaryotic HSP70, has been resolved [27].

### 12.1.3
### HSPs are Adjuvants

HSPs can interact specifically with antigen-presenting cells (APCs), such as dendritic cells (DCs), through receptor-dependent mechanism [28–32]. Such interaction leads to DC activation evidenced by the production of pro-inflammatory cytokines, and up-regulation of the surface expression of a number of co-stimulatory molecules such as CD80 and CD86 [33–39]. Most of the attention has been focused on the role of HSPs in productive immune responses. It should be kept in mind that HSPs could also play roles in tolerance induction by inducing DCs to produce anti-inflammatory cytokines. For example, it has been reported that small molecular weight HSPs such as HSP27 could stimulate human monocytes to produce IL-10, which is an anti-inflammatory cytokine [40].

### 12.1.4
### HSPs are Involved in Cross-Priming

It has been commonly accepted that tumor antigens have to be cross-presented from tumor cells to the MHC class I and class II molecules of APC for the priming of respective CD8$^+$ and CD4$^+$ T cells due to lack of co-stimulatory molecules on tumor cells. This is known as cross-presentation. The activation of naïve T cells through cross-presentation is defined as cross-priming [41, 42]. It has been observed that HSP-chaperoned peptides can be presented to MHC class I through their common receptor CD91 on the surface of APCs *in vitro* [43, 44]. Furthermore, immunization with HSP-peptide complexes can clearly lead to the activation of CD8$^+$ CTLs *in vivo*, supporting the roles of HSPs in cross priming.

## 12.1.5
## Other Roles

Additionally, HSPs have been found to be expressed on the cell surface, and in various scenarios HSPs can serve as direct targets for γδ T cells [45, 46], NK cells [47] and CD4⁻CD8⁻ T cells [48]. These intriguing findings illustrate the plasticity of HSPs in immune responses, and certainly prompt more research into the structural and mechanistic basis of their actions.

## 12.2
## Cancer Immunotherapy Strategies with HSPs

The emerging immunological principles of HSPs have stimulated interests in the development of HSPs as tumor vaccines. There are generally three strategies (Fig. 12.2). First, purified autologous tumor-derived HSPs can be used as tumor vaccines based on the fact that tumor-derived HSPs chaperone antigenic peptides and prime adaptive immunity. Second, defined tumor antigens can be fused either covalently or non-covalently to HSPs and used as a T cell vaccine due to the adjuvanticity of HSPs. Third, manipulation of the site and level of HSP expression in the tumor cells have been shown to stimulate tumor-specific immunity.

## 12.2.1
## Strategy 1: Autologous HSPs as Tumor-Specific Vaccines

Extensive transplantation experiments with syngeneic tumors in the 1950s [49–53] have demonstrated that tumor rejection antigens responsible for tumor-protective immunity are private, or individually distinct. Thus tumor A cannot immunize against tumor B and *vice versa* even though tumor A and B are derived from the same histological types, induced by the same carcinogen or even developed in the same host. This phenomenon revealed one fundamentally important obstacle of cancer immunotherapy, i.e. immunotherapy of cancer has to be individualized. Shared antigens that are conserved among cancers such as differentiation antigen and genes involved in tumorigenesis (oncogene or tumor suppressor genes) are probably not effective tumor rejection antigens.

This argument suggests that antigenic composition is different among tumors, and predicts that the effective cancer vaccine has to be derived from autologous tumors. Since HSPs can bind to peptides with broad specificity and there are no free-flowing peptides inside the cells [54], it has been suggested that peptides bound to HSPs represent a total cellular peptide pool [3, 55], which forms a basis for tumor vaccines with autologous tumor-derived HSPs.

The phenomenology of tumor-specific protection by immunization with tumor-specific HSPs in experimental animals is widespread [3, 9]. In addition, purified tumor-derived HSP–peptide complexes are potent vaccines for pre-established cancers such as lung, melanoma, lymphoma, fibrosarcoma, adenocarcinoma of the colon, sar-

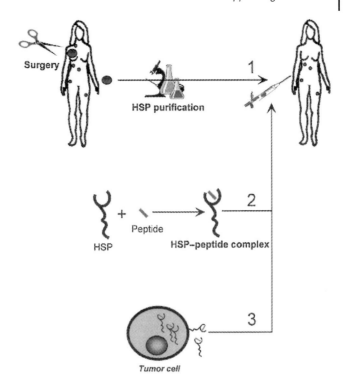

**Fig. 12.2**   Cancer immunotherapy strategies with HSPs. Three general strategies are explored for immunotherapy of cancer by HSPs. (1) Autologous tumor-derived HSPs can be purified and re-injected into a patient to elicit tumor-specific immunity. (2) If the tumor antigen is defined, the HSP–tumor antigen complex can be generated either covalently or non-covalently and used as a vaccine to generate antigen-specific immunity. (3) Whole tumor cells engineered to express high levels of HSPs or express HSPs ectopically (secretion or cell surface expression) are used as tumor vaccines.

coma, prostate or breast cancers (Tab. 12.1). The first pilot trial for the treatment of human malignancy showed that this approach is safe and feasible [56]. In this trial, 16 patients with various advanced malignancies (seven gastrointestinal tract, one pancreatic, two hepatocellular, three thyroid, one breast, one mesothelioma and one unknown primary), which had become refractory to established therapies, were treated with autologous tumor-derived gp96. Patients were injected subcutaneously (s.c.) with 25 µg autologous gp96 once a week for 4 weeks. After each vaccination, patients were carefully monitored clinically and serologically. No unacceptable toxicities or autoimmune phenomenon were observed. Three patients reported mild hot flashes between 30 and 48 min after immunization, without the need for medical intervention. Of these, two experienced hot flashes after each immunization, while one ex-

**Tab. 12.1**   Immunotherapy of cancers with tumor-derived HSP–peptide complexes

| Host | Tumor model | HSP | Reference |
|------|-------------|-----|-----------|
| Mouse | Meth A fibrosarcoma | gp96, HSP90, HSP70 | 93–95 |
| | | CRT | 96 |
| | | HSP110, GRP170 | 97 |
| | UV-induced sarcoma | gp96, HSP70 | 98 |
| | colon cancer | gp96, HSP70 | 99 |
| | leukemia | HSP70, gp96, HSP90, CRT | 100 |
| | melanoma | gp96, HSP70 | 99 |
| | lung cancer | gp96, HSP70 | 99 |
| Rat | prostate cancer | gp96 | 101 |
| | hepatoma | gp96 | 102 |
| Xenopus | lymphoma | gp96, HSP70 | 103 |
| Human | a variety of tumors | gp96 | 57 |

perienced them again only after the second immunization. In four patients, pain or fever occurred during the immunization period; however, their onset was unrelated to the timing of immunization and the events were attributed to tumor progression. None of these patients mounted significant titer of the following antoantibodies: anti-nucleoprotein antibody, antibody to double- or single-stranded DNA, antibodies to mitochondria, thyroglobulin, microsome, perinuclear, or cytoplasmic antigens after gp96 immunization. One patient died 4 days after the second immunization, which was determined to be due to the progression of his disease. Thus, there is no evidence of acute gp96 induced side effects due to self-destructive immune reactions.

The efficacy of gp96 in the treatment of stage III renal cell carcinoma after surgical resection is now being studied by a phase III randomized, multi-center trial around the world. The phase I and II data in the treatment of various malignancies by gp96 have been reviewed recently [57, 58].

## 12.2.2
### Strategy 2: HSPs as Adjuvant

While the peptide-binding property of HSP is predictable in light of the protein chaperoning function of HSPs in general, the recent discovery of the immunomodulating properties of HSPs was entirely unexpected. It was found that gp96, HSP90, HSP60, calreticulin and HSP70 can all bind to the surface of APCs in a receptor-dependent manner. They share a common receptor CD91 [43, 44]. The interaction of HSPs with APCs results in two functional consequences: the activation of APCs to increase the expression of antigen-presenting and co-stimulatory molecules, and the cross-presentation of HSP-associated peptides to MHC class I for the priming of CTLs (Fig. 11.1). The modulating function of HSPs is not dependent on the ability of them to bind to peptides, which suggest that HSPs can also serve as adjuvants.

**Tab. 12.2**   T cell immunity against defined antigens induced by HSP–peptide complexes

| Antigen | HSP | Reference |
|---|---|---|
| Intracellular bacteria (*L.monocytogenes*, MTB) | gp96 | 104 |
| Bovine herpes virus 1 | gp96 | 105 |
| Adenovirus type 5 E1B | gp96 | 37 |
| Ovalbumin | CRT, gp96 | 16 |
|  | HSP70, gp96 | 15 |
| Mouse leukemia RL symbol 1 | HSP90, gp96 and HSP70 | 17 |
| Influenza virus nucleoprotein | gp96 | 106 |
| VSV nucleoprotein | gp96 | 13 |
| β-Galactosidase | gp96 | 14 |
| Minor H antigens | gp96 | 14 |
| LCMV antigen | HSP70 | 107 |

#### 12.2.2.1  Non-covalent complex between HSP and antigenic peptides

The immunomodulating function of HSPs in the application of cancer therapy has not been thoroughly explored. One reason is probably the observation that the optimal immunity is elicited when antigen is physically complexed with HSPs [59]. Mixing of the two alone without complexing is clearly suboptimal. Therefore, the effort currently for using the adjuvanticity of HSPs is to complex HSPs with a known target (antigen).

Gp96 can associate with peptides reproducibly *in vitro* by a simple heat-dependent refolding assay. Such an interaction between gp96 and peptides has no apparent bias or selectivity towards the sequence and length of the peptides [59]. Therefore, if a tumor-associated peptide is defined, it can be easily complexed with gp96 and be used as a tumor vaccine. The reconstituted gp96 peptide complex is efficient in priming CD8$^+$ T cells [59]. Using this strategy, it was demonstrated that immunization with gp96–VSV peptide complex leads to rejection of thymoma that are made to express VSV.

To further prove the concept, gp96 and other HSPs have been complexed with various infectious agents , and used successfully for generating pathogen-specific T cell responses against lymphocytic choriomeningitis virus (LCMV), *Listeria monocytogenes*, influenza A virus and SV-40 virus large T antigen (Tab. 12.2).

HSP–peptide complex reconstituted *in vitro* retains other immunological functions such as in cross-presentation. For example, pulsing of APCs with gp96 complexed with a retroviral antigen, AH-1, can stimulate AH-1-specific CTLs to release IFN-γ [43]. This re-presentation pathway is dependent on the receptor CD91.

#### 12.2.2.2  Covalent complex between HSP and antigenic peptides

Recombinant *Mycobacterium tuberculosis* (MTB) HSP70 fused covalently with a model peptide has also been found to be highly immunogenic against the peptide [60–62]. Using this system, it was found that the immunogenicity associated with HSP70 fusion protein was dependent on a discrete 200-amino acid protein fragment at the N-terminal ATP-binding domain [63]. The implication for the function of HSP70 is unclear, since the fusion protein may have adopted a different conforma-

**Tab. 12.3**   T cell immunity against defined antigens induced by HSP–peptide fusion proteins

| Antigen | Fusion partners (HSP) | Reference |
|---|---|---|
| Human papillomavirus type 16 E7 | BCG Hsp65 | 108 |
| | *M. tuberculosis* HSP70 | 109 |
| Ovalbumin | Mycobacterial HSP65 | 64 |
| | *M. tuberculosis* HSP70 | 61, 63 |
| Influenza virus nucleoprotein | *M. bovis* BCG Hsp65 | 110 |
| HIV-1 p24 | *M. tuberculosis* HSP70 | 60 |

tion. However, from a practical standpoint, recombinant HSP–antigen fusion protein guarantees coupling and can be manufactured with ease in larger quantities. Moreover, HSP70 fused with a target antigen has also been used successfully in the format of a DNA vaccine. Therefore, in the case when antigen is defined, HSP–antigen fusion vaccine is an attractive approach for immunotherapy (Tab. 12.3).

The mechanism governing the ability of HSP–antigen fusion protein to prime adaptive immunity appears similar to native HSPs. A recombinant mycobacterial HSP65 fused to a polypeptide that contains an octapeptide (SIYRYYGL) can stimulate C57BL/6 mice, as well as CD4$^+$ T cell-deficient mice, to produce CD8$^+$ CTLs to the fusion partner's octapeptide [64]. Moreover, this fusion protein itself stimulated DCs *in vitro* and *in vivo* to up-regulate the levels of MHC (class I and II) and co-stimulatory molecules.

### 12.2.3
### Strategy 3: Whole Cell Vaccine based on the Modulation of the Expression of HSPs

Autologous, or allogeneic, whole tumor cell vaccines continue to be the most common tumor vaccines tested clinically [65]. In addition to being safe and easy to manufacture, there are several unique reasons:

(1) Most tumor antigens are not known, therefore specific antigen-based vaccines are not applicable to a vast majority of patients.
(2) Whole cell vaccines deliver multivalent antigens of both MHC class I and class II epitopes for the activation of multivalent tumor immunities.
(3) When carefully controlled and titrated, the efficacy of whole cell vaccines have been consistently demonstrated in pre-clinical models.

Whole cell vaccines have been tried in numerous clinical settings such as in colorectal cancer, melanoma, sarcoma, renal cell carcinoma, pancreatic cancer, breast cancer and others. In order to increase the efficiency of whole-cell-based vaccines, efforts have been in modifying tumor cells genetically to express immunologically important molecules such as MHC class I and II molecules, co-stimulatory proteins, chemokines or cytokines. More recently, fusion of autologous tumor cells with DCs has shown some clinical promise in the treatment of stage IV renal cell carcinoma [66].

Most HSPs are constitutively expressed, although under stress conditions their expression can be up-regulated to different degrees. For example, the inducible HSP70 in the cytosol seems to be strictly regulated by stress and not expressed at the basal level, whereas the endoplasmic reticulum (ER) homolog of HSP70, grp78 or Bip, is expressed at high levels under non-stress conditions. Moreover, there seem to be "no rules" governing the subcellular localization of HSPs. ER HSPs including gp96 can be displayed on the cell surface during stress and under certain physiological conditions [67–70]. Mechanistic studies of gp96 in cross-presentation of antigens suggested that extracellular gp96 gains access to the cytosolic compartment [37, 43, 44, 71]. Moreover, secretion, surface expression and transport across the plasma membrane of a cytosolic HSP70 have been demonstrated [47, 72, 73]. Surface HSP70 can also serve as a direct target for the immune system [47]. Recently, it has been suggested that the surface forms of supposedly cytosolic HSP70 and HSP90 might participate in the receptor clustering for CD14-independent lipopolysaccharide (LPS) signaling [74].

Due to the emerging knowledge about HSPs in the immune response, whole cells engineered to express HSPs at different levels and different sites have now been tested for immunotherapy of cancer. Such effort has also challenged cell biologists for the basis of plasticity of subcellular transport of HSPs, and immunologists for the significance of "ectopic" expression of HSPs in immunoregulation in both physiological and pathophysiological conditions.

### 12.2.3.1 Modulation of the level of HSPs for cancer immunotherapy

The attempt to modulate the expression of HSPs, knowingly or unknowingly, has been an ancient practice. Induction of local heat by way of moxibustion by the Chinese for the treatment of infections or other diseases is as old as human civilization. Systemic heat can also be induced by herbs and other natural substances to change the balance of "Ying" and "Yang" for man's health and longevity. Despite this long practice and phenomenology, the experience and mechanism of thermotherapy as an established modality for treatment of cancers is still very limited [75].

Repasky's group has begun, systemically, the examination of the role and mechanism of fever in modulating immune responses and anti-tumor effects by a mild fever-range hyperthermia protocol. They found that hyperthermia (i) increases the homing of lymphocytes (Langerhans cells) to the draining lymph nodes, resulting in increased contact hypersensitivity [76] and decreases the number of lymphocytes in the circulation, peritoneal cavity and spleen [77]; (ii) potentiates LPS-induced interleukin (IL)-6 and tumor necrosis factor (TNF)-$\alpha$ production [78]; (iii) induces a reorganization of protein kinase C, spectrin and HSP70 into a large cytoplasmic aggregate [79]; and (iv) causes increased tumor infiltration and function of NK cells [80].

The effect of heat shock on tumor immunogenicity has been investigated. Heat treatment of colon-26 cells induced HSP70, but not other HSPs. Immunization of BALB/cJ mice with heat-treated colon-26 cell extract, which was enriched in HSP70, elicited anti-tumor immunity against s.c. injected colon-26 cells [81]. Furthermore, combination therapy of heat treatment and immunization with heat-treated colon-26 cell extract significantly reduced tumor volumes compared with heat treatment alone. Similar immunization enhanced the cytotoxic activity of mouse splenic lymphocytes against untreated and heat-treated colon-26 cells in an *in vitro* assay. Clark and Menoret have found that pretreatment of tumor cells with heat shock led to increased immunogenicity [82]. Surprisingly, immunization with heat-shocked cells, but not with untreated cells, induced TNF-α-producing cells in the spleen in an antigen-independent manner. Recently, it was found that heat-shocked apoptotic tumor cells are effective tumor vaccines [83]. It is unclear from all the above studies, however, how much of the changes are due to the result of increased HSP production versus a "non-specific" effect of heat alone.

Studies of naturally arising tumor variants from a rat colon carcinoma clone suggested that tumor regression is associated with their ability to synthesis the strictly heat inducible HSP70 [84]. Furthermore, inducible HSP70, induced during non-apoptotic cell death increases tumor immunogenicity *in vivo* [85]. Increasing HSP expression in tumor cells alone by transfection of HSP70 genes under different promoters indicated that (i) HSP70 augments antigen presentation through the MHC class I pathway as revealed by increased lysis of the engineered cells by the cognate CTL clone [86], and (ii) induces an infiltrate of T cells, macrophages and predominantly DCs into the tumors as well as an intratumoral profile of $T_h1$ cytokine expression (interferon, TNF and IL-12) [87].

Thus whole cells with increasing level of HSPs, particularly the inducible HSP70, should be examined clinically for the immunotherapy of human malignancies.

### 12.2.3.2 Modulation of the site of HSP expression for cancer immunotherapy

The appreciation of immunological properties of HSPs has inspired an effort in exposing endogenous HSPs extracellularly to stimulate effective anti-tumor immunity. This is best represented by gp96. gp96 is predominantly a lumenal protein of the ER, although both secretion and surface expression of gp96 have been observed (see above). Since the cell biological basis of "ectopic" trafficking of gp96 is unknown, two groups have adopted a genetic approach to understand the immunological significance of extracellular gp96. Gp96 contains an ER retention motif, Lys–Asp–Glu–Leu (KDEL), at its C-terminus. By deleting KDEL and replacing it with the hinge, $C_H2$ and $C_H3$ domains of murine IgG1, Yamazaki *et al.* have created a secretory form of gp96, gp96–Ig [88]. Transfection of tumor cells with gp96–Ig led to active secretion of it without evidence of intracellular accumulation. Gp96-secreting tumor cells are able to prime tumor-specific $CD8^+$ T cell immunity in a $CD4^+$ T cell-independent manner.

Similarly, Zheng *et al.* [111] have replaced the C-terminal KDEL motif of gp96 with a transmembrane domain of murine platelet-derived growth factor receptor. High levels of cell surface expression of gp96 in type I orientation was achieved consistently. By using the gp96 surface-expressing target cells, two questions are examined. First, can tumor cells, by virtue of its surface expression, stimulate DCs to mature? Secondly, can gp96 surface-expressing tumor cells prime T cells more effectively? It was found that direct access of gp96 to DCs, by cell surface expression, induces DC maturation resulting in secretion of proinflammatory cytokines IL-1â, IL-12, chemokine monocyte chemoattractant protein (MCP)-1, and up-regulation of the expression of MHC I, MHC II, CD80, CD86 and CD40. Furthermore, surface expression of gp96 on tumor cells renders them regressive via a T lymphocyte-dependent mechanism. This work not only demonstrated that surface expression of gp96 has a profound influence on immunity, but also reinforced the notion that gp96 is an endogenous DC activator.

Therefore, extracellular expression of HSPs might be an effective way to bridge innate and adaptive immunity for cancer immunotherapy.

## 12.3
## Conclusion and Perspectives

Although the immunological features of HSPs have been discovered in the context of defining tumor antigens, it is now clear that HSPs play far-reaching roles in the immune responses. The story of HSPs is somewhat analogous to that of MHC molecules. The MHC was discovered as a major transplant barrier, but its "natural" role actually lies in antigen presentation. Different from HSPs, the function of MHC is almost exclusively immunological with a few exceptions [89, 90], which permits the creation of innovative animal models and sophisticated genetic studies. The study of HSPs so far still relies on biochemistry, i.e. purification of HSPs and testing the immunological properties of purified materials. This situation must change in order to address the fundamental roles of HSPs in the physiological context. There are still many unanswered questions.

(1) *What are the roles of HSPs in antigen presentation?* It has been proposed that various HSPs constitute a relay line for peptide transfer from proteasome to MHC I molecules [91]. However, this point has not been firmly proven even though HSPs are peptide-binding proteins and there are generally no free-flowing peptides in the cells [54]. Inhibition of peptide binding of HSP70 by 15-deoxyspergualin inhibits antigen presentation to MHC class I [92], which is consistent with the roles of HSP70 in antigen presentation; however, the finding could also be explained by the roles of HSP70 in other cellular processes unrelated to peptide binding. The major obstacles are lack of systems where each member of the HSPs can be specifically manipulated and examined, and the fact that HSPs are essential for life.

(2) *Are HSPs involved in cross-presenting peptides to thymic T cells for positive or negative selection?* This is a logical question since if HSPs are indeed involved in the priming of T cells, it should be expected that distal release of HSP–peptide complexes (as a result of cell death or active secretion) in the neonatal period might contribute to thymic T cell selection. This question has never been examined, perhaps due to lack of a good experimental model.

(3) *What are the contributions of HSPs to peripheral tolerance?* The proponents for the roles of HSPs in priming adaptive immunity have not examined this issue in conditions where HSPs are released constantly, such as in patients with burns, trauma, peripheral vascular diseases and infections. Similarly, the roles of HSPs in immunopathology have not been carefully studied.

Despite all of these questions, the clinical development of HSPs in the treatment of malignancies is already in full swing. This effort must be encouraged in closely monitored settings since there are limited treatment modalities for most human cancers. However, one must be cautious that unless the roles and mechanisms of HSPs in immune response are well defined, it is certain that the clinical translations will face many uncertainties.

### References

1 F. M. BURNET, *Prog Exp Tumor Res* 1970; **13**: 1–27.

2 H. SCHREIBER, in *Fundamental Immunology*, 4th edn (W. E. Paul, Ed.). Lippincott-Raven, Philadelphia, PA 1999: 1237–1270.

3 P. K. SRIVASTAVA, A. MENORET, S. BASU, R. J. BINDER and K. L. McQUADE, *Immunity* 1998; **8**: 657–665.

4 S. LINDQUIST and E. A. CRAIG, *Annu Rev Genet* 1988; **22**: 631–677.

5 M. E. FEDER and G. E. HOFMANN, *Annu Rev Physiol* 1999; **61**: 243–282.

6 P. CSERMELY, T. SCHNAIDER, C. SOTI, Z. PROHASZKA and G. NARDAI, *Pharmacol Ther* 1998; **79**: 129–168.

7 J. FRYDMAN, *Annu Rev Biochem* 2001; **70**: 603–647.

8 R. I. MORIMOTO, *Genes Dev* 1998; **12**: 3788–3796.

9 Z. LI, *Semin Immunol* 1997; **9**: 315–322.

10 C. GAUDIN, F. KREMER, E. ANGEVIN, V. SCOTT and F. TRIEBEL, *J Immunol* 1999; **162**: 1730–1738.

11 P. K. SRIVASTAVA and M. HEIKE, *Semin Immunol* 1991; **3**: 57–64.

12 P. K. SRIVASTAVA and R. G. MAKI, *Curr Topics Microbiol Immunol* 1991; **167**: 109–123.

13 T. J. NIELAND, M. C. TAN, M. MONNE-VAN MUIJEN, F. KONING, A. M. KRUIS-BEEK and G. M. VAN BLEEK, *Proc Natl Acad Sci USA* 1996; **93**: 6135–6139.

14 D. ARNOLD, S. FAATH, H. RAMMENSEE and H. SCHILD, *J Exp Med* 1995; **182**: 885–889.

15 M. BRELOER, T. MARTI, B. FLEISCHER and A. VON BONIN, *Eur J Immunol* 1998; **28**: 1016–1021.

16 S. NAIR, P. A. WEARSCH, D. A. MITCHELL, J. J. WASSENBERG, E. GILBOA and C. V. NICCHITTA, *J Immunol* 1999; **162**: 6426–6423.

17 T. ISHII, H. UDONO, T. YAMANO, H. OHTA, A. UENAKA, T. ONO, A. HIZUTA, N. TANAKA, P. K. SRIVASTAVA and E. NAKAYAMA, *J Immunol* 1999; **162**: 1303–1309.

18 S. D. MENG, T. GAO, G. F. GAO and P. TIEN, *Lancet* 2001; **357**: 528–529.

19 P. A. WEARSCH, L. VOGLINO and C. V. NICCHITTA, *Biochemistry* 1998; **37**: 5709–5719.

20 S. SASTRY and N. LINDEROTH, *J Biol Chem* 1999; **274**: 12023–12035.

21 N. A. LINDEROTH, A. POPOWICZ and S. SASTRY, *J Biol Chem* 2000; **275**: 5472–5477.

22 N. A. LINDEROTH, M. N. SIMON, J. F. HAINFELD and S. SASTRY, *J Biol Chem* 2001; **276**: 11049–11054.

23 N. A. LINDEROTH, M. N. SIMON, N. A. RODIONOVA, M. CADENE, W. R. LAWS, B. T. CHAIT and S. SASTRY, *Biochemistry* 2001; **40**: 1483–1495.

24 G. C. FLYNN, T. G. CHAPPELL and J. E. ROTHMAN, *Science* 1989; **245**: 385–390.

25 H. UDONO and P. K. SRIVASTAVA, *J Exp Med* 1993; **178**: 1391–1396.

26 C. CASTELLI, A. M. CIUPITU, F. RINI, L. RIVOLTINI, A. MAZZOCCHI, R. KIESSLING and G. PARMIANI, *Cancer Res* 2001; **61**: 222–227.

27 X. ZHU, X. ZHAO, W. F. BURKHOLDER, A. GRAGEROV, C. M. OGATA, M. E. GOTTESMAN and W. A. HENDRICKSON, *Science* 1996; **272**: 1606–1614.

28 D. ARNOLD-SCHILD, D. HANAU, D. SPEHNER, C. SCHMID, H. G. RAMMENSEE, H. DE LA SALLE and H. SCHILD, *J Immunol* 1999; **162**: 3757–3760.

29 J. J. WASSENBERG, C. DEZFULIAN and

C. V. Nicchitta, *J Cell Sci* 1999; **112**: 2167–2175.

30 R. J. Binder, M. L. Harris, A. Menoret and P. K. Srivastava, *J Immunol* 2000; **165**: 2582–2587.

31 A. Asea, S. K. Kraeft, E. A. Kurt-Jones, M. A. Stevenson, L. B. Chen, R. W. Finberg, G. C. Koo and S. K. Calderwood, *Nat Med* 2000; **6**: 435–442.

32 F. Castellino, P. E. Boucher, K. Eichelberg, M. Mayhew, J. E. Rothman, A. N. Houghton and R. N. Germain, *J Exp Med* 2000; **191**: 1957–1964.

33 S. Basu, R. J. Binder, R. Suto, K. M. Anderson and P. K. Srivastava, *Int Immunol* 2000; **12**: 1539–1546.

34 R. J. Binder, K. M. Anderson, S. Basu and P. K. Srivastava, *J Immunol* 2000; **165**: 6029–6035.

35 H. Singh-Jasuja, N. Hilf, H. U. Scherer, D. Arnold-Schild, H. G. Rammensee, R. E. Toes and H. Schild, *Cell Stress Chaperones* 2000; **5**: 462–470.

36 H. Singh-Jasuja, H. U. Scherer, N. Hilf, D. Arnold-Schild, H. G. Rammensee, R. E. Toes and H. Schild, *Eur J Immunol* 2000; **30**: 2211–2215.

37 H. Singh-Jasuja, R. E. Toes, P. Spee, C. Munz, N. Hilf, S. P. Schoenberger, P. Ricciardi-Castagnoli, J. Neefjes, H. G. Rammensee, D. Arnold-Schild and H. Schild, *J Exp Med* 2000; **191**: 1965–1974.

38 Y. Moroi, M. Mayhew, J. Trcka, M. H. Hoe, Y. Takechi, F. U. Hartl, J. E. Rothman and A. N. Houghton, *Proc Natl Acad Sci USA* 2000; **97**: 3485–3490.

39 A. Kol, A. H. Lichtman, R. W. Finberg, P. Libby and E. A. Kurt-Jones, *J Immunol* 2000; **164**: 13–17.

40 A. K. De, K. M. Kodys, B. S. Yeh and C. Miller-Graziano, *J Immunol* 2000; **165**: 3951–3958.

41 M. J. Bevan, *J Exp Med* 1976; **143**: 1283–1288.

42 M. J. Bevan, *J Immunol* 1976; **117**: 2233–2238.

43 R. J. Binder, D. K. Han and P. K. Srivastava, *Nat Immunol* 2000; **1**: 151–155.

44 S. Basu, R. J. Binder, T. Ramalingam

and P. K. Srivastava, *Immunity* 2001; **14**: 303–313.

45 I. Kaur, S. D. Voss, R. S. Gupta, K. Schell, P. Fisch and P. M. Sondel, *J Immunol* 1993; **150**: 2046–2055.

46 Y. Wei, X. Zhao, Y. Kariya, H. Fukata, K. Teshigawara and A. Uchida, *Cancer Res* 1996; **56**: 1104–1110.

47 G. Multhoff, C. Botzler, L. Jennen, J. Schmidt, J. Ellwart and R. Issels, *J Immunol* 1997; **158**: 4341–4350.

48 Y. Tamura, N. Tsuboi, N. Sato and K. Kikuchi, *J Immunol* 1993; **151**: 5516–5524.

49 L. Gross, *Cancer Res* 1943; **3**: 323–326.

50 R. W. Baldwin, *Br J Cancer* 1955; **9**: 652–657.

51 R. T. Prehn and J. M. Main, *J Natl Cancer Inst* 1957; **18**: 769–778.

52 G. Klein, H. O. Sjogren, E. Klein and K. E. Hellstrom, *Cancer Res* 1960; **20**: 1561–1572.

53 L. J. Old, E. A. Boyse, D. A. Clarke and E. A. Carswell, *Ann NY Acad Sci* 1962; **101**: 80–106.

54 A. Menoret, P. Peng and P. K. Srivastava, *Biochem Biophys Res Commun* 1999; **262**: 813–818.

55 D. Arnold, C. Wahl, S. Faath, H. G. Rammensee and H. Schild, *J Exp Med* 1997; **186**: 461–466.

56 S. Janetzki, D. Palla, V. Rosenhauer, H. Lochs, J. J. Lewis and P. K. Srivastava, *Int J Cancer* 2000; **88**: 232–238.

57 M. Caudill and Z. Li, *Exp Opin Biol Ther* 2001; **1**: 539–547

58 P. K. Srivastava, *Nat Immunol* 2000; **1**: 363–366.

59 N. E. Blachere, Z. Li, R. Y. Chandawarkar, R. Suto, N. S. Jaikaria, S. Basu, H. Udono and P. K. Srivastava, *J Exp Med* 1997; **186**: 1315–1322.

60 K. Suzue and R. A. Young, *J Immunol* 1996; **156**: 873–879.

61 K. Suzue, X. Zhou, H. N. Eisen and R. A. Young, *Proc Natl Acad Sci USA* 1997; **94**: 13146–13151.

62 D. W. Liu, Y. P. Tsao, J. T. Kung, Y. A. Ding, H. K. Sytwu, X. Xiao and S. L. Chen, *J Virol* 2000; **74**: 2888–2894.

63 Q. Huang, J. F. Richmond, K. Suzue, H. N. Eisen and R. A. Young, *J Exp Med* 2000; **191**: 403–408.

**64** B. K. Cho, D. Palliser, E. Guillen, J. Wisniewski, R. A. Young, J. Chen and H. N. Eisen, *Immunity* 2000; **12**: 263–272.

**65** T. F. Greten and E. M. Jaffee, *J Clin Oncol* 1999; **17**: 1047–1060.

**66** A. Kugler, G. Stuhler, P. Walden, G. Zoller, A. Zobywalski, P. Brossart, U. Trefzer, S. Ullrich, C. A. Muller, V. Becker, A. J. Gross, B. Hemmerlein, L. Kanz, G. A. Muller and R. H. Ringert, *Nat Med* 2000; **6**: 332–336.

**67** A. Altmeyer, R. G. Maki, A. M. Feldweg, M. Heike, V. P. Protopopov, S. K. Masur and P. K. Srivastava, *Int J Cancer* 1996; **69**: 340–349.

**68** C. Booth and G. L. Koch, *Cell* 1989; **59**: 729–737.

**69** D. L. Wiest, A. Bhandoola, J. Punt, G. Kreibich, D. McKean and A. Singer, *Proc Natl Acad Sci USA* 1997; **94**: 1884–1889.

**70** N. Seddiki, F. Nato, P. Lafaye, Z. Amoura, J. C. Piette and J. C. Mazie, *J Immunol* 2001; **166**: 6423–6429.

**71** R. Suto and P. K. Srivastava, *Science* 1995; **269**: 1585–1588.

**72** L. E. Hightower and P. T. Guidon, Jr, *J Cell Physiol* 1989; **138**: 257–266.

**73** S. M. Fujihara and S. G. Nadler, *EMBO J* 1999; **18**: 411449.

**74** K. Triantafilou, M. Triantafilou and R. L. Dedrick, *Nat Immunol* 2001; **2**: 338–345.

**75** M. H. Falk and R. D. Issels, *Int J Hypertherm* 2001; **17**: 1–18.

**76** J. R. Ostberg, C. Gellin, R. Patel and E. A. Repasky, *J Immunol* 2001; **167**: 2666–2670.

**77** J. R. Ostberg, R. Patel and E. A. Repasky, *Cell Stress Chaperones* 2000; **5**: 458–461.

**78** J. R. Ostberg, S. L. Taylor, H. Baumann and E. A. Repasky, *J Leuk Biol* 2000; **68**: 815–820.

**79** Y. P. Di, E. A. Repasky and J. R. Subjeck, *J Cell Physiol* 1997; **172**: 44–54.

**80** R. Burd, T. S. Dziedzic, Y. Xu, M. A. Caligiuri, J. R. Subjeck and E. A. Repasky, *J Cell Physiol* 1998; **177**: 137–147.

**81** M. Okamoto, K. Tazawa, T. Kawagoshi, M. Maeda, T. Honda, T. Sakamoto and K. Tsukada, *Int J Hypertherm.* 2000; **16**: 263–273.

**82** P. R. M. Clark, A., *Cell Stress Chaperones* 2001; **6**: 121–125.

**83** H. Feng, Y. Zeng, L. Whitesell and E. Katsanis, *Blood* 2001; **97**: 3505–3512.

**84** A. Menoret, Y. Patry, C. Burg and J. Le Pendu, *J Immunol* 1995; **155**: 740–747.

**85** A. Melcher, S. Todryk, N. Hardwick, M. Ford, M. Jacobson and R. G. Vile, *Nat Med* 1998; **4**: 581–587.

**86** A. D. Wells, S. K. Rai, M. S. Salvato, H. Band and M. Malkovsky, *Int Immunol* 1998; **10**: 609–617.

**87** S. Todryk, A. A. Melcher, N. Hardwick, E. Linardakis, A. Bateman, M. P. Colombo, A. Stoppacciaro and R. G. Vile, *J Immunol* 1999; **163**: 1398–1408.

**88** K. Yamazaki, T. Nguyen and E. R. Podack, *J Immunol* 1999; **163**: 5178–5182.

**89** C. Ober, L. R. Weitkamp, N. Cox, H. Dytch, D. Kostyu and S. Elias, *Am J Hum Genet* 1997; **61**: 497–504.

**90** G. S. Huh, L. M. Boulanger, H. Du, P. A. Riquelme, T. M. Brotz and C. J. Shatz, *Science* 2000; **290**: 2155–2159.

**91** P. K. Srivastava, H. Udono, N. E. Blachere and Z. Li, *Immunogenetics* 1994; **39**: 93–98.

**92** R. J. Binder, N. E. Blachere and P. K. Srivastava, *J Biol Chem* 2001; **18**: 17163–17171.

**93** P. K. Srivastava, A. B. DeLeo and L. J. Old, *Proc Natl Acad Sci USA* 1986; **83**: 3407–3411.

**94** S. J. Ullrich, E. A. Robinson, L. W. Law, M. Willingham and E. Appella, *Proc Natl Acad Sci USA* 1986; **83**: 3121–3125.

**95** H. Udono and P. K. Srivastava, *J Immunol* 1994; **152**: 5398–5403.

**96** S. Basu and P. K. Srivastava, *J Exp Med* 1999; **189**: 797–802.

**97** X. Y. Wang, L. Kazim, E. A. Repasky and J. R. Subjeck, *J Immunol* 2001; **166**: 490–497.

**98** S. Janetzki, N. E. Blachere and P. K. Srivastava, *J Immunother* 1998; **21**: 269–276.

**99** Y. Tamura, P. Peng, K. Liu, M. Daou and P. K. Srivastava, *Science* 1997; **278**: 117–120.

**100** M. Graner, A. Raymond, D. Romney, L. He, L. Whitesell and E. Katsanis, *Clin Cancer Res* 2000; **6**: 909–915.

**101** S. P. Yedavelli, L. Guo, M. E. Daou, P. K. Srivastava, A. Mittelman and R. K. Tiwari, *Int J Mol Med* 1999; **4**: 243–248.

**102** P. K. Srivastava and M. R. Das, *Int J Cancer* 1984; **33**: 417–422.

**103** J. Robert, A. Menoret, S. Basu, N. Cohen and P. R. Srivastava, *Eur J Immunol* 2001; **31**: 186–195.

**104** U. Zugel, A. M. Sponaas, J. Neckermann, B. Schoel and S. H. Kaufmann, *Infect Immun* 2001; **69**: 4164–4167.

**105** M. Navaratnam, M. S. Deshpande, M. J. Hariharan, D. S. Zatechka, Jr and S. Srikumaran, *Vaccine* 2001; **19**: 1425–1434.

**106** A. Heikema, E. Agsteribbe, J. Wilschut and A. Huckriede, *Immunol Lett* 1997; **57**: 69–74.

**107** A. M. Ciupitu, M. Petersson, C. L. O'Donnell, K. Williams, S. Jindal, R. Kiessling and R. M. Welsh, *J Exp Med* 1998; **187**: 685–691.

**108** N. R. Chu, H. B. Wu, T. Wu, L. J. Boux, M. I. Siegel and L. A. Mizzen, *Clin Exp Immunol* 2000; **121**: 216–225.

**109** C. H. Chen, T. L. Wang, C. F. Hung, Y. Yang, R. A. Young, D. M. Pardoll and T. C. Wu, *Cancer Res* 2000; **60**: 1035–1042.

**110** L. S. Anthony, H. Wu, H. Sweet, C. Turnnir, L. J. Boux and L. A. Mizzen, *Vaccine* 1999; **17**: 373–383.

**111** H. Zheng, J. Dai, D. Stoilova and Z. Li, *J Immunol* 2001; **167**: 6731–6735.

# 13

# Applications of CpG Motifs from Bacterial DNA
# in Cancer Immunotherapy

Arthur M. Krieg

## 13.1
### History of Cancer Immunotherapy with Bacterial Extracts and Nucleic Acids

For centuries there have been sporadic reports of patients with advanced malignancy who underwent spontaneous regression following a bacterial infection (reviewed in [1]). However, there was no systematic effort to investigate this phenomenon until the 1890s, when a New York surgeon, William B. Coley, became aware of a patient with a widely metastatic sarcoma who had experienced a remarkable and complete tumor regression following a streptococcal infection in the region of the tumor. Suspecting that the streptococcal infection may have triggered the regression, Coley took the heroic step of injecting a live streptococcal culture into an unresectable sarcoma in a patient with hopelessly advanced disease. Although the patient almost succumbed to the infection, he too experienced a complete regression [2]. In order to reduce the toxicity of this new form of treatment, William Coley then began treating many sarcoma patients with a mixture of killed bacteria including *Streptococcus* and *Proteus*, which became known as "Coley's toxins". Over the next decades, Coley treated close to 1000 patients with his toxin and achieved an astonishing response rate of more than 40% in these advanced malignancies, some of which persisted for decades [2, 3] Despite his impressive success rate and the success of some other investigators using his toxins, this form of cancer immunotherapy was not widely pursued in the years following Coley's death. Nevertheless, bacterial immunotherapy for cancer lives on in the use of the attenuated mycobacteria Bacillus Calmette-Guerin (BCG) as a therapy for human bladder cancer [4, 5]

Perhaps the most important lesson to be gained from this brief history of immunotherapy with bacteria is that by activating the immune system with bacterial components, it is possible to induce sustained remissions in at least some humans with advanced malignancies. It is now clear that the "Coley's toxins" did not in fact contain toxins as originally assumed, but rather that bacterial products activate innate and acquired immune defense mechanisms that can kill tumor cells. In the century that has passed since Coley's initial therapeutic successes, we have gained a much better understanding of the immune system, which allows us to provide a better answer to the question of what may be the microbial products that induce these antitumor responses. Endotoxin became an obvious candidate for mediating this toxicity, especially as it was recognized to be a trigger for the production of the hopefully named tumor necrosis factor (TNF). Although lipopolysaccharides (LPSs) have many remarkable immune effects, they clearly cannot be the sole explanation for the antitumor activities of "Coley's toxins". One reason is simply that the first patient treated by Coley was treated only with streptococcus, which of course has no endotoxin. Second, endotoxins are very toxic, which appears to preclude their human clinical development, with the exception of detoxified forms such as monophosphorylipid, which has shown activity as an adjuvant.

In order to determine the active component of BCG, Tokunaga *et al.* fractionated it into the various components and assayed each of these for their antitumor activity [6]. Surprisingly, these studies demonstrated that only the DNA fraction of BCG contained antitumor activity. BCG DNA was further shown to induce natural killer (NK) cell activity, and the production of type 1 and type 2 interferons (IFNs) [7]. Tokunaga's discovery led to human clinical trials of a BCG DNA preparation in Japan, with some encouraging responses, but no further clinical development [8]. By cloning mycobacterial genes and synthesizing constituent oligodeoxynucleotides (ODN), these investigators concluded that the immune stimulatory effects of BCG DNA could be attributed to the presence of certain self-complementary palindromes in these ODN [9]. All of the active palindromes were noted to contain at least one CpG dinucleotide and to be more common in the genomes of bacteria compared to humans [10]. The mechanism of immune recognition of the palindromes was thought to depend on their secondary or tertiary structure and methylation of the CpGs was reported to have no influence on the immune stimulatory activities of the DNA [10].

In independent studies, Pisetsky *et al.* reported that bacterial DNA (bDNA) induced murine B cell proliferation and immunoglobulin secretion, but vertebrate DNA did not [11]. This effect was shown to be independent of any LPS contamination of the bDNA because it was abolished by nuclease digestion of the DNAs and was not affected by polymixin. bDNA was not unique in being immune stimulatory – Pisetsky *et al.* also demonstrated that synthetic poly(dC · dG) was a B cell mitogen and that this mitogenicity was abolished by methylation of the cytosines [12]. However, these investigators also did not associate CpG methylation with different immune activities of bacterial and vertebrate DNAs. Instead, they suggested that the immune stimulatory effects resulted from unique higher-ordered structures of the DNA molecules that were disrupted by methylation.

While the immune stimulatory effects of these DNA molecules were unexpected, they should not be totally surprising. After all, nucleic acids are polyanions, and can form hydrogen bonds with other biological molecules, which in principle could give them drug-like effects. In fact, certain double-stranded RNA structures have been known for many years to have immune stimulatory effects, which are thought to result from an immune defense mechanism triggered by viral double-stranded RNAs [13]. This immune activation can be mimicked by poly(rI · rC), which induces NK cell activity and $T_h1$-like immune activation with interleukin (IL)-12, IFN-$\alpha$ and IFN-$\gamma$ production in both murine and human cells [14, 15]. In mice and primates, poly(rI · rC) has prophylactic and therapeutic activity against otherwise lethal viral infections [16, 17], and is an effective vaccine adjuvant [18]. In fact, several human clinical trials in cancer were performed with various formulations of poly(rI · rC), but the clinical activity was disappointing in comparison to the substantial toxicity [19, 20] The immune activation triggered by this polynucleotide is thought to be mediated by the double-stranded RNA-dependent protein kinase, PKR [21].

Another polynucleotide which has also been shown to have immune stimulatory effects is poly(A · U). Like poly(rI · rC), poly(A) · poly(U) has been shown to have immune stimulatory activity in animal models [22]. Although it has some similar properties to poly(rI · rC) in terms of its ability to promote production of IFNs and activate NK cells, poly(A · U) has been proposed to be less toxic. Poly(A · U) has also been shown to have adjuvant effects when administered in combination with hepatitis B surface antigen to mice [23]. In human clinical trials, poly(A · U) has shown some encouraging signs of efficacy in patients with breast cancer [24, 25]. Poly(A · U) has also been reported to have substantial therapeutic activity without significant side effects when used as an immune modulator for the treatment of chronic active hepatitis B [26]. NK cell activation has also been reported to be triggered by poly(dG · dC) [27]. DNA containing runs of consecutive guanines, termed poly(G) sequences or G-quartets, can induce B cell proliferation [28]. Fragments of double-stranded DNA or RNA as short as 25 bp have been reported to induce non-immune cells to induce or activate STAT1, STAT3, NF-κB and mitogen-activated protein kinases (MAPKs), and to express MHC and co-stimulatory molecules in a sequence-independent manner that required the DNA or RNA to be introduced into the cell cytoplasm, which could possibly occur during a viral infection [29]. In contrast to bDNA, which is active in either double- or single-stranded form, vertebrate DNA is only active in the double-stranded form [29]. Introduction of host DNA into the cytoplasm of dendritic cells (DCs) induces them to mature, with enhanced functional activity [30]. It is unclear whether these different immune stimulatory polynucleotides exert their effects through the same or different mechanisms.

## 13.2
### CpG Motifs in bDNA Explain its Immune Stimulatory Activity

As reviewed above, Tokunaga *et al.* and Pisetsky *et al.* demonstrated that bDNA activated NK and B cells, but that vertebrate DNA was inactive. Although Tokunaga proposed that palindromes in the bDNA were responsible for its immune stimulatory activity [9], further studies demonstrated that a sufficient sequence element was a CpG dinucleotide in particular base contexts, termed "CpG motifs" [reviewed in 31]. Elimination of the CpG dinucleotides from ODN abolished their stimulatory activities [32]. The role of the CpG motif as the active element in bDNA provides a new insight into the old observation that vertebrate and bDNAs differ markedly in their CpG content and methylation [33]. Bacterial DNA generally contains the expected frequency of about one CpG dinucleotide per 16 bases. However, CpG dinucleotides are known to be markedly suppressed in vertebrate genomes: they occur only about a quarter as frequently as would be predicted if base utilization was random [33].

Furthermore, the bases flanking CpGs in vertebrate genomes are not random: the most common base preceding a CpG is a C and the most common base following a CpG is a G [34]. It is therefore noteworthy that these types of CpG motifs (CCG and CGG) do not support strong immune stimulation, but can actually neutralize other immune stimulatory CpG motifs [35]. Thus, vertebrate DNA inhibits the immune stimulatory effects of bDNA [36]. In addition to these differences in CpG content, CpG dinucleotides are not methylated in bDNA, but are routinely methylated at the 5 position of about 70% of the cytosines in vertebrate DNAs [33], which increases their immune inhibitory effects [36].

The immune stimulatory effects of bDNA are due to the unmethylated CpG motifs, since methylation with CpG methylase completely abolished its activity [32]. Extracts of *Babesia bovis*, like those of many other microbes, are immune stimulatory. These effects result from the DNA, since they are abolished by treatment of the extracts with nuclease and can be reproduced with purified *B. bovis* DNA [37]. Immune-stimulatory DNA is not unique to microbes; *Drosophila* extracts are also immune stimulatory, due to the unmethylated CpG motifs in insect DNA [38]. A survey of different genomic DNAs has shown immune stimulation by nematode and mollusk DNAs and confirmed that hypomethylation of CpG is required for immune stimulation [39].

## 13.3
## Identification of a Specific Receptor for CpG motifs, Toll-like Receptor (TLR)-9

"Pattern recognition receptors" (PRRs) give the innate immune system a general ability to detect certain molecular structures that are conserved among pathogens, but are not present in self tissues [21, 40]. Examples of PRR ligands include endotoxins, high manose proteins, double-stranded viral RNAs and, most recently, CpG motifs [21, 40, 41] The immune system uses specific PRRs to detect the presence of particular types of pathogens, coupling this detection to the activation of appropriate defense pathways. A major group of PRRs is the TLR family, named for their homology to the fruit fly Toll protein, that coordinates insect innate immune responses to infection [42, 43] This family of proteins appears to have at least 10 members in the human, that couple the detection of microbial or viral products to cell activation via the adaptor molecule MyD88 and TRAF6, that are linked to the IκB kinase complex and to the MAPKs.

Some PRRs are expressed on the cell surface, where they may easily detect pathogens. For example, some peptidoglycans are detected by TLR-2, most LPS are detected via TLR-4 and flagellin is detected via TLR-5 [42]. In contrast, it appears that CpG ODN must be taken up by cells and bind to an intracellular receptor [32, 44–47].

Drugs that interfere with the endosomal acidification/processing of ODN, such as chloroquine, specifically block the immune stimulatory effects of CpG DNA, but not those of LPS [45, 48, 49]. These data suggest that an endosomal step is required for the CpG-induced signal transduction pathways [45, 49]. Recently, mice deficient in a member of the TLR family, TLR-9, were shown to be unresponsive to a phosphorothioate CpG ODN despite normal activation by LPS [50]. It is therefore intriguing that TLR-9 appears to be localized within the endosome [51]. Human 293 (embryonic kidney) cells do not express TLR-9, and normally are not activated by a CpG ODN. However, these cells become CpG responsive when they are transfected to express TLR-9 [51]. Among human cell types, TLR-9 expression is highest in B cells and plasmacytoid DC, which are also the only cell types that have been reproducibly shown to be directly activated by phosphorothioate CpG ODN [51, 52]. Perhaps the most direct evidence for the role of TLR-9 in the direct recognition of a CpG motif is the fact that 293 cells transfected to express the mouse TLR-9 protein become optimally responsive to the preferred mouse CpG motif, GACGTT, while 293 cells transfected to express the human TLR-9 protein become optimally responsive to the preferred human CpG motif, GTCGTT. Thus, the TLR-9 protein determines the species specificity of CpG motifs and presumably either binds to the CpG motif directly or in close association with some unidentified cofactor.

CpG DNA activates the MAPK pathways and NFκB within minutes of exposure in B cells, DCs and mouse macrophage-like cell lines [45, 53–55] Although these signaling pathways are also used in responses to LPS, differences in their biologic effects demonstrate that there must be some additional specific signal(s) provided by LPS and/or CpG [56–59] Independent signaling activities are also suggested by the observations that CpG DNA and LPS synergize for inducing macrophage NO production [60] and TNF-α expression *in vitro* [61], and for inducing the systemic inflammatory response syndrome (SIRS; "cytokine storm") *in vivo* [62].

## 13.4
### Backbone-dependent Immune Effects of CpG Motifs and Delineation of CpG-A versus CpG-B Classes of ODN

The immune effects of a CpG ODN are determined not only by the bases flanking the CpG dinucleotide, but also by the backbone of the ODN. ODN synthesized with the normal phosphodiester DNA backbone (PO) are rapidly degraded inside lymphocytes [63]. The susceptibility of phosphodiester ODN to degradation not only reduces their ability to drive B cell proliferation, but can even result in an artifact in studies using a [$^3$H]thymidine incorporation assay to measure B cell proliferation. Degradation of the phosphodiester DNA releases free thymidine which competes for the [$^3$H]thymidine, causing an apparent decrease in cell proliferation [64]. This non-specific effect is most marked if thymidine nucleotides are present at the 3¢ end of an ODN, but can also be observed with high-molecular-weight DNA such as bacterial genomic DNA. At least one exonuclease is specifically expressed in B lymphocytes, indicating that results obtained using phosphodiester DNA in one cell type cannot necessarily be extrapolated to other cell types [65]. Moreover, nuclease activities appear to be higher in human than in mouse cells, with the result that phosphodiester DNA can appear non-stimulatory unless it is added repeatedly [66, 67].

Replacement of one of the non-bridging oxygen atoms around the phosphodiester linkage with a sulfur atom, which is called a phosphorothioate (PS) linkage, provides an extremely high degree of nuclease resistance and greatly stabilizes the ODN against degradation [68]. The phosphorothioate ODN backbone dramatically increases the non-specific ODN binding to a wide variety of proteins [69, 70] Phosphorothioate ODN bind much more avidly to cell membranes, and generally have a much higher degree of cell uptake [63, 71, 72] The phosphorothioate backbone results in sequence-independent activities including the activation of SP1 transcription factor activity [73], inhibition of smooth muscle cell proliferation and migration [74, 75] inhibition of basic fibroblast growth factor binding to its receptor [76, 77] and angiogenic activity [78], reduction of the sequence specific binding of transcription factors to their binding sites [79], inhibition of cellular adhesion to extracellular matrix [80], enhancement of LPS-induced TNF production [81], and some degree of non-sequence specific immune stimulation [82]. The immune stimulatory effects of PS ODN are reduced by further modification with 2' methoxyethoxy modifications [83]. Finally, the PS backbone enhances certain effects of poly(G) sequences, which may form G-quartets, including the ability to inhibit CD28 expression and *in vivo* contact hypersensitivity responses [84].

PS ODN are approximately 200 times more potent at activating B cells than the same sequence with a PO backbone [32, 63, 85, 86] However, the immune-stimulatory effects of CpG motifs in PS ODN are qualitatively different from PO ODN. PS ODN bearing suboptimal CpG motifs are less likely than PO ODN to drive B cell proliferation, especially if the CpG is followed by a G. PS ODN without CG motifs are also frequently observed to non-specifically drive the proliferation of murine and human B cells, although to a more limited degree than that which occurs with CpG ODN [87, 66, 82, 88] PS non-CpG ODN can synergize with strong signals for B cell stimulation [89]. In contrast to their powerful B cell-stimulating activity, PS ODN are less active than ODN in which the CpG motif is PO when assayed for their ability to activate macrophages or NK cells [90–92].

As a result of the effects reviewed above, ODN with different backbones and different sequence motifs induce dramatically different profiles and kinetics of immune activation [90, 93–99]. The term "CpG DNA" should therefore be used with care, since not all of the effects described in the literature are seen with all ODN, bacterial genomic DNAs or plasmids containing CpG motifs. Throughout this chapter effort will be made to clarify when the effects described are unique to one or another form of CpG DNA.

ODN containing PO backbones, or in which the CpG motifs are PO, are referred to as CpG-A ODN, based on their potent activity at inducing IFN-α production from plasmacytoid DC precursors and activating NK cells [86, 90, 98, 100–102]. The NK cell activation and induction of plasmacytoid DC IFN-α expression that is induced by an optimal CpG-A ODN is far higher than that induced by bDNA and the level of B cell activation is generally lower. Even in comparing bDNA from different bacteria, there are striking differences in the levels of immune activation; *E. coli* DNA tending to be much more stimulatory than that from *C. perfringens*, a kind of bacteria or *Streptococcal* or *Staphylococcal* sp. [8, 9, 39, 103]. ODN in which the 5' and 3' ends are phosphorothioate-modified and the center portion is phosphodiester, have a high degree of nuclease resistance provided by the phosphorothioate-modified ends, and also have enhanced ability to activate NK cells since the CpG motif is PO [90, 86] The addition of poly(G) motifs to the 5′ and 3′ ends of the ODN enhance the cellular uptake, and substantially improve its ability to activate NK cells [90, 104] and to induce IFN-α production from human plasmacytoid DC precursors [102]. The uptake and activity of bDNA or PO ODN without poly(G) motifs can be similarly enhanced using cationic lipids [47] or antibodies [100], in which case the cytokine induction can be increased to a level comparable to that seen with a poly(G) CpG-A ODN.

In contrast to CpG-A ODN, CpG motifs in nuclease-resistant phosphorothioate backbones have dramatically enhanced B cell stimulatory properties but reduced NK stimulation, despite being much more stable than phosphodiester ODN [53, 90, 92, 93]. ODN in which the CpG motif has a PS backbone are therefore termed CpG-B ODN [101], to reflect this enhanced B cell activation. Even though CpG-B ODN as a family have similar properties, there can still be qualitative differences in their effects, and some are substantially more effective at inducing the expression of TNF-α than others [105].

## 13.5
## Applications of CpG DNA in Immunotherapy of Cancer

### 13.5.1
### CpG-A or CpG-B DNA as a Monotherapy

As reviewed in the Introduction, the antitumor effects of infections have been recognized for hundreds of years, effectively demonstrating that immune activation can result in tumor eradication. This point is consistent with the recently rediscovered role of "cancer immunosurveillance", mediated by IFN-γ and lymphocytes, in suppressing tumor growth [106]. By inducing IFN-γ production and activating lymphocytes CpG-induced innate immune activation might enhance cancer immunosurveillance, and prevent tumor development.

The efficacy of CpG-A DNA in treating tumor-bearing mice has been examined in several experimental models. In some models, plasmids containing CpG motifs were stabilized by the formation of complexes with cationic lipids, which enables them to induce systemic NK cell activation and $T_h1$ cytokine production [107]. Methylation of the plasmids reduced their immune stimulatory effects, demonstrating the CpG-specificity. Such cationic lipid–DNA complexes are taken up in the pulmonary vascular bed and trigger the local accumulation of activated NK cells that produce IFN-γ. Mice were given tumors by i.v. injection with experimental fibrosarcoma, melanoma or colon carcinoma cell lines, and then treated with i.v. cationic lipid–DNA complexes 3 and 10 days later [107]. Mice with intact immune systems had a marked decrease in the number of pulmonary metastases, compared to mice given lipid or DNA alone [107]. However, these CpG-A molecules had no protective effects in mice depleted of NK cells with anti-asialo-$GM_1$ antiserum or in mice genetically deficient in IFN-γ [107]. Similar cationic lipid–plasmid DNA complexes have been demonstrated effective in two murine mesothelioma models, AC29 and AB12 [108].

In the less aggressive model, AC29, treatment with CpG-A resulted in a greater than 90% long-term survival rate, while in the more aggressive AB 12 model, treatment still gave greater than 40% long-term survival [108]. In both models, CpG treatment led to a protective memory response, since surviving mice resisted repeat tumor challenge. CD8$^+$ T cells and NK cells were absolutely required, and CD4$^+$ T cells contributed to the CpG-induced protective effect [108].

Using systemic or local therapy with an NK-optimized CpG-A ODN, we prevented death in 80% of syngeneic C57 BL/6 mice after an otherwise lethal challenge of poorly immunogenic B16 melanoma [109]. Even when treatment was begun 3 days after tumor challenge, 60% of mice could still be cured of disease with CpG-A treatment. Of interest, CpG-B ODN treatment was less effective in this tumor model [109]. SCID mice were also protected against tumor challenge by CpG DNA, indicating that neither B nor T cells are required. In contrast to the mesothelioma models described in the preceding paragraph, specific immunity was not generated, since CpG-treated mice that had survived a tumor challenge were not protected against subsequent tumor challenges [109].

CpG-B ODN also have therapeutic activity in several mouse tumor models as monotherapy, with either local or systemic administration. Injection of CpG DNA directly into a tumor lesion may activate DCs in or around the tumor, inducing a T$_h$1-like cytokine environment which may overcome the normal immune suppressive effects of the tumor and result in an effective antitumor immune response. In support of this hypothesis, Carpentier *et al.* have demonstrated that daily injection of CpG-B ODN for 15 days into syngeneic neuroblastoma tumor nodules results in complete tumor regression in about 50% of the mice [110]. Animals cured with CpG treatment were protected against further tumor challenge, suggesting the development of an antigen-specific T cell response, in contrast to the lack of a role for T cells in the case of the B16 model described in the previous paragraph. These results demonstrating the development of an active antitumor response following treatment with CpG-B ODN have recently been extended to a glioblastoma model [111] and a T cell lymphoma model [109].

In the C1498 mouse AML model, a CpG-A ODN was ineffective when used alone, but a CpG-B ODN had both preventive and therapeutic activity [112]. NK cells were required for the CpG-induced protective effect, but neither T nor B cells contributed and no memory response appeared to be induced. In a post bone marrow transplantation AML model CpG ODN alone had little effect, but either CpG-A or CpG-B ODN substantially improved the efficacy of donor lymphocyte infusion (DLI) [112]. A combination of a CpG-A ODN together with a CpG-B ODN synergized strongly with DLI in this model, giving 90% long-term survival when DLI alone gave 0% [112]. In summary, monotherapy of tumors with either CpG-A or CpG-B ODN alone or in combinations of the two or with other immunotherapies may be useful, depending on the tumor type. It appears that CpG-A may be most effective against NK-sensitive tumors, and CpG-B may be most effective when broader immune activation and an adaptive immune response can enhance the efficacy of therapy.

13.5.2
**CpG DNA as an Adjuvant for Cancer Vaccines**

Numerous studies have demonstrated the strong activity of CpG-B ODN as adjuvants for vaccines against infectious disease in mouse models, as well as in nonhuman primates ([88, 113–115] and reviewed in [116]). An important factor in their activity in tumor vaccines may be that CpG-B ODN promote cross-priming with strong cytolytic T cell and antibody responses to peptides and protein antigens independently of T cell help [ 95, 117–122]. CpG-B ODN appear to be more effective $T_h1$-like adjuvants than complete Freund's [119, 123, 124] or any other adjuvant to which they have been compared [125].

Both CpG-B and CpG-A ODN are highly effective adjuvants for tumor vaccines, although most studies have been performed with CpG-B ODN. The first demonstration of the efficacy of CpG DNA as an adjuvant for a tumor antigen was accidental. In studies of *Drosophila* cells that were engineered to function as antigen-presenting cells (APCs) and present tumor antigens, Sprent *et al.* made the surprising observation that untransfected *Drosophila* cells were highly stimulatory to murine B cells, which up-regulated co-stimulatory molecules and could provide bystander co-stimulation for $CD8^+$ T cells [38]. They further showed that the *Drosophila* DNA is unmethylated and immune stimulatory, but loses this property after treatment with CpG methylase. *Drosophila* cells transfected to express a tumor antigen in the context of the appropriate class I MHC could induce MHC compatible spleen cells to respond to a tumor antigen *in vitro* and to mediate tumor rejection *in vivo* [38].

We have evaluated the antitumor adjuvant properties of CpG DNA in the 38C13 murine B cell lymphoma model, in which the idiotype (Id) of the 38C13 surface IgM serves as the tumor-associated antigen. A CpG-B ODN induced the production of high levels of Id-specific antibody in mice immunized with the CpG together with a conjugate of the Id to keyhole limpet hemocyanin (KLH) [123]. The CpG ODN was highly effective when used to immunize via the intradermal or subcutaneous routes, but was slightly less effective through the intraperitoneal route. A dose of 25 µg of the ODN was highly effective, but a maximal response was seen at doses of 50–100 µg. Control mice challenged with a lethal dose of tumor cells all died within 1 month of challenge, but mice immunized together with the CpG-B ODN had 40% long-term survival [123]. The efficacy of the CpG-B ODN was further improved when the Id was conjugated to GMCSF [126]. A GMCSF-Id fusion protein, used as an immunogen without an adjuvant, was an extremely effective immunogen for inducing anti-Id antibodies. However, almost all of the antibody response was of the IgG1 isotype, and only 30% of mice were long-term survivors of a tumor challenge given 3 days after a single immunization. In contrast, when a CpG ODN was combined with the granulocyte macrophage colony stimulating factor (GM-CSF)–Id fusion protein, the antibody response was largely IgG2a, the magnitude of the antibody response was increased approximately 5-fold and the long-term survival of the mice was improved from 30 to 70% [126]. In a different model system, Celis *et al.* showed that repeated immunization of mice with ovalbumin (OVA) protein or peptide together with a CpG-B ODN resulted in a 10- to 100-

fold increase in CTL responses and substantial therapeutic activity even when vaccination was delayed until day 7 after injection of mice with a B16 melanoma that expressed OVA [127].

CpG-B ODN have also been shown to enhance tumor immunotherapy with adoptive transfer of T cells primed against the tumor cells. Donor mice are immunized against a tumor such as the A20 lymphoma, and then stimulated *in vitro* with APCs and irradiated tumor cells. The addition of a CpG-B ODN to the *in vitro* culture improved CD4 T cell recovery by 12- to 70-fold and the recovered cells were effective at eliminating an established A20 lymphoma in recipient mice without apparent induction of autoimmune disease [128]. There has been much recent interest in the use of DC vaccines for tumor immunotherapy. CpG is an effective adjuvant for DC co-cultured with irradiated tumor cells, providing a substantial increase in both prophylactic and therapeutic activity in a murine colon cancer model [129].

### 13.5.3
### Application of CpG DNA to Enhance ADCC for Treating Cancer

Passive immunotherapy with monoclonal antibodies (mAbs) against tumor antigens has not been as effective in humans as originally hoped. Nevertheless, three mAbs, Rituximab, Herceptin and Alemtuzumab, have been approved by the US Food and Drug Administration. Multiple mechanisms probably contribute to the antitumor activity of mAbs, but one of their major mechanisms is probably antibody-dependent cellular cytotoxicity (ADCC). mAbs specific for tumor cell surface antigens bind to the tumor cell, which can then be recognized by lymphocytes such as NK cells and neutrophils which express Fc receptors. To test the hypothesis that the efficacy of antitumor mAbs could be improved by activation of ADCC with CpG-B ODN, we used the 38C13 B cell lymphoma in syngeneic immunocompetent C3H mice [130]. Several days after tumor implantation, the mice were injected with a dose of CpG-B ODN sufficient to cause systemic immune activation and enhanced Fc receptor function. They were then treated with a standard dose of the mAb. Although treatment with mAb alone gave only a 10% long-term survival, mice pretreated with CpG-B ODN had 70–80% survival [130]. The CpG-B ODN was equally effective at promoting survival when administered before the mAb, on the same day, or up to 2 days after the mAb. However, delayed administration of CpG-B ODN until 4 days after mAb resulted in survival that was indistinguishable from mAb alone. Dose–response studies showed that high doses of CpG-B ODN (up to 200 μg) enhanced the antitumor activity of mAb more effectively than lower doses, but some activity was apparent even at doses of just 2 μg/mouse [131]. With repeated administration of CpG and mAb, even large established tumors could be cured in this model [131].

CpG-B ODN have pronounced phenotypic effects on normal and primary human malignant B cells from patients with various histologies, inducing expression of class I and II MHC, CD20, CD40, CD54, CD58, CD80 and CD86 and improved activation of T cells in an allogeneic MLR [132–134] Interestingly, the CpG-B ODN appeared less effective at inducing normal B cells to express increased levels of CD20.

Such changes would be expected to make the malignant cells better targets for Rituximab, as well as for immunotherapy in general. Human clinical trials of this form of combination immunotherapy have recently been initiated.

## 13.6
## Conclusion

The early days of cancer immunotherapy were marked by the use of crude bacterial extracts such as "Coley's toxins", which were remarkably effective despite their eventual fall from favor. Even though BCG continues to be used in the treatment of superficial bladder cancer, in today's regulatory climate it would be effectively impossible to resurrect immune therapy with bacterial extracts on a widespread basis. With the advent of recombinant cytokines, there was much hope that these would offer a less toxic and more effective form of immunotherapy. Unfortunately, despite some successes, immunotherapy using recombinant cytokines has not lived up to its initial promise. Perhaps the use of a pharmacologic dose of a recombinant cytokine can never reproduce the complexity of a multifaceted therapeutic antitumor immune response in more than occasional cases. However, the field of immunology has advanced to the point that we may now reasonably hope to achieve the same sustained remissions in established advanced malignancy as were seen with the use of "Coley's toxins" by using molecular mimics of microbial molecules, instead of the bacterial extracts themselves. CpG DNA, provides a way to induce the immune system to produce a whole panoply of cytokines and chemokines in a coordinated manner, which may be more effective and less toxic than the administration of individual recombinant cytokines or chemokines in pharmacologic quantities. Synthetic CpG ODN are essentially mimics of bDNA that "trick" the immune system into thinking that an infection has occurred, leading to the initiation of remarkably effective immune defense mechanisms. The orchestrated stimulation of the immune system with resulting therapeutic power unleashed by CpG DNA has already been demonstrated in a variety of mouse models, with encouraging results as reviewed above. Results from initial human clinical trials with a CpG-B ODN suggest this approach may be reasonably well tolerated in humans, but the full therapeutic benefit of these approaches remains to be determined.

## Acknowledgments

We thank Denise Arsenault for excellent secretarial assistance. Financial support was provided through DARPA and the Coley Pharmaceutical Group.

## References

1 HALL, S. S. A commotion in the blood: Life, death, and the immune system. *Sloan Technology Series* 1997; Henry Holland Company, New York.

2 COLEY, W. B. The treatment of malignant tumors by repeated inoculations of erysipelas: with a report of ten original cases. *Am J Med Sci* 1893; **105**: 487–511.

3 WIEMANN, B. and STARNES, C. O. Coley's toxins, tumor necrosis factor and cancer research: a historical perspective. *Pharmacol Ther* 1994; **64**: 529–564.

4 BAST, R. C., JR, ZBAR, B., BORSOS, T. and RAPP, H. J. BCG and cancer. *N Engl J Med* 1974; **290**: 1458–1469.

5 MORALES, A. Adjuvant immunotherapy in superficial bladder cancer. *Natl Cancer Inst Monogr* 1978; **49**: 315–319.

6 TOKUNAGA, T., YAMAMOTO, H., SHIMADA, S., *et al*. Antitumor activity of deoxyribonucleic acid fraction from *Mycobacterium bovis* BCG. I. Isolation, physicochemical characterization, and antitumor activity. *J Natl Cancer Inst* 1984; **72**: 955–962.

7 YAMAMOTO, S., KURAMOTO, E., SHIMADA, S. and TOKUNAGA, T. *In vitro* augmentation of natural killer cell activity and production of interferon-$\alpha/\beta$ and -$\gamma$ with deoxyribonucleic acid fraction from *Mycobacterium bovis* BCG. *Jpn J Cancer Res* 1988; **79**: 866–873.

8 TOKUNAGA, T., YAMAMOTO, T. and YAMAMOTO, S. How BCG led to the discovery of immunostimulatory DNA. *Jpn J Infect Dis* 1999; **52**: 1–11.

9 YAMAMOTO, S., YAMAMOTO, T., SHIMADA, S., *et al*. DNA from bacteria, but not from vertebrates, induces interferons, activates natural killer cells and inhibits tumor growth. *Microbiol Immunol* 1992; **36**: 983–997.

10 KURAMOTO, E., YANO, O., KIMURA, Y., *et al*. Oligonucleotide sequences required for natural killer cell activation. *Jpn J Cancer Res* 1992; **83**: 1128–1131.

11 MESSINA, J. P., GILKESON, G. S. and PISETSKY, D. S. Stimulation of *in vitro* murine lymphocyte proliferation by bacterial DNA. *J Immunol* 1991; **147**: 1759–1764.

12 MESSINA, J. P., GILKESON, G. S. and PISETSKY, D. S. The influence of DNA structure on the *in vitro* stimulation of murine lymphocytes by natural and synthetic polynucleotide antigens. *Cell Immunol* 1993; **147**: 148–157.

13 JACOBS, B. L. and LANGLAND, J. O. When two strands are better than one: the mediators and modulators of the cellular responses to double-stranded RNA. *Virology* 1996; **219**: 339–349.

14 TALMADGE, J. E., ADAMS, J., PHILLIPS, H., *et al*. Immunomodulatory effects in mice of polyinosinic–polycytidylic acid complexed with poly-l-lysine and carboxymethylcellulose. *Cancer Res* 1985; **45**: 1058–1065.

15 MANETTI, R., ANNUNZIATO, F., TOMASEVIC, L., *et al*. Polyinosinic acid: polycytidylic acid promotes T helper type 1-specific immune responses by stimulating macrophage production of interferon-$\alpha$ and interleukin-12. *Eur J Immunol* 1995; **25**: 2656–2660.

16 KERN, E. R., OVERALL, J. C., JR and GLASGOW, L. A. Herpesvirus hominis infection in newborn mice: treatment with interferon inducer polyinosinic-polycytidylic acid. *Antimicrob Ag Chemother* 1975; **7**: 793–800.

17 LEVY, H. B., LONDON, W., FUCCILLO, D. A., BARON, S. and RICE, J. Prophylactic control of simian hemorrhagic fever in monkeys by an interferon inducer, polyriboinosinic–polyribocytidylic acid-poly-l-lysine. *J Infect Dis* 1976; **133** (Suppl.): A256–A259.

18 HARRINGTON, D. G., CRABBS, C. L., HILMAS, D. E., *et al*. Adjuvant effects of low doses of a nuclease-resistant derivative of polyinosinic acid.polycytidylic acid on antibody responses of monkeys to inactivated Venezuelan equine encephalomyelitis virus vaccine. *Infect Immun* 1979; **24**: 160–166.

19 LEVINE, A. S. and LEVY, H. B. Phase I–II trials of poly IC stabilized with poly-l-lysine. *Cancer Treat Rep* 1978; **62**: 1907–1912.

**20** KROWN, S. E., FRIDEN, G. B., KHAN-SUR, T., *et al.* Phase I trial with the inter-feron inducer polyI:C/poly-l-lysine (Poly ICL). *J Interferon Res* 1983; **3**: 281–290.

**21** KUMAR, A., YANG, Y. L., FLATI, V., *et al.* Deficient cytokine signaling in mouse embryo fibroblasts with a targeted dele-tion in the PKR gene: role of IRF-1 and NF-κB. *EMBO J* 1997; **16**: 406–416.

**22** MICHELSON, A. M., SHAOOL, D. and LACOUR, F. Poly(A).poly(U) as adjuvant in cancer treatment distribution and pharmacokinetics in rabbits. *Proc Soc Exp Biol Med* 1985; **179**: 180–186.

**23** PARK, S. J., KIM, W. H., HAN, K. H., *et al.* Adjuvant effect of polyadenylic.po-lyuridylic acid on antibody production of recombinant hepatitis B surface anti-gen in mice. *Int J Immunopharmacol* 1995; **17**: 513–516.

**24** LACOUR, J. Clinical trials using polya-denylic–polyuridylic acid as an adjuvant to surgery in treating different human tumors. *J Biol Response Mod* 1985; **4**: 538–543.

**25** KHAN, A. L., RICHARDSON, S., DREW, J., *et al.* Polyadenylic–polyuridylic acid en-hances the natural cell-mediated cyto-toxicity in patients with breast cancer undergoing mastectomy. *Surgery* 1995; **118**: 531–538.

**26** HAHM, K. B., HAN, K. Y., KIM, W. H., *et al.* Efficacy of polyadenylic.polyur-idylic acid in the treatment of chronic active hepatitis B. *Int J Immunopharma-col* 1994; **16**: 217–225.

**27** TOKUNAGA, T., YAMAMOTO, S. and NAMBA, K. A synthetic single-stranded DNA, poly(dG,dC), induces interferon-α/β and -γ, augments natural killer ac-tivity, and suppresses tumor growth. *Jpn J Cancer Res* 1988; **79**: 682–686.

**28** PISETSKY, D. S. and REICH, C. F., III. The influence of base sequence on the immunological properties of defined oligonucleotides. *Immunopharmacology* 1998; **40**: 199–208.

**29** SUZUKI, K., MORI, A., ISHII, K. J., *et al.* Activation of target-tissue immune-re-cognition molecules by double-stranded polynucleotides. *Proc Natl Acad Sci USA* 1999; **96**: 2285–2290.

**30** ISHII, K. J., SUZUKI, K., COBAN, C., *et al.* Genomic DNA released by dying cells induces the maturation of APCs. *J Im-munol* 2001; **167**: 2602–2607.

**31** KRIEG, A. M. CpG motifs in bacterial DNA and their immune effects. *Annu. Rev. Immunol.* 2002; **20**: 709–760.

**32** KRIEG, A. M., YI, A. K., MATSON, S., *et al.* CpG motifs in bacterial DNA trigger di-rect B-cell activation. *Nature* 1995; **374**: 546–549.

**33** BIRD, A. P. CpG islands as gene mar-kers in the vertebrate nucleus. *Trends Genet* 1987; **3**: 342–347.

**34** HAN, J., ZHU, Z., HSU, C. and FIN-LEY, W. H. Selection of antisense oligo-nucleotides on the basis of genomic fre-quency of the target sequence. *Antisense Res Dev* 1994; **4**: 53–65.

**35** KRIEG, A. M., WU, T., WEERATNA, R., *et al.* Sequence motifs in adenoviral DNA block immune activation by sti-mulatory CpG motifs. *Proc Natl Acad Sci USA* 1998; **95**: 12631–12636.

**36** CHEN, Y., LENERT, P., WEERANTA, R., *et al.* Identification of methylated CpG motifs as inhibitors of the immune sti-mulatory CpG motifs. *Gene Ther* 2001; **8**: 1024–1032.

**37** BROWN, W. C., ESTES, D. M., CHANT-LER, S. E., KEGERREIS, K. A. and SUAREZ, C. E. DNA and a CpG oligonu-cleotide derived from *Babesia bovis* are mitogenic for bovine B cells. *Infect Im-mun* 1998; **66**: 5423–5432.

**38** SUN, S., CAI, Z., LANGLADE-DEMOYEN, P., *et al.* Dual function of *Drosophila* cells as APCs for naive CD8+ T cells: implica-tions for tumor immunotherapy. *Immu-nity* 1996; **4**: 555–564.

**39** SUN, S., BEARD, C., JAENISCH, R., JONES, P. and SPRENT, J. Mitogenicity of DNA from different organisms for murine B cells. *J Immunol* 1997; **159**: 3119–3125.

**40** DEMPSEY, P. W., ALLISON, M. E., AKKA-RAJU, S., GOODNOW, C. C. and FEARON, D. T. C3d of complement as a molecular adjuvant: bridging innate and acquired immunity. *Science* 1996; **271**: 348–350.

**41** MEDZHITOV, R. and JANEWAY, C. A., JR. Innate immunity: impact on the adaptive immune response. *Curr Opin Immunol* 1997; **9**: 4–9.

**42** ADEREM, A. and ULEVITCH, R. J. Toll-like receptors in the induction of the innate immune response. *Nature* 2000; **406**: 782–787.

**43** MEDZHITOV, R. and JANEWAY, C. The toll receptor family and microbial recognition. *Trends Microbiol* 2000; **8**: 452–456.

**44** YAMAMOTO, T., YAMAMOTO, S., KATAOKA, T. and TOKUNAGA, T. Lipofection of synthetic oligodeoxyribonucleotide having a palindromic sequence of AACGTT to murine splenocytes enhances interferon production and natural killer activity. *Microbiol Immunol* 1994; **38**: 831–836.

**45** HACKER, H., MISCHAK, H., MIETHKE, T., *et al.* CpG-DNA-specific activation of antigen-presenting cells requires stress kinase activity and is preceded by nonspecific endocytosis and endosomal maturation. *EMBO J* 1998; **17**: 6230–6240.

**46** MANZEL, L. and MACFARLANE, D. E. Lack of immune stimulation by immobilized CpG-oligodeoxynucleotide. *Antisense Nucleic Acid Drug Dev* 1999; **9**: 459–464.

**47** MUI, B., RANEY, S. G., SEMPLE, S. C. and HOPE, M. J. Immune stimulation by a CpG-containing oligodeoxynucleotide is enhanced when encapsulated and delivered in lipid particles. *J Pharmacol Exp Ther* 2001; **298**: 1185–1192.

**48** MACFARLANE, D. E. and MANZEL, L. Antagonism of immunostimulatory CpG-oligodeoxynucleotides by quinacrine, chloroquine, and structurally related compounds. *J Immunol* 1998; **160**: 1122–1131.

**49** YI, A. K., TUETKEN, R., REDFORD, T., *et al.* CpG motifs in bacterial DNA activate leukocytes through the pH-dependent generation of reactive oxygen species. *J Immunol* 1998; **160**: 4755–4761.

**50** HEMMI, H., TAKEUCHI, O., KAWAI, T., *et al.* A Toll-like receptor recognizes bacterial DNA [In process citation]. *Nature* 2000; **408**: 740–745.

**51** BAUER, S., KIRSCHNING, C. J., HACKER, H., *et al.* Human TLR9 confers responsiveness to bacterial DNA via species-specific CpG motif recognition.

*Proc Natl Acad Sci USA* 2001; **98**: 9237–9242.

**52** KRUG, A., TOWAROWSKI, A., BRITSCH, S., *et al.* Toll-like receptor expression reveals CpG DNA as a unique microbial stimulus for plasmacytoid dendritic cells which synergizes with CD40 ligand to induce high amounts of IL-12. *Eur J Immunol* 2001;

**53** STACEY, K. J., SWEET, M. J. and HUME, D. A. Macrophages ingest and are activated by bacterial DNA. *J Immunol* 1996; **157**: 2116–2122.

**54** HACKER, H., MISCHAK, H., HACKER, G., *et al.* Cell type-specific activation of mitogen-activated protein kinases by CpG-DNA controls interleukin-12 release from antigen-presenting cells. *EMBO J* 1999; **18**: 6973–6982.

**55** YI, A. K. and KRIEG, A. M. Rapid induction of mitogen-activated protein kinases by immune stimulatory CpG DNA. *J Immunol* 1998; **161**: 4493–4497.

**56** JAKOB, T., WALKER, P. S., KRIEG, A. M., UDEY, M. C. and VOGEL, J. C. Activation of cutaneous dendritic cells by CpG-containing oligodeoxynucleotides: a role for dendritic cells in the augmentation of $T_h1$ responses by immunostimulatory DNA. *J Immunol* 1998; **161**: 3042–3049.

**57** COWDERY, J. S., BOERTH, N. J., NORIAN, L. A., MYUNG, P. S. and KORETZKY, G. A. Differential regulation of the IL-12 p40 promoter and of p40 secretion by CpG DNA and lipopolysaccharide. *J Immunol* 1999; **162**: 6770–6775.

**58** HARTMANN, G. and KRIEG, A. M. CpG DNA and LPS induce distinct patterns of activation in human monocytes. *Gene Ther* 1999; **6**: 893–903.

**59** SWEET, M. J., STACEY, K. J., KAKUDA, D. K., MARKOVICH, D. and HUME, D. A. IFN-γ primes macrophage responses to bacterial DNA. *J Interferon Cytokine Res* 1998; **18**: 263–271.

**60** GAO, J. J., ZUVANICH, E. G., XUE, Q., *et al.* Cutting edge: bacterial DNA and LPS act in synergy in inducing nitric oxide production in RAW 264.7 macrophages. *J Immunol* 1999; **163**: 4095–4099.

**61** GAO, J. J., XUE, Q., PAPASIAN, C. J. and MORRISON, D. C. Bacterial DNA and lipopolysaccharide induce synergistic production of TNF-α through a post-transcriptional mechanism. *J Immunol* 2001; **166**: 6855–6860.

**62** COWDERY, J. S., CHACE, J. H., YI, A. K. and KRIEG, A. M. Bacterial DNA induces NK cells to produce IFN-γ *in vivo* and increases the toxicity of lipopolysaccharides. *J Immunol* 1996; **156**: 4570–4575.

**63** ZHAO, Q., MATSON, S., HERRERA, C. J., *et al.* Comparison of cellular binding and uptake of antisense phosphodiester, phosphorothioate, and mixed phosphorothioate and methylphosphonate oligonucleotides. *Antisense Res Dev* 1993; **3**: 53–66.

**64** MATSON, S. and KRIEG, A. M. Nonspecific suppression of [³H]thymidine incorporation by "control" oligonucleotides. *Antisense Res Dev* 1992; **2**: 325–330.

**65** KENTER, A. L. and TREDUP, J. High expression of a 3′–5′ exonuclease activity is specific to B lymphocytes. *Mol Cell Biol* 1991; **11**: 4398–4404.

**66** LIANG, H., NISHIOKA, Y., REICH, C. F., PISETSKY, D. S. and LIPSKY, P. E. Activation of human B cells by phosphorothioate oligodeoxynucleotides. *J Clin Invest* 1996; **98**: 1119–1129.

**67** HARTMANN, G., WEINER, G. J. and KRIEG, A. M. CpG DNA: a potent signal for growth, activation, and maturation of human dendritic cells. *Proc Natl Acad Sci USA* 1999; **96**: 9305–9310.

**68** STEIN, C. A., SUBASINGHE, C., SHINOZUKA, K. and COHEN, J. S. Physicochemical properties of phosphorothioate oligodeoxynucleotides. *Nucleic Acids Res* 1988; **16**: 3209–3221.

**69** STEIN, C. A. and CHENG, Y. C. Antisense oligonucleotides as therapeutic agents–is the bullet really magical? *Science* 1993; **261**: 1004–1012.

**70** STEIN, C. A. and KRIEG, A. M. Problems in interpretation of data derived from *in vitro* and *in vivo* use of antisense oligodeoxynucleotides [Editorial]. *Antisense Res Dev* 1994; **4**: 67–69.

**71** ZHAO, Q., WALDSCHMIDT, T., FISHER, E., HERRERA, C. J. and KRIEG, A. M. Stage-specific oligonucleotide uptake in murine bone marrow B-cell precursors. *Blood* 1994; **84**: 3660–3666.

**72** CROOKE, R. M. *In vitro* cellular uptake, distribution, and metabolism of oligonucleotides. In: *Antisense Research and Application.*, ed. S. T. Crooke, Springer, Berlin 1998; 103–140.

**73** PEREZ, J. R., LI, Y., STEIN, C. A., *et al.* Sequence-independent induction of Sp1 transcription factor activity by phosphorothioate oligodeoxynucleotides. *Proc Natl Acad Sci USA* 1994; **91**: 5957–5961.

**74** WANG, X. Z. and RON, D. Stress-induced phosphorylation and activation of the transcription factor CHOP (GADD153) by p38 MAP Kinase. *Science* 1996; **272**: 1347–1349.

**75** BURGESS, T. L., FISHER, E. F., ROSS, S. L., *et al.* The antiproliferative activity of c-*myb* and c-*myc* antisense oligonucleotides in smooth muscle cells is caused by a nonantisense mechanism. *Proc Natl Acad Sci USA* 1995; **92**: 4051–4055.

**76** FENNEWALD, S. M. and RANDO, R. F. Inhibition of high affinity basic fibroblast growth factor binding by oligonucleotides. *J Biol Chem* 1995; **270**: 21718–21721.

**77** GUVAKOVA, M. A., YAKUBOV, L. A., VLODAVSKY, I., TONKINSON, J. L. and STEIN, C. A. Phosphorothioate oligodeoxynucleotides bind to basic fibroblast growth factor, inhibit its binding to cell surface receptors, and remove it from low affinity binding sites on extracellular matrix. *J Biol Chem* 1995; **270**: 2620–2627.

**78** KITAJIMA, I., UNOKI, K. and MARUYAMA, I. Phosphorothioate oligodeoxynucleotides inhibit basic fibroblast growth factor-induced angiogenesis *in vitro* and *in vivo*. *Antisense Nucleic Acid Drug Dev* 1999; **9**: 233–239.

**79** BROWN, D. A., KANG, S. H., GRYAZNOV, S. M., *et al.* Effect of phosphorothioate modification of oligodeoxynucleotides on specific protein binding. *J Biol Chem* 1994; **269**: 26801–26805.

**80** KHALED, Z., BENIMETSKAYA, L., ZELTSER, R., *et al.* Multiple mechanisms may contribute to the cellular anti-adhesive effects of phosphorothioate oligodeoxynucleotides. *Nucleic Acids Res* 1996; **24**: 737–745.

81 HARTMANN, G., KRUG, A., WALLER-FONTAINE, K. and ENDRES, S. Oligodeoxynucleotides enhance lipopolysaccharide-stimulated synthesis of tumor necrosis factor: dependence on phosphorothioate modification and reversal by heparin. *Mol Med* 1996; **2**: 429–438.

82 MONTEITH, D. K., HENRY, S. P., HOWARD, R. B., *et al.* Immune stimulation – a class effect of phosphorothioate oligodeoxynucleotides in rodents. *Anticancer Drug Des* 1997; **12**: 421–432.

83 HENRY, S., STECKER, K., BROOKS, D., *et al.* Chemically modified oligonucleotides exhibit decreased immune stimulation in mice. *J Pharmacol Exp Ther* 2000; **292**: 468–479.

84 TAM, R. C., WU-PONG, S., PAI, B., *et al.* Increased potency of an aptameric G-rich oligonucleotide is associated with novel functional properties of phosphorothioate linkages. *Antisense Nucleic Acid Drug Dev* 1999; **9**: 289–300.

85 ZHAO, Q., TEMSAMANI, J., IADAROLA, P. L., JIANG, Z. and AGRAWAL, S. Effect of different chemically modified oligodeoxynucleotides on immune stimulation. *Biochem Pharmacol* 1996; **51**: 173–182.

86 KRIEG, A. M., MATSON, S. and FISHER, E. Oligodeoxynucleotide modifications determine the magnitude of B cell stimulation by CpG motifs. *Antisense Nucleic Acid Drug Dev* 1996; **6**: 133–139.

87 YI, A. K., CHANG, M., PECKHAM, D. W., KRIEG, A. M. and ASHMAN, R. F. CpG oligodeoxyribonucleotides rescue mature spleen B cells from spontaneous apoptosis and promote cell cycle entry [published erratum appears in *J Immunol* 1999; **163**(2): 1093]. *J Immunol* 1998; **160**: 5898–5906.

88 HARTMANN, G., WEERATNA, R. D., BALLAS, Z. K., *et al.* Delineation of a CpG phosphorothioate oligodeoxynucleotide for activating primate immune responses *in vitro* and *in vivo*. *J Immunol* 2000; **164**: 1617–1624.

89 GOECKERITZ, B. E., FLORA, M., WITHERSPOON, K., *et al.* Multivalent cross-linking of membrane Ig sensitizes murine B cells to a broader spectrum of CpG-containing oligodeoxynucleotide motifs, including their methylated counterparts, for stimulation of proliferation and Ig secretion. *Int Immunol* 1999; **11**: 1693–1700.

90 BALLAS, Z. K., RASMUSSEN, W. L. and KRIEG, A. M. Induction of NK activity in murine and human cells by CpG motifs in oligodeoxynucleotides and bacterial DNA. *J Immunol* 1996; **157**: 1840–1845.

91 SESTER, D. P., BEASLEY, S. J., SWEET, M. J., *et al.* Bacterial/CpG DNA down-modulates colony stimulating factor-1 receptor surface expression on murine bone marrow-derived macrophages with concomitant growth arrest and factor-independent survival. *J Immunol* 1999; **163**: 6541–6550.

92 BOGGS, R. T., McGRAW, K., CONDON, T., *et al.* Characterization and modulation of immune stimulation by modified oligonucleotides. *Antisense Nucleic Acid Drug Dev* 1997; **7**: 461–471.

93 YAMAMOTO, S., YAMAMOTO, T., KATAOKA, T., *et al.* Unique palindromic sequences in synthetic oligonucleotides are required to induce INF and augment INF-mediated natural killer activity. *J Immunol* 1992; **148**: 4072–4076.

94 SUN, S., ZHANG, X., TOUGH, D. F. and SPRENT, J. Type I interferon-mediated stimulation of T cells by CpG DNA. *J Exp Med* 1998; **188**: 2335–2342.

95 LIPFORD, G. B., BAUER, M., BLANK, C., *et al.* CpG-containing synthetic oligonucleotides promote B and cytotoxic T cell responses to protein antigen: a new class of vaccine adjuvants. *Eur J Immunol* 1997; **27**: 2340–2344.

96 LIPFORD, G. B., BENDIGS, S., HEEG, K. and WAGNER, H. Poly-guanosine motifs costimulate antigen-reactive CD8 T cells while bacterial CpG-DNA affect T-cell activation via antigen-presenting cell-derived cytokines. *Immunology* 2000; **101**: 46–52.

97 VERTHELYI, D., ISHII, K. J., GURSEL, M., TAKESHITA, F. and KLINMAN, D. M. Human peripheral blood cells differentially recognize and respond to two distinct CpG motifs. *J Immunol* 2001; **166**: 2372–2377.

**98** Kadowaki, N., Antonenko, S. and Liu, Y. J. Distinct CpG DNA and polyinosinic–polycytidylic acid double-stranded RNA, respectively, stimulate CD11 c(–) type 2 dendritic cell precursors and CD11 c(+) dendritic cells to produce type I IFN. *J Immunol* 2001; **166**: 2291–2295.

**99** Sester, D. P., Naik, S., Beasley, S. J., Hume, D. A. and Stacey, K. J. Phosphorothioate backbone modification modulates macrophage activation by CpG DNA. *J Immunol* 2000; **165**: 4165–4173.

**100** Vallin, H., Perers, A., Alm, G. V. and Ronnblom, L. Anti-double-stranded DNA antibodies and immunostimulatory plasmid DNA in combination mimic the endogenous IFN-α inducer in systemic lupus erythematosus. *J Immunol* 1999; **163**: 6306–6313.

**101** Krieg, A. M. Now I know my CpGs. *Trends Microbiol* 2001; **9**: 249–252.

**102** Krug, A., Rothenfusser, S., Hornung, V., *et al.* Identification of CpG oligonucleotide sequences with high induction of IFN-αβ in plasmacytoid dendritic cells. *Eur J Immunol* 2001; **31**: 2154–2163.

**103** Neujahr, D. C., Reich, C. F. and Pisetsky, D. S. Immunostimulatory properties of genomic DNA from different bacterial species. *Immunobiology* 1999; **200**: 106–119.

**104** Kimura, Y., Sonehara, K., Kuramoto, E., *et al.* Binding of oligoguanylate to scavenger receptors is required for oligonucleotides to augment NK cell activity and induce IFN. *J Biochem (Tokyo)* 1994; **116**: 991–994.

**105** Lipford, G. B., Sparwasser, T., Bauer, M., *et al.* Immunostimulatory DNA: sequence-dependent production of potentially harmful or useful cytokines. *Eur J Immunol* 1997; **27**: 3420–3426.

**106** Shankaran, V., Ikeda, H., Bruce, A. T., *et al.* IFNγ and lymphocytes prevent primary tumour development and shape tumour immunogenicity. *Nature* 2001; **410**: 1107–1111.

**107** Dow, S. W., Fradkin, L. G., Liggitt, D. H., *et al.* Lipid–DNA complexes induce potent activation of innate immune responses and antitumor activity when administered intravenously. *J Immunol* 1999; **163**: 1552–1561.

**108** Lanuti, M., Rudginsky, S., Force, S. D., *et al.* Cationic lipid:bacterial DNA complexes elicit adaptive cellular immunity in murine intraperitoneal tumor models. *Cancer Res* 2000; **60**: 2955–2963.

**109** Ballas, Z. K., Krieg, A. M., Warren, T., *et al.* Divergent therapeutic and immunologic effects of oligodeoxynucleotides with distinct CpG motifs. *J Immunol* 2001; **167**: 4878–4886.

**110** Carpentier, A. F., Chen, L., Maltonti, F. and Delattre, J. Y. Oligodeoxynucleotides containing CpG motifs can induce rejection of a neuroblastoma in mice. *Cancer Res* 1999; **59**: 5429–5432.

**111** Carpentier, A. F., Xie, J., Mokhtari, K. and Delattre, J. Y. Successful treatment of intracranial gliomas in rat by oligodeoxynucleotides containing CpG motifs. *Clin Cancer Res* 2000; **6**: 2469–2473.

**112** Blazar, B. R., Krieg, A. M. and Taylor, P. A. Synthetic unmethylated cytosine–phosphate–guanosine oligodeoxynucleotides are potent stimulators of antileukemia responses in naive and bone marrow transplant recipients. *Blood* 2001; **98**: 1217–1225.

**113** Hartmann, G. and Krieg, A. M. Mechanism and function of a newly identified CpG DNA motif in human primary B cells. *J Immunol* 2000; **164**: 944–953.

**114** Davis, H. L., Suparto, I. I., Weeratna, R. R., *et al.* CpG DNA overcomes hyporesponsiveness to hepatitis B vaccine in orangutans [In process citation]. *Vaccine* 2000; **18**: 1920–1924.

**115** Jones, T. R., Obaldia, N., III, Gramzinski, R. A., *et al.* Synthetic oligodeoxynucleotides containing CpG motifs enhance immunogenicity of a peptide malaria vaccine in *Aotus* monkeys. *Vaccine* 1999; **17**: 3065–3071.

**116** Krieg, A. M. and Davis, H. L. Enhancing vaccines with immune stimulatory CpG DNA. *Curr Opin Mol Ther* 2001; **3**: 15–24.

**117** Sparwasser, T., Vabulas, R. M., Villmow, B., Lipford, G. B. and Wagner, H.

Bacterial CpG-DNA activates dendritic cells *in vivo*: T helper cell-independent cytotoxic T cell responses to soluble proteins. *Eur J Immunol* 2000; **30**: 3591–3597.

118 VABULAS, R. M., PIRCHER, H., LIPFORD, G. B., HACKER, H. and WAGNER, H. CpG-DNA activates *in vivo* T cell epitope presenting dendritic cells to trigger protective antiviral cytotoxic T cell responses. *J Immunol* 2000; **164**: 2372–2378.

119 CHU, R. S., TARGONI, O. S., KRIEG, A. M., LEHMANN, P. V. and HARDING, C. V. CpG oligodeoxynucleotides act as adjuvants that switch on T helper 1 (T$_h$1) immunity. *J Exp Med* 1997; **186**: 1623–1631.

120 ROMAN, M., MARTIN-OROZCO, E., GOODMAN, J. S., *et al.* Immunostimulatory DNA sequences function as T helper-1-promoting adjuvants [see Comments]. *Nat Med* 1997; **3**: 849–854.

121 WILD, J., GRUSBY, M. J., SCHIRMBECK, R. and REIMANN, J. Priming MHC-I-restricted cytotoxic T lymphocyte responses to exogenous hepatitis B surface antigen is CD4$^+$ T cell dependent. *J Immunol* 1999; **163**: 1880–1887.

122 DAVIS, H. L., WEERATNA, R., WALDSCHMIDT, T. J., *et al.* CpG DNA is a potent enhancer of specific immunity in mice immunized with recombinant hepatitis B surface antigen [published erratum appears in *J Immunol* 1999; **162**(5): 3103]. *J Immunol* 1998; **160**: 870–876.

123 WEINER, G. J., LIU, H. M., WOOLDRIDGE, J. E., DAHLE, C. E. and KRIEG, A. M. Immunostimulatory oligodeoxynucleotides containing the CpG motif are effective as immune adjuvants in tumor antigen immunization. *Proc Natl Acad Sci USA* 1997; **94**: 10833–10837.

124 SUN, S., KISHIMOTO, H. and SPRENT, J. DNA as an adjuvant: capacity of insect DNA and synthetic oligodeoxynucleotides to augment T cell responses to specific antigen. *J Exp Med* 1998; **187**: 1145–1150.

125 KIM, S. K., RAGUPATHI, G., MUSSELLI, C., *et al.* Comparison of the effect of different immunological adjuvants on the antibody and T-cell response to immunization with MUC1–KLH and GD3–KLH conjugate cancer vaccines. *Vaccine* 1999; **18**: 597–603.

126 LIU, H. M., NEWBROUGH, S. E., BHATIA, S. K., *et al.* Immunostimulatory CpG oligodeoxynucleotides enhance the immune response to vaccine strategies involving granulocyte-macrophage colony-stimulating factor. *Blood* 1998; **92**: 3730–3736.

127 DAVILA, E. and CELIS, E. Repeated administration of cytosine-phosphorothiolated guanine-containing oligonucleotides together with peptide/protein immunization results in enhanced CTL responses with anti-tumor activity. *J Immunol* 2000; **165**: 539–547.

128 EGETER, O., MOCIKAT, R., GHORESCHI, K., DIECKMANN, A. and ROCKEN, M. Eradication of disseminated lymphomas with CpG-DNA activated T helper type 1 cells from nontransgenic mice. *Cancer Res* 2000; **60**: 1515–1520.

129 BRUNNER, C., SEIDERER, J., SCHLAMP, A., *et al.* Enhanced dendritic cell maturation by TNF-α or cytidine-phosphate-guanosine DNA drives T cell activation *in vitro* and therapeutic anti-tumor immune responses *in vivo*. *J Immunol* 2000; **165**: 6278–6286.

130 WOOLDRIDGE, J. E., BALLAS, Z., KRIEG, A. M. and WEINER, G. J. Immunostimulatory oligodeoxynucleotides containing CpG motifs enhance the efficacy of monoclonal antibody therapy of lymphoma. *Blood* 1997; **89**: 2994–2998.

131 WARREN, T. L., DAHLE, C. E. and WEINER, G. J. CpG oligodeoxynucleotides enhance monoclonal antibody therapy of a murine lymphoma. *Clin Lymphoma* 2000; **1**: 57–61.

132 JAHRSDORFER, B., HARTMANN, G., RACILA, E., *et al.* CpG DNA increases primary malignant B cell expression of costimulatory molecules and target antigens. *J Leuk Biol* 2001; **69**: 81–88.

133 DECKER, T., SCHNELLER, F., SPARWASSER, T., *et al.* Immunostimulatory CpG-oligonucleotides cause proliferation, cytokine production, and an immunogenic phenotype in chronic lym-

phocytic leukemia B cells. _Blood_ 2000; 95: 999–1006.

**134** DECKER, T., SCHNELLER, F., KRONSCH- NABL, M., _et al._ Immunostimulatory CpG-oligonucleotides induce functional high affinity IL-2 receptors on B-CLL cells: costimulation with IL-2 results in a highly immunogenic phenotype. _Exp Hematol_ 2000; 28: 558–568.

# 14

# The T-Body Approach: Towards Cancer Immuno-Gene Therapy

Jehonathan H. Pinthus and Zelig Eshhar

## 14.1
## Background

The T-body approach employs T cells redirected with antibody specificity using chimeric receptors (CRs). In this chapter we use the term T-bodies to define T cells bearing surface CRs. In functional terms, the CR combines antibody specificity in the form of Fv (variable region fragment) linked to a T cell stimulatory molecule. Primarily, we developed the T-body approach in order to endow T cells with predefined antibody specificity in order to study some physicochemical parameters involved in T cell activation (for review, see [1]). In the first design of the CR, we took advantage of the similarity in structure and genetic organization between the T cell receptor (TCR) and the antibody molecules, and replaced the variable (V) region of the TCR $\alpha$ and $\beta$ chains with the antibody $V_H$ and $V_L$ [2]. Using the V region of antihapten antibodies we demonstrated that T cell hybridoma expressing such chimeric TCR genes could recognize antigen in an MHC-unrestricted manner, and could undergo activation for IL-2 production and target cell killing in a non-MHC-dependent manner [1].

Quite readily, we and others have appreciated that T-bodies with antitumor specificity hold promise for cancer immunotherapy (for reviews, see [3, 4]). The idea behind this assumption was to combine the availability of monoclonal antibodies (mAbs) towards tumor-associated antigens with the efficacy of tumor penetration and rejection of T cells. Using this combination we expected to overcome the inefficiency of antibodies in rejecting solid tumors, on the one hand, and difficulties in obtaining tumor-specific T cells, on the other.

**14.2**
**CRs with Antitumor Specificity**

**14.2.1**
**Optimizing the CR Design**

#### 14.2.1.1 The single-chain CR

The original chimeric TCR configuration did not comply with the practical requirements for its application in tumor therapy. In order to express it in the patient's lymphocytes, one has to deliver two genes – each encoding one of the two TCR chains.
Such an undertaking was very inefficient considering the state of the art of gene delivery in the early 1990s. We therefore introduced and developed the single-chain
CR, where we took advantage of the ability to express the antibody binding in the
form of single-chain Fv (scFv) [5, 6]. Here we joined the scFv to receptor chains, such
as the CD3 ζ chain or FcR γ chain, which are capable of directly triggering T cell activation [7]. Such a single-chain configuration now enabled the expression of the CR
following only one gene transfer. This innovation opened a new era in the development of T-bodies towards the adoptive immunotherapy of cancer. It was indeed reflected by the many research groups that joined the effort and many CRs were developed to cancers of various histologies (see Tab. 14.2 below). Combined with the advent in gene transfer into lymphocytes it became a valid option for clinical trials. The
single-chain configuration also expanded the choice of T cell triggering molecules
that could be used in the CR context, thereby extending the repertoire of effector
cells whose specificity could be redirected by this genetic manipulation (Tab. 14.1).
We have shown, for example, that the CR can redirect the specificity of a natural
killer (NK)-like cell line [8].

#### 14.2.1.2 Direct recruitment of intracellular triggering molecules

In the clinic the CRs will have to be expressed in lymphocytes of tumor patients and
it is likely that the first clinical trials will be performed in patients with advanced disease that has resisted common therapeutic treatments. It has been known for a while
now that lymphocytes derived from patients with a heavy tumor burden are often defective in their signaling pathway due to impaired protein tyrosine kinases (PTKs)

**Tab. 14.1**  Molecules and cells employed in the scFcR context

| Receptor | Subunit chain | Cells |
|---|---|---|
| TCR | α, β, γ, δ | T cells |
| CD3 | ζ, η, γ | T cells |
| FcγRIII | CD16α, γ | NK, lymphokine-activated killer (LAK) cells |
| IL-2R | α, β, γ | lymphocytes |
| IL-nR | various chains | lymphocytes |
| Cytoplasmic + transmembrane | PTK | lymphocytes |

that participate in the receptor-proximal stage of the chain of events leading to T cell activation [9]. In order to bypass these defective steps, we tried to directly link soluble, cytoplasmic PTKs of the ZAP-70 family such as ZAP-70 and Syk, known to be recruited to the phosphorylated immuno receptor tyrosine activation motifs (ITAMs) of lymphocyte receptors. After testing different combinations of these PTKs with various transmembranal and extracellular spacer domains [10, 11], we found that Syk is the preferable cytoplasmic PTK. Whether Syk-based CR performs better in cancer patients' lymphocytes has still to be shown.

### 14.2.1.3 Combining stimulatory and co-stimulatory signals

Redirection of the specificity of effector lymphocytes, using single-chain CR composed of an antibody linked to a lymphocyte triggering receptor subunit, has become a valid option for adoptive cancer therapy. Although the CR can stimulate effector functions in pre-activated T cells, it has been shown that this CR, lacking the capacity to provide critical co-stimulatory signaling, cannot activate resting lymphocytes, such as T cells derived from genetically modified stem cells or from CR transgenic mice [12]. It is well established that, in the absence of co-stimulatory signaling by CD28, resting T lymphocytes typically undergo anergy or apoptosis [13] and pre-activated T lymphocytes may also display suboptimal effector responses in response to CR engagement [14].

To overcome these obstacles, several groups have constructed CRs made of scFv linked to the intracellular part of CD28 and have shown that co-expression of two CR genes, each made of the same scFv linked to CD3ζ in the one and CD28 in the second, could provide both stimulatory and co-stimulatory signals for T cell activation [15–17]. Nevertheless, this approach required co-expression of two genes. A better design included the two signaling moieties on a single CR [18]. We have designed a novel tripartite CR composed of a scFv recognition moiety fused to the non-ligand binding part of the extracellular and the entire transmembrane and intracellular domains of the CD28 co-stimulatory molecule and the intracellular domain of FcRγ (scFv–CD28–γ) [19]. Human peripheral blood lymphocytes (PBLs) transduced with such a CR gene demonstrated specific stimulation of IL-2 production and target cell killing [19]. This was dependent on CD28 co-stimulatory activity as evidenced by IL-2 secretion profiles in the presence of the certain signal transduction inhibitors (A. Bendavid *et al.*, unpublished). Moreover, we have recently generated lines of transgenic mice expressing CR under the control of T cell-specific regulatory sequences. Unprimed naive T lymphocytes from mice transgenic for scFv–CD28–γ undergo high levels of proliferation, IL-2 secretion and rescue from apoptosis as a result of stimulation by plastic-bound cognate antigen (A. Bendavid *et al.*, unpublished).

In these studies we have demonstrated for the first time that FcRγ and CD28 can cooperate in providing co-stimulatory signaling to human T lymphocytes and activation of unprimed naive T lymphocytes via an engineered single-chain receptor of predefined specificity. For clinical application, these results point to a critical advantage for the tripartite configuration of CR in the generation of persistent and functional redirected T cells.

14.2.2
**Anticancer Specificities of CRs**

14.2.2.1 **Cancer-specific antibodies**
Since the development of the single-chain CR in 1993 [7], many anticancer antibodies have served to generate T-bodies specific to a broad variety of tumors. Table 14.2 lists the various specificities employed by different groups.

Our group has focused on targeting the erbB2 molecule, a member of the erbB growth factor receptors. Like others, we believe that the erbB2 is an excellent target for immunotherapy, not only because of its over-expression, but also because it serves, for certain tumors, as an oncoreceptor on which the transformed phenotype is dependent [20]. This implies a growth disadvantage for tumor variants that will escape immunotherapy by not expressing erbB2. The principal anti-erbB2 antibody we used throughout these studies was N29, generated in Professor Yarden's laboratory and was found to inhibit the growth of human cancer cell lines in nude mice [21].

Using erbB2-specific scFv–γ or –ζ CRs we [22] and others [23] have shown that T cell lines and hybridomas, as well as NK cells, could specifically kill a variety of erb-expressing human cells and undergo stimulation for interleukin production following *in vitro* interaction with these tumors. Moreover, Groner's group was the first to report that erbB2-specific T-bodies could prevent the growth of syngeneic erbB2-transfected NIH 3T3 tumors in mice [23, 24]. We demonstrated in a human prostate cancer xenograft model in SCID mice that human lymphocytes, expressing the erbB2-specific tripartite receptor, could slow the progression of the human tumors and even cure a significant number of mice (detailed in Section 14.2.3). Several other tumor-specific T-body systems have been thoroughly studied *in vitro*, some of which have been tested *in vivo* (see Tab. 14.2) and a few have reached the stage of clinical trials and are discussed in Sections 14.2.3 and 14.2.4.

14.2.2.2 **Ligands and receptors recognition units**
In the previous section we have focused on the anticancer activities of lymphocytes redirected with CRs with antibody specificity. Other molecules, such as receptors whose ligands are selectively expressed on tumor cells, or ligands to receptors over-expressed on certain cancers, can even serve as the specific recognition unit of CR. In fact, the first single-chain CRs used to activate lymphocytes employed ectodomains of the CD16 [25] and CD4 [26] (which was later used to target HIV infected cells [27]). Certain groups have reported on CRs made of TCR [28]; however, only recently a single-chain CR made with scFv of TCR specific to tumor peptide was expressed on cancer cells. We have collaborated with the group of Professor Bolhuis in designing the first of such single-chain CRs specific to the human melanoma MAGE-1 peptide in association with HLA.A2 [29]. Further configurations of this TCR-based CR were also shown to be functionally expressed in human T cells [29]. The advantage of this CR with TCR specificity is that such a recognition unit has been naturally selected in terms of affinity and specificity to function in the T cell milieu. However, since the repertoire of tumor-specific-defined TCRs is limited and their scope of function is restricted to a certain HLA haplotype, it is likely to target

**Tab. 14.2** Tumor-specific T-bodies

| Antigen | Tumor | Model | Group[a] | Reference |
|---|---|---|---|---|
| Angiogenic endothelial cell receptor: kinase insert domain receptor (KDR) | tumor neovasculature | *in vitro* | Kershaw, M. H. and Hwu, P. | 43 |
| CEA | colon | *in vitro* | Darcy, P. R. and Smyth, M. J. | 17, 44–49 |
| | | *in vivo* | Haynes, N. M. and Darcy, P. K. | 50 |
| CD20 | B cell lymphoma | *in vitro* | Jensen, M. and Raubitschek, A. | 51 |
| CD30 | Hodgkin's lymphoma | *in vitro* | Hombach, A. and Abken. H. | 52, 53 |
| CD33 | leukemia | *in vitro* | Finney, H. M. and Lawson, A. D. G. | 18 |
| CD44 | pancreatic carcinoma | *in vitro/ in vivo* | Henke, A. and Ponta, H. | 54, 55 |
| EGP40 | colorectal cancer | *in vitro* | Daly, T. and Hwu, P. | 56 |
| Epithelial glycoprotein 2 (EGP-2) | many human carcinomas (breast, colon, lung, renal, pancreatic) | *in vitro* | Ren-Heidenreich, L. and Trevor, K. T. | 57 |
| erbB2 (HER2/Neu) | adenocarcinomas: breast, prostate and others | *in vitro* | Stankovski, I. and Eshhar, Z. | 22, 30 |
| | | *in vivo* | Moritz, D. and Groner, B. | 23, 24 |
| erbB3 and erbB4 | various carcinomas | *in vitro* | Altenschmidt, U. and Groner, B. | 30 |
| FBP | ovarian carcinoma | *in vitro* | Hwu, P. and Shafer, G. E. | 58, 59 |
| | | *in vivo* | Hwu, P. and Eshhar, Z. | 32, 33 |
| G250 | renal cell carcinoma | *in vitro* | Weijtens, M. E. M. and Bolhuis, R. L. H. | 60–62 |
| GD3 | melanoma | *in vitro* | Yun, C. O. and Junghans, R. P. | 63 |
| High-molecular-weight melanoma-associated antigen (HMW-MAA) | melanoma | *in vitro* | Reinhold, U. and Abken, H. | 64 |
| Lewis$^Y$ (Le$^Y$) | several human carcinomas | *in vitro* | Mezzanzanica, D. and Canevari, S. | 65 |
| MAGE-A1/HLA-A1 | melanoma | *in vitro* | Willemsen, R. A. and Bolhuis, R. L. H. | 29 |
| Prostate-specific membrane antigen (PSMA) | prostate cancer | *in vitro* | Gong, M. C. and Sadelain, M. | 34 |
| TAG72 | gastrointestinal adenocarcinoma and pan-adenocarcinoma | *in vitro* | Hombach, A. and Abken, H. | 66, 67 |

[a] Names of first author and corresponding author of the first relevant publication.

only those tumor cells which express the given HLA peptide, which is often not expressed in tumors that escape the host immune system.

As to ligand-based CR, we have developed CRs using the erbB ligand Heregulin [also known as Neuregulin differentiation factor (NDF)] (Feigelson *et al.*, submitted). We and others [30] used NDF to target adenocarcinoma cells over-expressing the *erbB* family of oncogenic receptors. NDF is known to bind to homodimers of erbB3 and erbB4, and with higher affinity to heterodimers of these molecules with the erbB2 [20]. In our study the CR was made of the EGF (epidermal growth factor), cysteine-rich domain of NDF that encompasses all the binding ability of NDF. T cells expressing such NDF-based CR indeed demonstrated functional specificity of NDF – they underwent activation by human breast and ovarian carcinoma cells expressing erbB3 and erB4, with and without erbB2, and not with targets expressing only the erbB2. These results suggest a different targeting specificity than the anti-erbB antibodies, which may be advantageous towards certain types of cancers and may provide a higher level of selectivity over normal tissue, and as such may serve as a valid option for therapy.

### 14.2.3.
### Pre-Clinical Experimental Models

*In vitro*, the CR approach has proved helpful in conferring antitumor specificity to effector lymphocytes, stimulating these cells for cytokines production and target cell killing. However, although promising, the information derived under such conditions is not sufficient to provide us with important information as to the potential therapeutic potential of T-bodies. Without entering into the legitimate argument whether there is an appropriate *in vivo* experimental system that can equal or mimic with high fidelity the human situation, we strongly believe that some critical elements related to the T-body therapy can be tested and evaluated in experimental animal models, provided that the artificial conditions are controlled and taken into account.

Several *in vivo* models have been employed to evaluate the anticancer potential of the T-body approach. In the first one [23], mouse T cells expressing erbB2-specific CR were injected (together with its target transfected with the human erbB2 gene) subcutaneously (s.c.) into nude mice. In such a model it was observed that the tumor development was significantly delayed. In a more recent study by the same group [24], it was shown that erbB2-specific splenic T cells directly and repeatedly administered into erbB2-expressing mouse mammary tumors resulted in a total tumor regression.

Using carcinoembryonic antigen (CEA)-specific CR-expressing cytotoxic T lymphocytes (CTLs) from different mice [31], Smith's group showed an *in vivo* anticolon carcinoma effect. The CTLs used in this study required perforin and interferon (IFN)-$\gamma$ and were independent of Fas ligand or tumor necrosis factor. In a more clinically relevant experiment [32], Hwu, in collaboration with us, used murine tumor-infiltrating lymphocytes transduced with the folate binding protein (FBP)-specific CR. The tumor target was a syngeneic metastatic sarcoma, transduced with the human FBP gene. When injected intravenously into mice, with a systemic daily supply of IL-2, it was clearly shown that the only group of mice that developed a significantly lower number of lung metastasis was the one treated with the FBP-specific T cells plus IL-2. Another *in vivo* study by the same group [33] evaluated the potency of bone marrow stem cells, transduced with FBP-specific CR gene, to differentiate and mature into specific effector cells. Indeed, in mice whose hematopoietic system was reconstituted by FBP-expressing bone marrow a retardation of the growth of FBP-expressing tumor was observed. Interestingly, T cells were not directly involved in this process. Depletion of CD4 and CD8 cells did not diminish the antitumor activity, and it was suggested that NK cells and/or macrophages expressing the anti-FBP CR are responsible for this effect. These experiments highlighted an extension of the T-body approach by the administration of effector cells into patients undergoing systemic cyto-ablative therapy. Immediate possible candidates for such a treatment are leukemic patients receiving stem cells grafts. The tripartite CR is the construct of choice for such treatment because of the support of the built-in co-stimulatory signaling function to the priming and activation of naive T cells to mature specific effector cells.

Recently we have evaluated the therapeutic efficacy of anti-erbB2 CR-bearing human lymphocytes on human prostate cancer xenografts in a SCID mouse model (Pinthus *et al.*, submitted). Local delivery of erbB2-specific human lymphocytes to well-established subcutaneously and orthotopic tumors resulted in retardation of tumor growth and prostate-specific antigen (PSA) secretion, prolongation of survival and, importantly, tumor elimination in a significant number of mice. Concurrent administration of IL-2 was required for effective rejection of the prostate cancer xenograft. We believe that prostate cancer is an excellent candidate for T-body therapy not only because it expresses a variety of tissue- and tumor-specific antigens that can serve as targets (e. g. PSMA [34], PSCA [35], STEAP [36], PCTA-1 [37] and erbB2 [38, 39]) and for monitoring disease progression (such as PSA), but also because direct trans-rectal ultrasound guided intratumoral administration of the T-bodies into localized tumors is a valid therapeutic option.

## 14.2.4.
### Clinical Trials

The T-body approach has already been used in clinical trials. So far, several phase I trials have been initiated. Because of the lack of published information it is impossible to objectively evaluate these trials. Therefore, most of the information provided below is based on a recent review by Junghans [4] who has also conducted one of these trials. The most documented phase I trial was conducted in HIV-infected subjects receiving $3 \times 10^{10}$ autologous lymphocytes bearing the CD4$\zeta$ CR [40]. Out of 24 patients, 11 also received concurrent $6 \times 10^7$ IU/24 h IL-2 infusions for 5 days. The treatment was well tolerated with grade 3 or 4 adverse events predominantly associated with the IL-2 infusion. In some patients a transient decrease of the viral load was observed in the plasma and the rectal mucosa, the tissue reservoir for HIV. All 24 subjects tested negative for replication-competent retrovirus for up to 1 year after infusion. Cell Genesys, the company which carried out this study, also conducted phase I clinical trials in colorectal patients using the anti-TAG72-$\zeta$ CR made from the humanized CC49 mAb [41]. However, this trial was terminated due to the devel-

opment of anti-idiotypic antibodies in the patients' sera that caused misleading interpretation of the results. Junghans' group applied 24 doses of CEA-specific R-bearing
lymphocytes, totaling to up to $10^{11}$ per patient. The treatment was reported to be ade-
quately tolerated with only two minor responses observed in two patients [42]. Hwu
and colleagues at the NCI are conducting a phase I clinical trial in ovarian patients
using T-bodies made of the FBP-specific CR described below. Escalated doses of the
modified cells are infused into the patients together with controlled administration
of IL-2. So far no adverse side effects have been seen, neither was there any improvement in the patient status. In some of the patients' sera neutralizing antibodies were
found, specific to the murine MoV18 mAb from which the scFv was derived.

Although not unexpected in the category of patients in which these trials were carried out, some warning signals emerge that need our attention in further developing
this approach to effective therapy. These are related in part to the formation of neutralizing antibodies (following either murine or humanized scFv CR administration), to the low number of engineered cells that eventually reach the tumor and to
the relative short survival of the patients, reflecting their end-stage disease.

Altogether these results are encouraging with respect to the lack of adverse effects related to the T-body administration.

## 14.3
## Conclusions and Perspectives

As described in this chapter, great progress has been already accomplished along the
road of application of the T-body approach to cancer immunotherapy. We have at our
disposal a large repertoire of antibodies that can selectively recognize tumor-associated antigens in human cancer, we know how to optimally design the CR configuration to fit a certain disease or cell, and the advent of gene delivery and lymphocyte
culture technologies allows us to obtain very large quantities of genetically engineered, designer lymphocytes, stably expressing functional receptors. In the few
clinical trials done so far, these lymphocytes appear safe even after the administration of $10^{11}$ cells per patient. Yet, we lack sufficient information to optimize the effect
of these lymphocytes in the patient. From the classical adoptive immunotherapy
using unarmed lymphocytes such as tumor-infiltrating lymphocytes or LAK cells,
and from more recent pre-clinical studies using T-bodies in experimental systems,
we know that continuous supply of IL-2 supports the effector function of T cells. We
are now starting to understand the contribution of supplementing CR-bearing $CD4^+$
cells to the redirected, CR-bearing $CD8^+$ CTLs. Apparently, the PBL-derived T cells,
following to their activation, transduction and prolonged propagation *in vitro*, alter
their homing properties and do not behave like the good "old" splenocytes that can
faithfully transfer T cell immunity to their syngeneic mouse host.

We want the T-bodies to home to the tumor site after their systemic administration,
and, upon interaction with the target antigen, to kill the tumor and undergo activation and induce local inflammation that will result in complete tumor elimination.
Apparently, not too many CR bearing lymphocytes reach the tumor after their ad-

ministration and most of them appear to be stuck in the lungs and liver. To obtain efficient antitumor activity, we believe that more research should be focused on two issues. How to bring more T-bodies to the tumor, and how to maintain the ones that get stuck in the reticulo-endothelial system so that they will leave the liver and lungs and seek their tumor targets. Lessons learned from lymphocyte migration should be adopted and may prove useful here. In the meantime, we may elect to focus on clinical conditions where direct, intralesional administration of the engineered lymphocytes is clinically reasonable and feasible, and may prove helpful as a neoadjuvant or adjuvant treatment modality. The intratumoral administration of T-bodies into localized prostate cancer, as we have practiced in the pre-clinical model described above, is one of the favorable targets for such treatment.

Another issue that has been considered as crucial for optimal therapeutic performance of the T bodies is to prolong their survival as functional cells in the patient. We believe that the issue of immunogenicity of the scFv can be solved and the accumulated experience in obtaining fully human or optimally humanized mAb will answer the problem. Alternatively, a supply of moderate immunosuppressants can decrease the tendency of generating anti-idiotypic antibodies in the patients. The issue of antigen-induced cell death and the lack of long-term expansion of pre-activated T cells can be solved by using tripartite CR that provides the CD28 co-stimulatory signal to the programmed cells. Again, external cytokines such as IL-2 or optimal mixtures of antigen-specific $CD4^+$ and $CD8^+$ cells can contribute to sustain and prolong the survival of functional lymphocytes.

Altogether, we believe that the optimization of the T-body preparation and administration, along the lines discussed above, combined with the experience that will be acquired in phase I and II clinical trials, will allow the testing of the therapeutic effect of T bodies in more realistic situations (in contrast to end-stage cases as currently applied) and will put the T-body approach amongst the modalities for cancer therapy.

## Acknowledgments

We are indebted to a group of devoted past and present members of our group and colleagues who contributed to the studies described in this chapter. Recent studies from our group were supported by the US Army Breast and Prostate Cancer Fellowships, the European Union Life Science program, and CaP-CURE Israel.

## References

1 Gross, G. and Eshhar, Z. *FASEB J* 1992; **6**: 3370–8.

2 Gross, G., Waks, T. and Eshhar, Z. *Proc Natl Acad Sci USA* 1989; **86**: 10024–8.

3 Eshhar, Z. *Cancer Immunol Immunother* 1997; **45**: 131–6.

4 Ma, Q. Z., Gonzalo-Daganzo, R. and Junghans, R. P. In *Cancer Chemotherapy & Biological Response Modifiers*, Giaccone, G., Schilsky, R., Sondel, P. (eds.). Elsevier Science, Oxford 2002; **20**: 319–45.

5 HUSTON, J. S., LEVINSON, D., MUDGETT-HUNTER, M., TAI, M. S., NOVOTNY, J., MARGOLIES, M. N., RIDGE, R. J., BRUCCOLERI, R. E., HABER, E., CREA, R. and OPPERMANN, H. *Proc Natl Acad Sci USA* 1988; **85**: 5879–83.

6 BIRD, R. E., HARDMAN, K. D., JACOBSON, J. W., JOHNSON, S., KAUFMAN, B. M., LEE, S. M., LEE, T., POPE, S. H., RIORDAN, G. S. and WHITLOW, M. *Science* 1988; **242**: 423–6.

7 ESHHAR, Z., WAKS, T., GROSS, G. and SCHINDLER, D. G. *Proc Natl Acad Sci USA* 1993; **90**: 720–4.

8 BACH, N., WAKS, T. and ESHHAR, Z. *Tumor Target* 1995; **1**: 203.

9 ZIER, K., GANSBACHER, B. and SALVADORI, S. *Immunol Today* 1996; **17**: 39–45.

10 FITZER-ATTAS, C. J., SCHINDLER, D. G., WAKS, T. and ESHHAR, Z. *J Biol Chem* 1997; **272**: 8551–7.

11 FITZER-ATTAS, C. J., SCHINDLER, D. G., WAKS, T. and ESHHAR, Z. *J Immunol* 1998; **160**: 145–54.

12 BROCKER, T., PETER, A., TRAUNECKER, A. and KARJALAINEN, K. *Eur J Immunol* 1993; **23**: 1435–9.

13 BOUSSIOTIS, V. A., FREEMAN, G. J., GRIBBEN, J. G. and NADLER, L. M. *Immunol Rev* 1996; **153**: 5–26.

14 CHAMBERS, C. A. *Trends Immunol* 2001; **22**: 217–23.

15 ALVAREZ-VALLINA, L. and HAWKINS, R. E. *Eur J Immunol* 1996; **26**: 2304–9.

16 KRAUSE, A., GUO, H. F., LATOUCHE, J. B., TAN, C., CHEUNG, N. K. and SADELAIN, M. *J Exp Med* 1998; **188**: 619–26.

17 BEECHAM, E., ORTIZ-PUJOLS, S. and JUNGHANS, R. *J Immunother* 2000; **23**: 332–343.

18 FINNEY, H. M., LAWSON, A. D., BEBBINGTON, C. R. and WEIR, A. N. *J Immunol* 1998; **161**: 2791–7.

19 ESHHAR, Z., WAKS, T., BENDAVID, A. and SCHINDLER, D. G. *J Immunol Methods* 2001; **248**: 67–76.

20 KLAPPER, L. N., KIRSCHBAUM, M. H., SELA, M. and YARDEN, Y. *Adv Cancer Res* 2000; **77**: 25–79.

21 STANCOVSKI, I., HURWITZ, E., LEITNER, O., ULLRICH, A., YARDEN, Y. and SELA, M. *Proc Natl Acad Sci USA* 1991; **88**: 8691–5.

22 STANCOVSKI, I., SCHINDLER, D. G., WAKS, T., YARDEN, Y., SELA, M. and ESHHAR, Z. *J Immunol* 1993; **151**: 6577–82.

23 MORITZ, D., WELS, W., MATTERN, J. and GRONER, B. *Proc Natl Acad Sci USA* 1994; **91**: 4318–22.

24 ALTENSCHMIDT, U., KLUNDT, E. and GRONER, B. *J Immunol* 1997; **159**: 5509–15.

25 IRVING, B. A. and WEISS, A. *Cell* 1991; **64**: 891–901.

26 ROMEO, C. and SEED, B. *Cell* 1991; **64**: 1037–46.

27 ROBERTS, M. R., QIN, L., ZHANG, D., SMITH, D. H., TRAN, A. C., DULL, T. J., GROOPMAN, J. E., CAPON, D. J., BYRN, R. A. and FINER, M. H. *Blood* 1994; **84**: 2878–89.

28 CHUNG, S., WUCHERPFENNIG, K. W., FRIEDMAN, S. M., HAFLER, D. A. and STROMINGER, J. L. *Proc Natl Acad Sci USA* 1994; **91**: 12654–8.

29 WILLEMSEN, R., WEIJTENS, M., RONTELTAP, C., ESHHAR, Z., GRATAMA, J., CHAMES, P. and BOLHUIS, R. *Gene Ther* 2000; **7**: 1369–77.

30 ALTENSCHMIDT, U., KAHL, R., MORITZ, D., SCHNIERLE, B. S., GERSTMAYER, B., WELS, W. and GRONER, B. *Clin Cancer Res* 1996; **2**: 1001–8.

31 DARCY, P. K., HAYNES, N. M., SNOOK, M. B., TRAPANI, J. A., CERRUTI, L., JANE, S. M. and SMYTH, M. J. *J Immunol* 2000; **164**: 3705–12.

32 HWU, P., YANG, J. C., COWHERD, R., TREISMAN, J., SHAFER, G. E., ESHHAR, Z. and ROSENBERG, S. A. *Cancer Res* 1995; **55**: 3369–73.

33 WANG, G., CHOPRA, R. K., ROYAL, R. E., YANG, J. C., ROSENBERG, S. A. and HWU, P. *Nat Med* 1998; **4**: 168–72.

34 GONG, M. C., LATOUCHE, J. B., KRAUSE, A., HESTON, W. D., BANDER, N. H. and SADELAIN, M. *Neoplasia* 1999; **1**: 123–7.

35 REITER, R. E., GU, Z., WATABE, T., THOMAS, G., SZIGETI, K., DAVIS, E., WAHL, M., NISITANI, S., YAMASHIRO, J., LE BEAU, M. M., LODA, M. and WITTE, O. N. *Proc Natl Acad Sci USA* 1998; **95**: 1735–40.

36 HUBERT, R. S., VIVANCO, I., CHEN, E., RASTEGAR, S., LEONG, K., MITCHELL, S. C., MADRASWALA, R., ZHOU, Y., KUO, J., RAITANO, A. B., JAKOBOVITS, A.,

Saffran, D. C. and Afar, D. E. *Proc Natl Acad Sci USA* 1999; **96**: 14523–8.

37 Su, Z. Z., Lin, J., Shen, R., Fisher, P. E., Goldstein, N. I. and Fisher, P. B. *Proc Natl Acad Sci USA* 1996; **93**: 7252–7.

38 Lyne, J. C., Melhem, M. F., Finley, G. G., Wen, D., Liu, N., Deng, D. H. and Salup, R., *Cancer J Sci Am* 1997; **3**: 21–30.

39 Signoretti, S., Montironi, R., Manola, J., Altimari, A., Tam, C., Bubley, G., Balk, S., Thomas, G., Kaplan, I., Hlatky, L., Hahnfeldt, P., Kantoff, P. and Loda, M. *J Natl Cancer Inst* 2000; **92**: 1918–25.

40 Mitsuyasu, R. T., Anton, P. A., Deeks, S. G., Scadden, D. T., Connick, E., Downs, M. T., Bakker, A., Roberts, M. R., June, C. H., Jalali, S., Lin, A. A., Pennathur-Das, R. and Hege, K. M. *Blood* 2000; **96**: 785–93.

41 Warren, R., Fisher, G. and Bergaland, E. *Abstracts of the 7th Int Conf on Gene Therapy of Cancer* 1998. *Cancer Gene Therapy* 1998; **5**: Suppl. 6, 1–35.

42 Junghans, R., Safa, M. and Huberman, M. *Proc Am Ass Cancer Res* 2000; **41**: 543.

43 Kershaw, M. H., Westwood, J. A., Zhu, Z., Witte, L., Libutti, S. K. and Hwu, P. *Hum Gene Ther* 2000; **11**: 2445–52.

44 Darcy, P. K., Kershaw, M. H., Trapani, J. A. and Smyth, M. J. *Eur J Immunol* 1998; **28**: 1663–72.

45 Hombach, A., Koch, D., Sircar, R., Heuser, C., Diehl, V., Kruis, W., Pohl, C. and Abken, H. *Gene Ther* 1999; **6**: 300–4.

46 Nolan, K., Yun, C., Akamatsu, Y., Murphy, J., Leung, S., Beecham, E. and Junghans, R. *Clin Cancer Res* 1999; **5**: 3928–3941.

47 Hombach, A., Schneider, C., Sent, D., Koch, D., Willemsen, R. A., Diehl, V., Kruis, W., Bolhuis, R. L., Pohl, C. and Abken, H. *Int J Cancer* 2000; **88**: 115–20.

48 Beecham, E. J., Ma, Q., Ripley, R. and Junghans, R. P. *J Immunother* 2000; **23**: 631–42.

49 Kuroki, M., Arakawa, F., Khare, P. D., Liao, S., Matsumoto, H., Abe, H. and Imakiire, T. *Anticancer Res* 2000; **20**: 4067–71.

50 Haynes, N. M., Snook, M. B., Trapani, J. A., Cerruti, L., Jane, S. M., Smyth, M. J. and Darcy, P. K. *J Immunol* 2001; **166**: 182–7.

51 Jensen, M., Tan, G., Forman, S., Wu, A. M. and Raubitschek, A. *Biol Blood Marrow Transplant* 1998; **4**: 75–83.

52 Hombach, A., Heuser, C., Sircar, R., Tillmann, T., Diehl, V., Pohl, C. and Abken, H. *Cancer Res* 1998; **58**: 1116–9.

53 Hombach, A., Heuser, C., Sircar, R., Tillmann, T., Diehl, V., Pohl, C. and Abken, H. *J Immunother* 1999; **22**: 473–80.

54 Hekele, A., Dall, P., Moritz, D., Wels, W., Groner, B., Herrlich, P. and Ponta, H. *Int J Cancer* 1996; **68**: 232–8.

55 Dall, P., Hekele, A., Beckmann, M. W., Bender, H. G., Herrlich, P. and Ponta, H. *Gynecol Oncol* 1997; **66**: 209–16.

56 Daly, T., Royal, R. E., Kershaw, M. H., Treisman, J., Wang, G., Li, W., Herlyn, D., Eshhar, Z. and Hwu, P. *Cancer Gene Ther* 2000; **7**: 284–91.

57 Ren-Heidenreich, L., Hayman, G. T. and Trevor, K. T. *Hum Gene Ther* 2000; **11**: 9–19.

58 Hwu, P., Shafer, G., Treisman, J., Schindler, D., Gross, G., Cowherd, R., Rosenberg, S. and Eshhar, Z. *J Exp Med* 1993; **178**: 361–366.

59 Parker, L. L., Do, M. T., Westwood, J. A., Wunderlich, J. R., Dudley, M. E., Rosenberg, S. A. and Hwu, P. *Hum Gene Ther* 2000; **11**: 2377–87.

60 Weijtens, M. E., Willemsen, R. A., Valerio, D., Stam, K. and Bolhuis, R. L. *J Immunol* 1996; **157**: 836–43.

61 Weijtens, M. E., Hart, E. H. and Bolhuis, R. L. *Gene Ther* 2000; **7**: 35–42.

62 Weijtens, M. E., Willemsen, R. A., Hart, E. H. and Bolhuis, R. L. *Gene Ther* 1998; **5**: 1195–203.

63 Yun, C. O., Nolan, K. F., Beecham, E. J., Reisfeld, R. A. and Junghans, R. P., *Neoplasia* 2000; **2**: 449–59.

64 Reinhold, U., Liu, L., Ludtke-Handjery, H. C., Heuser, C., Hombach, A., Wang, X., Tilgen, W., Ferrone, S. and

ABKEN, H. *J Invest Dermatol* 1999; **112**: 744–50.

**65** MEZZANZANICA, D., CANEVARI, S., MAZ-ZONI, A., FIGINI, M., COLNAGHI, M. I., WAKS, T., SCHINDLER, D. G. and ESHHAR, Z. *Cancer Gene Ther* 1998; **5**: 401–7.

**66** HOMBACH, A., HEUSER, C., SIRCAR, R., TILLMANN, T., DIEHL, V., KRUIS, W., POHL, C. and ABKEN, H. *Gastroenterology* 1997; **113**: 1163–70.

**67** PATEL, S. D., GE, Y., MOSKALENKO, M. and McARTHUR, J. G. *J Immunother* 2000; **23**: 661–8.

# 15

# Bone Marrow Transplantation for Immune Therapy

Fabio Ciceri and Claudio Bordignon

## 15.1
## Introduction

Allogeneic bone marrow transplantation (BMT), now otherwise defined as hematopoietic cell transplantation (HCT), was initially considered for the treatment of malignancy as a means to deliver supralethal doses of chemotherapy and total body radiation [1–3]. Many malignancies exhibit a steep dose–response relationship to chemo- or radiotherapy, with higher doses producing greater cytoreduction. BMT allows escalation of doses of many agents beyond those producing severe bone marrow toxicity. The marrow transplant was considered a supportive care modality to restore hematopoiesis. It has become clear, however, that the high-dose therapy does not eradicate the malignancy in many patients and that the therapeutic benefit of allogeneic BMT is largely related to an associated immune-mediated graft-versus-malignancy effect. In the last few years, the focus has shifted away from attempts at eradicating malignant cells through high-dose chemoradiation therapy toward using immunocompetent cells transplanted with the donor's stem cells, or arising from them, to exert a potent graft-versus-tumor (GvT) effect. HCT is now definitely accepted as an immunotherapeutic approach, rather than solely a vehicle to deliver high-dose therapy [4].

## 15.2
## Graft-versus-Host (GvH) Reactions

Two immunologic barriers must be crossed to establish successful HCT allografts. The first consists of host-versus-graft (HvG) rejection and the second is made up of GvH reactions. The immunosoppressive regimens used to overcome the HvG rejection are administered before transplantation and are integrated into the high-dose conditioning therapy. The regimens for overcoming GvH reactions deal with the grafted donor immune cells and, accordingly, these treatments are delivered after transplantation in order to prevent graft-versus-host disease (GvHD). This potentially lethal complication of HCT occurs in 30–50% of patients undergoing HLA-matched-related allograft, despite standard immunosoppressive prophylaxis. Acute and chronic GvHD are commonly graded as outlined in Tabs 15.1–15.3. When GvHD occurs, immunosoppressive treatment is mandatory; in the case of steroid-resistant GvHD, the association of antithymocyte globulin, anticytokine monoclonal antibodies, mycophenolate and many others immunosoppressive agents is frequently unsatisfactory for the control of disease [5]. The direct effect of GvH tissues damage and infections secondary to immunosuppression, largely contribute to transplant-related mortality (TRM) [6].

**Tab. 15.1**   Clinical staging of acute GvHD

| Stage | Skin | Liver | Gut |
|-------|------|-------|-----|
| 0 | no rash | bilirubin <2 mg/dl | diarrhea <500 ml/day |
| 1 | maculopapular eruption involving <25% of body surface | bilirubin 2–3 mg/dl | diarrhea 500–1000 ml/day |
| 2 | maculopapular eruption involving 25–50% of body surface | bilirubin 3–6 mg/dl | diarrhea 1000–1500 ml/day |
| 3 | generalized erythroderma | bilirubin 6–15 mg/dl | diarrhea >1500 ml/day |
| 4 | generalized erythroderma with desquamation and bullae | bilirubin >15 mg/dl | diarrhea >2000 ml/day; pain or ileus |

**Tab. 15.2**   Glucksberg grade of acute GvHD

| Grade | Organ stage (S= skin, G = gut, L = liver) | Clinical performance |
|-------|-------------------------------------------|----------------------|
| 0 none | S = 0, G = 0, L = 0 | no decrease |
| I mild | S = 1–2, G = 0, L = 0 | no decrease |
| II moderate | S = 1–3, G = 1 and/or L = 1 | mild decrease |
| III severe | S = 2–3, G = 2–3 and/or L = 2–4 | marked decrease |
| IV life threatening | S = 2–4, G = 2–4 and/or L = 2–4 | extreme decrease |

**Tab. 15.3**   International Bone Marrow Transplant Registry GvHD severity index

| Code | Maximum organ stage (S= skin, G = gut, L = liver) | Index |
|------|---------------------------------------------------|-------|
| 0 | S = 0, G = 0, L = 0 | 0 |
| 1 | S = 1, G = 0, L = 0 | A |
| 2 | S, G = 1 and/or L = 2; or G and/or L =1 | B |
| 3 | S, G and/or L = 3 | C |
| 4 | S, G and/or L = 4 | D |

## 15.3
## Graft-versus-Tumor (GvT) Effect

Barnes in 1956 first suggested the existence of a GvT effect in experimental models, which Mathé termed "adoptive immunotherapy" in 1965 [7]. Landmark articles describing graft-versus-leukemia (GvL) effects in human marrow allograft recipients were published by Weiden in 1979 and 1981 [8]. In these studies, the Seattle group reported that leukemia relapse rates following allogeneic BMT were markedly less in patients who developed GvHD as compared with those who did not. Horowitz studies on relapse rates following allogeneic and syngeneic BMT, showed that relapse rates are lower in patients who develop both acute and chronic GvHD, higher in those who develop no clinically evident GvHD, and higher still if T cells are depleted from the marrow graft or in recipients of twin transplants [9]. These observations led to the hypothesis that the GvT response is mediated by immunologically competent donor cells and that these cells could be used therapeutically to induce a direct GvT reaction. The strongest evidence of GvT came from the observation that many patients who relapse after allogeneic BMT can be reinduced into long-term remission by simply infusing additional donor lymphocytes [10]. Table 15.4 summarizes the evidence supporting an allogeneic GvL effect.

## 15.4
## Donor Lymphocyte Infusions (DLIs)

Since the first report of Kolb in 1990, DLIs have been widely used as treatment of disease recurrence after allogeneic BMT [11–14]. From these large series of DLIs, major differences emerged among malignancies in their susceptibility to GvL effects. Table 15.5 shows results from the European Blood and Marrow Transplantation Group (EBMT) DLI study. Chronic myelogenous leukemia (CML) is the most sensitive leukemia, with a probability of complete cytogenetic remission after DLI of 80% with an overall survival at 5 years of 80%, in patients with cytogenetic relapse; in the case of disease recurring in transformed phase, the response rate to DLI and 5-year probability of survival are 36 and 25%, respectively. In the study reported by Collins et al. [13], the response rate and actuarial probability of long-term complete remissions (CRs) are comparable to the EBMT study. Remissions have been reported in patients who relapse soon after undergoing transplantation because of discontinuation of immunosuppressive therapy without DLI; the discontinuation of immuno-

**Tab. 15.4**   Evidence supporting an allogeneic GvL effect

Demonstration of minimal residual disease present early after high-dose therapy
Reduced risk of relapse in patients with acute and chronic GvHD
Increased risk of relapse after syngeneic and T cell-depleted transplants
Induction of remission by DLIs in patients relapsing post-BMT
Demonstration of reactivity of donor-derived T cell clones against malignant cells

suppression triggers GvHD in some patients, with an associated decline in leukemic cells. Abrupt discontinuation of cyclosporin may be indicated as a first step before DLI in patients without severe GvHD. In many patients, the leukemia does not respond immediately and leukocytosis may even increase before a response occurs. The median time to cytogenetic negativity being observed was 4.5 months, with responses as late as 12 months. The latency of the immunotherapeutic effect in a disease with a so-marked susceptibility to GvL may justify the lower response rate of DLI in diseases other than CML; in particular, acute leukemias, in which a rapid growing tumor mass overcomes the alloreactivity of donor T cells (Tab. 15.5) [13, 15]. Furthermore, responses have not been as durable in patients with recurrent acute leukemia, with overall actuarial survival not exceeding 10–15% at 3 years. Most patients with acute leukemias and transformed-phase CML recurring after marrow transplantation need cytotoxic chemotherapy to obtain a transient control of the disease, before the infusion of donor lymphocytes; the use of chemotherapy in acute lymphocytic leukemia (ALL) and acute myelocytic leukemia (AML) increases the rate and durability of responses. Recently, the response of AML to donor lymphocytes has been shown to be improved by the combination of donor lymphocytes with stem cells and granulocyte macrophage colony stimulating factor (GM-CSF) [16]. Treatment with stem cells and GM-CSF may improve antigen presentation, and favor cross-priming of donor-derived dendritic cells with antigens of the host.

DLI has limited benefit in ALL. Approximately 75% of patients treated with DLI, either alone or in the nadir after chemotherapy, did not achieve CR in registry studies, showing a likelihood of survival of less than 15% at 3 years [15] and 0% at 4.5 years [17]. The reason for the low efficacy of DLI in ALL patients is uncertain: it is likely that the leukemia burden is too high in patients with hematologic relapse – patients might die from rapid disease progression before GvT effects have a chance to evolve. However, a large retrospective analysis has shown that the GvL effect in ALL is particularly associated with GvHD [9]. Based on this observation in acute leukemias, the response rate to DLI is not to be considered as an absolute predictor of long-term disease eradication after allogeneic transplantation; in particular, a poor response rate to DLI should not discourage candidate patients with advanced disease from allogeneic transplantation as salvage treatment.

**Tab. 15.5** GvL effect of DLIs – EBMT study

| Diagnosis | No. of patients studied | Evaluable[a] | CRs (%) |
|---|---|---|---|
| CML | | | |
|    cytogenetic relapse | 57 | 50 | 40 (80%) |
|    hematological relapse | 124 | 114 | 88 (77%) |
|    transformed phase | 42 | 36 | 13 (36%) |
| Polycythemia vera/myelodyslastic syndrome | 2 | 1 | 1 (100%) |
| AML/myelodyslastic syndrome | 97 | 59 | 15 (25%) |
| ALL | 55 | 18 | 2 (11%) |
| Multiple myeloma | 25 | 17 | 5 (29%) |

[a] Patients surviving less than 30 days after DLIs were excluded from analysis.

The existence of a graft-versus-myeloma (GvM) and GvL effect has been shown directly by remissions occurring after DLI; a GvM effect is obtained in 20–40% of patients after cumulative doses of T cells higher than those currently needed in CML [18, 19].

## 15.5
## Complications of DLI: GvHD and Marrow Aplasia

About 50–60% of patients treated with DLI develop GvHD. The rates of acute GvHD reported in EBMT registry are 18% for grade I, 24% for grade II and 13% for grade III-IV.

## 15.6
## Strategies to reduce GvHD while preserving GvT

In recent years, different strategies have been investigated in order to prevent GvHD without losing the GvL effect. Mackinnon *et al.* focused on the infusion of small doses of cells, increasing the amount in a stepwise fashion until the disease responds or GvHD develops [12]. In a series of 22 patients with CML, the incidence of GvHD was correlated with the total dose of T cells administered: only one of the eight patients who achieved remission at a T cell dose of $1 \times 10^7$/kg developed GvHD, whereas this complication developed in eight of the 11 responders who achieved a T cell dose of $5 \times 10^7$/kg or higher. Unfortunately, the GvL reactions may require several weeks or even months for the elimination of the leukemic clone; given the slow rate of response in some patients, it is impossible to know when to discontinue the increasing cell doses of DLI unless GvHD occurs. The escalating doses regimen (EDR) has been extensively tested in CML patients by Dazzi *et al.*; EDR has been shown to give an equal GvL rate with a significant reduction in GvHD [20]. Another approach to decrease the risk of GvHD is the depletion of $CD8^+$ T cells from the inoculum [21]. The transfer of specific effector cells rather than a heterogeneous lymphocyte population should significantly reduce the risk of GvHD; *in vitro* cultured leukemia-reactive CTL lines have been successfully used to treat a patient with accelerated phase CML, without inducing GvHD [22].

However, the therapeutic usage of a heterogeneous T cell population with a wide range of antigen specificity carries some advantages over the usage of specific CTLs [23]. First, such a population can provide a more complete immunologic reconstitution to immunocompromised transplanted patients. Moreover, since the antigen specificity of the GvL effector cells is not completely clear, the usage of the entire T cell repertoire is up to now considered the best option to obtain a GvL effect. In this complex context, we investigated the genetic manipulation of donor lymphocytes with a suicide gene which could enable their selective elimination in the case of severe GvHD.

**15.7**
**The Suicide Gene Strategy**

A suicide gene codes for a protein able to convert a non toxic pro-drug into a toxic product. Therefore, cells expressing the suicide gene become selectively sensitive to the pro-drug. The transfer of a suicide gene into donor lymphocytes could allow the *in vivo* selective elimination of transduced lymphocytes and therefore switch off the GvHD.

Different suicide genes have been investigated and described in recent years. At present, the thymidine kinase of Herpes Simplex virus (HSV-*tk*) seems to be the most effective, and it is the first one proposed and used in clinical trials [24, 25]. The HSV-*tk* protein converts the pro-drug gancyclovir (GCV) to its monophosphate intermediate derivative. Cellular kinases phosphorylate it to a triphosphate (GCV-3P) compound, which is the toxic form. GCV-3P can be incorporated into DNA, replacing deoxyguanosine triphosphate, resulting in inhibition of DNA chain elongation.

The safety of gene transfer into peripheral blood lymphocytes (PBLs) has been evaluated both in animal models and in previous clinical protocols of somatic gene therapy [26–30].

The vectors that we used to modulate GvL in the context of allogeneic BMT and the transduction procedure of human PBLs have been described previously [31]. For patient 1–8, we used the SFCMM-2 vector encoding for the truncated form of the low-affinity receptor for the nerve growth factor (ΔNGFR) and a bifunctional protein carrying both the HSV-*tk* activity, conferring GCV sensitivity to transduced cells, and neomycin phosphotransferase (*neo*$^R$) activity, conferring resistance to the antibiotic neomycin and to its analogue G418. For patient 9–23, we removed the *neo*$^R$ gene in order to reduce the immunogenicity of the transgene. The SFCMM-3 vector confers higher GCV sensitivity to transduced cells: almost 100% of cells are killed by GCV concentrations reached *in vivo*. The cell surface molecule allows a rapid *in vitro* selection of transduced cells by the use of magnetic beads conjugated with an antibody directed to ΔNGFR; this selection requires a shorter culture time, an important variable in order to preserve the immune repertoire. In addition, a surface marker allows easy *ex vivo* detection and characterization of the transduced cells by FACS analysis. Moreover, since NGFR is a human protein, it is not expected to be a target of a specific immune response.

A phase I–II clinical study for the infusion of HSV-*tk*-transduced donor lymphocytes to patients affected by severe complications after allogeneic BMT began in 1993 at H. S. Raffaele (Milano). Two protocols were designed to evaluate the infusions of donor lymphocytes transduced with a suicide retroviral vector in the context of allogeneic BMT. In the Add-back protocol, $1 \times 10^7$ CD3$^+$ HSV-*tk* transduced lymphocytes were infused 6 weeks after transplant; the primary end-point of the Add-back protocol was the immune reconstitution obtained by HSV-*tk* cells after T-depleted transplants. In the Treatment protocol, patients received a mean dose of $4.4 \times 10^7$ CD3$^+$ HSV-*tk* cells for the treatment of disease relapse. More than 95% of transduced cells infused were CD3$^+$ and ΔNGFR$^+$, and most were CD8$^+$ with an activated phenotype. The *in vivo* functional properties of transduced lymphocytes were evaluated by asses-

sing immune reconstitution after T-depleted transplants, i.e. antitumor (GvL) and al-
loreactive (GvHD) responses; the GCV sensitivity of transduced cells was assessed *in vivo*. Patients surviving less than 30 days after lymphocyte infusion were excluded from response analysis; patients surviving less than 90 days after infusion were ex-cluded from GvHD analysis.

Thirty-three patients were enrolled in the study, 24 were been infused and 16 were evaluable for response. Eight patients were not evaluable because of early death after infusion.

The clinical results obtained in the evaluable patients of the Treatment protocol are summarized in Tab. 15.6. The clinical responses were directly associated with survi-val and *in vivo* expansion of transduced lymphocytes. GvHD followed transduced cell infusions in three out of 16 patients evaluable for this complication. The *in vivo* effi-cacy of the suicide system was evaluable in five patients. GCV was administered for GvHD in three patients and resulted in complete clinical remission of GvHD signs in two cases; in one patient with chronic extensive GvHD, an amelioration of lung and skin signs was registered, but a complete elimination of transduced lymphocytes could not be obtained despite extended GCV treatment. The *in vivo* administration of GCV has been required as a protocol violation for cytomegalovirus (CMV) infection-unresponsive to foscarnet in two patients treated with SFCMM-3-transduced donor lymphocytes. In both patients, the selective elimination of transduced cells was docu-mented within a few days from the first GCV administration, when HSV-*tk* cells dropped from $10^{-3}$ to levels undetectable by polymerase chain reaction (below $10^{-4}$).

The major side effect of the strategy was the development of an immunization against the transduced cells in six out of 15 evaluable patients that resulted in com-plete disappearance of cells from circulation. In these patients, an immune response against HSV-*tk*/Neo fusion protein (SFCMM-2) or HSV-*tk* (SFCMM-3) was docu-mented; no immunity to the cell surface marker ΔNGFR was detected in any pa-tient. The clinical outcome of patients after immune elimination of HSV-*tk* cells has been analyzed. The two patients who achieved a complete tumor remission after HSV-*tk* lymphocytes infusions maintained the state of long-lasting remission after immunization. On the contrary, the two patients who were in partial remission at the moment of immune elimination of transduced cells had a disease relapse. In one patient with CML, a complete cytogenetic remission was stabilized after a sec-ond unmanipulated DLI. No local or systemic toxicity related to the gene transfer

**Tab. 15.6** Antileukemia effect of HSV-*tk* engineered donor lymphocytes after allogeneic SCT at San Raffaele Scientific Institute

| Diagnosis | Studied | Evaluable | CR | Partial remission |
|---|---|---|---|---|
| CML/chronic myelomonocytic leukemia | 5 | 5 | 2 | 2 |
| AML | 8 | 3 | 1 | 1 |
| ALL | 1 | 1 | 0 | 0 |
| Non-Hodgkin's lymphoma | 5 | 4 | 2 | 1 |
| Hodgkin's disease | 2 | 1 | 0 | 0 |
| Multiple myeloma | 2 | 2 | 1 | 1 |

procedure was observed. These data confirm the therapeutic potential and safety of HSV-*tk*-modified T cells in the context of allografting. The immunologic *in vivo* potential of transduced lymphocytes is maintained in terms of immune reconstitution early after transplantation, antitumor effect and alloreactivity. GCV *in vivo* administration has been confirmed as a specific method for the elimination of HSV-*tk* cells and modulation of DLI effects.

## 15.8
### HSV-*tk* Lymphocyte Add-backs after Haploidentical Transplantation

The program of reinfusion of *tk*-engineered donor lymphocytes has been extended to haploidentical transplantation for hematological malignancies. Haploidentical transplantation remains the only option available for a number of individuals who lack a HLA-compatible family or unrelated donor [32]. However, there is a reluctance to undertake such a procedure due to the high rates of morbidity and mortality. The depletion of T cells from the initial graft results in an increased frequency of infective complications and allows disease relapse or progression. A strategy whereby donor T cells are added back in an incremental fashion at specific time points after haplo-cell transplantation may permit enhanced immune recovery with protection from infection and prevent relapse of malignancy, but obviously runs the risk of severe GvHD. The incorporation of a suicide gene into these cells would provide the ability to control GvHD should this complication arise. We recently designed a clinical protocol for programmed *tk*-DLI for immune reconstitution and relapse prevention after haplo-stem cell transplantation (SCT). Seven patients with high-risk hematologic malignancies who underwent haplo-SCT (four chemorefractory AML, one CR2 ALL, one multiple myeloma and one CR2 AML) received escalating doses of *tk*-DLI starting from 42 days after SCT (dose escalation: $5 \times 10^4 - 10^7$/kg). At the time of infusion, no circulating CD3$^+$ cells could be detected. Infused lymphocytes were 100% CD3$^+$ and 13–50% CD4$^+$. Circulating *tk*-transduced cells were documented in six of seven patients (peak 2–63 cells/µl, median day of engraftment +28, range +12–43). Two of seven patients reached 50 CD3$^+$/µl by day 30, increasing steadily thereafter. Functional analysis of *ex vivo* PBLs showed that engrafted T cells were fully functional, being able to proliferate and produce high levels of interferon-γ after polyclonal stimulation. Moreover, when immune reconstitution was achieved, T cells specific for allogeneic and viral antigens could be demonstrated *ex vivo*. One out of four of the chemorefractory AML patients maintained CR for over 3 months after the infusion, while the other three patients relapsed during the first month after *tk*-DLI before *tk* cells engraftment. Two of two chemorefractory AL and one of one multiple myeloma maintained CR for over 6 months after *tk*-DLI. No acute GvHD was observed in this initial series of patients. In those patients who achieved immune reconstitution after *tk*-DLI, no additional anti-CMV treatment was required. However, four of seven patients had to be treated with GCV within the first 30 days after infusion, before immune reconstitution was achieved, to control CMV infection resistant to foscarnet. This resulted in the rapid *in vivo* elimination of *tk* cells. Three patients received a second *tk*-DLI after GCV discontinuation. T cell engraftment was documented in all patients, with a kinetic comparable to the first infusion. Two patients of this series received unmodified DLI and died of refractory GvHD.

## 15.9
### Reduced Intensity versus Conventional Conditioning Regimens

The use of allogeneic BMT is limited by the high treatment-related mortality. The toxicity of the conditioning regimen plays a crucial role in the development of most of the transplant-related complications. The intensity of conditioning regimen is critical in determining organ toxicity and damage to the mucosal barrier; both these side effects of conventional intensity conditioning regimen have also been correlated with an increased incidence of acute GvHD. The occurrence of GvHD plays a crucial role in influencing treatment-related morbidity/mortality. The incidence of GvHD in patients older than 45 years undergoing allogeneic transplantation with conventional conditioning is around 50–60% [33]. In addition, it should emphasized that treatment mortality as high as 80% has been reported after conventional allografting in patients failing a previous autograft [34].

Very recently, the use of non-ablative regimens has been proposed as an alternative strategy for selected patients with advanced hematologic malignancies. The relatively low toxicity profile of this approach has allowed the treatment of older patients with concomitant organ dysfunction. Analysis of preliminary data has shown that such a strategy has proven to be effective in giving a sustained engraftment and in producing some complete responses; in particular, in low-grade, mantle cell lymphomas, Hodgkin's disease and multiple myeloma. In cohorts of high-risk patients, many authors have shown that treatment-related mortality was lower than expected with conventional conditioning regimens [35–43].

Solid tumors represent an area of major interest in which the antitumor effect is under investigation. After sporadic reports of GvT after allogeneic transplants in breast cancer, some phase II trials are ongoing in metastatic renal, ovarian, colon and prostate cancer [44, 45]. More than 150 patients have been reported to the EBMT registry and the first available results in renal carcinomas are encouraging. However, the efficacy of this procedure remains uncertain for other potential indications.

### References

1 RINGDEN O, HOROWITZ MM, GALE RP, et al. Outcome after allogeneic bone marrow transplant for leukemia in older adults. *J Am Med Ass* 1993; **270**: 57–60.

2 ARMITAGE JO. Bone marrow transplantation. *N Engl J Med* 1994; **330**: 827–838.

3 KLINGEMANN HG, STORB R, FEFER A, et al. Bone marrow transplantation in patients aged 45 years and older. *Blood* 1986; **67**: 770–776.

4 APPELBAUM FR. Hematopoietic cell transplantations immunotherapy. *Nature* 2001; **411**: 385–389.

5 Basara N, Blau IW, Willenbacher W, Kiehl MG, Fauser AA. New strategies in the treatment of graft-versus-host disease. *Bone Marrow Transplant* 2000; **25** (suppl 2): S12–S15.

6 Gaziev D, Galimberti M, Lucarelli G, Polchi P. Chronic graft-versus-host disease: is there an alternative to the conventional treatment? [Review]. *Bone Marrow Transplant* 2000; **25**: 689–696.

7 Barnes DWH, et al. Treatment of murine leukemia with X-rays and homologous bone marro. Preliminary communications. *Br Med J* 1956; **2**: 626–627.

8 Weiden PL, Flournoy N, Thomas ED, et al. Antileukemic effect of graft versus host disease in human recipients of allogeneic marrow grafts. *N Engl J Med* 1979; **300**: 1068–1073.

9 Horowitz MM, Gale RP, Sondel PM, et al. Graft-versus-leukemia reactions after bone marrow transplantation. *Blood* 1990; **75**: 555–562.

10 Kolb HJ, Mittermuller J, Clemm CH, et al. Donor leukocyte transfusions for treatment of recurrent chronic myelogenous leukemia in marrow transplant patients. *Blood* 1990; **76**: 2462–2465.

11 Kolb HJ, Schattenberg A, Goldman JM, et al. Graft-versus-leukemia effect of donor lymphocytes transfusions in marrow grafted patients. European Group for Blood and Marrow Transplantation Chronic Leukemia Working Party. *Blood* 1995; **86**: 2041–2050.

12 Mackinnon S, Papadopoulos EP, Carabasi MH, et al. Adoptive immunotherapy evaluating escalating doses of donor leukocytes for relapse of chronic myeloid leukemia following bone marrow transplantation: separation of graft-versus-leukemia responses from graft-versus-host disease. *Blood* 1995; **86**: 1261–1268.

13 Collins RH, Shpilberg OJ, Drobyski WR, et al. Donor leukocyte infusions in 140 patients with relapsed malignancy after allogeneic bone marrow transplantation. *J Clin Oncol* 1997; **15**: 433–444.

14 Porter DL, Connors JM, Van Deerlin VM, et al. Graft-versus-tumor induction with donor leukocyte infusions as primary therapy for patients with malignancies. *J Clin Oncol* 1999; **17**: 1234.

15 Collins RH Jr, Goldstein S, Giralt S, et al. Donor leukocyte infusions in acute lymphocytic leukemia. *Bone Marrow Transplant* 2000; **26**: 511–516.

16 Schmid C, Lange C, Salat C, et al. Treatment of recurrent acute leukemia after marrow transplantation with donor cells and GM-CSF. *Blood* 1999; **94** (10 suppl 1), 668 a (abstr 2965).

17 Porter DL, Collins RH Jr, Shpilberg O, et al. Long-term follow-up of patients who achieved complete remission after donor leukocyte infusions. *Biol Blood Marrow Transplant* 1999; **5**: 253–261.

18 Lokhorst HM, Schattenberg A, Cornelissen JJ, et al. Donor leukocyte infusions are effective in relapsed multiple myeloma after allogeneic bone marrow transplantation. *Blood* 1997; **90**: 4206–4212.

19 Mandigers CM, Meijerink JP, Raemaekers JM, Schattenberg AV, Mensink EJ. Graft-versus-lymphoma effect of donor leucocyte infusion shown by real-time quantitative PCR analysis of t(14;18). *Lancet* 1998; **352**: 1522–1523.

20 Dazzi F, Szydlo RM, Craddock C, et al. Comparison of single-dose and escalating-dose regimens of donor lymphocyte infusion for relapse after allografting for chronic myeloid leukemia. *Blood* 2000; **95**: 67–71.

21 Giralt S, Hester J, Huh Y, et al. CD8-depleted donor lymphocyte infusion as treatment for relapsed chronic myelogenous leukemia after allogeneic BMT. *Blood* 1995; **86**: 4337–4343.

22 Falkenburg JHF, Wafelman AR, Joosten P, et al. Complete remission of accelerated phase CML by treatment with leukemia-reactive cytotoxic T lymphocytes. *Blood*, 1999; **94**: 1201–1208.

23 Bordignon C, Carlostella C, Colombo MP, et al. Cell therapy: achievements and perspectives. *Haematologica* 1999; **84**: 1100–1149.

24 Bordignon C, Bonini C. A clinical protocol for gene transfer into peripheral blood lymphocytes for *in vivo* immunomodulation of donor anti-tumor

immunity in patients affected by recurrent disease after allogeneic bone marrow transplantation. *Hum Gen Ther* 1995; **2**: 813–819.

25 BONINI C, FERRARI G, VERZELETTI S, *et al*. HSV-*TK* gene transfer into donor lymphocytes for control of allogeneic graft-versus-leukemia. *Science* 1997; **276**: 1719–1724.

26 BORDIGNON C, NOTARANGELO LD, NOBILI N, *et al*. Gene therapy in peripheral blood lymphocytes and bone marrow for ADA-immunodeficient patients. *Science* 1995; **270**: 470–475.

27 BONINI C, CICERI F, MARKTEL S, BORDIGNON C. Suicide-gene-transduced T-cells for the regulation of the graft-versus-leukemia effect [Review]. *Vox Sang* 1998; **74** (suppl 2): 341–343.

28 TIBERGHIEN P. Use of donor T-lymphocytes expressing herpes-simplex thymidine kinase in allogeneic bone marrow transplantation: a phase I–II study. *Hum Gene Ther* 1997; **8**: 615–624.

29 TIBERGHIEN P, FERRAND C, LIOURE B, *et al*. Administration of herpes simplex-thymidine kinase-expressing donor T cells with a T-cell depleted allogeneic marrow graft. *Blood* 2001; **97**: 63–72.

30 CHAMPLIN R, BESINGER W, HENSLEE-DOWNEY J, *et al*. Phase I/II study of thymidine kinase (TK)-transduced donor lymphocyte infusions (DLI) in patients with hematologic malignancies. *Blood* 1999; **94**: 1448a.

31 VERZELLETTI S, BONINI C, MARKTEL S, *et al*. Herpes simplex virus thymidine kinase gene transfer for controlled graft-versus-host disease and graft-versus-leukemia: clinical follow-up and improved new vectors. *Hum Gene Ther* 1998; **9**: 2243–2251.

32 AVERSA F, TABILIO A, VELARDI A, *et al*. Treatment of high risk acute leukemia with T-cell-depleted stem cells from related donors with one fully mismatched HLA haplotype. *N Engl J Med* 1998; **339**: 1186–1193.

33 KLINGEMANN HG, STORB R, FEFER A, *et al*. Bone marrow transplantation in patients aged 45 years and older. *Blood* 1986; **67**: 770.

34 TSAI T, GOODMAN S, SAEZ R, *et al*. Allogeneic bone marrow transplantation in

patients who relapse after autologous transplantation. *Bone Marrow Transplant* 1997; **20**: 859.

35 GIRALT S, THALL PF, KHOURI I, *et al*. Engraftment of allogeneic hematopoietic progenitor cells with purine analog-containing chemotherapy: harnessing graft-versus-leukemia without myeloablative therapy. *Blood* 1997; **89**: 4531–4536.

36 SLAVIN S, NAGLER A, NAPARSTEK E, *et al*. Nonmyeloablative stem cell transplantation and cell therapy as an alternative to conventional bone marrow transplantation with lethal cytoreduction for the treatment of malignant and nonmalignant hematologic diseases. *Blood* 1998; **91**: 756–763.

37 KHOURI IF, KEATING M, KORBLING M, *et al*. Transplant-lite: induction of graft-versus-malignancy using fludarabine-based nonablative chemotherapy and allogeneic blood progenitor-cell transplantation as treatment for lymphoid malignancies. *J Clin Oncol* 1998; **16**: 2817–2824.

38 McSWEENEY PA, NIEDERWIESER D, SHIZURU JA, *et al*. Hematopoietic cell transplantation in older patients with hematologic malignancies: replacing high-dose cytotoxic therapy with graft-versus-tumor effect. *Blood* 2001; **97**: 3390–3400.

39 CARELLA AM, CAVALIERE M, LERMA E, *et al*. Autografting followed by nonmyeloablative immunosuppressive chemotherapy and allogeneic peripheral-blood hematopoietic stem-cell transplantation as treatment of resistant Hodgkin's disease and non-Hodgkin's lymphoma. *J Clin Oncol* 1000; **18**: 3918.

40 NAGLER A, SLAVIN S, VARADI G, *et al*. Allogeneic peripheral blood stem cell transplantation using fludarabine-based low intensity conditioning regimen for malignant lymphoma. *Bone Marrow Transplant* 2000; **25**: 1021.

41 RAIOLA AM, VAN LINT MT, LAMPARELLI T, *et al*. Reduced intensity thiotepa-cyclophosphamide conditioning for allogeneic haemopoietic stem cell transplants (HSCT) in patients up to 60 years of age. *Br J Haematol* **109**: 716, 2000.

**42** KOTTARIDIS PD, MILLIGAN DW, CHO-PRA R, *et al*. *In vivo* CAMPATH-1H prevents graft-versus-host disease following nonmyeloablative stem cell transplantation. *Blood* 2000; **96**: 2419–2425.

**43** CORRADINI P, TARELLA C, OLIVIERI A, *et al*. Reduced intensity conditioning followed by allografting of hematopoietic cells can produce clinical and molecular remissions in patients with poor-risk hematologic malignancies. *Blood*, in press. vupdate?v

**44** CHILDS R, DRACHENBERG D. Allogeneic stem cell transplantation for renal cell carcinoma [Review]. *Curr Opin Urol* 2001; **11**: 495–502.

**45** CHILDS R, CHERNOFF A, CONTENTIN N, *et al*. Regression of metastatic renal-cell carcinoma after nonmyeloablative allogeneic peripheral-blood stem-cell transplantation. *N Engl J Med* 2000; **343**: 750–758.

# 16

## Immunocytokines: Versatile Molecules for Biotherapy of Malignant Disease

Holger N. Lode, Rong Xiang, Jürgen C. Becker, Andreas G. Niethammer, F. James Primus, Stephen D. Gillies and Ralph A. Reisfeld

## 16.1
### Introduction

Sixteen years after the discovery of antibodies by Emil von Behring in 1890, Paul Ehrlich proposed their use as "magic bullets and poisoned arrows" to specifically target toxic substances to pathogenic targets [1]. However, it required almost another century before such antibody-based therapies were applied to the management of residual disease that remains a major problem in the treatment of cancer. This strategy was made possible by the discovery of monoclonal antibodies (mAbs) directed against well-characterized antigens by Köhler and Milstein in 1975 [2]. It was further accelerated and extended by the subsequent introduction of DNA technologies and their rapidly developing advances which facilitated the development of an ever-increasing array of bioengineered antibodies and their fragments during the last 25 years. This chapter deals with one such product of bioengineered antibodies, recombinant antibody–cytokine fusion proteins, and focuses entirely on data obtained with these immunocytokines in preclinical studies in the authors' laboratories with emphasis on evaluating their efficacy in eradicating established tumors and metastases in syngeneic mice. In addition, we will describe extended applications of immunocytokines in combination with gene therapies, anti-angiogenesis treatment modalities and DNA-based cancer vaccines to prevent or eradicate tumor metastases.

### 16.1.1
#### Immunocytokines

Recombinant antibody–cytokine fusion proteins are immunocytokines designed to achieve sufficient concentrations in the tumor microenvironment to effectively stimulate a cell-mediated immune response against tumors. This approach differs from passive immunotherapy by antibodies directed against tumor-associated antigens (TAAs), which utilizes the natural effector mechanisms of antibodies to destroy tumor cells. A key feature of immunocytokines is to provide a tool for active cancer immunotherapy by increasing the cytokine concentration in the tumor microenvironment, thereby potentiating immunogenicity of syngeneic tumors, followed in some cases by activation and expansion of T cells, and a subsequent memory immune response. Importantly, immunocytokines are not limited by either a patient-specific *modus operandi* nor by heterogeneity of TAAs, since only a relatively limited number of antigen sites are required as their docking sites. Immunocytokines placed in the tumor microenvironment can activate and expand such immune effectors as T lymphocytes, natural killer cells, macrophages and granuloctyes, and thereby eradicate tumor cells and their metastases. This same effect can amplify insufficient T cell immune responses previously induced by cytokine gene therapy or DNA-based cancer vaccines and lead to effective tumor eradication with subsequent long-lasting protective immunity.

### 16.1.2
### Construction of Immunocytokines

The immunocytokines used in the preclinical evaluations of our laboratories described here were constructed by following one common strategy. Thus, Gillies *et al.* [3, 4] generated the coding sequences for the cytokines by reverse transcriptase polymerase chain reaction (RT-PCR) with primers that include designated restriction sites used for cloning purposes. Once generated, these cytokines were fused with the human $C_\gamma 1$ gene at the Cl end of the heavy chain of an antibody. Specifically, Gillies *et al.* [5, 6] inserted the fused gene of a chimeric human/mouse antiganglioside $GD_2$ antibody (ch14.18) and recombinant human interleukin (rhIL)-2 into the vector pdHL2, which also encodes the dihydrofolate reductase gene. The same vector carried the gene encoding for the light chain of the ch14.18 antibody in a separate expression unit. Both expression units were driven by a metallothionine promotor. The expression plasmid was transduced into the immunoglobulin-non-producer murine hybridoma cell line Sp2/0Ag14 cells by protoplast fusion and selected in the presence of increasing concentrations of methotrexate (100 nM to 5μM). The same strategy was employed for the construction of an antibody–cytokine fusion protein that specifically recognizes a well-characterized human epithelial cell adhesion molecule Ep-CAM/KS antigen (KSA) [7], which is extensively expressed on epithelial cell-derived carcinomas including colon, breast, prostate and non-small cell lung carcinoma. In contrast to ch14.18, a humanized antibody (huKS1/4) directed against KSA was produced by grafting of the CDR-binding regions of the murine KS1/4 antibody onto a human IgG1 or IgG4 framework. The heavy chain was subsequently fused to IL-2. In this case, the expression vector pdhL7s was used in which the cytomegalovirus promotor drives the expression of each antibody chain [7].

All the fusion proteins described were purified by making use of the Fc portion of the antibody molecule, which selectively binds Protein A–Sepharose. Following elution at low pH, pure preparations of the antibody–cytokine fusion protein were obtained and used for further characterization. This article focuses mainly on antibody–IL-2 and lymphotoxin (LT)-α fusion proteins and the preclinical *in vivo* results obtained in the authors' laboratories. Functional characterizations are described mainly for ch14.18–IL-2 and huKS1/4–IL-2 immunocytokines, which were used to critically evaluate antitumor responses in syngeneic and SCID mouse models.

**Binding and Cytokine Activity of IL-2 Immunocytokines**

Evaluation of biological activities of IL-2 fusion proteins indicated that fusion of rhIL-2 to the C-terminal of the immunoglobulin heavy chain did not reduce IL-2 activity when measured in proliferation assays with IL-2-dependent mouse or human T cell lines. In these assays the IL-2 activity of both constructs, ch14.18–IL-2 and huKS1/4–IL-2, was compared to that of commercially available rhIL-2. These fusion proteins proved remarkably stable throughout their purification and during subsequent storage for over 4 years at –20 °C or lyophilized. The effector functions of the fusion proteins, i.e. their ability to mediate antibody-dependent cellular cytotoxicity and complement-dependent cytotoxicity *in vitro*, were found to be maintained in a similar range as those of the parental antibodies.

A comparison of the binding activity of the ch14.18–IL-2 fusion protein with that of the ch14.18 antibody revealed essentially identical $GD_2$ binding as determined by both direct and competitive binding assays [6, 8]. Dissociation constants ($K_d$), calculated from Scatchard analysis of saturation binding curves, were 18 and 24 nM for ch14.18 and its IL-2 fusion protein, respectively. A $K_d$ of 1.15 nM was determined for the humanized KS1/4 antibody (huKS1/4), which was identical to that of the huKS1/4–IL-2 fusion protein.

In summary, these findings indicated that these immunocytokines were biologically functional and combine the unique targeting ability of antibodies with the immuno-modulatory properties of multi-functional cytokines. These data encouraged us to critically evaluate the antitumor activity of these immunocytokines as tools to deliver effective amounts of IL-2 to the tumor microenvironment capable of local activation of suitable effector cells. The following sections are devoted exclusively to treatment effects and mechanisms of immunocytokines in tumor models of colon carcinoma, non-small cell lung carcinoma, prostate carcinoma, melanoma and neuroblastoma.

**16.2**
**Treatment of Tumor Metastases with Immunocytokines**

16.2.1
**Colorectal Carcinoma**

Colon carcinoma kills almost 55 000 people each year in the US [9]. Efforts were made by Riethmüller *et al.* [10] to improve this situation by exploiting the over-expression of the human epithelial cell adhesion molecule Ep-CAM/GA733–2 on the surface of colon carcinoma cells recognized by the murine antibody 17–1A. In a randomized clinical trial of 189 patients with minimal residual disease after complete resection of Dukes' C colon carcinoma, a follow-up after 5 years indicated that treatment with 17–1A reduced the death rate by 30% and the recurrence rate by 27%. A 7-year median follow-up confirmed these data and suggested that treatment with 17–1A may have actually cured colon carcinoma patients with no recurrence after

7 years. Mechanisms proposed for this antibody-induced antitumor effect were antibody-dependent or complement-dependent cytotoxicity and phagocytosis [10].

Based on these encouraging clinical data we addressed the question whether an immunocytokine, retaining all properties of another Ep-CAM-specific mAb with additional immunostimulatory capabilities of IL-2, might be equally or more effective in eliciting an antitumor response. For this purpose a huKS1/4–IL-2 immunocytokine was constructed recognizing KSA, an Ep-CAM essentially identical in amino acid sequence to that detected by the 17–1A antibody with only one amino acid difference in the transmembrane portion of the protein antigen. This construct was used to determine efficacy and mechanism of action of its antitumor activity in a syngeneic mouse colon tumor model.

Because colon carcinoma is most likely to metastasize to liver in humans, an experimental liver metastasis model was developed in BALB/c mice in order to establish efficacy of immunocytokine therapy against the major metastatic site of this disease. This was achieved by intrasplenic injection of CT26 colon carcinoma cells, which were transduced with the gene encoding human KSA that served as a docking site for the huKS1/4–IL-2 immunocytokine. Treatment of microscopically established hepatic micrometastases resulted in a complete eradication of macroscopic liver metastases. This was in contrast to controls that either received equivalent mixtures of antibody and cytokine or a non-specific immunocytokine, such as ch14.18–IL-2, resulting in both cases in the same massive tumor growth as in mice that received only PBS and no other treatment. These findings are illustrated in Tab. 16.1. Proof of complete absence of micrometastasis was extended beyond that commonly established for other tumor models by establishing a highly sensitive detection system for CT26-KSA cells. This was accomplished by RT-PCR of the human cDNA encoding the KS A expressed only by CT26-KSA cells in contrast to naive murine hepatocytes. This assay detected

**Tab. 16.1** Eradication of murine colorectal carcinoma liver and lung metastases by the huKS1/4–IL 2 fusion protein

| Treatment[a] | Metastatic score | Organ weight (g) |
|---|---|---|
| Liver metastasis | | |
| PBS | 3333333 | 3.78±0.71 |
| huKS1/4+IL-2 | 2233333 | 3.74±0.78 |
| ch14.18–IL-2 | 2223333 | 3.11±0.55 |
| huKS1/4–IL-2 | 0000000 | 1.07±0.07 |
| Lung metastasis | | |
| PBS | 333333 | 0.80±0.07 |
| huKS1/4+IL-2 | 122233 | 0.58±0.18 |
| huKS1/4–IL-2 | 000000 | 0.19±0.02 |

[a] Experimental liver and lung metastases were induced by intrasplenic injection of $3 \times 10^4$ or i. v. injection of $5 \times 10^4$ CT26 KSA cells, respectively. Treatment was started 4 days thereafter, and consisted of daily i. v. administration of PBS, 15 μg huKS1/4 and 45 000 I. U. recombinant IL 2 or 15 μg of either the non-specific fusion protein, ch14.18–IL 2, or the tumor-specific fusion protein, huKS1/4–IL 2, as indicated for 7 consecutive days.

one CT26-KSA tumor cell in $10^6$ hepatocytes. Using this detection system, only liver specimens of mice that received the immunocytokine therapy revealed a complete absence of a KSA signal, indicating no detectable micrometastasis at this high sensitivity [12]. Additional evidence for the absence of metastatic disease was obtained by prolonged survival analyses. Thus, mice that received successful immunocytokine therapy that eradicated hepatic colon carcinoma metastasis did reveal more than a tripling in lifespan (over 120 days) as compared to control groups that either received an equivalent mixture of antibody and cytokine or the non-specific fusion protein. In fact, all control mice died prior to day 40 after tumor cell inoculation [12].

To delineate the immune mechanism involved in the eradication of established colon carcinoma metastases, pulmonary metastases were induced by intravenous (i.v.) injection of CT26-KSA cells, in order to keep the spleen *in situ* for further *in vitro* analyses. The ability of the huKS1/4–IL-2 immunocytokine to also eradicate established pulmonary metastases was demonstrated in contrast to equivalent mixtures of antibody and cytokine. Thus, mice with pulmonary metastases receiving the immunocytokine survived more than 6 months after tumor induction, which is defined as "cure" by Kaplan–Meier standards. When such mice were sacrificed and their lungs analyzed by RT-PCR for expression of the KS antigen none of them revealed its presence, thus clearly indicating a persistent absence of colon carcinoma metastasis [12].

The first line of evidence for T cell-mediated immunity in the colorectal carcinoma model was established by using immune-deficient BALB/c *scid/scid* and BALB/c *beige/beige* mice. Treatment of established pulmonary metastases with the huKS1/4–IL-2 immunocytokine in NK cell-deficient *beige/beige* mice proved completely effective. In contrast, in T cell-deficient *scid/scid* mice, this therapeutic effect was abrogated. These results were further supported by *in vivo* depletion of NK cells or CD4$^+$ and/or CD8$^+$ T cells in immunocompetent BALB/c mice. The absence of NK cells again had no impact on the therapeutic efficacy of the immunocytokine. This finding was in contrast to those obtained in mice that were depleted of CD8$^+$ or both CD8$^+$ and CD4$^+$ T cells which presented with extensive metastases following immunocytokine therapy. Interestingly, depletion of CD4$^+$ T cells only partially reduced the therapeutic efficacy of the immunocytokine, because three of five mice thus depleted revealed macroscopic metastases following treatment with immunocytokine. This phenomenon possibly indicates a helper function for the CD4$^+$ T cell subpopulation. However, CD8$^+$ T cells clearly are the major effector cells in this system as demonstrated by these *in vivo* experiments [11].

A second line of evidence for T cell-mediated immune mechanisms was provided by *in vitro* analyses of splenic effector cells 3 days after completion of treatment. In this case, both CT26-KSA and CT26 wild-type cells were used as targets in cytotoxicity assays. Importantly, both target cells were killed to a similar extent by freshly isolated splenocytes of immunocytokine-treated animals. This clearly indicated that the cytotoxic response observed in these assays is quite independent of the presence or absence of KSA which only serves as a docking site to direct the immunocytokine into the tumor microenvironment. Subsequent purification of CD8$^+$ and CD4$^+$ T cells revealed a cytotoxic activity only in the CD8$^+$ T cell population. This response was demonstrated to be MHC class I antigen-restricted since only addition of anti-MHC class I antibodies (H-2K$^d$/H-2D$^d$) completely suppressed CD8$^+$ T cell-mediated cytotoxicity *in vitro*. In fact, MHC class I antigen restriction was demonstrated for both CT26-KSA and CT26 target cells, emphasizing that the cytotoxic response occurs independent of the KS antigen which clearly is not the antigen recognized by the T cells. Actually the origin of the T cell antigen in this system remains to be elucidated. In this regard, it is well known that T cells recognize peptides presented in the binding groove of MHC class I antigens. Since both CT26-KSA and CT26 cells were killed by CD8$^+$ T cells *in vitro*, these cells apparently share an antigen peptide present on both related cell lines. Interestingly, it was reported previously that CT26 colon carcinoma cells engineered to secrete granulocyte macrophage colony stimulating factor (GM-CSF) generated several tumor-specific cytotoxic T cell lines that recognized a single immunodominant tumor-associated, MHC class I-restricted peptide antigen (SPSYVYHQF) [13]. This particular antigen was derived as a non-mutated nonamer from the gp70 envelope protein of an endogenous ectotropic murine leukemia provirus. However, this same immunodominant peptide was apparently not recognized by CD8$^+$ T cells in our experiments. In fact, our data indicated that SPSYVYHQF-pulsed RENCA tumor cells, syngeneic with BALB/c mice, could not be lysed *in vitro* by CT26-KSA-specific cytotoxic T lymphocytes (CTLs) [11, 12].

A third line of evidence for a cellular immune response mediated by CD8$^+$ T lymphocytes was provided by histological and immunohistochemical analyses. These studies were performed on liver tissues of tumor-bearing mice following treatment with the huKS1/4–IL-2 immunocytokine and compared to that of control animals receiving either phosphate-buffered saline (PBS) injections or an equivalent mixture of antibody and cytokine. Only those mice that received immunocytokine treatment revealed a strong, predominantly lymphocytic infiltrate in micrometastasis-bearing livers, in contrast to all control mice. Subsequent analysis of these infiltrates by immunohistochemical methods indicated strong positive staining for both, CD8$^+$ and CD4$^+$ T cells. These findings clearly illustrated the presence of an intense local immune response largely consisting of CD8$^+$ and CD4$^+$ T lymphocytes in tumor-bearing livers of only immunocytokine-treated mice [14].

### 16.2.2
### Long-lived Tumor-Protective Immunity is Boosted by Non-curative Doses of huKS1/4–IL-2 Immunocytokine

Further proof for an induction of CD8$^+$ T cell-mediated immunity was provided by demonstrating a persistent tumor-protective memory immune response. In fact, mice cured of established pulmonary micrometastases following treatment with tumor-specific huKS1/4–IL-2 immunocytokine revealed a complete absence of hepatic metastases in 50% of the animals upon a lethal challenge with colon carcinoma cells up to 20 weeks after initial vaccination. The remaining 50% showed a decrease in metastases. Since there were always several animals that completely failed to reject the tumor cells, we tested the hypothesis that boosting with non-curative doses of huKS1/4–IL-2 will result in tumor rejection in all experimental animals after tumor challenge. The data shown in Tab. 16.2 indicate that this was indeed the case when

**Tab. 16.2** Boost of tumor-protective immunity after tumor challenge of mice cured of established pulmonary colon cancer metastases

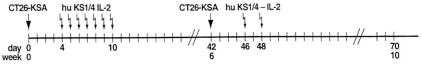

| Initial tumor | Treatment | Interval (weaks) | Tumor challenge | Boost | Metastatic score | Lung weight (g) |
|---|---|---|---|---|---|---|
| CT26-KSA | huKS1/4–IL-2 | 6 | CT26-KSA | – | 0,0,0,0,1,1,2,3 | 0.28±0.1 |
| CT26-KSA | huKS1/4–IL-2 | 6 | CT26-KSA | huKS1/4–IL 2[a] | 0,0,0,0,0,0,0,0 | 0.19±0.01 |
| None | none | none | CT26-KSA | PBS | 2,2,2,3,3,3,3,3 | 0.51±0.11 |
| None | none | none | CT26-KSA | huKS1/4–IL-2[a] | 2,2,3,3,3,3,3,3 | 0.62±0.10 |

[a] A boost of tumor-protective immunity was attempted 4 days after tumor challenge by two i. v. injections of 5 μg huKS1/4–IL-2 each on days 4 and 6.

BALB/c mice ($n$ = 8) that had been tumor free for 6 weeks after treatment with huKS1/4–IL-2 were challenged at this time point with CT26-KSA, followed after 4 days with two non-curative doses of huKS1/4–IL-2 fusion protein. Thus, 4 weeks after this boost, all eight mice completely rejected the tumor cell challenge. In contrast, a control group of mice ($n$ = 8) that was challenged with CT26-KSA tumor cells after 6 weeks, but received PBS instead of the huKS1/4–IL-2 fusion protein, exhibited metastases in all eight mice, 4 weeks after tumor cell challenge [12].

The finding of a long-lasting tumor-protective immunity was always consistent with the appearance of CD8$^+$ memory T cells in secondary lymphoid organs as determined by flow cytometry. Furthermore, mice with established pulmonary metastases successfully treated with huKS1/4–IL-2 immunocytokine showed a 10% increase in CD44$^{hi}$, Ly-6C$^{hi}$, CD45RB$^{lo}$ and CD62L$^{lo}$ CD8$^+$ T cells in contrast to naive mice 6 weeks after tumor inoculation. This represents a well-accepted memory phenotype [15, 16].

T cell memory was further analyzed by assessing CTL precursor (pCTL) frequency by limiting dilutions. In this case, the huKS1/4–IL-2 immunocytokine-treated mice revealed an approximately 30-fold increase in pCTL frequency over PBS controls, which further documented the development of a CD8$^+$ T cell memory immune response [15]. Significantly, this memory immune response was maintained in the absence of tumor antigen. This was demonstrated by using CD8$^+$ T cells from huKS1/4–IL-2-treated animals which were horizontally transferred into syngeneic *scid/scid* mice. These CD8$^+$ T cells were literally parked for 6 weeks in these immune-deficient mice, lacking mature T and B lymphocytes, to allow activated CD8$^+$ T cells to apoptose and CD8$^+$ memory T cells to survive. In fact, there was a continuous decrease in the number of CD8$^+$ T cells, until 5 weeks later less than 5% of CD8$^+$ T cells were detectable by FACS analysis, suggesting that the majority of these T effector cells apoptosed. Thus, the continuous presence of tumor antigen or naive T cells was not required to maintain a long-lived CD8$^+$ T cell memory among CD8$^+$ T cells that were adoptively transferred into syngeneic mice and left there for 6 weeks. In fact, when these SCID mice were challenged with CT26-KSA tumor cells at the 6-week time point and then received a boost with huKS1/4–IL-2 immunocytokine 4 days later, the putative memory remaining in these mice again recognized the tumor antigen as indicated by a markedly increased generation of CD8$^+$ T cells. Importantly, only those CD8$^+$ T cells specifically lysed CT26-KSA tumor target cells *in vitro*. Further evidence for strong priming of these very same CD8$^+$ T cells was indicated by their strong expression of CD25, a marker for the high-affinity IL-2 receptor $\alpha$ chain, and CD69, an early T cell activation marker. Further evidence for effective priming of these CD8$^+$ T cells was provided by their substantial release of IL-2 and of pro-inflammatory cytokines IL-12 and GM-CSF measured by a sandwich ELISA [15].

The data obtained in our colorectal carcinoma model demonstrated independence of the immunologic response from the target antigen used for directing IL-2 into the tumor microenvironment. Specifically, the direction of IL-2 into the tumor microenvironment was followed by the induction of a CD8$^+$ T cell response in conjunction with antigen peptides presented via MHC class I antigens on the surface of tumor cells and via MHC class II antigens by antigen-presenting cells (APC), which are both well-established requirements for T cell priming [16]. The localization of these events occurring in our tumor model was suggested to be in the draining lymph nodes. In fact, activation of T cells was indicated by FACS analysis of single-cell suspensions obtained from draining lymph nodes at the termination of immunocytokine treatment. In this case, expression of both the early T cell activation marker CD69 and the CD25 marker indicating the high-affinity IL-2 receptor $\alpha$ chain were markedly elevated [15]. There is also evidence from the literature that the actual presentation of tumor-derived peptides via MHC class II antigens on APCs occurs in the draining lymph nodes rather than in the tumor microenvironment. Thus, Maass *et al.* [17] reported that IL-2 transduced tumor cells are eliminated from the inoculation site by macrophages and granulocytes followed by an invasion of APCs at the tumor cell inoculation site, which travel to the locoregional lymph nodes, where T cell activation then occurs. This contention was based on the presence of T cell activation markers only in the draining lymph node system, but not at the site of vaccination. Once effective priming of a CD8$^+$ T cell response was induced in our colon carcinoma model system, further proliferation and expansion of such T cells was required for an optimal antitumor effect. This was facilitated in the presence of both the T cell growth factor IL-2 and the peptide antigen(s) presented via MHC class I antigens on tumor cells, which provided an effective growth stimulus via IL-2 and T cell receptors, respectively. The expansion of CD8$^+$ effector T cells induced effective eradication of micrometastases which was accomplished 5 days after the end of treatment with the IL-2 immunocytokine. After tumor cell eradication was achieved, most of these effector T cells did undergo apoptotic elimination and only a small number persisted as memory cells that, once properly reactivated, elicited the long-lived tumor-protective immune responses observed in our colon carcinoma model [15].

16.2.3
**Carcinoembryonic Antigen (CEA)-based DNA Vaccines for Colon Carcinoma Boosted by IL-2 Immunocytokine**

A new area of cancer immunotherapy emerged during the last decade based on the recognition that some tumors encode rejection antigens capable of inducing a tumor-protective immune response primarily by activating the cellular arm of the immune response [18]. This approach was based on the finding that CTLs are particularly effective in recognizing tumor cells as foreign and eradicating them [19]. Recent efforts focused on the development of DNA-based cancer vaccines designed to overcome peripheral T cell tolerance against tumor-self antigens, such as human CEA [20]. This well-characterized oncofetal glycoprotein of $M_r$ 180 000–200 000 which is encoded by 29 genes and part of the immunoglobulin supergene family [21–23] has already served as a useful target for CEA-specific radioimmunoconjugates in clinical detection and therapy protocols [24–26], and was used more recently to construct DNA vaccines for cancer immunotherapy [27]. A real advantage for these immunotherapy studies was the availability of a mouse line that carriers the genomic DNA transgene for human CEA [28]. This CEA transgenic mouse also expresses CEA in a tissue-specific manner, similar to that observed in humans, in which the colon is the major site for CEA production. Importantly for our purposes, anti-CEA CD8$^+$ T cells were elicited in these CEA-transgenic mice after *in vivo* priming with CEA-transfected fibroblasts [29]. However, anti-CEA antibody responses were not detected in such transgenic mice unless an independent carrier was used, suggesting tolerance to CEA in the CD4$^+$ T cell compartment [29]. Importantly, recent studies indicated that CEA-based vaccines can induce CEA-specific immune responses in transgenic mice and in humans [30]. In fact, a wide range of CEA immunogens, including cDNA encoding the entire CEA gene or a variety of CEA peptides with dominant MHC class I antigen anchor residues, carried by a replication-deficient vaccinia virus, induced CEA-specific MHC-restricted CTL responses, T cell proliferation, as well as CD4$^+$ T cell and antibody responses in both CEA-transgenic mice [31, 32] and cancer patients [30].

We determined in a series of experiments whether peripheral T cell tolerance to CEA, a human tumor self-antigen, could be overcome by a DNA vaccine containing the entire gene encoding CEA delivered *per os* by an attenuated *Salmonella typhimurium* carrier to CEA-transgenic mice [33]. It was of particular interest to assess whether this vaccine could induce a T cell-mediated, tumor-protective immune response that was effective in rejecting a lethal challenge of murine MC38 colon carcinoma cells, stably transduced to express CEA and the human epithelial cell adhesion molecule (Ep-CAM/KSA). In view of our encouraging results obtained in effectively boosting tumor-protective immunity against murine colon carcinoma induced by the huKS1/4–IL-2 immunocytokines with small, non-curative doses of huKS1/4–IL-2 [12], it was important to determine whether the protective immunity induced by the CEA-based DNA vaccine could also be further improved by such immunocytokine boosts.

In initial experiments, scanning confocal microscopy and Western blotting demonstrated that we could selectively obtain subcellular localization of CEA by designing two expression plasmids with completely opposite characteristics. One, pW-CEA, encoded the intact CEA gene that ultimately achieved expression of CEA epitopes on the cell surface. The other, pER-CEA, served as a control as it lacked both the endogenous leader and C-terminal anchor sequences, contained an endoplasmic reticulum (ER) targeting signal and the ER-retention signal, SEKDEL, thus causing its complete retention in the ER. Consequently, this truncated molecule could not be processed in the cytoplasm and proteasome, and was retained in the ER, thus preventing suitable peptide epitopes from combining with MHC class I antigen heavy and light chains for transport to the cell surface. Additionally, lysis of COS-7 cells transfected with either of these two expression vectors and subsequent Western blotting indicated that both expressed CEA protein of the correct molecular size of 180 kDa [33].

Importantly, it was evident from our experiments that the pW-CEA vaccine, when administered by oral gavage with attenuated *S. typhimurium* was effective in eliciting an MHC class I antigen-restricted T cell-mediated tumor-protective immune response. This resulted in the complete rejection of a lethal MC38-CEA-KSA tumor cell challenge in 50% of C57BL/6J mice transgenic for CEA, while the remaining animals revealed a marked, three-fold suppression in tumor size compared to controls. All three control groups exhibited rapid and uniform tumor growth in all CEA-transgenic mice. In this regard, a prior report by Schlom *et al.* [32] indicated that treatment of CEA-transgenic mice with a recombinant vaccinia virus expressing CEA (rV-CEA) also caused the rejection of MC38 tumor cells expressing CEA in 50% of experimental animals; however, in contrast to our data, the remaining 50% of mice did not display a 3-fold reduction in tumor size, but exhibited large, subcutaneous (s.c.) tumors that were generally indistinguishable from controls [32]. Also, the rV-CEA vaccine induced anti-CEA IgG antibody titers in CEA transgenic mice which developed $T_h1$-type CEA-specific $CD4^+$ T cell responses. In contrast, our oral CEA vaccine delivered by attenuated *S. typhimurium* failed to elicit any detectable anti-CEA IgM or IgG antibody titers, but induced MHC class I antigen-restricted $CD8^+$ T cell responses in CEA transgenic mice, resulting in effective tumor-protective immunity.

Significantly, our data suggested immunological mechanisms responsible for the effective immunization with the pW-CEA vaccine. Thus, marked activation of T cells and dendritic-like cells ($B220^-$, $CD11c^+$) was indicated by the decisive up-regulation in expression of the T cell integrin, LFA-1, and the intercellular adhesion molecule (ICAM)-1 (CD54). These two molecules are known to synergize in the binding of lymphocytes to APCs [34]. In fact, the transient binding of naive T cells to APCs is crucial in providing time for T cells to sample large numbers of MHC molecules on the surface of each APC for the presence of specific peptides. This might increase the chance of a naive T cell recognizing its specific peptide/MHC ligand, followed by signaling through the TCR and induction of a conformational change in LFA-1. This, in turn, will greatly increase its affinity for ICAM-1 and stabilize the association between the antigen-specific T cell and the cell presenting antigen [35, 36].

In addition, we observed a marked increase in the expression of CD28 on T cells and the B7–1 and B7–2 co-stimulatory molecules on dendritic-like cells following vaccination and tumor cell challenge. This is of key importance, particularly since the activation of naive T cells requires two independent signals. First, binding of the peptide/MHC complex by the TCR which transmits signals to T cells indicating antigen recognition and second, ligation of CD28 with B7–1 or B7–2 which produces a second signal and thereby initiates T cell responses and production of armed effector T cells [37, 38].

A marked increase over controls observed in expression of CD25, i.e. the high-affinity IL-2 receptor α chain, and CD69, an early T cell activation antigen, indicated that T cell activation took place in secondary lymphoid tissues following vaccination and tumor cell challenge. Furthermore, we observed a specific and decisive elevation in the production of pro-inflammatory cytokines, interferon (IFN)-γ and IL-12 by such T cells as shown in Fig. 16.1 which is known to be a key feature of their activation [17]. The notion that secondary lymphoid tissue of mice that exhibited protective tumor immunity contained tumor-specific CD8⁺ T cells was further supported by the finding that splenocytes isolated from such mice specifically lysed MC38-CEA-KSA tumor target cells *in vitro* in an MHC class I antigen-restricted manner. In contrast, splenocytes isolated from mice in all control groups failed to lyse these tumor target cells.

As mentioned above, the rationale for using small boosts with huKS1/4–IL-2 fusion protein to improve tumor-protective immune responses induced by our CEA-based DNA vaccine was based on results of our prior work where this approach completely eradicated CT26 lung tumor metastases in 100 % of syngeneic BALB/c mice [11, 12]. In fact, injection of small, non-curative doses of huKS1/4–IL-2 fusion protein shortly

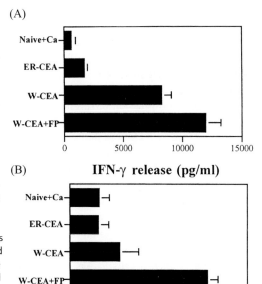

**Fig. 16.1** Induction of pro-inflammatory cytokines. C57BL/6J mice transgenic for CEA were immunized, challenged with MC38-CEA-KSA tumor cells and boosted with huKS1/4–IL-2 fusion protein. Splenocytes were obtained 1 week after tumor cell challenge and cells were plated in the presence of irradiated MC38 cells; cultured supernatants were harvested after 24 h and either analyzed for release of IFN-γ (A) or IL-12 (B) by a solid-phase sandwich ELISA. Each value represents the mean for four animals; bars, SD.

after tumor cell challenge also markedly improved the tumor-protective effect of our CEA-based DNA vaccine in CEA transgenic mice. Thus, six of eight vaccinated mice now completely rejected the tumor cell challenge and the remaining two animals exhibited a marked suppression in tumor growth. These results are illustrated in Fig. 16.2.

Taken together the results of these studies demonstrated that our orally administered, CEA-based DNA vaccine induced effective tumor-protective immunity mediated by MHC class I antigen-restricted CTLs. This antitumor effect correlated with the marked up-regulation of co-stimulatory molecules on APCs, markers of activation on T lymphocytes and increased release of pro-inflammatory cytokines. Small, non-curative suboptimal doses of huKS1/4–IL-2 immunocytokine administered after tumor cell challenge further increased these antitumor effects.

## 16.2.4
### T Cell-mediated Protective Immunity against Colon Carcinoma Induced by a DNA Vaccine encoding CEA and CD40 Ligand Trimer (CD40LT)

Since we achieved at best a partial tumor-protective response against a lethal challenge of MC38 murine colon carcinoma cells with a CEA-based, DNA vaccine, boosted with the huKS1/4–IL-2 immunocytokine [33], we determined whether these results could be improved by achieving complete tumor-protection in 100% of experimental animals. To this end, we constructed and tested a CEA-based DNA vaccine encoding both CEA and CD40LT, and again boosted with suboptimal doses of huKS1/4–IL-2 immunocytokine. This dual-function vaccine indeed achieved this objective as eight out of eight CEA-transgenic mice completely rejected a lethal challenge of MC38-CEA-KSA colon carcinoma cells following three immunization with this DNA vaccine at 2-week intervals [39]. We attribute this success to the combined action of the unique dual-function DNA vaccine and the huKS1/4–IL-2 fusion protein, which accomplished the concurrent activation of both antigen-presenting dendritic cells (DCs) and naive T cells. Possible mechanisms of action were suggested by the up-regulated expression of several receptor/ligand pairs known to critically impact effective activation of T cells following their interaction with DCs which present them with MHC/peptide complexes. These included CD40/CD40LT, LFA-1/ICAM-1, CD28/B7–1 and B7–2 and CD25/IL-2, as well as the increased secretion of pro-inflammatory cytokines IFN-$\gamma$ and IL-12. Several lines of evidence pointed to effective priming of CD8$^+$ T cells *in vivo* following immunization with the pCD40LT-CEA dual-function DNA vaccine and challenge with colon carcinoma cells. First, a marked activation of T cells and CD11c$^+$ dendritic-like cells was indicated by the decisive up-regulation in expression of T cell integrins LFA-1 and ICAM-1, which are known to synergize in the binding of lymphocytes to APCs [34]. In fact, this transient binding of naive T cells to APCs is crucial in providing time for these cells to sample large numbers of MHC molecules on the surface of each APC for the presence of specific peptides. This mechanism may increase the chance of a naive T cell recognizing its specific MHC/peptide ligand, followed by signaling through the TCR and induction of a conformational change in LFA-1. This, in turn, will greatly in-

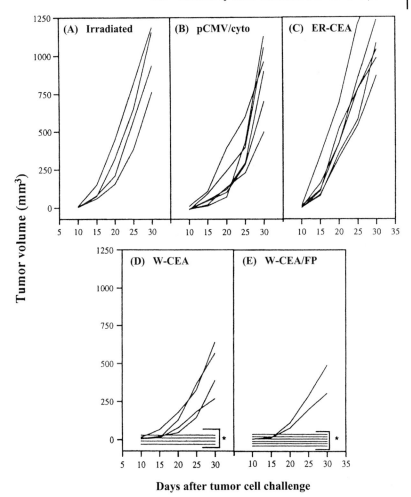

**Days after tumor cell challenge**

**Fig. 16.2** Tumor-protective immune response elicited by oral DNA vaccine and boosts of huKS1/4–IL-2 fusion protein. A control group of female C57BL/6J mice transgenic for CEA were immunized with $2.5 \times 10^5$ irradiated MC38-CEA-KSA colon carcinoma cells on days 0 and 7, and then challenged after 2 weeks s.c. with a lethal dose of $2.5 \times 10^5$ MC38-CEA-KSA cells. Experimental groups of CEA-transgenic mice ($n = 8$) were each immunized by oral gavage 3 times at 2-week intervals with $10^8$ attenuated *S. typhimurium* harboring either pW-CEA or pER-CEA plasmids. Control groups received the attenuated bacteria with either PBS or the empty vector (pCMV/cyto). Two weeks after the last immunization, all mice were challenged s.c. in the right front flank with a lethal dose of $2.5 \times 10^5$ MC38-KSA-CEA colon cancer cells. Mice immunized with pW-CEA were boosted i.v. with five doses (5 μg each) of huKS1/4–IL-2 fusion protein (pW-CEA + FP) and an additional group of naive mice was treated with fusion protein alone as a control (FP). Animals were examined daily until the tumor became palpable, after which its diameter was measured with microcalipers in two dimensions every other day. The tumor growth of each mouse is depicted by a solid line. (*) differences are statistically significant $P < 0.01$.

crease LFA-1's affinity for ICAM-1, and stabilize the association between the antigen-specific T cell and the APC [35, 36]. Second, the marked increase in expression of CD28 on T cells as well as the co-stimulatory molecules B7–1 and B7–2 on DCs, following vaccination and tumor cell challenge is particularly significant since it provides the two signals required for activation of naive T cells. Third, a clear indication of T cell activation in secondary lymphoid tissues was provided by marked increases in expression of CD25, the high-affinity IL-2 receptor α chain, and CD69, an early T cell activation antigen.

The significant elevation in the production of pro-inflammatory cytokines IFN-γ and IL-12 by T cells induced by our dual-function DNA vaccine suggested that a third signal may act directly on T cells [40]. This "danger signal", was reported to be required for $T_h1$ differentiation leading to clonal expansion of T cells [40]. In fact, whenever T cell help is required to generate an effective CD8$^+$ T cell response against a tumor-self antigen like CEA, triggering of DCs is necessary prior to their encounter with an antigen-specific CD8$^+$ T cell [41]. This effect is mediated by ligation of CD40 on the surface of APCs [35] with CD40L expressed on activated CD4$^+$ T cells. CD40LT expressed by our DNA vaccine likely acted as a surrogate for activated CD4$^+$ T cells, leading to maturation of DCs as indicated by their decisive up-regulation of B7–1 and B7–2 co-stimulatory molecules [42]. Taken together our results indicated that the orally administered dual-function DNA vaccine containing genes encoding for both CEA and CD40LT induced a highly efficient tumor-protective immunity against CEA self-antigen in all experimental CEA-transgenic mice. It is anticipated that this strategy may ultimately aid in improving the efficacy of DNA vaccines for colon cancer therapy.

## 16.3
## Non-small Cell Lung Carcinoma

### 16.3.1
### Boost of a CEA-based DNA Vaccine by the huKS1/4–IL-2 Immunocytokine

We asked whether a CEA-based DNA vaccine also could overcome peripheral T cell tolerance toward this human tumor-self antigen when expressed by highly tumorigenic murine non-small cell lung carcinoma cells. To this end, we used Lewis lung carcinoma cells, stably transduced with CEA and Ep-CAM/KSA (LLC-CEA-KSA), and injected them both s.c. and i.v. into CEA-transgenic mice [43]. We were particularly interested to assess whether this vaccine could induce a T cell-mediated, tumor-protective immunity which was sufficiently effective to eradicate not only s.c. tumor growth, but also prevented the dissemination of experimental pulmonary metastases. Since, as discussed above, boosts of suboptimal doses of IL-2 specifically targeted to the tumor microenvironment by an IL-2 immunocytokine markedly enhanced the tumor-protective immunity induced by a DNA vaccine against colon carcinoma, we determined whether this concept was also applicable in a highly aggressive non-small cell lung carcinoma model and examined some of its mechanisms of action.

Effective vaccination was demonstrated in a prophylactic setting when immunization with the pW-CEA vaccine, followed by a lethal challenge with LLC-CEA-KSA cells, reduced s.c. tumor growth to about 25% of that observed in control animals injected only with PBS. Control vaccinations with attenuated *S. typhimurium* carrying only the control expression vector pER-CEA which was anchored in the ER did not inhibit s.c. tumor growth [43]. These findings have several implications. First, attenuated *S. typhimurium per se* failed to induce tumor-protective immunity in our animal model. Second, using this carrier with the pW-CEA vaccine accomplished targeting to secondary lymphoid tissue since this attenuated strain of *S. typhimurium* was reported previously to serve as a useful oral carrier which effectively transported DNA through the gastrointestinal tract and then through the M cells into the Peyer's patches of the small intestine [44–46]. From there, the attenuated bacteria enter APCs such as macrophages and DCs, where they die because of their mutation rendering then unable to synthesize aromatic amino acids, thereby liberating multiple copies of DNA inside the phagocytes. Third, aside from providing a "danger signal" that stimulates the innate immune system by producing IL-12 and NO [44–46], the attenuated bacteria carrier provided for an intralymphatic vaccination with naked DNA [47–49] which was recently reported to be far more effective than either intramuscular, intradermal, s.c. or intrasplenical routes of vaccination [50]. Importantly, the pER-CEA vaccine provided an important negative control because it lacked both the endogenous leader and C-terminal anchor sequences, while also containing an ER targeting and an ER-retention signal, SEKDEL, thus causing its complete retention in the ER. Thus, this truncated molecule could not enter the cytoplasm to be processed in the proteasome. Consequently this prevented suitable peptide epitopes from combining with MHC class I molecules for transport to the cell surface. However, this very same sequence of antigen processing and presentation worked very well indeed in our tumor model as indicated by the effective protective immunity induced by the pW-CEA vaccine encoding the intact CEA gene that ultimately achieved expression of CEA epitopes on the cell surface [43].

Significantly, our results indicated that the pW-CEA vaccine elicited an effective MHC class I antigen-restricted and T cell-mediated, tumor-protective immune response. This resulted in a 75% reduction of s.c. tumor growth and completely prevented the dissemination of experimental pulmonary metastases in two of eight CEA-transgenic mice. Importantly, however, i.v. boosts with non-curative doses of huKS1/4–IL-2 immunocytokine ($5 \times 5$ µg) completely eradicated s.c. tumor growth in 100% of experimental animals and prevented dissemination of pulmonary metastases in 75% of these mice. In contrast, in a control experiment, an equal dose of the huKS1/4–IL-2 immunocytokine used to boost the control vaccine pER-CEA proved ineffective. The results of our experiment preventing experimental pulmonary metastases of Lewis lung carcinoma are depicted in Fig. 16.3.

Significantly, our results suggested some of the immunological mechanisms responsible for the effective vaccination with the pW-CEA vaccine. Thus, marked activation of both T cells and DCs was indicated by a decisive up-regulation in expression of the T cell integrin LFA-2 (CD2) on CD8[+] T cells and the CD48 adhesion molecule on DCs. These two molecules are known to synergize in the binding of T lymphocytes

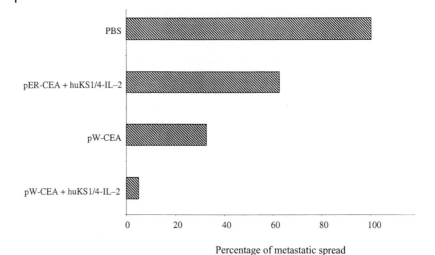

Percentage of metastatic spread

**Fig. 16.3** Prevention of pulmonary Lewis lung metastases by an oral, CEA-based DNA vaccine boosted by huKS1/4–IL-2 immunocytokine C57BL/6J mice transgenic for CEA ($n$ = 8) were immunized 3 times at 2-week intervals by oral gavage with 100 µl PBS containing $10^8$ attenuated *S. typhimurium* harboring either pW-CEA or the control vector pER-CEA. Additional controls were naive mice that received only PBS. Experimental pulmonary metastases were induced 2 weeks after the last immunization by i.v. injection of $5 \times 10^5$ LLC-CEA-KSA cells suspended in 100 µl PBS into the lateral tail vein. Mice were sacrificed 4 weeks after i.v. tumor cell challenge. Tumor burden was determined as the percentage of lung surface covered by tumor nodules.

to APCs by providing sufficient time for T cells to sample large numbers of MHC molecules on the surface of APCs for the presence of specific peptides. This prolonged sampling increases the chances of a naive T cell recognizing its specific peptide/MHC ligand, followed by signaling through the TCR, and induction of a conformational change in LFA-2. In turn, the increased affinity of LFA-2 for CD48 stabilizes the association between the antigen-specific T cell and the APC [51].

We also observed a marked increase in expression of CD28 on T cells and of the co-stimulatory CD80 molecule on DCs, both of which are of considerable importance in providing the two independent signals required for effective activation of naive T cells: (1) antigen recognition and binding of the peptide/MHC complex to the TCR providing the first signal, and (2) ligation of CD28 with CD80 and/or CD86 to initiate T cell responses and production of armed effector cells providing the second signal [52, 53].

A pronounced increase in expression of the high-affinity IL-2 receptor α chain CD25 over controls indicated that T cell activation took place in secondary lymphoid tissues after vaccination and tumor cell challenge. The notion that such lymphoid tissues from mice exhibiting tumor-protective immunity contained tumor antigen-specific CD8⁺ T cells was further supported by the finding that splenocytes isolated from such mice could specifically lyse LLC-CEA-KSA tumor target cells *in vitro* in an MHC class I antigen-restricted manner. Furthermore, this effect proved to be specific since splenocytes isolated from mice in all control groups failed to lyse these tumor target cells. It was quite evident from these results that the boost of IL-2 targeted to the tumor microenvironment by the IL-2 immunocytokine was highly effective in up-regulating several receptor ligand pairs critically important for activation of T cells and their interaction with APCs. Importantly, the up-regulation of these activation markers correlated completely with the increase in tumor-protective immunity induced by the CEA-based DNA vaccine.

Taken together, these results demonstrated that breaking of peripheral T cell tolerance toward the human CEA self-antigen by a CEA-based DNA vaccine was also achieved in an aggressive model of Lewis lung carcinoma which lead to eradication of s.c. tumor growth and prevented dissemination of pulmonary metastases in CEA-transgenic mice. In this prophylactic setting, tumor-protective immunity was induced by MHC class I antigen-restricted CTLs, a finding which correlated with the up-regulated expression of receptor/ligand pairs critical for the activation of T lymphocytes and DCs. Importantly, boosts with small, non-curative doses of an IL-2 immunocytokine resulted in increased efficacy of this therapy, suggesting that combinations of DNA vaccines with such immunocytokines may lead to improved treatments for non-small cell lung cancer.

## 16.4
## Prostate Carcinoma

### 16.4.1
### Suppression of Human Prostate Cancer Metastases by an IL-2 Immunocytokine

Prostate cancer, the most frequent cancer in men in the US, with an estimated 184 500 new cases, is being projected with an annual death rate of 39 000 [54]. One of the most common immunological therapies applied to treat this malignancy is the use of local immunotherapy with immunoregulatory cytokines, which is referred to as cytokine gene therapy. The effectiveness of such an approach for prostate carcinoma was established in studies involving the challenge of the Copenhagen rat with syngeneic Dunning rat prostate carcinoma cells modified to secrete xenotypic murine cytokines, IL-2 [55, 56], IFN-γ [56] and GM-CSF [56, 57], indicating an anti-prostate cancer immune response. The role for IL-2 in the induction of this antitumor immune response was further supported by the finding that Dunning rat prostate carcinoma cells, genetically modified *ex vivo* to express IL-2, produced a local inflammatory response, resulting in the elimination of the injected tumor cells, even when mixed with wild-type parental cells [55]. This gene transfer is consistent with the paracrine nature of IL-2 working physiologically at high concentrations within a few cell diameters from its cell of origin. We applied an alternative approach for directing cytokines preferentially to the tumor microenvironment by a simple *modus operandi*, which complies with the paracrine nature of most cytokines. This was based on our already established proof of concept for this approach with several immunocytokines that combine the unique targeting ability of antibodies with the multifunctional activities of cytokines. The immunocytokines which have been described in this article achieved sufficient local concentrations of cytokines, such as IL-2, to induce the T cell-mediated eradication of colon carcinoma metastases [11, 12] in a syngeneic mouse tumor model.

Consequently, we determined whether the humanized immunocytokine, huKS/4–IL-2, directed against Ep-CAM/KSA and extensively expressed on biopsy specimens of metastatic human prostate carcinoma and on most epithelial cell-derived tumors [58] could effectively suppresses growth and dissemination of lung and bone marrow metastases of human prostate carcinoma in SCID mice. We could indeed demonstrate that targeting IL-2 to the tumor microenvironment of human prostate carcinoma cells (PC-3.MM2) with an immunocytokine (huKS1/4–IL-2) effectively suppressed growth and dissemination of pulmonary and bone marrow metastases, and significantly prolonged the lifespan of immunodeficient C57BL/6 *scid/scid* mice. The antitumor effect achieved by the huKS1/4–IL-2 immunocytokine was found to be specific since another immunocytokine, ch14.18–IL-2, directed against ganglioside $GD_2$ absent from PC-3.MM2 tumor cells, was ineffective. Targeting IL-2 to the KSA docking site for huKS1/4–IL-2 in the tumor microenvironment proved critical for its effectiveness in suppressing dissemination of metastases, since a mixture of rhIL-2 and mAb huKS1/4 at equivalent dose levels was ineffective in this regard. The efficacy of huKS1/4–IL-2 in eliminating bone marrow metastases was demonstrated by a sensitive RT-PCR assay for human β-actin, detecting one tumor cell in 10 000 naive bone marrow cells. All mice treated with huKS1/4–IL-2 at two different dose levels revealed an absence of tumor cells. The prevention of disseminated metastases by treatment with the huKS1/4–IL-2 immunocytokine was further demonstrated by a 4-fold increase in lifespan of these mice when compared to animals that received only PBS or a mixture of rhIL-2 and mAb huKS1/4 at dose levels equivalent to the immunocytokine.

Importantly, the antitumor effect of the immunocytokine against human prostate carcinoma cells was achieved in C57BL/6 *scid/scid* mice that are deficient in mature B and T lymphocytes [59]. Because these immune-deficient animals have a normal compartment of NK cells, granulocytes and macrophages, we identified the effector cell(s) involved in the antitumor effect of the immunocytokine. Thus, when we performed the treatment experiments in C57BL/6 *scid/beige* mice deficient in B, T and NK cells, the immunocytokine still induced a pronounced suppression of pulmonary metastases in all mice compared to animals treated with PBS. Because the prevention of metastases was not complete in four of six mice that still revealed less than 5% of lung surfaces covered with metastases, NK cells were considered to be only partially involved in the antitumor effects induced by the immunocytokine. Further evidence for an NK cell-independent treatment effect was provided by the failure of inducing an increased antitumor effect with the immunocytokine following reconstitution of C57BL/6 *scid/scid* mice with human lymphokine-activated killer cells (LAK) cells, which are largely composed of NK cells. Furthermore, granulocyte depletion of NK cell-deficient C57BL/6 *scid/beige* mice during the period of immunocytokine treatment did not measurably change the antitumor efficacy of the immunocytokine. These findings implied macrophages as the key effector cells involved in the suppression of disseminated metastases induced by huKS1/4–IL-2 in this particular xenograft model of human prostate carcinoma [59].

Taken together, our preclinical findings were of interest when considering the future clinical application of the huKS1/4–IL-2 immunocytokine for the treatment of human prostate carcinoma. Thus, several phase I clinical trials have been ongoing that evaluate the efficacy of certain cytokine gene therapies [60], as well as the presentation of prostate carcinoma antigens by individual patients' DCs to induce a T cell-mediated immunity against prostate carcinoma. However, there are also some doubts about the ultimate success of such approaches. One limiting factor of these therapies is their need for autologous tumor or DCs requiring customization of treatment for individual patients. However, immunocytokines containing IL-2 are capable of activating potent T cell-dependent antitumor immune responses [11, 12] without solely depending on this type of immune response for cancer therapy. In fact, as demonstrated in this prostate cancer model, we found effective suppression of bone marrow and pulmonary metastases of human prostate carcinoma in SCID mice to be mediated by immune effector cells other than B, T or NK cells. Since the same huKS1/4–IL-2 immunocytokine used in these experiments will be entered into phase I clinical trials of prostate carcinoma, it is certainly of interest that this immunocytokine was capable of inducing suppression of metastases by activating and proliferating various effector cells. In this regard, we also showed, as described above, that the huKS1/4–IL-2 immunocytokine is able to induce antitumor effects via CD8$^+$ T cells in a murine colon carcinoma metastases model [11, 12]. Clearly, the induction of a T cell-mediated immune response has the advantage of memory T cells inducing a long-lived protective tumor immunity and thus performing as a tumor vaccine. However, a T cell-mediated immune response also has clearly defined requirements that cannot always be met, particularly by cancer patients who are highly immunosuppressed following extensive chemo- and radiotherapies. The huKS1/4–IL-2 immunocytokine, on the other hand, provides an approach for the treatment of human prostate carcinoma that is not limited by customization of treatment to individual patients like cytokine gene therapies and other cell-based immunotherapies. In fact, IL-2 immunocytokines have the added advantage of being able to activate and expand a variety of effector cells, thus providing a broader base for a potentially effective treatment of prostate carcinoma in an adjuvant setting for patients with minimal residual disease.

**16.5**
**Melanoma**

**16.5.1**
**Treatment of Tumor Metastases with Immunocytokines**

Human melanoma tumors reveal up-regulated expression of an array of ganglio-sides, including disialoganglioside $GD_2$. However, even though gangliosides can cross species barriers, murine B16 melanoma cells failed to express ganglioside $GD_2$ and were thus transfected with human genes encoding for two enzymes catalyzing the last steps of $GD_2$ biosynthesis, β-1,4-N-acetylgalactosaminyltransferase and α-2,8-siatyltransferase. These transduced B16 melanoma cells stably expressed $GD_2$, bound the ch14.18–IL-2 fusion protein, and formed experimental hepatic and pulmonary metastases in syngeneic C57BL/6 mice following intrasplenic or i.v. injection [61].

Immunotherapy of established hepatic and pulmonary melanoma metastases in C57BL/6J mice with ch14.18–IL-2 fusion protein 1 week after tumor cell inoculation completely eradicated established metastases in the vast majority of mice. A typical example depicting the eradication of established pulmonary metastases shown in Tab. 16.3. This was also indicated by histologic examination of tissue sections. More-over, the treatment effect was specific since a non-specific fusion protein directed against the human epidermal growth factor receptor, ch225–IL-2, not expressed on B16 cells or its subline B78-pD3T-31, did not show any antitumor effect [61]. The efficacy of fusion protein therapy in eradicating established hepatic metastases of melanoma was further demonstrated by a 2-fold increase in lifespan of only ch14.18–IL-2 immunocytokine-treated mice. This is illustrated in Fig. 16.4.

Immunocytokine therapy also overcame heterogeneity of the tumor docking sites as indicated by a successful eradication of melanoma metastases achieved when a small percentage of tumor cells expressing the $GD_2$ docking site were admixed with $GD_2$-negative cells and could still be successfully employed as *in vivo* targets [62]. This tumor cell killing was dependent on CD8[+] T cells. In fact, we demonstrated the presence of clonotypic T cells in tumor lesions in both IL-2 immunocytokine-treated

**Tab. 16.3** Effect of the tumor-specific antibody-IL-2 fusion protein on established pulmonary metastases

| Treatment | No. of foci | Lung weight (g) |
|---|---|---|
| None | > 500, > 500, > 500, > 500, > 500, > 500, > 500 | 0.39 ± 0.16 |
| rIL-2 + ch14.18 | 82, 151, 154, 163, > 500, > 500, > 500, > 500 | 0.37 ± 0.10 |
| ch14.18–IL-2 | 0,0,0,0,0,0,0,0 | 0.19 ± 0.09 |

Experimental pulmonary metastases were induced by i.v. injection of $5 \times 10^6$ B78-pD3T-31 cells. Treatment was started 1 week thereafter and consisted of daily i.v. administration of 8 μg chimeric mAb ch14.18 + 24 000 IU recombinant IL-2, of 8 μg of the tumor-specific fusion protein ch14.18–IL-2 for 7 consecutive days.

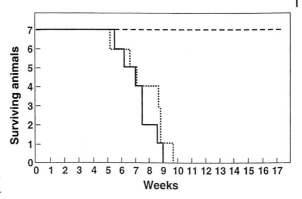

**Fig. 16.4** Kaplan–Meier Plot depicting survival of mice bearing hepatic melanoma metastases. C57BL/6 mice were injected intrasplenically with $2.5 \times 10^6$ murine melanoma cells. After 1 week, animals received i.v. injections of either PBS (solid line), 8 µg ch14.18 + 24 000 IU IL-2 (dashed line) or 8 µg of ch14.18–IL-2 (dotted line) for 7 consecutive days. Surviving animals were sacrificed on day 122.

and non-treated control mice. Taken together, these data indicated that such clonotypic T cells are activated and expanded by IL-2 in the tumor microenvironment, and subsequently are capable of controlling tumor growth [63]. Alternatively, $GD_2$-positive B78-D14 murine melanoma tumors and $GD_2$-negative wild-type B16 melanoma tumors were induced by separate s.c. injection of these respective tumor cells on the left and the right side of the animal, resulting in individual tumors either expressing or lacking the $GD_2$ target antigen of the IL-2 immunocytokine. Boosting the immune response by targeting IL-2 to one localized tumor proved sufficient to promote a powerful response against non-targeted tumors. This experimental design definitely excluded the possibility that the curative response against the wild-type B16 tumor was a bystander effect of the response against the B78-D14 cells. This finding is also highly significant for future clinical trials, since heterogeneity of gene expression is a characteristic of many tumors and their subsequent metastases. In fact, loss of antigen was suggested to be a major mechanism of immune escape in melanoma [64]. The eradication of tumor masses achieved despite the lack of targeting due to lack of the $GD_2$ antigen expression strongly emphasizes the curative potential of this therapy in a clinical setting.

Since T cells are the main effector cells induced by the IL-2 immunocytokine in our animal model, the eradication of distant wild-type B16 tumors strongly indicated a systemic involvement of this T cell response. Thus, T cells were activated either at the tumor site which was targeted by ch14.18–IL-2 or at the lymph node draining the tumor [65] where T cells entered the periphery and migrated to the $GD_2$-negative wild-type B16 tumors. Importantly, analyses of T cell infiltrates by quantitative RT-PCR indicated the presence of highly expressed TCR $V_\beta$ regions in both tumor variants. TCR clonotype mapping revealed the high expression of these regions to be caused by clonal expansion and also indicated that these specific clonotype TCR transcripts were identical in both tumors. Taken together, these data suggested that T cell clones, activated locally by targeted IL-2 therapy actually recirculate and mediate the eradication of distant tumor sites not subjected to *in situ* immunocytokine therapy [66].

Treatment of melanoma with the ch14.18–IL-2 immunocytokine induced a T cell-dependent immune response, followed by a long-lasting protective tumor immunity against a lethal challenge with wild-type tumor cells. Importantly, immunocytokine-treated animals exhibited an inflammatory response indicated by heavy infiltrates of lymphocytes intermixed with a few granulocytes and macrophages. Strong staining of CD8[+] T cells, and to a lesser extent CD4[+] T cells, infiltrating the tumor microenvironment was observed while occasional NK cells were located primarily in the tumor periphery [62]. More rigorous proof for a T cell-mediated mechanism was obtained in C57BL/6 *scid/scid* mice that lack mature T and B cells, and in C57BL/6 *beige/beige* devoid of functional NK cells. Significantly, an absence of NK cells did not hinder the successful treatment of established pulmonary melanoma metastases; however, a lack of T lymphocytes abrogated this effect. This was further demonstrated by selective *in vivo* depletion of distinctive T cell subpopulations and *in vitro* cytotoxicity assays indicating that CD8[+] T cells are mediators of the ch14.18–IL-2-induced, MHC class I antigen-restricted immune response in this tumor model [61, 62]. Interestingly, the depletion of CD4[+] T cells partially diminished the efficacy of the immunocytokine-mediated immune response. In fact, the absence of cytolytic activity in the CD4[+] T cell compartment against melanoma target cells *in vitro* suggested a helper function of CD4[+] T cells for the most optimal activation of CD8[+] T cell response. The mechanism of help provided by CD4[+] T cells was mediated by CD40/CD40L interactions and not by the release of IL-2 from this T cell subpopulation. This conclusion was based on the observation that ch14.18–IL-2-mediated anti-melanoma activity was partially abrogated in CD40L knockout (KO) mice, but not in IL-2 KO mice in which the immunocytokine was completely effective. Partial abrogation of the antitumor effect was induced with anti-CD40L antibody to the same extent as with CD4[+] T cell depletion. Also, a complete antitumor response induced by hu14.18–IL-2 could be reconstituted in CD40L KO mice by simultaneous stimulation with anti-CD40 antibody [65].

Successful therapy with the ch14.18–IL-2 immunocytokine also resulted in long-lived, transferable tumor immunity. Consequently, mice cured of established s.c. melanoma or pulmonary metastases by the immunocytokine completely rejected a subsequent lethal i.v. challenge with melanoma cells in at least 50 % of all animals up to 4 months after the initial treatment [67]. Significantly, challenges with an unrelated syngeneic thymoma cell line (EL4), expressing the GD$_2$ docking site, induced fulminant metastases in the same mice that could, however, be fully protected against challenges with murine melanoma cells. These findings suggested that as yet undefined tumor antigens recognized by T cells are required to induce a tumor-protective immunity. Importantly, this is completely independent of the GD$_2$ docking site that simply serves to deliver IL-2 to the tumor microenvironment [67].

Taken together, the findings obtained in the melanoma model provided proof of concept for an immunocytokine to direct IL-2 to the tumor microenvironment, eradicate established metastases and induce a T cell-mediated memory immune response, suggesting that this approach may be used as a non individualized tumor vaccine.

16.5.2
**Tumor Targeting of LT-α Induces a Peripheral Lymphoid-like Tissue Leading to an Efficient Immune Response against Melanoma**

Initial studies of a tumor-specific ch14.18–LT-α immunocytokine were performed in a xenograft melanoma model where this treatment was effective in eliminating pulmonary metastases [68]. Additional experiments in mice with different immune defects demonstrated a dependence of the therapeutic effect on B lymphocytes and NK cells. Based on these results, we further examined the effect of ch14.18–LT-α in an autologous murine melanoma model and thereby scrutinized the working mechanisms of directed LT-α therapy.

The LT-α immunocytokine-mediated therapy proved to be an effective treatment resulting in the eradication of established pulmonary murine melanoma metastases and s.c. tumors. Furthermore, our results suggested an improved T cell immune response, which is most likely evoked by the induction of peripheral lymphoid tissue at the tumor site. In fact, the functional significance of this tertiary lymphoid tissue at tumor sites was confirmed by immunohistologic and electron microscopic analysis of endothelial/lymphocyte interactions as well as TCR clonotype mapping, providing evidence for the induction of new T cell clones among tumor-infiltrating lymphocytes (TIL), which were shown to specifically lyse melanoma cells and to produce IFN-γ in response to a TRP-$2_{180-188}$-derived peptide [69].

Importantly, the lymphoid-like tissue induced at the site of LT-α accumulation in the tumor provided a prime environment for initiating T cell responses [70]. Consequently, we determined whether this lymphoid tissue could promote the clonal expansion of infiltrating T cells. In fact, analysis of the T cell clonality by RT-PCR/DGGE (denaturing gradient gel electrophoresis) clonotype mapping revealed a specific increase in the number of clones over the course of treatment. Comparative clonotype analysis demonstrated that this increase in the number of clonally expanded T cells was due to both the persistence as well as the occurrence of new clones. Significantly, T cell clones detected in lymph nodes draining the tumor were never detected recurrently in the tumor. This observation, together with the immunohistological and electron microscopical evidence for the occurrence of high endothelial venules and interaction of lymphocytes with the endothelia, provided strong presumptive evidence that the therapy-induced tertiary lymphoid organ was functional and allowed for priming of naive lymphocytes at the tumor site. Thus, the effects of ch14.18–LT-α therapy differed substantially from the effects induced by the ch14.18–IL-2 fusion protein therapy that only boosted a pre-existing T cell response [71]. Nevertheless, for both therapies the eradication of B78-D14 melanoma tumors was mediated via clonally expanded tumor-specific T cells rather than a polyclonal, nonspecific T cell population. As in the case of ch14.18–IL-2 treatment, targeted ch14.18–LT-α therapy was closely linked to tumor regression, raising the question whether the emergence of new clones was directly related to the treatment or a secondary phenomenon reflecting the immunological rejection. However, separate analysis of regressive and progressive parts of human melanoma lesions did not reveal differences in the numbers of clonotypic T cells, indicating that immunological rejection was not coupled to the presence of higher numbers of clonotypic T cells [71]. Moreover the last tumor samples for TCR clonotype mapping were obtained at day 21, a time when the progressive growth of the tumor just started to level off; thus, the presence of clonally expanded T cells was at least not caused by tumor necrosis but rather was a therapy-induced immune response.

The finding that almost no clones were discovered in the draining lymph nodes further suggested that priming occurred in the tumor and not in the lymph node. Furthermore, even when we were able to detect an occasional clonal expansion within these lymph nodes, none of these were identical to those present in the tumor. The induction of lymphoid tissues at the tumor site will overcome two of the major obstacles to prolonged immune responses to weakly immunogenic tumors, i.e. clonal anergy and clonal exhaustion [72]. Thus it may avoid T cell anergy by providing a suitable cytokine and cellular environment together with a high antigen load. Clonal exhaustion may also be prevented, since naive T cells can be continuously primed. Actually, immunocytokine LT-α-dependent lymphoid neogenesis may improve antitumor responses in several ways and the possibility that naive T cells can be primed next to the tumor by a tertiary lymphoid organ has several advantages for immunotherapy. First, a larger number of primed tumor-specific T cells will become available since tumor-specific antigens predominate [73]. Second, a reduction will occur in the time between priming and expansion thus decreasing the risk of primed T cells not reaching the tumor. Third, ongoing T cell responses will react more readily and quickly to changes in the antigen expression profile of the tumor. In addition, this may stop lymphocytes from leaving the tumor microenvironment, which is beneficial since effective immunotherapy depends more on sustaining an immune response at the appropriate location than on its initiation [74]. Taken together, our results suggested that the effectiveness of tumor-targeted LT-α therapy was due to direct clonal expansion of tumor-specific T cells through the formation of peritumoral lymphoid tissue [69].

### 16.5.3
### ch14.18–IL-2 Immunocytokine Boosts Protective Immunity Induced by an Autologous Oral DNA Vaccine against Murine Melanoma

Initial experiments designed to develop an autologous oral DNA vaccine protecting against murine melanoma indicated that peripheral tolerance toward melanoma self-antigens gp100 and TRP-2 could be broken by such a vaccine in CD57BL/6J mice. Specifically, this was accomplished by a DNA vaccine containing the murine ubiquitin gene fused to minigenes encoding peptide epitopes $gp100_{25-33}$ and $TRP-2_{181-188}$. Characteristically, these epitopes contained dominant anchor residues for MHC class I antigen alleles $H-2D^b$ and $H-2K^b$, respectively. Delivery of this vaccine was by oral gavage using an attenuated strain of *S. typhimurium* as carrier that delivered the DNA to a secondary lymphoid tissues, i.e. the Peyer's patch. Three vaccinations with $10^8$ bacteria at 2-week intervals induced effective tumor-protective immunity in a prophylactic setting since a lethal s.c. challenge of wild-type B16 melanoma cells 1 week after the last vaccination, resulted in complete tumor rejection in 25% of experimental mice.

The remaining animals exhibited a 5-fold reduction in tumor growth compared to controls receiving PBS, the empty vector, or the DNA vaccine lacking ubiquitin. All animals in the three control groups grew large tumors (800–900 mm$^3$) and failed to reject the wild-type tumor cell challenge [75].

Two lines of evidence indicated that the tumor-protective immunity induced by the DNA vaccine was mediated by MHC class I antigen-restricted CD8$^+$ T cells secreting increased amounts of the pro-inflammatory cytokine IFN-$\gamma$. First, adoptive transfer of CD8$^+$ T cells from mice successfully immunized by the DNA vaccine to syngeneic *scid/scid* mice resulted in more than 60% reduction in s.c. tumor growth after challenge with wild-type B16 melanoma cells when compared with control animals that received CD8$^+$ T cells from mice vaccinated with only the empty ubiquitin vector. Second, only CD8$^+$ T cells isolated from splenocytes of successfully vaccinated mice induced MHC class I antigen-restricted CTL-mediated cytolytic killing of melanoma target cells *in vitro*. Significantly, the presence of ubiquitin upstream of the minigene proved to be essential for achieving this tumor-protective immunity, suggesting that more effective antigen processing in the proteasome and presentation by antigen-presenting cells made it possible to break peripheral T cell tolerance to tumor self-antigens [76, 77].

Although these findings obtained with the DNA vaccine encoding melanoma mini-genes were encouraging, we attempted to improve its efficacy by combining it with small boosts by sub-optimal doses of ch14.18–IL-2 immunocytokine. Actually, three lines of prior evidence provided the rationale for this approach. First, we demonstrate previously that immunocytokines targeted to the tumor microenvironment where they actively activated and expanded CD8$^+$ T cell. In fact, combined with CD4$^+$ T cell help, this approach induced effective antitumor responses and eradicated established metastases of murine colon carcinoma [11, 12] and murine melanoma [61, 62]. Second, we already demonstrated that the humanized huKS1/4–IL-2 immunocytokine (huKS1/4–IL-2) elicited a long-lived cellular-mediated memory immune response against murine colon carcinoma which, importantly, was substantially amplified by additional boosts with non-curative, suboptimal doses of this same immunocytokine targeted to the tumor microenvironment. Third, systemically administered IL-2 was shown to be of key importance for boosting the efficacy of a variety of malignancies tested in the clinic [78, 79]. In fact, modified gp100$_{209-217}$ peptide-induced T cell responses resulted in a striking objective clinical response rate of 42% among melanoma patients only when these individuals received concurrent boosts with high systemic doses of IL-2 [79]. Thus, IL-2 may actually be essential for breaking peripheral T cell tolerance against melanoma self-antigens.

To prove this point, C57BL6/J mice immunized three times with the DNA vaccine encoding ubiquitin and the gp100$_{25-53}$ and TRP-2$_{181-189}$ minigenes, were challenged s.c. with wild-type murine melanoma cells, 1 week after the last immunization and 24 h later received i.v. boosts with 5 µg ch14.18–IL-2 for 4 consecutive days. This resulted in complete tumor rejection in 75% of experimental animals with the remaining mice revealing an almost 10-fold reduction in tumor growth when compared with control animals. These fusion-protein boosts markedly enhanced tumor-protective immunity when compared to the vaccine alone ($P > 0.01$), which resulted in tumor rejection in only 25% of experimental animals. An important control experiment combining the same amount of ch14.18–IL-2 immunocytokine used for boosting with the empty ubiquitin vector showed no antitumor effect, and was equal to that of controls receiving PBS and a s.c. tumor cell challenge. Significantly, we also found that only one vaccination coupled with the immunocytokine boost was equally as effective as three such vaccinations and ch14.18–IL-2 boosts [80].

The immunological mechanisms involved in these antitumor effects were indicated by experiments in CD8 KO and CD4 KO mice demonstrating that CD8$^+$ T cells were essential together with CD4$^+$ T cell help. However, the latter was shown by *in vivo* immunodepletion experiments to be required for tumor cell killing only in the effector phase of the immune response. The involvement of additional immunological mechanisms was suggested by a decisively increased secretion of tumor necrosis factor (TNF)-α and IFN-γ from CD4$^+$ and CD8$^+$ T cells, demonstrated by intracellular cytokine staining experiments. FACS analyses indicated a markedly up-regulated expression on CD8$^+$ T cells of the high affinity IL-2-receptor α chain (CD25), co-stimulatory molecule CD28 and adhesion molecule LFA-2 (CD2). These FACS analyses of splenocytes from successfully immunized mice also showed that the combination therapy induced increased expression of co-stimulatory molecules B7–1 and CD48 on murine APCs [80].

The data indicating CD4$^+$ T cell help to be required for optimal efficacy of the DNA vaccine are not entirely surprising; however, the finding indicating that this help is needed only in the effector phase but not required for CD8$^+$ T cell priming in the immunization phase was new and extended our previous observations. Thus, we previously found that eradication of hepatic and pulmonary metastases of murine melanoma achieved by multiple injection of ch14.18–IL-2 immunocytokine was impaired in part by *in vivo* depletion of CD4$^+$ T cells [12]. Subsequent findings indicated that tumor-protective immunity induced by this immunocytokine required CD4$^+$ T cell help which was mediated by CD40/CD40L interaction without requiring production of endogenous IL-2 by T cells [65]. The requirement of CD4$^+$ T cell help for adaptive immunity is well established and was initially described for the B cell compartment. Subsequent reports also indicated the need for CD4$^+$ T cell help in the induction of CD8$^+$ T cell-mediated immune responses [80]. The fact that our DNA vaccine doubled the number of T$_h$1 CD4$^+$ T cells expressing IFN-γ and that this number was increased 3-fold by ch14.18–IL-2 boosts underlined the need for CD4$^+$ T cell help for optimal tumor-protective immunity. Taken together, our data in this prophylactic melanoma model clearly indicated that a minigene-based DNA vaccine plus ch14.18–IL-2 immunocytokine boosts were highly effective in inducing tumor-protective immunity against murine melanoma.

# 16.6
# Neuroblastoma

## 16.6.1
## Treatment with ch14.18–IL-2 Immunocytokine

The rationale for constructing an IL-2 immunocytokine with a human/mouse chimeric antiganglioside $GD_2$ antibody (ch14.18–IL-2) was based on encouraging data obtained in clinical trials of passive immunotherapy of neuroblastoma patients with human/mouse chimeric antibody ch14.18 and with murine antiganglioside $GD_2$ antibody 14G2a plus rhIL-2. Specifically, passive immunotherapy in adjuvant settings with ch14.18 antibody resulted in a response rate of over 50% in phase I and phase I/II clinical trials, including several long-term and complete remissions of stage four patients [81]. Data from a phase I/Ib clinical trial using a combination therapy with murine anti-$GD_2$ mAb 14.G2a and rhIL-2 also showed antitumor activity [82]. Thus, preclinical experiments with a recombinant ch14.18–IL-2 immunocytokine in a syngeneic immunocompetent mouse model were a logical sequel, which was established by using $GD_2$-positive NXS2 murine neuroblastoma cells in syngeneic A/J mice [83]. Importantly, following s.c. and i.v. injections, NXS2 cells metastasized both spontaneously and experimentally to sites typical for human neuroblastoma, including bone marrow, liver, lymph nodes and adrenal glands. The characterization of this model was further extended by two findings. First, MYCN, a very important oncogene for neuroblastoma used as a most predictive prognostic marker [84–86] with a proven involvement in neuroblastoma pathogenesis [87], was found in NXS2 cells. Second, the expression of the noradrenaline transporter was established in NXS2 cells which was previously characterized as the intracellular uptake system for *meta*-iodobenzylguanidine ($[^{131}I]mIBG$) [49], an experimental radionuclide currently under clinical evaluation for the adjuvant treatment of neuroblastoma [88–91]. The positive signal for this transporter in NXS2 cells suggested that this model might be a useful tool for the evaluation of this type of radiotherapy as a single modality or in combination with other adjuvant therapies including immunotherapy or anti-angiogenesis.

## 16.6.2
## Immunocytokine Treatment of Bone Marrow and Liver Metastases

The therapeutic effect of the ch14.18–IL-2 immunocytokine observed in both, spontaneous and experimental bone marrow and liver metastasis models was achieved only in A/J mice that received this immunocytokine [83]. Significantly, these animals had no macroscopic liver disease and revealed a lack of detectable metastasis to the bone marrow, determined by tyrosine hydroxylase RT-PCR detecting one tumor cell in 100 000 naive bone marrow cells. A Kaplan–Meier analysis of mice following induction of spontaneous bone marrow and liver metastases indicated a tripling in lifespan in 50% of the animals only when treated with the immunocytokine. This was in contrast to the lack of increased survival in control groups, which received an equivalent mixture of antibody and rhIL-2 or PBS. In fact at least a doubling in life-span was seen following induction of experimental liver metastasis only in mice trea-ted with the immunocytokine [92]. The specificity of ch14.18–IL-2 immunotherapy was demonstrated by ineffective treatment of liver metastases of $GD_2$-negative TBJ cells with the ch14.18–IL-2 immunocytokine [92]. Taken together, these data indi-cated that therapy with an immunocytokine directed against ganglioside $GD_2$, that is a naturally occurring and heterogeneously expressed antigen in this tumor model, can effectively eradicate disseminated metastasis in at least two different metastatic sites. It is noteworthy that similar situations are to be expected in humans, where TAAs are distributed heterogeneously and metastasis is usually not limited to a sin-gle organ system. Due to the various similarities of this murine neuroblastoma model with human neuroblastoma, the therapeutic effect observed with the ch14.18–IL-2 immunocytokine could thus be indicative of a potentially successful clinical application.

### 16.6.3
### Mechanism of Immunocytokine-mediated Immune Responses

In contrast to previously reported T cell-mediated immune responses following ther-apy with immunocytokines in animal models for murine colorectal carcinoma [11, 12] and melanoma [61], several lines of evidence indicated that the effector mechan-ism in the syngeneic neuroblastoma model was exclusively mediated by NK cells. First, the treatment of liver and bone marrow metastases with ch14.18–IL-2 immu-nocytokine proved completely effective in T cell-deficient *scid/scid* mice. This treat-ment effect was only abrogated in *scid/beige* mice that lack both T and NK cells. How-ever, reconstitution of NK cells in this mouse strain by injection of $3 \times 10^7$ NK cells per mouse re-established the therapeutic efficacy of the immunocytokine. Second, depletion of NK cells and $CD8^+$ T cells in immunocompetent A/J mice eliminated the therapeutic effect only in NK cell depleted mice [92]. A role for $CD8^+$ T cells was further excluded by s.c. injection of $1 \times 10^6$ NXS2 cells into mice with established li-ver and bone marrow metastases that had been successfully treated with ch14.18–IL-2 immunocytokine. Thus, s.c. tumor growth 11 days after this challenge of immu-nocytokine-treated animals was the same as that of naive mice, untreated tumor-bearing mice or mice that received an equivalent mixture of antibody and cytokine. These results indicated the absence of a memory immune response, a typical feature of NK cells. Third, immunohistochemical analyses of inflammatory infiltrates in livers of mice successfully treated with ch14.18–IL-2 indicated positive staining for NK cells, but not for $CD8^+$ T cells. This was in contrast to livers of mice that received PBS injections or the equivalent antibody/IL-2 mixture, and showed no detectable in-flammatory cells [92].

Based on these *in vivo* data, strong evidence for an NK cell-mediated mechanism was established which was further supported by *in vitro* analyses of NK cell activation and killing of NXS2 target cells. Specifically, treatment of tumor-bearing mice with ch14.18–IL-2 increased NK cell activity of freshly isolated splenocytes in contrast to PBS and antibody/IL-2 mixture controls. Only splenocytes of mice receiving the immunocytokine showed a drastic increase in their lysis of NK cell-sensitive YAC-1 target cells. In contrast, only a marginal increase in NK cell activation over the natural NK cell activity was detected in splenocytes of mice treated with a combination of antibody and IL-2. When cytotoxic activity of splenocytes obtained from mice treated with the ch14.18–IL-2 immunocytokine was determined with NXS2 target cells, the separation into NK cell and CD8$^+$ T cell subpopulations indicated effective killing only in the NK cell fraction whereas CD8$^+$ T cells were completely ineffective. These data provided further proof for an NK cell-mediated cellular immune response in this model [92].

The dichotomy of immune mechanisms involved in ch14.18–IL-2 immunocytokine-mediated antitumor responses lead to the question as to whether low expression of major MHC class I antigens could favor NK cells over T cells in the syngeneic neuroblastoma tumor model. Therefore, MHC class I antigens were up-regulated by additional s.c. application of recombinant murine IFN-γ (mIFN-γ). In this case, a combination therapy of ch14.18–IL-2 immunocytokine and mIFN-γ was more effective in eradicating established bone marrow and liver metastasis. Although mIFN-γ strongly up-regulated MHC class I expression, splenocytes of mice successfully treated with the immunocytokine/mIFN-γ combination were incapable of MHC class I antigen-restricted killing of NXS2 target cells. Thus, a switch from an NK- to a T cell-mediated mechanism did not occur. In fact, quite the opposite was observed as the addition of anti-MHC class I antibodies increased the cytolytic activity of splenocytes obtained from mice after completion of the immunocytokine/mIFN-γ combination treatment. This is typical for NK cell-mediated killing of tumor cells, since NK cells activity is down-regulated by stimulated lectin type C inhibitory NK cell receptors of the LY49 family that are specific for MHC class I antigen molecules [93–95] We did overcome this down-regulation by addition of MHC class I antigen blocking antibodies. Consequently, the increase achieved in antitumor activity of the ch14.18–IL-2 fusion protein by addition of mIFN-γ *in vivo* could be attributed to a further activation of NK cells. This contention was further supported by the finding that splenocytes from mice treated with the ch14.18–IL-2/mIFN-γ combination achieved the highest lysis of YAC1 cells, when compared with mIFN-γ and ch14.18–IL-2 controls [92].

The absence of a T cell-mediated immune response in the NSX-2 model and its concomitant replacement by NK cells may be due to factors secreted by the tumor cells that suppress T cells but stimulate NK cells. In fact, NXS2 cells were shown to produce transforming growth factor (TGF)-β1 and IL-10 *in vitro* and *in vivo*, both immunomodulators being associated with T cell anergy [96–101]. However, IL-10 was also reported to stimulate NK cells [102] and to inhibit tumor metastasis via NK cell mediated mechanisms [103]. Thus, it is feasible that the presence of TGF-β1 and IL-10 in our model could favor NK cell dependent antitumor mechanisms by causing NK cell stimulation and concomitant T cell-anergy.

16.6.4
**Amplification of Suboptimal CD8$^+$ T Memory Cells by a Cellular Vaccine**

Based on the superior efficacy of tumor targeted IL-2 as outlined in this chapter and its role as an effective adjuvant for cancer vaccines emerging from clinical trials, we hypothesized that tumor-specific targeting of IL-2 into the tumor microenvironment is more effective in amplifying a cancer vaccine-induced T cell-mediated immune responses than systemic IL-2.

This hypothesis was tested in two independent experimental systems with a cellular vaccine consisting of NXS2 neuroblastoma cells genetically engineered to produce single-chain IL-12 [104] and, as described above, in the CT26-KSA colon carcinoma model, following induction of a vaccination effect by targeted IL-2 using huKS1/4–IL-2 fusion protein. We could demonstrate in both systems that the initial T cell response is effectively amplified by tumor-specific targeting of IL-2 into the tumor microenvironment with tumor-specific immunocytokines ch14.18–IL-2 [105] and huKS1/4–IL-2 [15], respectively. This was clearly indicated in the NSX2 neuroblastoma model by the complete absence of metastases in the majority of animals that were challenged by lethal i.v. injection with wild-type tumor cells up to 90 days after the initial vaccination and followed by injections with non-curative doses of tumor-specific immunocytokines. However, administration of non-specific immunocytokines or equivalent mixtures of tumor-specific antibody and IL-2 were completely ineffective [15, 105]. This is illustrated by the data shown in Tab. 16.4. In this case, A/J mice were vaccinated by s.c. injection of $5 \times 10^6$ NXS2 cells genetically engineered to produce scIL-12 and challenged by a lethal i.v. injection of $5 \times 10^4$ NXS2 wild-type cells 90 days after initial vaccination. Treatment was initiated at day 5 after tumor cell challenge by 5 daily i.v. injections of PBS; 10 µg of ch14.18 antibody plus 30 000 units of rhIL-2, 10 µg of the non-specific ch225–IL-2 fusion protein or 10 µg of the tumor-specific ch14.18–IL-2 fusion protein. Liver metastases were staged according to the percentage of metastatic liver surface as follows: 0, 0%; 1, <25%; 2, 25–50%; 3, 50–75%; 4, >75%. Data for liver weight were the mean $\pm$ SD. Differences in bone marrow staging, liver metastasis and liver weights between fusion-protein-treated mice and all control groups were statistically significant ($P < 0.01$).

Increases in CD25$^+$/CD8$^+$ T cells, MHC class I-restricted target cell killing, and V$_\beta$11 and V$_\beta$13 T cell receptor usage suggested a mechanism for reactivation of CD8$^+$ memory T cells induced by the vaccine effectively boosted with ch14.18–IL-2 [105].

**Tab. 16.4** Boost of gene therapy-induced immunoprotection with recombinant ch14.18–IL-2 fusion protein

| Vaccine | Treatment | Metastatic score | Liver weight (mg) |
|---------|-----------|------------------|-------------------|
| scIL 12 NXS2 | PBS | 4,4,3,2,1,1 | 2011 ± 986 |
| scIL 12 NXS2 | ch14.18 + IL-2 | 3,2,2,1 | 1530 ± 320 |
| scIL 12 NXS2 | ch225–IL-2 | 4,3,2,2,1,1 | 1610 ± 357 |
| scIL 12 NXS2 | ch14.18–IL-2 | 0,0,0,0,0,0 | 912 ± 126 |

Similar findings were reported for the colorectal carcinoma model, as described above, Taken together, the results of these studies clearly demonstrated a superior role for tumor targeted IL-2 as an adjuvant for cancer vaccines.

## 16.6.5
### Synergy between Targeted IL-2 and Antiangiogensis

The generation of new blood vessels, or angiogenesis, plays a key role in tumor growth and has generated much interest in developing agents that inhibit angiogenesis [106–111]. However, the identification of well-characterized, vasculature-specific inhibitors of angiogenesis that are synergistic with therapies specifically targeting the tumor compartment may be critical for achieving optimally effective cancer treatment.

Angiogenesis is characterized by invasion, migration and proliferation of endothelial cells, processes that depend on cell interactions with extracellular matrix components. In this regard, the endothelial adhesion receptor integrin $\alpha_v\beta_3$ was shown to be a key player [112, 113] by providing a vasculature-specific target for anti-angiogenic treatment strategies. The requirement for vascular integrin $\alpha_v\beta_3$ in angiogenesis was demonstrated by several *in vivo* models where the generation of new blood vessels by transplanted human tumors was entirely inhibited either by systemic administration of peptide antagonists of integrin $\alpha_v\beta_3$ or anti-$\alpha_v\beta_3$ antibody LM609 [112, 114] Such antagonists block the ligation of integrin $\alpha_v\beta_3$ which promotes apoptosis of the proliferative angiogenic vascular cells and thereby disrupt the maturation of newly forming blood vessels, an event essential for the proliferation of tumors.

A major obstacle for effective treatment of disseminated malignancies includes minimal residual disease characterized by micrometastases that lack a well-established vascular supply. In this regard, immunocytokines proved to be a very efficient tumor compartment-specific approach as summarized in the previous sections of this chapter. Although quite effective at early stages of tumor metastasis, this tumor compartment-directed approach could only delay growth of metastases at later stages of tumor growth characterized by a fully developed vascular compartment. Consequently, we addressed the question of whether there is a complementary advantage of such specific vascular and tumor compartment-directed treatment strategies being synergistic when used in sequential and simultaneous combinations.

We tested this hypothesis in three syngeneic murine tumor models of colon carcinoma, melanoma and neuroblastoma. The ganglioside $GD_2$ and Ep-CAM antigens specifically delineate the tumor compartments in these models targeted by the respective IL-2 immunocytokines ch14.18–IL-2 and huKS1/4–IL-2. The vascular compartment of these tumor models was defined by expression of integrin $\alpha_v\beta_3$ on newly formed blood vessels [112] as described for several animal models. Targeting of integrin $\alpha_v\beta_3$ on endothelial cells of the tumor vasculature facilitated successful treatment. Thus, we could show that a peptide antagonist, targeting the vasculature through interaction with $\alpha_v$ integrins expressed on angiogenic blood vessels [112, 113] effectively suppressed blood vessel formation and dramatically regressed subsequent tumor growth. This was also demonstrated by treating three aggressively growing primary tumors and one spontaneously metastasizing tumor [115] These data indicated such a vascular targeting approach to be effective in clinically relevant tumor models. Importantly, the antitumor effect of targeting the tumor vasculature was amplified by a simultaneous attack on the tumor compartment, which was effective against both primary tumors and spontaneous metastases [115]. In fact, the simultaneous targeting of the vascular and tumor compartments proved very effective, since it combined a decrease in tumor cell nourishment with the active destruction of tumor cells, leading to a regression of primary tumors and the eradication of distant metastases. This finding was in contrast to a single vascular compartment-directed approach using two different anti-angiogenic treatment strategies that resulted only in suppression of s.c. tumor growth in a syngeneic model [116]. In contrast, in our strategy, the tumor compartment-specific response was mediated by inflammatory cells that were activated and directed to the tumor microenvironment by the tumor-specific immunocytokines. Significantly, the anti-angiogenic strategy, although quite effective in growth suppression of primary tumors with a well-established vascular supply, lacked a similar efficacy against distant micrometastases when used as monotherapy. However, in such a minimal residual disease setting with small tumor loads characterized by poor vascularization, the antitumor compartment treatment arm used in our combination therapies was quite effective when used as monotherapy [11, 92] In this situation, the role of anti-angiogenic treatment strategies could be to suppress micrometastasis-induced neovascularization and subsequent enlargement of metastatic foci [111]. This, in turn, would facilitate eradication of such micrometastases by tumor compartment-directed therapies, which are optimally effective in the minimal residual disease setting.

## 16.7
## Conclusions and Perspectives

The effective adjuvant treatment of solid tumors remains a major challenge in clinical oncology. Although, a variety of novel therapeutic strategies have became available for biotherapeutic treatment, most of these were evaluated as monotherapies and often resulted in diminished enthusiasm due to poor clinical response rates. In view of the increased success of cancer chemotherapy due to sophisticated combination of drugs with distinct modes of action, a similar approach may be called for in the adjuvant treatment of cancer. Consequently, the preclinical evaluation of the presence or absence of synergystic effects in the combined adjuvant treatment strategies described in this chapter may aid in providing the critical information necessary to design successful adjuvant treatments for cancer. Such efforts combined with rapid clinical evaluations may provide the key to markedly advance cancer therapy in the 21st century.

# References

1 A. M. Silverstein, *A History of Immunology*. Academic Press, San Diego, CA, 1988.

2 G. Kohler and C. Milstein, *Nature* 1975; **256**: 495–497.

3 S. D. Gillies, K.-M. Lo and J. Wesolowski, *J Immunol Methods* 1989; **125**: 191–202.

4 S. D. Gillies, H. Dorai, G. Wesolowski, G. Majeau, D. Young, J. Boyd, J. Gardner and K. James, *BioTechnology* 1989; **7**: 799–804.

5 S. D. Gillies, D. Young, K.-M. Lo, S. F. Foley and R. A. Reisfeld, *Hybridoma* 1991; **10**: 347–356.

6 S. D. Gillies, E. B. Reilly, K.-M. Lo and R. A. Reisfeld, *Proc Natl Acad Sci USA* 1992; **89**: 1428–1432.

7 S. D. Gillies, Y. Lau, J. Wesolowski, X. Qian, R. A. Reisfeld, S. Holden, M. Super and K.-M. Lo, *J Immunol.* 1998; **160**: 6195–6203.

8 H. Sabzevari, S. D. Gillies, B. M. Mueller, J. D. Pancook and R. A. Reisfeld, *Proc Natl Acad Sci USA* 1994; **91**: 9626–9630.

9 S. Steimle, *J Natl Cancer Inst* 1997; **89**: 415–416.

10 G. Riethmuller, E. Schneider-Gadicke and G. Schlimok, German Cancer Aid 17–1A Study Group, *Lancet* 1994; **343**: 1177–1183.

11 R. Xiang, H. N. Lode, C. S. Dolman, T. Dreier, N. M. Varki, X. Qian, K.-M. Lo, Y. Lan, M. Super, S. D. Gillies and R. A. Reisfeld, *Cancer Res* 1997; **57**: 4948–4955.

12 R. Xiang, H. N. Lode, T. Dreier, S. D. Gillies and R. A. Reisfeld, *Cancer Res* 1998; **58**: 3918–3925.

13 A. Y. Huang, P. H. Gulden, A. S. Woods, C. Matthew, C. Thomas, C. D. Tong, W. Wang, V. H. Engelhard, G. Pasternack, R. Cotter, D. Hunt, D. M. Pardoll and E. M. Jaffee, *Proc Natl Acad Sci USA* 1996; **93**: 9730–9735.

14 H. N. Lode, R. Xiang, J. C. Becker, S. D. Gillies and R. A. Reisfeld, *Pharmacol Ther* 1998; **80**: 277–292.

15 R. Xiang, H. N. Lode, T. Dreier, S. D. Gillies and R. A. Reisfeld, *J Immunol* 1999; **163**: 3676–3683.

16 J. Sprent, *Curr Biol* 1995; **5**: 1095–1097.

17 G. Maass, W. Schmidt, M. Berger, F. Schilcher, F. Koszik, A. Schneeberger, G. Stingl, M. L. Birnstiel and T. Schweighoffer, *Proc Natl Acad Sci USA* 1995; **92**: 5540–5544.

18 T. Boon, J.-C. Cerottini, B. Van den Eynde, P. van der Bruggen and A. Van Pel, *Annu Rev Immunol* 1994; **12**: 337–365.

19 A. N. Houghton, *J Exp Med* 1994; **180**: 1–4.

20 J. Schlom, Carcinoembryonic antigen (CEA) peptides and vaccines for carcinoma. In *Peptide-based Cancer Vaccines*, M. Kast (Ed.). Landes Bioscience, Austin, TX, 2000.

21 J. E. Shively and J. D. Beatty, *Crit Rev Oncol Hematol* 1985; **2**: 355–399.

22 J. Thompson and W. Zimmerman, *Tumor Biol* 1988; **9**: 63–83.

23 H. Schrewe, J. Thompson, M. Bona, L. J. F. Hefta, A. Maruya, M. Hassauer, J. E. Shively, S. von Kleist and W. Zimmerman, *Mol Cell Biol* 1990; **10**: 2738–2748.

24 S. Von Kleist, I. Migule and B. Halla, *Anticancer Res* 1995; **15**: 1889–1894.

25 R. M. Sharkey, D. M. Goldenberg, H. Goldenberg, R. E. Lee, C. Balance, D. Powlyk, D. Varga and H. J. Hansen, *Cancer Res* 1990; **50**: 2823–2831.

26 J. Y. Wong, L. E. Williams, D. M. Yamauchi, E. Odon-Maryon, J. M. Esteban, M. Neumaier, A. M. Wu, D. K. Johson, F. J. Primus, J. E. Shively and A. Raubitschek, *Cancer Res* 1995; **55**: 5929s–5934s.

27 J. Kantor, K. Irvine, S. Abrams, H. Kaufmann, J. DiPetro and J. Schlom, *J Natl Cancer Inst* 1992; **84**: 1084–1091.

28 P. Clarke, J. Mann, J. F. Simpson, K. J. Ricard-Dickson and F. J. Primus, *Cancer Res* 1998; **58**: 1469–1477.

29 S. Mizobata, K. Tompkins, J. F. Simpson, Y. Shyr and F. J. Primus, *Cancer*

*Immunol Immunother* 2000; **49**: 285–295.

30  K. Y. TSANG, S. ZAREMBA, C. A. NIE-RODA, M. Z. ZHU, J. M. HAMILTON and J. SCHLOM, *J Natl Cancer Inst* 1995; **87**: 982–990.

31  J. P. McLAUGHLIN, J. SCHLOM, J. A. KANTOR and J. W. GREINER, *Cancer Res* 1996; 2361–2367.

32  E. KASS, J. SCHLOM, J. THOMPSON, F. GUADAGNI, P. GRAZIANO and J. W. GREINER, *Cancer Res* 1999; **59**: 676–683.

33  R. XIANG, S. SILLETTI, H. N. LODE, C. S. DOLMAN, J. M. RUEHLMANN, A. G. NIETHAMMER, U. PERTL, S. D. GILLIES, F. J. PRIMUS and R. A. REISFELD, *Clin Cancer Res* 2001; **7**: 856s–864s.

34  M. L. DUSTIN and T. A. SPRINGER, *Annu Rev Immunol* 1993; **9**: 27–66.

35  M. L. DUSTIN and T. A. SPRINGER, *Nature* 1989; **341**: 619–624.

36  N. HOGG and R. C. LANDIS, *Curr Opin Immunol* 1993; **5**: 383–390.

37  P. S. LINSLEY, W. BRADY, L. GROSMAIRE, A. ARUFFO, N. K. DAMLE and J. A. LEDBETTER, *J Exp Med* 1991; **173**: 721–730.

38  J. D. FRASER, B. A. IRVING, G. R. GRABTEE and A. WEISS, *Science* 1991; **251**: 313–316.

39  R. XIANG, F. J. PRIMUS, J. M. RUEHLMANN, A. G. NIETHAMMER, S. SILLETTI, H. N. LODE, C. S. DOLMAN, S. D. GILLIES and R. A. REISFELD, *J Immunol* 2001; **167**: 4560–4565.

40  J. M. CURTSINGER, C. S. SCHMIDT, A. MONDINO, D. C. LINS, R. M. KEDL, M. K. JENKINS and M. F. MESCHER, *J Immunol* 1999; **162**: 3256–3262.

41  C. A. CHAMBERS and J. P. ALLISON, *Curr Opin Cell Biol* 1999; **11**: 203–210.

42  S. P. SCHOENBERGER, R. E. TOES, E. I. VAN DER VOORT, R. OFFRINGA and C. J. M. MELIEF, *Nature* 1998; **393**: 480–483.

43  A. G. NIETHAMMER, F. J. PRIMUS, R. XIANG, C. S. DOLMAN, J. M. RUEHLMANN, S. D. GILLIES and R. A. REISFELD, *Vaccine* 2001; **20**: 421–429.

44  Z. K. PAN, G. IKONOMIDIS, D. PARDOLL and Y. PATERSON, *Cancer Res* 1999; **55**: 4776–4779.

45  A. DARJI, C. A. GUZMAN, B. GERSTEL, P. WACHHOLZ, K. N. TIMMIS, J. WEH-LAND, J. CHAKRABORTY and S. WEISS, *Cell* 1997; **91**: 765–775.

46  A. DARJI, L. S.-A. I. ZUR GARBE, T. CHAKRABORTY and S. WEISS, *Immunol Med Microbiol* 2000; **27**: 341–349.

47  E. MEDINA, C. A. GUZMAN, L. H. STAENDNER, M. P. COLOMBO and P. PAGLIA, *Eur J Immunol* 1999; **29**: 693–699.

48  E. MEDINA, P. PAGLIA, M. ROHDE, M. P. COLOMBO and C. A. GUZMAN, *Eur J Immunol* 2000; **30**: 768–777.

49  P. PAGLIA, E. MEDINA, I. ARIOLI, C. A. GUZMAN and M. P. COLOMBO, *Blood* 1998; **92**: 3172–3176.

50  K. J. MALOY, I. ERDMANN, V. BASCH, S. SIERRO, T. A. KRAMPS, R. M. ZINKERNAGEL, S. OEHEN and T. M. KÜNDIG, *Proc Natl Acad Sci USA* 2001; **98**: 3299–3303.

51  F. S. WONG, I. VICINITIN, L. WEN, R. A. FLAVELL and C. A. JANEWAY, JR, *J Exp Med* 1996; **183**: 67–76.

52  Y. LIU and C. A. JANEWAY, JR, *Proc Natl Acad Sci USA* 1992; **89**: 3845–3849.

53  C. E. RUDD, *Immunity* 1996; **4**: 527–534.

54  S. H. LANDIS, T. MURRAY, S. BOLDEN and P. A. WINGO, *CA Cancer J Clin* 1998; **48**: 6–29.

55  D. B. MOODY, J. C. ROBINSON, C. M. EWING, A. J. LAZENBY and W. B. ISAACS, *Prostate* 1994; **24**: 244–251.

56  J. VIEWEG, F. M. ROSENTHAL, R. BANNERJI, W. D. HESTON, W. R. FAIR, B. GANSBACHER and E. GILBOA, *Cancer Res* 1994; **54**: 1760–1765.

57  M. G. SANDA, S. R. AYYAGARI, E. M. JAFFEE, J. I. EPSTEIN, S. L. CLIFT, L. K. COHEN, G. DRANOFF, D. M. PARDOLL, R. C. MULLIGAN and J. W. SIMONS, *J Urol* 1994; **151**: 622–628.

58  S. ZHANG, H. S. ZHANG, V. E. REUTER, S. F. SLOVIN, H. I. SCHER and P. O. LIVINGSTON, *Clin Cancer Res* 1998; **4**: 295–302.

59  C. S. DOLMAN, B. M. MUELLER, H. N. LODE, R. XIANG, S. D. GILLIES and R. A. REISFELD, *Clin Cancer Res* 1998; **4**: 2551–2557.

60  J. A. ROTH and R. J. CRISTIANO, *J Natl Cancer Inst* 1997; **89**: 21–39.

**61** J. C. Becker, J. D. Pancook, S. D. Gillies, K. Furukawa and R. A. Reisfeld, *J Exp Med* 1996; **183**: 2361–2366.

**62** J. C. Becker, N. M. Varki, S. D. Gillies, K. Furukawa and R. A. Reisfeld, *Proc Natl Acad Sci USA* 1996; **93**: 7826–7831.

**63** P. thor Straten, P. Guldberg, T. Seremet, R. A. Reisfeld, J. Zeuthen and J. C. Becker, *Proc Natl Acad Sci USA* 1998; **95**: 8785–8790.

**64** G. Pawelec, J. Zeuthen and R. Kiessling, *Crit Rev Oncog* 1997; **8**: 111–141.

**65** H. N. Lode, R. Xiang, U. Pertl, E. Forster, S. P. Schoenberger, S. D. Gillies and R. A. Reisfeld, *J Clin Invest* 2000; **105**: 1623–1630.

**66** P. thor Straten, P. Guldberg, D. Schrama, M. H. Anderson, U. Moerch, T. Seremet, C. Siedel, R. A. Reisfeld and J. C. Becker, *Eur J Immunol* 2001; **31**: 250–258.

**67** J. C. Becker, N. M. Varki, S. D. Gillies, K. Furukawa and R. A. Reisfeld, *J Clin Invest* 1997; **98**: 2801–2804.

**68** R. A. Reisfeld, S. D. Gillies, J. Mendelsohn, N. M. Varki and J. C. Becker, *Cancer Res* 1996; **56**: 1707–1712.

**69** D. Schrama, P. thor Straten, W. H. Fischer, A. D. Mc Lellan, E.-B. Bröcker, R. A. Reisfeld and J. C. Becker, *Immunity* 2001; **14**: 111–121.

**70** F. G. Lakkis, A. Arakelov, B. T. Konieczny and Y. Inoue, *Nat Med* 2000; **6**: 686–688.

**71** P. thor Straten, J. C. Becker, T. Seremet, E.-B. Bröcker and J. Zeuthen, *J Clin Invest* 1996; **98**: 279–284.

**72** P. Fields, F. W. Fitch and T. F. Gajewski, *J Mol Med* 1996; **74**: 673–683.

**73** K. J. Flynn, G. T. Belz, J. D. Altman, R. Ahmed, D. L. Woodland and P. C. Doherty, *Immunity* 1998; **8**: 683–691.

**74** P. Shrikant and M. F. Mescher, *J Immunol* 1999; **162**: 2858–2866.

**75** R. Xiang, H. N. Lode, T.-H. Chao, J. M. Ruehlmann, C. S. Dolman, F. Rodriguez, J. L. Whitton, W. W. Overwijk, N. P. Restifo and R. A. Reisfeld, *Proc Natl Acad Sci USA* 2000; **97**: 5492–5497.

**76** F. Rodriguez, J. Zhang and J. L. Whitton, *J Virol* 1997; **71**: 8497–8503.

**77** F. Rodriguez, A. Ling Ling, S. Harkins, J. Zhang, M. Yokoyama, G. Widera, J. T. Fuller, C. Kincaid, I. L. Campbell and J. L. Whitton, *J Virol* 1998; **72**: 5174–5181.

**78** R. F. Wang and S. A. Rosenberg, *Immunol Rev* 1999; **170**: 85–100.

**79** S. A. Rosenberg, J. C. Yang, D. J. Schwartzentruber, P. Hwu, F. M. Marincola, S. L. Topalian, N. P. Restifo, M. Sznol, S. L. Schwarz, P. J. Spiess, J. R. Wunderlich, C. A. Seipp, J. H. Einhorn, L. Rogers-Freezer and D. E. White, *J Immunol* 1999; **163**: 1690–1695.

**80** A. G. Niethammer, R. Xiang, J. M. Ruehlmann, H. N. Lode, C. S. Dolman, S. D. Gillies and R. A. Reisfeld, *Cancer Res* 2001; **61**: 6178–6184.

**81** R. Handgretinger, K. Anderson, P. Lang, R. Dopfer, T. Klingebiel, M. Schrappe, P. Reuland, S. D. Gillies, R. A. Reisfeld and D. Neithammer, *Eur J Cancer* 1995; **31A**: 261–267.

**82** J. D. Frost, J. A. Hank, G. H. Reaman, S. R. N. Frierdich, R. C. Seeger, J. Gan, P. M. Anderson, L. J. Ettinger, M. S. Cairo, B. R. Blazar, M. D. Krailo, K. K. Matthay, R. A. Reisfeld and P. M. Sondel, *Cancer* 1997; **80**: 317–333.

**83** H. N. Lode, R. Xiang, N. M. Varki, C. S. Dolman, S. D. Gillies and R. A. Reisfeld, *J Natl Cancer Inst* 1997; **89**: 1586–1594.

**84** R. P. Castleberry, *N Engl J Med* 1999; **340**: 1992–1993.

**85** F. Berthold, K. Sahin, B. Hero, H. Christiansen, M. Gehring, D. Harms, Horz, F. Lampert, M. Schwab and J. Terpe, *Eur J Cancer* 1997; **33**: 2092–2097.

**86** G. M. Brodeur, R. C. Seeger, M. Schwab, H. E. Varmus and J. M. Bishop, *Science* 1984; **224**: 1121–1124.

**87** W. A. Weiss, K. Aldape, G. Mohapatra, B. G. Feuerstein and J. M. Bishop, *EMBO J* 1997; **16**: 2985–2995.

**88** S. Tepmongkol and S. Heyman, *Med Pediatr Oncol* 1999; **32**: 427–431.

**89** Y. Perel, J. Conway, M. Kletzel, J. Goldman, S. Weiss, A. Feyler and S. L. Cohn, *J Pediatr Hematol/Oncol* 1999; **21**: 13–18.

**90** T. Klingebiel, P. Bader, R. Bares, J. Beck, B. Hero, H. Jurgens, P. Lang, D. Niethammer, B. Rath and R. Handgretinger, *Eur J Cancer* 1998; **34**: 1398–1402.

**91** R. Mastrangelo, A. Tornesello and S. Mastrangelo, *Med Pediatr Oncol* 1998; **31**: 22–26.

**92** H. N. Lode, R. Xiang, T. Dreier, N. M. Varki, S. D. Gillies and R. A. Reisfeld, *Blood* 1998; **91**: 1706–1715.

**93** D. H. Raulet, *Curr Opin Immunol* 1996; **8**: 372–377.

**94** D. H. Raulet and W. Held, *Cell* 1995; **82**: 697–700.

**95** J. E. Gumperz and P. Parham, *Nature* 1995; **378**: 245–248.

**96** J. Massague, *Cell* 1987; **49**: 437–438.

**97** T. Roszman, L. Elliott and W. Brooks, *Immunol Today* 1991; **12**: 370–374.

**98** P. A. Ruffini, L. Rivoltini, A. Silvani, A. Boiardi and G. Parmiani, *Cancer Immunol Immunother* 1993; **36**: 409–416.

**99** R. H. Schwartz, *J Exp Med* 1996; **184**: 1–8.

**100** K. A. Smith, *Blood* 1993; **81**: 1414–1423.

**101** M. A. Tigges, L. S. Casey and M. E. Koshland, *Science* 1989; **243**: 781–786.

**102** W. E. Carson, M. J. Lindemann, R. Baiocchi, M. Linett, J. C. Tan, C. C. Chou, S. Narula and M. A. Caligiuri, *Blood* 1995; **85**: 3577–3585.

**103** L. M. Zheng, D. M. Ojcius, F. Garaud, C. Roth, E. Maxwell, Z. Li, H. Rong, J. Chen, X. Y. Wang, J. J. Catino and I. King, *J Exp Med* 1996; **184**: 579–584.

**104** H. N. Lode, T. Dreier, R. Xiang, N. M. Varki, A. S. Kang and R. A. Reisfeld, *Proc Natl Acad Sci USA* 1998; **95**: 2475–2480.

**105** H. N. Lode, R. Xiang, S. R. Duncan, A. N. Theofilopoulos, S. D. Gillies and R. A. Reisfeld, *Proc Natl Acad Sci USA* 1999; **96**: 8591–8596.

**106** L. Holmgren, M. S. O'Reilly and J. Folkman, *Nat Med* 1995; **1**: 149–153.

**107** J. Folkman, *Nat Med* 1995; **1**: 27–31.

**108** M. S. O'Reilly, L. Holmgren, Y. Shing, C. Chen, R. A. Rosenthal, M. Moses, W. S. Lane, Y. Cao, E. H. Sage and J. Folkman, *Cell* 1994; **79**: 315–328.

**109** R. S. Kerbel, *Nature* 1997; **390**: 335–336.

**110** T. Boehm, J. Folkman, T. Browder and M. S. O'Reilly, *Nature* 1997; **390**: 404–407.

**111** O. V. Volpert, J. Lawler and N. P. Bouck, *Proc Natl Acad Sci USA* 1998; **95**: 6343–6348.

**112** P. C. Brooks, R. A. Clark and D. A. Cheresh, *Science* 1994; **264**: 569–571.

**113** M. Friedlander, P. C. Brooks, R. W. Shaffer, C. M. Kincaid, J. A. Varner and D. A. Cheresh, *Science* 1995; **270**: 1500–1502.

**114** P. C. Brooks, A. M. Montgomery, M. Rosenfeld, R. A. Reisfeld, T. Hu, G. Klier and D. A. Cheresh, *Cell* 1994; **79**: 1157–1164.

**115** H. N. Lode, T. Moehler, R. Xiang, A. Jonczyk, S. D. Gillies, D. A. Cheresh and R. A. Reisfeld, *Proc Natl Acad Sci USA* 1999; **96**: 1591–1596.

**116** H. J. Mauceri, N. N. Hanna, M. A. Beckett, D. H. Gorski, M. Staba, K. A. Stellato, K. Bigelow, R. Heimann, S. Gately, M. Dhanabal, G. A. Soff, V. P. Sukhatme, D. W. Kufe and R. R. Weichselbaum, *Nature* 1998; **394**: 287–291.

# 17

# Immunotoxins and Recombinant Immunotoxins in Cancer Therapy

Yoram Reiter and Avital Lev

## 17.1
## Introduction

The rapid progress in the understanding the molecular biology of cancer cells has made a large impact on the design and development of novel therapeutic strategies. These have been developed because treatment of cancer by chemotherapy is limited by a number of factors, and usually fails in patients whose malignant cells are not sufficiently different from normal cells in their growth and metabolism. Other limiting factors are the low therapeutic index of most chemotherapeutic agents, the emergence of drug-resistant populations, tumor heterogeneity and the presence of metastatic disease.

The concept of targeted cancer therapy is thus an important means to improve the therapeutic potential of anticancer agents and a lead to the development of novel approaches such as immunotherapy. The approach of cancer immunotherapy and targeted cancer therapy combines rational drug design with the current advances in our understanding of cancer biology [1–4]. This approach takes advantage of some special properties of cancer cells – many of them contain mutant or over-expressed oncogenes on their surface and these proteins are attractive antigens for targeted therapy. The first cell surface receptor to be linked to cancer was the epidermal growth factor (EGF) receptor present in lung, brain, kidney, bladder, breast and ovarian cancer [5, 6]. Several other members of the EGF receptor family, i.e. erbB2, erbB3 and erbB4 receptors, appear to be abundant on breast and ovary tumors, and erbB2, for example, is the target for phase I and II immunotherapy clinical trials [7, 8].

Other promising candidates for targeted therapy are differentiation antigens that are expressed on the surface of mature cells, but not on the immature stem cells. The most widely studied examples of differentiation antigens currently being used for targeted therapy are expressed by hematopoietic malignancies, and include CD19, CD20 and CD22 on B cell lymphomas and leukemias, and the interleukin (IL-)-2 receptor on T cell leukemias [9–11]. Differentiation antigens have also been found on ovarian, breast and prostate cancer [12–14].

Another class of antigen, termed tumor-associated antigens (TAAs), is made up of molecules which are tightly bound to the surface of cancer cells and are associated with the transformed cancer cells. An example is the carbohydrate antigen Lewis Y

(LeY) that is found in many types of solid tumors [15]. Another class of TAAs includes cancer peptides that are presented by class I MHC molecules on the surface of tumor cells [16, 17].

It should be possible to use these molecular cell surface markers as targets to eliminate the cancer cells while sparing the normal cells. For this approach to be successful, we must generate a targeting moiety which will bind very specifically to the antigen or receptor expressed on the cancer cell surface and arm this targeting moiety with an effector cytotoxic moiety. The targeting moiety can be a specific antibody directed toward the cancer antigen or a ligand for a specific over-expressed receptor. The cytotoxic arm can be a radioisotope, a cytotoxic drug or a toxin. One strategy to

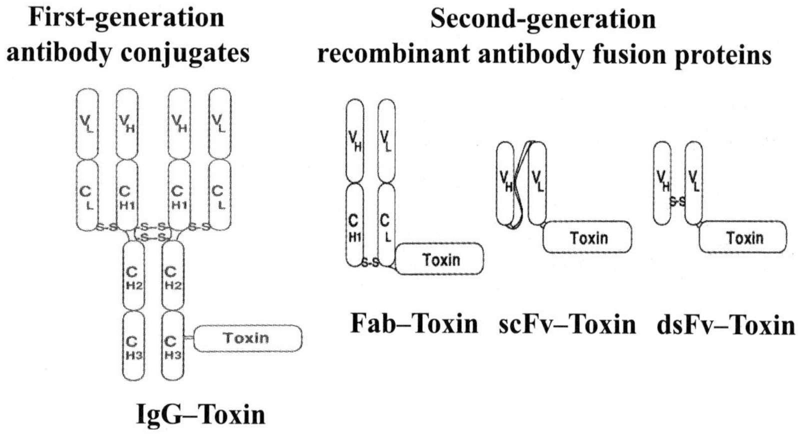

**First-generation antibody conjugates**

**IgG–Toxin**

**Second-generation recombinant antibody fusion proteins**

**Fab–Toxin  scFv–Toxin  dsFv–Toxin**

| | | | |
|---|---|---|---|
| MW: | 200 kDa | 90 kDa | 66 kDa | 64 kDa |
| Composition: | heterogeneous | -------------Homogeneous-------------------- | | |
| IC$_{50}$ in culture: | 3 ng/ml | | 1.5 ng/ml | 1.5 ng/ml |
| Dose for CR: | 0.75 mg/kg | | 0.063 mg/kg | 0.075 mg/kg |
| T$_{1/2}$ in circulation: | 8 h | | 20 min | 23 min |
| Tumor penetration: | fair | | good | good |

**Fig. 17.1** Immunotoxins for targeted cancer therapy. First-generation immunotoxins are whole mAbs to which the toxin is chemically conjugated. Second-generation immunotoxins are made by recombinant DNA technology by fusing recombinant antibody fragments to the toxin (usually a truncated or mutated form of the toxin). Three types of recombinant antibody fragments are used as the targeting moiety in recombinant immunotoxins. Fabs are composed of the light chain and the heavy chain Fd fragment (V$_H$ and C$_H$1), connected to each other via the interchain disulfide bond between C$_L$ and C$_H$1. scFv fragments are stabilized by a peptide linker which connects the C-terminus of V$_H$ or V$_L$ with the N-terminus of the other domain. The V$_H$ and V$_L$ heterodimer in dsFv is stabilized by engineering a disulfide bond between the two domains. The biochemical and biological properties described in the lower part of the figure are depicted for B3–lysPE38 (LMB-1) [89] (a first-generation antibody–PE chemical conjugate), B3(Fv)–PE38 (LMB-7) [67] (second-generation recombinant scFv–immunotoxin for a scFv–immunotoxin) and B3(dsFv)–PE38 (LMB-9) [74] (for a second-generation recombinant dsFv–immunotoxin].

achieve this is to arm antibodies that target cancer cells with powerful toxins that can originate from both plants and bacteria. The molecules generated are termed recombinant immunotoxins.

The goal of immunotoxin therapy is to target a very potent cytotoxic agent to cell surface molecules which will internalize then the cytotoxic agent, resulting in cell death. Developing this type of therapy has gained much interest in recent years. Since immunotoxins differ greatly from chemotherapy in their mode of action and toxicity profile, it is hoped that immunotoxins will have the potential to improve the systemic treatment of tumors incurable with existing modes of therapy.

As shown in Fig. 17.1, immunotoxins can be divided into two groups: chemical conjugates (or first-generation immunotoxins) and second-generation (or recombinant) immunotoxins. They both contain toxins that have their cell-binding domains either mutated or deleted to prevent them from binding to normal cells and are either fused or chemically conjugated to a ligand or an antibody specific for cancer cells (Tab. 17.1).

This chapter will summarize our current understanding of the design and application of second-generation recombinant Fv–immunotoxins, which utilize recombinant antibody fragments as the targeting moiety, in the treatment of cancer, and will also discuss briefly the use of recombinant antibody fragments for other modes of cancer therapy and diagnosis.

**Tab. 17.1**  Examples of recombinant immunotoxins against cancer

| Immunotoxin | Antigen | Toxin | Cancer | Clinical trial | Reference |
|---|---|---|---|---|---|
| Anti-CD7–dgA | CD7 | ricin | non-Hodgkin's lymphoma | phase I | 191 |
| DAB$_{389}$–IL-2 | IL-2 receptor | DT | T cell lymphoma, Hodgkin's disease | phase III | 136, 139 |
| Anti-Tac (Fv)–PE38 (LMB-2) | CD25 | PE | B and T lymphoma, leukemias | phase I | 80, 95 |
| DT–anti-Tac(Fv) | CD25 | DT | leukemias, lymphoma | – | 91 |
| RFB4(dsFv)–PE38 | CD22 | PE | B leukemias | phase I | 90 |
| Di-dgA–RFB4 | CD22 | ricin | leukemias, non-Hodgkin's lymphoma | – | 98 |
| B3–lysPE38 (LMB-1) | LeY | PE | carcinomas | phase I | 103 |
| B3(Fv)–PE38 (LMB-7) | LeY | PE | carcinomas | phase I | 81 |
| B3(dsFv)–PE38 (LMB-9) | LeY | PE | carcinoma | phase I | 88 |
| BR96(sFv)–PE40 | LeY | PE | carcinoma | – | 109 |
| e23(Fv)–PE38 | erbB2/HER2 | PE | breast cancer | phase I | 82 |
| FRP5(scFv)ETA | erbB2/HER2 | PE | breast cancer | – | 110 |
| Tf–CRM107 | transferrin receptor | DT | glioma | phase I | 117 |
| HB21(Fv)–PE40 | transferrin receptor | PE | various | – | 69 |
| MR1(Fv)–PE38 | mutant EGF receptor | PE | liver, brain tumors | – | 113 |
| SS1(Fv)–PE38 | mesothelin | PE | ovarian cancer | – | 114 |

## 17.2
## First- and Second-Generation Immunotoxins

First-generation immunotoxins were made in the early 1970s and were composed of cancer-specific monoclonal antibodies (mAbs) to which native bacterial or plant toxins were chemically conjugated. The understanding of toxin structure–function properties, and the advancement in recombinant DNA technology and antibody engineering lead to important breakthroughs in the late 1980s to construct second-generation recombinant immunotoxins that are composed of recombinant antibody fragments derived from cancer-specific antibodies or phage-display libraries and truncated forms of toxins. These molecules are produced in large amounts, needed for preclinical and clinical studies, in bacteria and feature better clinical properties.

As shown in Fig. 17.1, first- and second-generation immunotoxins contain toxins that have their cell-binding domains either mutated or deleted to prevent them from binding to normal cells, and are either chemically conjugated or fused to a ligand or an antibody specific for cancer cells.

First-generation immunotoxins, composed of whole antibodies chemically conjugated to toxins, demonstrated the feasibility of this concept. Cancer cells cultured *in vitro* could be killed under conditions in which the immunotoxin demonstrated low toxicity towards cultured normal cells. Clinical trials with these agents had some success; however, they also revealed several problems, such as non-specific toxicity towards some normal cells, difficulties in production and, particularly for the treatment of solid tumors, poor tumor penetration due to their large size.

Second-generation immunotoxins have overcome many of these problems. Progress in the elucidation of the toxin's structure and function combined with the techniques of protein engineering facilitated the design and construction of recombinant molecules with a higher specificity for cancer cells and reduced toxicity to normal cells. At the same time, advances in recombinant DNA technology and antibody engineering enabled the generation of small antibody fragments. Thus, it was possible to decrease the size of immunotoxins significantly and to improve their tumor-penetration potential *in vivo*. The development of advanced methods of recombinant protein production enabled the large-scale production of recombinant immunotoxins of high purity and quality for clinical use in sufficient quantities to perform clinical trials.

Another strategy to target cancer cells is to construct chimeric toxins in which the engineered truncated portion of the toxin [*Pseudomonas* exotoxin (PE) or diphtheria toxin (DT)] gene is fused to cDNA encoding growth factors or cytokines. These include transforming growth factor (TGF)-β [18], insulin-like growth factor (IGF)-1 [19], acidic and basic fibroblast growth factor (FGF) [20], IL-2 [21], IL-4 [22], and IL-6 [23]. These recombinant toxins (oncotoxins) are designed to target specific tumor cells that over-express these receptors (Fig. 17.1).

In the following sections we will summarize the rationale and current knowledge on the design and application of second-generation recombinant Fv–immunotoxins, which utilize recombinant antibody fragments as the targeting moiety. Recent results of clinical trials are summarized. We will also discuss the powerful new technologies for selecting new antibodies with unique specificities and improved properties.

## 17.3
## The Development of Recombinant DNA-based Immunotoxins: Design of Recombinant Immunotoxins

### 17.3.1
### The Toxin Moiety

The toxins that are most commonly used to make immunotoxins are ricin, DT and PE. These toxins belong to a group of polypeptide enzymes that catalytically inactivate protein synthesis leading to cell death. Some of these toxins have been shown to induce apoptosis [24, 25].

The genes for these toxins have been cloned and expressed in *Escherichia coli*, and the crystal structures of all three proteins have been solved [50, 55]. This information, in combination with mutational studies, has elucidated which toxin subunits are involved in their biological activity and, most importantly, the different steps of the cytocidal process. DT, PE, ricin and their derivatives have all been successfully used to prepare immunotoxin conjugates [3, 26], but only PE- and DT-containing fusion proteins generate active recombinant immunotoxins [1, 27]. This is because the toxic moiety must be separated from the binding moiety after internalization [28, 29]. PE and DT fusion proteins generate their free toxic moieties by proteolytic processing. Ricin does not possess such a proteolytic processing site and therefore cannot be attached to the targeting moiety with a peptide bond without losing cytotoxic activity. Recently, proteolytic processing sites were introduced into ricin by recombinant DNA techniques to try to overcome this problem [30].

#### 17.3.1.1  Plant toxins
Ricin, or the ricin A chain fragment, has been a commonly used toxin for conjugation to antibodies. Ricin is synthesized as single polypeptide chains and processed post-translationally into two subunits. A and B linked though a disulfide bond. Ricin is a 65-kDa glycoprotein purified from the seeds of the castor bean (*Ricinus communis*). It is composed of an A subunit which kills cells by catalytically inactivating ribosomes. The A subunit is linked by a disulfide bond to a B subunit which is responsible for cell binding. The B chain is a galactose-specific lectin that binds to galactose residues present on cell surface glycoproteins and glycolipids [31]. Once the B subunit of ricin binds to the cell membrane, the protein enters the cell through coated pits and endocytic vesicles. The A and B subunits of ricin are separated by a process involving disulfide bond reduction. The A subunit of ricin translocates across an intracellular membrane to the cell cytosol, probably with the assistance of the B subunit. In the cytosol, it arrests protein synthesis by enzymatically inactivating the 28S subunit of eukaryotic ribosomes [32, 33]. Because native ricin is highly toxic and lacks specificity, several modified forms of ricin have been developed to prepare immunotoxins that are better tolerated by patients.

To decrease the non-specific binding of whole ricin, the A chain alone has been coupled to antibodies. The A chain is obtained by reducing the disulfide bond that links it to the B chain. Immunotoxins composed of the ricin A chain coupled to well-internalized antibodies can be highly cytotoxic [34]. In the absence of the B chain (the binding subunit), however, immunotoxins made with poorly internalized antibodies are not cytotoxic.

Immunotoxins containing the ricin A chain are rapidly cleared from the circulation by the liver by the binding of mannose and fucose residues of the A chain to receptors present on the reticuloendothelial system and hepatocytes. To circumvent this problem, these carbohydrate residues were chemically modified [35], resulting in a deglycosylated A chain (dgA) molecule. In preclinical studies, dgA-containing immunotoxins were found to have longer half-lives in the circulation and better antitumor efficacy *in vivo* [36]. Also, recombinant A chain produced in *E. coli* can be used in place of dgA because it is devoid of carbohydrate and is not rapidly cleared by the liver.

Another strategy to decrease the non-specific toxicity of native ricin is to block the galactose-binding sites of the B chain by cross-linking with glycopeptide [37] or to use short cross-linkers to connect the antibody to the toxin so that the galactose-binding site is sterically blocked by the antibody [38]. Blocked ricin retains a low affinity for galactose-binding sites, which enhances internalization and cytotoxicity of an antibody that binds to a poorly internalized antigen.

Other plant toxins commonly used for clinical immunotoxin construction are saporin and pokeweed antiviral protein, which are single polypeptide chains that inactivate ribosomes in a similar fashion to ricin. Because these toxins lack the binding chain (B chain), they are relatively non-toxic to cells and are used for immunotoxin production [39–42].

### 17.3.1.2 Bacterial toxins: DT and DT derivatives

DT is a 58-kDa protein, secreted by pathogenic *Corynebacterium diphtheria*, which contains a lysogenic β phage [43]. DT ADP-ribosylates eukaryotic elongation factor (EF)-2 at a "diphthamide" residue located at His415, using $NAD^+$ as a cofactor [44]. This modification arrests protein synthesis and subsequently leads to cell death [45]. Only a few, and perhaps only one, DT molecules need to reach the cytosol in order to kill a cell. When DT is isolated from the culture medium of C. *diphtheria* it is composed of an N-terminal 21-kDa A subunit and a C-terminal 37-kDa B subunit held together by a disulfide bond. DT is the expression product of a single gene [43], which when secreted into the medium is processed into two fragments by extracellular proteases. When DT is produced as a recombinant single-chain protein in *E. coli*, it is not cleaved by the bacteria, but is instead cleaved by a protease in the target cells [46]. The A domain of DT contains its enzymatic activity. The N-terminus of the B subunit of DT (or the region between A and B in single-chain DT) mediates translocation of the A subunit into the cytoplasm. The B domain, especially its C-terminus, is responsible for the binding of DT to target cells. Deletions or mutations in this part of the molecule abolish or greatly diminish the binding and toxicity of DT [47–49]. DT enters cells via coated pits and is proteolytically cleaved within the endocytic compartment, if it is not already in the two-chain form, and reduced. It also undergoes a conformational change at the acidic pH present in endosomes, which probably assists translocation of the A chain into the cytosol, perhaps via a pore-like structure mediated by the B chain [50–52]. Derivatives of DT that are used to make immunotoxins have the C-terminus altered by mutations or partially deleted

(DAB486, DAB389 and DT388), but retain the translocation and ADP-ribosylation activity of DT [53]. Recombinant antibody fusion proteins with such derivatives target only cells that bind the antibody moiety of the immunotoxin.

### 17.3.1.3 Bacterial toxins: PE and PE derivatives

Two major research studies have enabled the use and genetic manipulation of PE for the design of immunotoxins [1–3]: (1) the elucidation of the crystal structure of PE, showing the toxin to be composed of three major structural domains, and (2) the finding that these domains are different functional modules of the toxin.

PE is a single-chain 66-kDa molecule secreted by *P. aeruginosa* that, like DT, irreversibly ADP-ribosylates the diphthamide residue of EF-2, using NAD$^+$ as cofactor [54]. As a consequence, protein synthesis is inhibited and cell death ensues. PE is composed of three major domains [55]. Different functions have been assigned to each domain by mutational analysis [56]. The N-terminal domain la mediates binding to the $\alpha_2$-macroglobulin receptor [57]. Domain lb is a small domain that lies between domains II and III, and has no known function [58]. Domain II mediates translocation of domain III, the C-terminal ADP-ribosylating domain, into the cytosol of target cells [59] (Fig. 17.2). Translocation occurs after internalization of the

**Fig. 17.2** The biological activity of PE A. The Fv portion of the immunotoxin targets domains II and III of PE to a cell surface receptor or other target molecule on the tumor cell (A). The immunotoxin enters the cell by internalization and is transferred into the endosome (B). Within the endosome the molecule unfolds due to a fall in pH. The conformational change exposes a proteolytic site, and a proteolytic cleavage occurs in the translocation domain between amino acids 279 and 280 (C). A disulfide bond is then broken, thus creating two fragments: the Fv moiety and a small part of domain II, and the rest of domain II connected to domain III (D). The C-terminal fragment containing the ADP-ribosylation domain (domain III) and most of the translocation domain (domain II) is carried into the endoplasmic reticulum (E), and translocation occurs from the endoplasmic reticulum into the cytosol (F). The enzymatically active domain ADP-ribosylates EF-2 at a diphtamide residue located at His415, using NAD$^+$ as a cofactor. This modification arrests protein synthesis and subsequently leads to cell death by apoptosis. In DT, the poteolytic processing occurs between residues 193 and 194. The catalytic A chain (amino acids 1–193) then translocates to the cytosol through the endosome with the help of translocation domain residues 326–347 and 358–376 which form an ion channel.

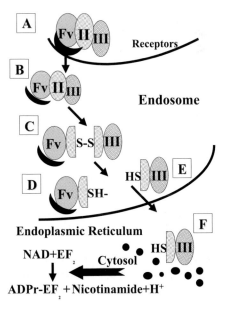

toxin and after a variety of other steps including a pH-induced conformational change [60–62], proteolytic cleavage at a specific site in domain II [29], and a reductive step that separates the amino and carboxyl fragments. Ultimately, the C-terminal portion of PE is translocated from the endoplasmic reticulum into the cytosol. Despite a similar mode of action of PE and DT, which is ADP-ribosylation, and a similar initial pathway of cell entry (internalization via coated pits and endocytic vesicles) and of processing (proteolytic cleavage and a reductive step), they share almost no sequence homology. The only similarity is the spatial arrangement of key residues in their active sites that are arranged around residue Glu553 in PE and Glu145 in DT [63–66].

When the whole toxin is used to make an immunotoxin, non-specific toxicity occurs mainly due to binding of the toxin portion to cells, mediated by the binding domain. Consequently, the goal of making improved derivatives of PE-based immunotoxins has been to inactivate or remove the binding domain. Molecules in which the binding domain has been retained but inactivated by mutations were made [67]; however, a better alternative to inactivating the cell-binding domain by mutations is to remove it from PE. The prototype molecule with this sort of deletion is PE40 (amino acids 253–613, MW 40 kDa]. Because PE40 and its derivatives described below lack the binding domain (amino acids 1–252), they have very low non-specific toxicity, but make very active and specific immunotoxins when fused to recombinant antibodies [68, 69]. Currently, almost all PE-derived recombinant immunotoxins are constructed with PE38 (MW 38 kDa), a PE40 derivative that has, in addition to the deletion of domain Ia, a second deletion encompassing a portion of domain Ib (amino acids 365–379) [58]. Another useful mutation is to change the C-terminal sequence of PE from REDLK to KDEL. This improves the cytotoxicity of PE and its derivatives, presumably by increasing their delivery to the endoplasmic reticulum where translocation takes place [70, 71].

## 17.3.2
### The Targeting Moiety – Recombinant Antibody Fragments

The antibody moiety of the recombinant immunotoxin is responsible for specifically directing the immunotoxin to the target cell, thus the usefulness of the immunotoxin depends on the specificity of the antibody or antibody fragment that is connected to the toxin. Consequently, for the construction of recombinant immunotoxins, the only antibodies that should be used are those that recognize antigens that are expressed on target cancer cells and are not present on normal cells, present at very low levels or are only present on less-essential cells (Tab. 17.1). Receptors for growth factors like EGF, IL-2, IL-4, IL-6 or erbB2 are common targets for targeted cancer therapy because they are highly expressed on many cancer cells. Other carcinoma-related antigens include developmental antigens such as complex carbohydrates, which are often highly abundant on the surface of cancer cells.

The use of antibodies for immunotoxin production also requires that the antibody–antigen complex be internalized, because the mechanism of PE-toxin killing requires endocytosis as a first step in the entry of the toxin into the cell.

Recombinant immunotoxins contain antibody fragments as the targeting moiety. These fragments can be produced in *E. coli*, and are the result of intensive research and development in recombinant-antibody technologies [72–74]. Several antibody fragments have been used to construct recombinant immunotoxins (Fig. 17.1). One type contains Fab fragments in which the light chain and the heavy chain Fd fragment ($V_H$ and $C_H1$) are connected to each other via an interchain disulfide bond between $C_L$ and $C_H1$. The toxin moiety can be fused to the carboxyl end of either $C_L$ or $C_H1$. Fabs can be produced in *E. coli*, either by secretion, with co-expression of light chains and Fd fragments or by expression of the chains in intracellular inclusion bodies in separate cultures; in the latter case, they are reconstituted by a refolding reaction using a redox-shuffling buffer system. Several immunotoxins with Fab fragments have been constructed and produced in this way [1–4, 75].

The smallest functional modules of antibodies required for antigen binding are Fv fragments. This makes them especially useful for clinical applications, not only for generating recombinant immunotoxins, but also for tumor imaging, because their small size improves tumor penetration. Fv fragments are heterodimers of the variable heavy chain ($V_H$) and the variable light chain ($V_L$) domains. Unlike whole IgG or Fab, in which the heterodimers are held together and stabilized by interchain disulfide bonds, the $V_H$ and $V_L$ of Fvs are not covalently connected and are consequently unstable; this instability can be overcome by making recombinant Fvs that have the $V_H$ and $V_L$ covalently connected by a peptide linker that fuses the C terminus of the $V_L$ or $V_H$ to the N-terminus of the other domain (Fig. 17.1). These molecules are termed single-chain Fvs (scFvs) [76, 77], and many retain the specificity and affinity of the original antibody. The cloning, construction and composition of recombinant Fv fragments of antibodies and Fv–immunotoxins are described in Fig. 17.3.

Many recombinant immunotoxins have been constructed using scFvs, in which molecules the scFv gene is fused to PE38 to generate a potent cytotoxic agent with targeted specificity [1–4, 78–84] (Figs 17.1 and 17.3).

Until recently, the construction of scFvs was the only general method available to make stable Fvs. However, many scFvs are unstable or have reduced affinity for the antigen compared with the parent antibody or Fab fragment. This is because the linker interferes with binding or because the linker does not sufficiently stabilize the Fv structure, leading to aggregation and loss of activity. This is particularly true at physiological temperatures (37 °C). To overcome these problems, an alternative strategy has been developed that involves generating stable Fvs by connecting the $V_H$ and $V_L$ domains by an interchain disulfide bond engineered between structurally conserved framework residues of the Fv; these molecules are termed disulfide-stabilized Fvs (dsFvs) [74, 85–87]. The positions at which the cysteine residues were to be placed were identified by computer-based molecular modeling; as they are located in the framework of each $V_H$ and $V_L$, this location can be used as a general method to stabilize almost all Fvs without the need for any structural information. Many dsFvs have been constructed in the past 3 years (mainly as dsFv–immunotoxins, in which the dsFv is fused to PE38) and they show several advantages over scFvs [74, 88–90]. In addition to their increased stability (due to a decreased tendency to aggregate), they

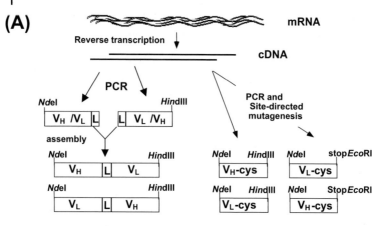

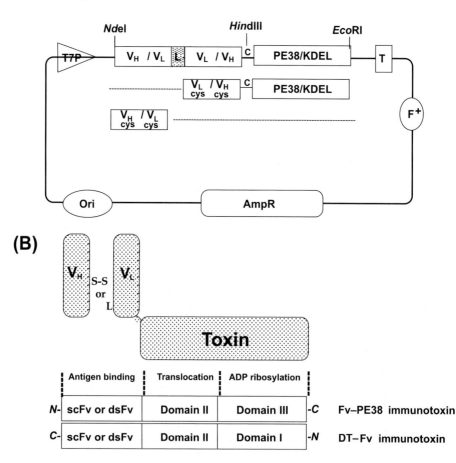

are often produced in higher yields than scFvs; in several cases, the binding affinity of the dsFv was significantly improved over that of the scFv.

## 17.4
## Construction and Production of Recombinant Immunotoxins

In the recombinant immunotoxins derived from PE, the recombinant antibody fragments are fused to the N-terminus of the truncated derivative of PE (with the cell-binding domain deleted, e.g. PE40 or PE38). This restores the original domain arrangement of PE, which consists of an N-terminal-binding domain followed by the translocation domain and the C-terminal ADP-ribosylation domain.

Only fusions of an antigen-binding domain (Fv) to the N-terminus of truncated PE are active; C-terminal fusions are not active because the bulky antigen-binding domain blocks translocation of the C-terminal fragment into the cytoplasm [1, 27].

DT immunotoxins are fusions of mutated DT with antigen-binding regions of a recombinant antibody. However, in this case the antigen-binding domain must be

---

◀ **Fig. 17.3** Cloning, construction and composition of scFv– and dsFv–immunotoxins. (A) Cloning and construction of recombinant scFv– and dsFv–immunotoxins. The genes encoding the $V_H$ and $V_L$ variable domains are cloned usually from hybridoma mRNA by reverse transcription, cDNA synthesis and subsequent PCR amplification using degenerate primers that are complementary to the 5′ or 3′ end of the $V_H$ and $V_L$ genes, or by primers which are designed according to the N-terminal amino acid sequence of the mAb to be cloned and conserved sequences at the N-terminal of the heavy and light constant regions. The variable genes can be also cloned by constant domains primers and using the RACE rapid amplification of cDNA ends (method). Restriction sites for assembling the peptide linker sequence which connects the $V_H$ and $V_L$ domains, and for cloning into the expression vector are also introduced by PCR. Construction of dsFv involves the generation of two expression plasmids which encode the two components of the dsFv $V_H$-Cys and $V_L$-Cys. The cysteines are introduced in position 44 in FR2 of $V_H$ and position 100 of FR4 of $V_L$ or position 105 of FR4 in $V_H$ and position 43 of FR2 in $V_L$ (numbering system of Kabat *et al.*) by site-directed mutagenesis using as template a uracil-containing single-stranded DNA of the scFv construct from the F+ origin present in the expression plasmid and co-transfection with M13 helper phage. In addition to the cysteines, cloning sites, ATG translation initiation codons and stop codons are introduced at the 5′ and 3′ ends and of the $V_H$ and $V_L$ genes as shown by site-directed mutagenesis or PCR. The antibody variable genes are subcloned into an expression vector which contains the gene for a truncated form of PE. This expression vector is controlled by the T7 promoter and upon induction of the T7 RNA polymerase, which is under the control of the *lac*UV5 promoter, in *E. coli* BL21 λDE3 by IPTG, large amounts of recombinant protein are produced. (B) Composition of recombinant immunotoxins. In PE-derived recombinant Fv–immunotoxins, the Fv region of the targeting antibody is fused to the N-terminus of a truncated form of PE which contains the translocation domain (domain II) and enzymatically active ADP-ribosylation domain (domain III). The cell-binding domain of whole PE (domain I) is replaced by the Fv targeting moiety thus, preserving the relative position of the binding domain function to the other functional domains of PE. In the dsFv–immunotoxins there are two components. In one, the $V_H$ or $V_L$ domains are fused to the N-terminus of the truncated PE and, in the other, the variable domain is covalently linked by the engineered disulfide bond. DT-derived immunotoxins are fused to the C-terminus due to the inverse arrangement of the functional modules of PE and DT.

fused to the C-terminus of DT [91, 92]. This corresponds to the inverse arrangement of the functional modules of PE and DT (see Fig. 17.3). DT immunotoxins are active only when the enzymatically active N-terminal domain is free to translocate into the cytosol.

The expression vectors used for DT immunotoxins are very similar to those used with PE with the exception that the DNA fragments encoding the binding moiety are ligated to the 3′-end of the DT coding region. The cloning of the antibody variable regions is performed using cloning techniques that are now well established (Fig. 17.3) [73]. The plasmid vector for the expression of scFv–immunotoxins or the components of dsFv–immunotoxins is a high-copy-number plasmid derived from vectors made and described by Studier and Moffatt [93]. These contain the T7 promoter, translation initiation signals and a transcription terminator, as well as an F+ phage replication origin to generate single-stranded DNA to be used for site-directed mutagenesis.

When these plasmids are transformed into *E. coli* BL21/DE3 (which contain the T7 RNA polymerase gene under the control of the *lac*UV5 promoter) they generate large amounts of recombinant protein upon IPTG induction. The recombinant scFv–immunotoxin or the components of the dsFv–immunotoxin accumulate in insoluble intracellular inclusion bodies. [dsFv–immunotoxins require two cultures, one expressing the $V_H$ and one expressing the $V_L$; the toxin moiety (PE38) can be fused to either the $V_H$ or the $V_L$.] The inclusion bodies are then isolated, purified, solubilized, reduced and subsequently used in a refolding reaction that is controlled for oxidation (redox shuffling). In the case of dsFv–immunotoxins, solubilized inclusion bodies of $V_H$ and $V_L$ (with the toxin fused to either) are mixed in a 1:1 molar ratio into the refolding solution. The formation of the interchain disulfide bond between the $V_H$ and $V_L$ domains is promoted by inducing oxidation using excess oxidized glutathione or by refolding at high pH. The immunotoxins are then purified from the refolding mixtures by ion-exchange and size-exclusion chromatography. Approximately 20 mg of clinical-grade active immunotoxin can be obtained from 1 l of a fermentor culture induced with IPTG.

## 17.5
### Preclinical Development of Recombinant Immunotoxins

A wide variety of recombinant immunotoxins have been made and tested against cancer target cells. If found to be active and are considered to be tested in clinical trials, they undergo several years of preclinical development to determine their efficacy and toxicity in several *in vitro* and *in vivo* experimental models (Tab. 17.2).

The initial phase is the characterization of the biological activity of the immunotoxin on cultured tumor cells. These assays include measurement of cell-free enzymatic activity, i.e. ADP-ribosylation activity in the case of bacterial toxins, and the binding affinity of the immunotoxin to the target antigen, which can be determined on purified antigen, on cells by binding displacement assays or by surface plasmon resonance assays. Cytotoxicity assays are performed on antigen-bearing cells and mea-

**Tab. 17.2** Functional properties *in vitro* and *in vivo* of PE-based recombinant Fv–immunotoxins

| Immunotoxin | Specificity | Activity in vitro (IC$_{50}$, ng/ml) | Binding affinity (K$_d$, nM) | Antitumor activity in vivo (xenograft model) |
|---|---|---|---|---|
| Anti-Tac(Fv)–PE38 (LMB-2) | CD25 | 0.15 | 1.4 | complete regressions/ cures (ATAC4) |
| B3(Fv)–PE38 (LMB-7) | LeY | 1.5 | 1300 | complete regressions/ cures (A431) |
| B3(dsFv)–PE38 (LMB-9) | LeY | 1.5 | 24000 | complete regressions/ cures (A431) |
| e23(Fv)–PE38 (erb-38) | erbB2/HER2 | 0.3 | 40 | partial regressions (A431) |
| RFB4(dsFv)–PE38 (BL22) | CD22 | 10 | 10 | partial and some complete regressions (CA46) |
| SS1(Fv)–PE38 | mesothelin | 0.5 | 11 | complete regressions/ cures (A431-K5) |
| MR1(Fv)–PE38 | mutant EGF receptor | 3.0 | 11 | partial regressions (glioblastoma) |
| 55.1(Fv)–PE38 | mucin carbohydrate | 0.3 | 80 | complete regressions (Colo205) |

sure either inhibition of protein synthesis, proliferation, colony counts or cell viability.

Cytotoxicity assays on malignant, single-cell suspensions directly obtained from patients are a very useful test, if available, since such cells contain the physiological numbers of receptor or target density which in many cases is lower than established cell lines [94–96]. The stability of recombinant immunotoxins *in vitro* in various physiological buffers or human serum is also an important test to predict their stability *in vivo* [74]. *In vivo* efficacy of recombinant immunotoxins is usually demonstrated in immunodeficient mice bearing xenografts of human tumor cells. The tumor xenografts can be established as subcutaneous solid tumors, orthotopic implants or disseminated leukemia [97–99].

Initial toxicity and pharmacokinetics studies have also been performed in mice; however, many target antigens are present at some level on some normal tissues, and thus toxicology and pharmacokinetics studies should be tested in an animal that has normal cells capable of binding the target antigen. For most immunotoxins, this requires studies in monkeys to test for targeted damage to normal tissues to predict whether such damage will occur in humans [100, 101].

**17.6**
**Application of Recombinant Immunotoxins**

17.6.1
**Recombinant Immunotoxins against Solid Tumors**

The treatment of solid tumors with immunotoxins is challenging due to their physiological nature of tight junctions between tumor cells, high interstitial pressure within tumors and heterogeneous blood supply, and also antigen expression [102]. The greatest need for new therapies is in the treatment of metastatic epithelial cancers, and immunotoxins can be a useful addition to the standard procedures of surgery, radiation and chemotherapy.

As already described, the use of recombinant fragments of antibodies for making recombinant immunotoxins is especially useful for the treatment of solid tumors because their small size improves tumor penetration. Over recent years, several recombinant immunotoxins that target solid tumors have been developed (Tab. 17.2); targets include breast, lung, gastric, bladder and central nervous system cancers. They are at different stages of clinical development and some are already employed in clinical trials [1–4].

mAb B3 is an antibody that reacts with the LeY antigen present on cancers of the colon, breast, stomach, lung and bladder [15]. Early trials with a first-generation immunotoxin (LMB-1) in which an antibody to LeY (mAb B3) was used to make a chemical conjugate with PE38 showed significant clinical activity, with responses in colon and breast cancer [103, 104]. The one complete response and one partial response observed in this trial were the first major responses to immunotoxins documented for metastatic breast and colon cancer, respectively.

The B3 antibody was then used to make a single-chain immunotoxin termed B3(Fv)–PE38 or LMB-7 [81]. LMB-7 has shown good activity against human cancer xenografts growing in mice [105] and it is also able to cure carcinomatous meningitis in rats when given by the intrathecal route [106]. A phase I clinical trial with LMB-7 began in 1995 and is nearing completion. During the trial, it became evident that LMB-7 lost activity when incubated at 37 °C because of aggregation [86, 107], which greatly limited its ability to penetrate solid tumors.

B3(dsFv)–PE38 (LMB-9) is the dsFv version of LMB-7 [107] with stability improved over that of LMB-7. This improved stability also allowed it to be used in a continuous-infusion mode in mice bearing human tumor xenografts; this route of administration showed an improved therapeutic window over a bolus injection [108]. Clinical trials with LMB-9 started in the middle of 1998. A different recombinant single-chain immunotoxin, BR96(scFv)–PE40 was derived from the anti-LeY mAb BR96 and is also currently undergoing clinical testing [109].

Monoclonal antibody e23 is directed at erbB2 (Her2/*neu*), which is highly expressed in many breast, lung, ovarian and stomach cancers. e23(dsFv)–PE38 is a dsFv–immunotoxin composed of the Fv portion of the e23 antibody and PE38 [68]. This dsFv–immunotoxin has a significantly improved binding affinity and stability compared with its scFv analogue, e23(Fv)–PE38 [75]. FRP5scFv–ETA is also a recombi-

nant immunotoxin targeting erbB2 [110]. Clinical trials with e23(Fv)–PE38 were initiated in early 1998. In a phase I study on breast cancer patients, hepatotoxicity was
observed in all patients. Immunohistochemistry showed the presence of erbB2 on
hepatocytes, explaining the liver toxicity of the immunotoxin. This study demonstrated that targeting of tumors with antibodies to erbB2 armed with toxic agents or
radioisotopes may result in unexpected organ toxicity due to the expression of the
target antigen on normal cells [111].

Other recombinant immunotoxins that have been constructed and have antitumor
activities *in vitro* and in mouse models *in vivo* include: B1(Fv)–PE38, also directed
against the LeY antigen [112]; 55.1(Fv)–PE38 and 55.1(dsFv)–PE38, which are directed at a carbohydrate mucin antigen over-expressed in colon cancers [84];
MR1(Fv)–PE38, constructed by antibody phage-display technology and directed to
a mutant EGF receptor over-expressed in liver and brain tumors [113]; and
SS(Fv)–PE38, a new recombinant immunotoxin specific for mesothelin, a differentiation antigen present on the surface of ovarian cancers, mesotheliomas and several other types of human cancers [114]. SS(Fv)–PE38 was constructed from an Fv
fragment that was isolated by antibody phage display from mice that underwent
DNA immunization with a plasmid expressing the cloned antigen [114]. This approach to antibody formation eliminates the need for the production of proteins
for immunization.

Immunotoxins were also used to target tumors of the central nervous system. Since
the transferrin receptor is expressed on tumor and normal hepatic cells, but not in
normal brain, several trials have targeted anti-transferrin receptor immunotoxins to
brain tumors. These include a conjugate of mAb 454A12 with a recombinant form
of ricin A (plant toxin) [115], a conjugate of human transferrin with a mutant form
of DT [116, 117] and chimeric toxin of recombinant IL-4–PE38 fusion [118, 119].

### 17.6.2
### Recombinant Immunotoxins against Leukemias and Lymphomas

Conventional immunotoxins, in which IgGs or Fabs are coupled to toxins, have also
been used to target leukemias and lymphomas. This approach should be quite effective because many of the tumor cells are in the blood and bone marrow, where they
are readily accessible to the drug. Moreover, fresh cells from patients may be easily
tested for immunotoxin binding and cytotoxic activity.

Immunotoxins have also been developed for indirect treatment of malignancies by
their killing of T cells that mediate graft-versus-host disease (GvHD) in the setting of
allogeneic transplantation. Clinical trials using ricin-based immunoconjugates for
treatment of leukemias have shown some promising results, but dose escalation has
been limited by the side effects of the toxin [2]. In addition, it is important to eliminate not only easily accessible tumor cells, but also malignant cells that are less accessible. Therefore, even for leukemias, there is a need to develop small recombinant
immunotoxins that will reach cells outside the circulation. Recombinant immunotoxins targeted at leukemia and lymphoma antigens have been made with antibody
fragments specific for the subunit of the IL-2 receptor (CD25) and for CD22. In addi-

tion, growth factor fusion proteins have been made that target the IL-2, IL-4, IL-6 and granulocyte macrophage colony stimulating factor (GM-CSF) receptors.

The most potent immunotoxin produced against leukemia cells is anti-Tac(Fv)–PE38 (LMB-2); this targets CD25, which is over-expressed on many T cell leukemias [11, 80]. LMB-2 is very active against leukemia cell lines *in vitro* and has very good activity in animal models [121]. It also selectively kills cells *in vitro* obtained from patients with adult T cell leukemia without harming hematopoietic stem cells [95, 96]. Phase I clinical trials with LMB-2 are showing promising results [108, 109]. The immuno-toxin was administered to 35 patients for a total of 59 treatment cycles. One hairy cell leukemia (HCL) patient achieved a complete remission, which is ongoing at 20 months. Seven partial responses were observed in cutaneous T cell lymphoma, HCL, chronic lymphocytic leukemia, Hodgkin's disease and adult T cell leukemia. Re-sponding patients had a 2–5 log reduction of circulating malignant cells, improve-ment in skin lesions, and regression of lymphomatous mass and splenomegally. All four patients with HCL responded to the treatment (one with complete responses and three had 98–99.8% reductions in malignant circulating cells). A phase II trial is planned in patients with CD25$^+$ hematologic malignancies and phase I trials are planned for the prevention of GvHD in patients undergoing high-risk allotransplan-tation [124].

The conventional immunotoxin RFT5–SMPT–dgA has also been developed to target CD25 and has resulted in several responses in Hodgkin's disease, one of which lasted over 2 years [125, 126]. It is already undergoing testing for the prevention of GvHD in patients undergoing allotransplantation and has recently been shown *ex vivo* to remove alloreactive donor T cells while preserving antileukemia and antiviral T cell responses [127].

A new agent, RFB4(dsFv)–PE38 (BL22), is a dsFv–immunotoxin directed at the CD22 differentiation antigen present on most B cell leukemias [90]. It has high cyto-toxic activity on cultured tumor cells as well as in animal models and preclinical tests have been completed. This recombinant immunotoxin recently entered clinical trials in patients with leukemias [128]. Initial phase I trials in 16 chemotherapy-resistant HCL patients resulted in 11 complete responses and two partial responses, including two partial responses in patients ineligible for LMB-2 because of CD25$^-$ HCL cells. Responses to BL22 were associated with at least a 99.5% reduction in circulating HCL cells [128]. BL22 also induced responses in chronic lymphocytic leukemia. These recent results demonstrate that recombinant Fv–immunotoxins containing truncated PE are particularly effective in patients with chemotherapy-refractory HCL and other hematological malignancies. Other targets for the development of B cell leukemia-specific recombinant immunotoxins include the CD19 and CD20 differen-tiation antigens in B cell tumors, and CD30 in Hodgkin's lymphoma.

The B cell lymphoma markers CD22 and CD19 were also targeted using conven-tional first-generation immunotoxins with dgA – IgG–RFB4–dgA (targeting CD22) and IgG–HD37–dgA (targeting CD19) [129–135]. Leukemias and lymphomas were also targeted with recombinant fusions of IL-2 with truncated DT [136–139].

## 17.7
## Isolation of New and Improved Antibody Fragments as Targeting Moieties: Display Technologies for the Improvement of Immunotoxin Activity

The generation of mAbs made by immunizing animals and allowing *in vivo* processes, such as immune tolerance and somatic hypermutation, to shape the antigen-combining site is a key issue for the generation of specific antibodies. The unique features required from these molecules were already described in the Introduction to this chapter. These antibodies created *in vivo* can be used for many research and diagnostic applications. Mouse mAbs might be made less immunogenic and more effective for human therapy by reformatting the binding site into chimeric or complementary-determining region (CDR)-grafted antibodies [73]. The advances in recombinant DNA technology and antibody engineering have also lead to the ability to manipulate the size of the antigen-binding domain as described in this chapter. The two variable domains of the binding site can be cloned and arranged into a large array of possible molecular formats and sizes, and expressed in a variety of hosts, ranging from bacteria, lower eukaryotes such as yeast and fungi, to the higher eukaryotes, including mammalian cells, transgenic animals and plants [140, 141]. Extraordinary progress in engineering and selecting small antibody fragments for immunotherapeutic approaches has been made over the past decade, when molecular display technologies have been developed that allow us to create very large repertoires of mouse or fully human antibodies that are displayed on filamentous phage or other molecular display systems. These technologies are now revolutionizing the way in which we can build high-affinity binding sites from scratch, from any species (including humans) and use them for clinical applications such as the targeting of a drug or toxin to cancer cells as in recombinant Fv–immunotoxins.

The concept of molecular display technology relays on the physical linkage between the genotype (the antibody variable region genes) and the phenotype (antigen-binding capability) to allow simultaneous selection of the genes that encode a protein with the desired binding function. This concept can be viewed as an *in vitro* mimicking system for the natural antibody response function of the immune system. This concept was first applied by George Smith in 1985 to small peptides [142]. The display of functional antibody repertoires on phages required several additional discoveries. First, a procedure for accessing large collections of antibody variable domains was needed; this was first described in 1989, when partially degenerate oligonucleotides priming to the 5′ and 3′ end of variable region genes and the polymerase chain reaction (PCR) were used to amplify hybridoma [143, 144] or large collections of variable genes [145, 146]. Second, as whole antibodies cannot yet be functionally expressed in bacteria, a crucial discovery was that antibody fragments (Fab or scFv) were functionally expressed in *E. coli* when they were secreted into the periplasm of the bacteria, which simulated the naturally oxidizing environment of the endoplasmic reticulum [147, 148]. By providing restriction sites in the oligonucleotides used for PCR amplification, antibody libraries could thus be cloned for expression in *E. coli*. Initially, such antibody libraries were expressed from phage λ vectors [146]; a plaque-screening assay with labeled antigen was then used to identify antigen-specific binding sites. Such time-consuming procedures were rapidly replaced by the third seminal development: the provision of a link between the phenotype and the genotype using phages. In 1990, McCafferty *et al.* showed that antibody fragments could be displayed on the surface of filamentous phage particles by fusion of the antibody variable genes to one of the phage coat proteins [149]. Multiple rounds of affinity selection could subsequently enrich antigen-specific phage antibodies, because the phage particle carries the gene encoding the displayed antibody. This was originally reported for scFv fragments [149], and later for Fab fragments [150–152] and other antibody derivatives such as diabodies [153], as well as extended to various display systems. With these advances in place, it became possible to make phage antibody libraries by PCR cloning of large collections of variable region genes expressing each of the binding sites on the surface of a different phage particle and harvesting the antigen-specific binding sites by *in vitro* selection of the phage mixture on a chosen antigen. In the early 1990s, Clackson *et al.* showed for the first time that phage-display technology could be used to select antigen-specific antibodies from libraries made from the spleen B cells of immunized mice [154], thereby bypassing the requirement to immortalize the antigen-specific B cells, as in the hybridoma technology. Similarly, libraries were made from human B cells taken from animals or individuals immunized with antigen [155], exposed to infectious agents [156], with autoimmune diseases [157] or with cancer [158]. Thus, phage-display technology in the early 1990s had already shown the potential to replace hybridoma technology by rescuing V genes from immune B cells. Further advances were reported in the mid-1990s that would bypass the use of immunization and animals altogether. First, it was shown that antibodies against many different antigens could be selected from non-immune libraries, made from the naive light chain and heavy chain IgM V gene pools of B cells of a non-immunized, healthy individual [159]. Second, libraries of synthetic antibody genes, with variable genes not harvested from immune sources but consisting of germline segments artificially provided with diversity by oligonucleotide cloning [150, 160], were shown to behave in a similar way to naive antibody libraries. It thus became possible to use primary antibody libraries, with huge collections of binding sites with different specificities, to select *in vitro* binding sites against most antigens, including non-immunogenic molecules, toxic substances and targets conserved between species [161].

Since these key discoveries, there have been numerous reports on applications of phage antibody libraries [162, 163], ranging from basic research to drug development. In addition, many novel, related molecular display methods for antibodies have been described, including display systems on ribosomes [164], bacteria [165] and yeast cells [166]. These technologies follow similar concepts for *in vitro* selection and improvement of binding sites. Novel selection strategies of phage-display libraries and other molecular display systems are being developed for the identification of novel antigen-binding fragments. These include selection for binding using purified or non-purified antigen, selection for function, selection based on display capability and phage infectivity, subtractive selection procedures, and also using high-throughput selection and screening [163, 167]. The use of phage-display systems will revolutionize the field of targeted drug therapy in general and the recombinant immunotoxin field in particular, because advances in this field are dependent not only on the identification of new targets on cancer cells, but also on the development of new and very specific targeting moieties such as antibody fragments (scFvs). Phage-display technology enables one now to select such molecules against unique targets, especially when hybridoma technology fails to produce antibodies against an antigen or when non-immunogenic or conserved targets between species are being used. Alternatives to phage display for making fully human antibodies are technologies developed using transgenic mice (xenomice). These transgenic mice have been engineered to lack the native murine immune repertoire and instead harbor most of the human immune system V genes in the germline [168, 169]. Injection of these "humanized" animals with a foreign antigen or hapten effectively evokes an immune response and a human-like antibody is produced in the B cells. The antibody genes can be recovered from B cells either by PCR and library selection or by fusion into a monoclonal cell line by classic hybridoma technology. Several examples of recombinant Fv–immunotoxins that were constructed from scFvs isolated by phage display have already been reported [113, 114, 170] and are being considered for use in clinical trials.

The phage-display approach has been used to isolate a scFv that binds with high affinity to a mutant form of the EGF receptor in which a deletion of a portion of the extracellular domain of the receptor generates a tumor-specific [113]. Another novel target for cancer therapy could be cancer-specific peptides presented on human leukocyte antigen (HLA) molecules on the surface of tumor cells. To accomplish this, it will be necessary to isolate antibodies that recognize tumor-specific peptides associated with class I MHC molecules on tumor cells. As a first step in this direction, a recombinant immunotoxin has been constructed using an antibody that was isolated by phage display and that binds specifically to peptide/MHC complexes found on virally infected cells [170–172]. This recombinant immunotoxin was cytotoxic only to cells specifically expressing hemagglutinin peptide HA255–262 in complex with H-2K$^k$ (mouse class I MHC) and was not cytotoxic to cells that express other peptides associated with H-2K$^k$ nor to cells not expressing H-2K$^k$. These studies indicate that, if antibodies that recognize tumor-specific peptides in the context of class I MHC molecules can be developed, they should be very useful agents for targeted cancer immunotherapy. Recently, the isolation of a human antibody directed against a peptide encoded by the melanoma-associated antigen MAGE-A1 presented by HLA-A1 molecules it was reported [173, 174]. A large phage Fab antibody repertoire was selected on a recombinant version of the complex. One of the selected phage antibodies shows binding to HLA-A1 complexed with the MAGE-A1 peptide, but does not show binding to HLA-A1 complexed with a peptide encoded by gene MAGE-A3 and differing from the MAGE-A1 peptide by only three residues. Phages carrying this recombinant antibody bind to HLA-A1$^+$ cells only after *in vitro* loading with MAGE-A1 peptide. It remains now to see if such human anti-MHC/peptide complexes may prove useful for monitoring the cell surface expression of these complexes and, eventually, as a targeting reagent for the specific killing of tumor cells expressing tumor peptide/MHC complexes. The isolation of such rare antibodies against unique tumor targets is a proof for the powerful abilities of antibody phage-display technology for the development of new generations of targeting molecules for cancer therapy and diagnosis.

Phage-display technology can be used not only to create new scFv antibodies, but also improve the properties of existing scFvs. Improvements in antibody stability, expression and binding affinity can be achieved by using a combination of strategies including random and directed mutagenesis of CDR regions, DNA shuffling, and error-prone PCR [175, 176]. These mutagenesis strategies combined with the powerful selection methods available to *screen* antibody phage-display libraries can yield scFv molecules with significantly improved properties for clinical applications. For example, phage display was used to improve antibody affinity by mimicking somatic hypermutation *in vitro* [177]. *In vivo* affinity maturation of antibodies involves mutation of hot spots in the DNA encoding the variable regions. This information was used to develop a strategy to improve antibody affinity *in vitro* using phage-display technology. The anti-mesothelin scFv, SS(scFv), was used to identify DNA sequences in the variable regions that are naturally prone to hypermutations. In a few selected hot spot regions encoding non-conserved amino acids, random mutations were introduced to make libraries with a size requirement between $10^3$ and $10^4$ independent clones. Panning of the hot spot libraries yielded several mutants with a 15- to 55-fold increase in affinity compared with a single clone with a 4-fold increased affinity from a library in which mutagenesis was done outside the hot spots (Tab. 17.2). This is an example of a powerful phage-display-based strategy that should be generally applicable for the rapid isolation of higher-affinity mutants of Fvs, Fabs and other recombinant antibodies from antibody phage libraries that are smaller in size.

In another example, random CDR mutagenesis to obtain mutants of MR1(Fv)–PE38, a single-chain recombinant immunotoxin that targets a mutant form of the EGF receptor, EGFRvIII, that is frequently over-expressed in malignant glioblastomas, was performed [178] (Tab. 17.2). Initially, nine residues of heavy chain CDR3 were randomly mutagenized and several mutants with increased binding affinity were isolated. All mutations were in regions which correspond to a DNA hot spot. The mutant MR1Fvs with an increased affinity for EGFRvIII had an increased activity when converted to recombinant immunotoxins. A specific region of the variable region of the antibody light chain CDR3 was mutagenized that corresponded to a hot spot, and a mutant antibody with an additional increase in affinity and cytotoxic activity was isolated. These studies further show that targeting hot spots in the CDRs of Fvs is an effective approach to obtaining Fvs with increased affinity.

## 17.8
### Improving the Therapeutic Window of Recombinant Immunotoxins: The Balance of Toxicity, Immunogenicity and Efficacy

Although some of the problems, including design, large-scale production and stability, associated with the initial recombinant immunotoxins have been solved, other fundamental problems need to be addressed that are relevant to much of the immunotherapy field. Specificity, toxicity and immunogenicity are major factors that will determine the usefulness and success of recombinant immunotoxins.

## 17.8.1
## Immune Responses and Dose-limiting Toxicity

As with any cytotoxic agent, side effects such as non-specific toxicity and immuno-genicity can occur when multiple injections of immunotoxins are given. One class of side effects is due to inappropriate targeting of the immunotoxin to normal cells be-cause of the poor specificity of the antibody. In addition, the toxin or the Fv portion of the antibody can bind non-specifically to various tissues. For example, in mice, which usually do not contain target antigens, liver damage occurs when large amounts of immunotoxins are given [179]. Molecular modeling combined with site-directed mutagenesis may help in the design of new versions of the toxin with de-creased toxicity caused by non-specific binding.

The development of neutralizing antibodies usually occurs after 10 days and limits the therapeutic application of immunotoxins to this 10-day period [4]. Recent data from clinical trials indicate that patients with solid tumors develop antibodies much more readily then those with hematologic tumors. It is speculated that some hema-tologic tumors may be associated with less immunogenicity than others. For exam-ple, none of 14 patients with chronic lymphocytic leukemia treated with LMB-2 or BL22 have shown any evidence of antibodies [4, 122, 128].

Several approaches have been taken to reduce immunogenicity. One is to make small molecules, which appear to be less immunogenic; another is to use immuno-suppressive agents such as deoxyspergualin or CTLA-4–Ig [180, 181], an inhibitor of the co-stimulation pathways required for T cell help and activation through the CD28/CTLA-4–CD80/CD86 complex. Another approach is to use the anti-CD20 mAb, Rituximab, which induces B cell depletion in the majority of patients and is it-self non-immunogenic [182].

The dose-limiting toxicity of many immunotoxins is vascular leak syndrome (VLS). Recent studies indicate that recombinant toxins, including those containing mutated forms of PE, produce VLS in rats and that inflammation, which can be suppressed by steroids or non-steroidal anti-inflammatory agents, mediates the VLS. VLS can also be mediated indirectly by the activation of endothelial cells and/or macrophages via cytokines such as tumor necrosis factor-$\alpha$ and interferon-$\gamma$. The activated cells produce NO which then can mediate oxidative damage to the endothelial cells and result in increased permeability [183].

Some studies demonstrate direct endothelial cell damage caused by binding the toxin to the cells. The direct damage to the cell is mediated by the enzymatic activ-ity of the toxin [181, 184, 185], while others show an indirect damage that is mediated by binding of the targeting moiety. For example, experiments with hu-man umbilical vein endothelial cells exposed to LMB-1 (antibody conjugate with truncated PE38) indicated that the mAb B3 rather than PE38 was binding to the LeY antigen on endothelial cells [184]. Recent experiments using an *in vivo* model composed of human neonatal foreskin xenografts in SCID immunodeficient mice identified a 3-amino-acid motif present in protein toxins and in IL-2 that causes VLS without other toxin activity [186–188]. Thus, VLS can be blocked in future trials with anti-inflammatory agents to block cytokine action, or by mutations or peptide inhibitors that will prevent the binding of the toxin or the targeting moiety to endothelial cells.

Toxicity can also be reduced by modifications in the scFv targeting moiety. For example, reduction of the non-specific animal toxicity of recombinant Fv–immunotoxin anti-Tac(Fv)–PE38 (which targets the IL-2 receptor) was achieved by introducing mutations in the framework regions of the Fv which lower the isoelectric point (p*I*) [189]. The dose escalation with this recombinant Fv–immunotoxin (that has produced eight responses, including a durable clinical complete remission in a recently completed phase I trial of leukemias and lymphomas) was limited by liver toxicity. It was noted that the Fv of anti-Tac has a p*I* of 10.2, which brought about the hypothesis that the overall positive charge on the Fv portion of anti-Tac(Fv)–PE38 contributes to non-specific binding to liver cells and results in dose-limiting liver toxicity. A mouse model was used to investigate the basis of this toxicity, and it was found that lowering the p*I* of the Fv of anti-Tac from 10.2 to 6. 82 by selective mutation of surface residues causes a 3-fold decrease in animal toxicity and hepatic necrosis. This change in p*I* did not significantly alter the CD25 binding affinity, the cytotoxic activity toward target cells, or antitumor activity, resulting in a 3-fold improvement in the therapeutic index. If this decreased toxicity occurs in humans, it should greatly increase the clinical utility of this immunotoxin.

Another strategy to overcome the problems of non-specific toxicity and antigenicity is by the chemical modification of the recombinant Fv–immunotoxins. An example for this was also demonstrated recently in which site-specific chemical modification with polyethylene glycol (PEGylation) of anti-Tac(Fv)–PE38 (LMB-2) improved its antitumor activity, and reduced animal toxicity and immunogenicity. PEGylation can increase plasma half-lives, stability and therapeutic potency. To produce a PEGylated recombinant immunotoxin with improved therapeutic properties, a mutant form of anti-Tac(Fv)–PE38 (LMB-2) in which one cysteine residue was introduced into the peptide connector (ASGCGPE) between the Fv and the toxin was constructed [190]. This mutant LMB-2 (Cys1-LMB-2), which retained full cytotoxic activity, was then site-specifically conjugated with 5 or 20 kDa of polyethylene glycol–maleimide. When compared with unmodified LMB-2, both PEGylated immunotoxins showed similar cytotoxic activities *in vitro*, but superior stability at 37 °C in mouse serum, a 5- to 8-fold increase in plasma half-lives in mice and a 3- to 4-fold increase in antitumor activity. This was accompanied by a substantial decrease in animal toxicity and immunogenicity. Site-specific PEGylation of recombinant immunotoxins may thus increase their therapeutic potency in humans.

17.8.2
**Specificity Dictated by the Targeting Moiety**

Specificity of the recombinant immunotoxin is determined by the distribution of the target antigens; several target antigens are relatively cancer specific, but are present on some normal cells in small amounts. For example, erbB2, although over-expressed on tumor cells, is also expressed on a limited number of normal cells. This reactivity with normal cells may cause side effects during immunotoxin therapy. It was discovered during a clinical trial that small amounts of the LeY antigen are expressed on the surface of endothelial cells and damage to these cells caused VLS. To overcome such problems, new specific targets and new reagents against the cancer antigens that will recognize only the tumor-associated molecules must be identified and developed. The construction of large phage-display antibody libraries may result in the isolation and characterization of new reagents with improved specificity and affinity for cancer-targeted therapy.

## 17.9
## Conclusions and Perspectives

Over the past decade, several second-generation recombinant immunotoxins with improved properties have been developed and are currently being evaluated in clinical trials. Several of these show clinical activity and promising results in phase I trials [4, 128]. The outcome of these clinical trials demonstrates that the promising preclinical results with these new agents can be translated into more substantial clinical responses and that similar agents that target other cancer antigens merit further clinical development. These accumulating results suggest that Fv–immunotoxins merit further development as a new modality for targeted cancer treatment.

### References

1 PASTAN I, CHAUDHARY V, FITZGERALD DJ (1992) Recombinant toxins as novel therapeutic agents. *Annu Rev Biochem* **61**: 331–54.

2 VITTETA ES (1994) From the basic science of B cells to biological missiles at the bedside. *J Immunol* **153**: 1407–20.

3 KREITAM RJ, PASTAN, I (1998) Immunotoxins for targeted cancer therapy. *Adv Drug Del Rev* **31**: 53–88.

4 KREITMAN RJ (1999) Immunotoxins in cancer therapy. *Curr Opin Immunol* **11**: 570–8.

5 VEALE D, KERR N, GIBSON GJ, HARRIS AL (1989) Characterization of epidermal growth factor receptor in primary human non-small cell lung cancer. *Cancer Res* **49**: 1313–7.

6 LAU JL, FOWLER J, GHOSH L (1988) Epidermal growth factor in normal and neoplastic kidney and bladder. *J Urol* **139**: 170–5.

7 HUNG MC, LAU YK (1999) Basic science of HER-2/*neu*: a review. *Semin Oncol* **26** (4 suppl 12): 51–9.

8 ROSS JS, FLETCHER JA (1999) HER-2/ *neu* (c-erb-B2) gene and protein in breast cancer. *Am J Clin Pathol* 1999; 112 (1 suppl 1): S53–67.

9 VITTETA ES, SONTE M, AMLOT P, *et al.* (1991) Phase I immunotoxin trial in patients with B-cell lymphoma. *Cancer Res* **51**: 4052–8.

10 GROSSBARD ML, LAMBERT JM, GOLDMACHER VS, *et al.* (1993) Anti-B4-blocked ricine: a phase I trial of 7-day continuous infusion in patients with B-cell neoplasms. *J Clin Oncol* **11**: 726–737.

11 WALDMANN TA, PASTAN, I, GANSOW OA, *et al.* (1992) The multichain interleukin-2 receptor: a target for immunotherapy. *Ann Intern Med* **116**: 148–60.

12 CHANG K, PAI LH, BATRA JK, PASTAN I, WILLINGHAM MC (1992) Characterization of the antigen (CAK1) recognized by monoclonal antibody K1 present on ovarian cancers and normal mesothelium. *Cancer Res* **52**: 181–6.

13 CHANG K, PASTAN I (1996) Molecular cloning of mesothelin, a differentiation

antigen present on mesothelium, mesotheliomas, and ovarian cancers. *Proc Natl Acad Sci USA* **93**: 136–40.

14 PASTAN I, LOVELACE E, RUTHERFORD AV, KUNWAR S, WILLINGHAM MC, PEEHL DM (1993) PR1 – a monoclonal antibody that reacts with an antigen on the surface of normal and malignant prostate cells. *J Natl Cancer Inst* **85**: 1149–54.

15 PASTAN I, LOVELACE ET, GALLO MG, RUTHERFORD AV, MAGNANI JL, WILLINGHAM MC (1991) Characterization of monoclonal antibodies B1 and B3 that react with mucinous adenocarcinomas. *Cancer Res* **51**: 3781–7.

16 WANG RF, ROSENBERG SA (1999) Human tumor antigens for cancer vaccine development. *Immunol Rev* **170**: 85–100.

17 ROSENBERG SA (1999) A new era for cancer immunotherapy based on the genes that encode cancer antigens. *Immunity* **10**: 281–7.

18 CHAUDHARY VK, FITZGERALD DJ, ADHYA S, PASTAN I (1987) Activity of a recombinant fusion protein between transforming growth factor type α and *Pseudomonas* toxin. *Proc Natl Acad Sci USA* **84**: 4538–42.

19 PRIOR TI, HELMAN LJ, FITZGERALD DJ, PASTAN I (1991) Cytotoxic activity of a recombinant fusion protein between insulin-like growth factor I and *Pseudomonas* exotoxin. *Cancer Res* **51**: 174–80.

20 SIEGALL CB, EPSTEIN S, SPEIR E, *et al.* (1991) Cytotoxic activity of chimeric proteins composed of acidic fibroblast growth factor and *Pseudomonas* exotoxin on a variety of cell types. *FASEB J* **13**: 2843–9.

21 LORBERBOUM-GALSKI H, FITZGERALD D, CHAUDHARY V, ADHYA S, PASTAN I (1988) Cytotoxic activity of an interleukin 2–*Pseudomonas* exotoxin chimeric protein produced in *Escherichia coli*. *Proc Natl Acad Sci USA* **85**: 1922–6.

22 DEBINSKI W, PURI RK, KREITMAN RJ, PASTAN I (1993) A wide range of human cancers express interleukin 4 (IL-4) receptors that can be targeted with chimeric toxin composed of IL-4 and *Pseudomonas* exotoxin. *J Biol Chem* **268**: 14065–70.

23 SIEGALL CB, SCHWAB G, NORDAN RP,

FITZGERALD DJ, PASTAN I (1990) Expression of the interleukin 6 receptor and interleukin 6 in prostate carcinoma cells. *Cancer Res* **50**: 7786–8.

24 KOMATSU N, ODA T, MURAMATSU T (1998) Involvement of both caspase-like proteases and serine proteases in apoptotic cell death induced by ricin, modeccin, diphtheria toxin, and *Pseudomonas* toxin. *J Biol Chem* **124**: 1038–44.

25 BOLOGNESI A, TAZZARI PL, OLIVIERI F, *et al.* (1996) Induction of apoptosis by ribosome-inactivating proteins and related immunotoxins. *Int J Cancer* **68**: 349–55.

26 VITETTA ES, FULTON RJ, MAY RD, TILL M, UHR JW (1987) Redesigning nature's poisons to create anti-tumor reagents. *Science* **238**: 1098–104.

27 PASTAN I, FITZGERALD D (1991) Recombinant toxins for cancer treatment. *Science* **254**: 1173–7.

28 MOSKAUG JO, SLETTEN K, SANDVIG K, OLSNES S (1989) Translocation of diphtheria toxin A-fragment to the cytosol. Role of the site of interfragment cleavage. *J Biol Chem* **264**: 15709–13.

29 OGATA M, CHAUDHARY VK, PASTAN I, FITZGERALD DJ (1990) Processing of *Pseudomonas* exotoxin by a cellular protease results in the generation of a 37,000-Da toxin fragment that is translocated to the cytosol. *J Biol Chem* **265**: 20678–85.

30 BRINKMANN U, PASTAN I (1995) Recombinant immunotoxins: from basic research to cancer therapy. *Methods: Methods Enzymol.* **8**: 143–56.

31 OLSNES S, PIHL A. (1982) Toxic lectins and related proteins. In: Cohen P, van Heyningen S, eds. *Molecular Action of Toxins and Viruses*. New York: Elsevier Science, p. 51.

32 EIKLID K, OLSNES S, PIHL A (1980) Entry of lethal doses of abrin, ricin and modeccin into the cytosol of HeLa cells. *Exp Cell Res* **126**: 321–9.

33 ENDO Y, TSURIGI K (1987) RNA *N*-glycosidase activity of ricin A-chain. Mechanism of action of the toxic lectin ricin on eukaryotic ribosomes. *J Biol Chem* **262**: 8128–30.

34 SHEN G-L, LI J-L, GHETIE MA, GHETIE V, *et al.* (1988) Evaluation of

four C022 antibodies as ricin A-chain containing immunotoxins for the *in vivo* therapy of human B-cell leukemias and lymphomas. *Int J Cancer* **42**: 792–7.

35 BLAKEY OS, WATSON GJ, KNOWLES PP, *et al.* (1987) Effect of chemical deglycosylation of ricin A-chain on the *in vivo* fate and cytotoxic activity of an immunotoxin composed of ricin A-chain and anti-Thy 1. 1 antibody. *Cancer Res* **47**: 947–52.

36 THORPE PE, WALLACE PM, KNOWLES PP, *et al.* (1988) Improved anti-tumor effects of immunotoxins prepared with deglycosylated ricin-A chain and hindered disulfide linkages. *Cancer Res* **48**: 6396–403.

37 MORONEY SE, O'ALARCAO LJ, GOLDMACHER VS, *et al.* (1987) Modification of the binding site(s) of lectins by an affinity column carrying an activated galactose-terminated ligand. *Biochemistry* **26**: 8390–8.

38 THORPE PE, Ross WCJ, BROWN ANF, *et al.* (1984) Blockade of the galactose-binding sites of ricin by its linkage to antibody. Specific cytotoxic effects of the conjugates. *Eur J Biochem* **140**: 63–71.

39 PASQUALUCCI L, WASIK M, TEICHER BA, *et al.* (1995) Antitumor activity of anti-CD30 immunotoxin (Ber-H2/saporin) *in vitro* and in severe combined immunodeficiency disease mice xenografted with human CD30⁺ anaplastic large-cell lymphoma. *Blood* **85**: 2139–46.

40 FLAVELL OJ (1998) Saporin immunotoxins. *Curr Topics Microbiol Immunol* **234**: 57–61.

41 UCKUN FM, REAMAN GH (1995) Immunotoxins for treatment of leukemia and lymphoma. *Leuk Lymph* **18**: 195–201.

42 IRVIN JO, UCKUN FM (1992) Pokeweed antiviral protein: ribosome inactivation and therapeutic applications. *Pharmacol Ther* **55**: 279–302.

43 GREENFIELD L, BJORN MJ, HORN G, *et al.* (1983) Nucleotide sequence of the structural gene for diphtheria toxin carried by corynebacteriophage β. *Proc Natl Acad Sci USA* **80**: 6853–7.

44 OMURA F, KOHNO K, UCHIDA T (1989) The histidine residue of codon 715 is essential for function of elongation factor 2. *Eur J Biochem* **180**: 1–8.

45 WILSON BA, COLLIER RJ (1992) Diphtheria toxin and *Pseudomonas aeruginosa* exotoxin A: active-site structure and enzymic mechanism. *Curr Topics Microbiol Immunol* **175**: 27–41.

46 WILLIAMS DP, WEN Z, WATSON RS, BOYD J, STROM TB, MURPHY JR (1990) Cellular processing of the interleukin-2 fusion toxin DAB486–IL-2 and efficient delivery of diphtheria fragment A to the cytosol of target cells requires Arg194. *J Biol Chem* **265**: 20673–7.

47 GIANNINI G, RAPPUOLI R, RATTI G (1984) The amino-acid sequence of two non-toxic mutants of diphtheria toxin: CRM45 and CRM197. *Nucleic Acids Res* **12**: 4063–9.

48 MYERS DA, VILLEMEZ CL (1988) Specific chemical cleavage of diphtheria toxin with hydroxylamine. Purification and characterization of the modified proteins. *J Biol Chem* **263**: 17122–7.

49 GREENFIELD L, JOHNSON VG, YOULE RJ (1987) Mutations in diphtheria toxin separate binding from entry and amplify immunotoxin selectivity. *Science* **238**: 536–9.

50 CHOE S, BENNETT MJ, FUJII G, *et al.* (1992) The crystal structure of diphtheria toxin. *Nature* **357**: 216–22.

51 SANDVIG K, OLSNES S (1980) Diphtheria toxin entry into cells is facilitated by low pH. *J Cell Biol* **87**: 828–32.

52 JOHNSON VG, YOULE RJ (1989) A point mutation of proline 308 in diphtheria toxin B chain inhibits membrane translocation of toxin conjugates. *J Biol Chem* **264**: 17739–44.

53 WILLIAMS DP, PARKER K, BACHA P, *et al.* (1987) Diphtheria toxin receptor binding domain substitution with interleukin-2: genetic construction and properties of a diphtheria toxin-related interleukin-2 fusion protein. *Protein Eng* **1**: 493–8.

54 IGLEWSKI BH, KABAT D (1975) NAD-dependent inhibition of protein synthesis by *Pseudomonas aeruginosa* toxin. *Proc Natl Acad Sci USA* **72**: 2284–8.

55 ALLURED VS, COLLIER RJ, CARROLL SF, McKAY DB (1986) Structure of exotoxin A of *Pseudomonas aeruginosa* at 3.0 Ang-

strom resolution. *Proc Natl Acad Sci USA* **83**: 1320–4.

**56** HWANG J, FITZGERALD DJ, ADHYA S, PASTAN I (1987) Functional domains of *Pseudomonas* exotoxin identified by deletion analysis of the gene expressed in *E. coli. Cell* **48**: 129–36.

**57** KOUNNAS MZ, MORRIS RE, THOMPSON MR, FITZGERALD DJ, STRICKLAND DK, SAELINGER CB (1992) The $\alpha_2$-macroglobulin receptor/low density lipoprotein receptor-related protein binds and internalizes *Pseudomonas* exotoxin A. *J Biol Chem* **267**: 12420–3.

**58** SIEGALL CB, CHAUDHARY VK, FITZGERALD DJ, PASTAN I (1989) Functional analysis of domains II, Ib, and III of *Pseudomonas* exotoxin. *J Biol Chem* **264**: 14256–61.

**59** JINNO Y, OGATA M, CHAUDHARY VK, WILLINGHAM MC, ADHYA S, FITZGERALD D, PASTAN I (1989) Domain II mutants of *Pseudomonas* exotoxin deficient in translocation. *J Biol Chem* **264**: 15953–9.

**60** IDZIOREK T, FITZGERALD D, PASTAN I (1990) Low pH-induced changes in *Pseudomonas* exotoxin and its domains: increased binding of Triton X-114. *Infect Immun* **58**: 1415–20.

**61** JIANG JX, LONDON E (1990) Involvement of denaturation-like changes in *Pseudomonas* exotoxin a hydrophobicity and membrane penetration determined by characterization of pH and thermal transitions. Roles of two distinct conformationally altered states. *J Biol Chem* **265**: 8636–41.

**62** OGATA M, PASTAN I, FITZGERALD D (1991) Analysis of *Pseudomonas* exotoxin activation and conformational changes by using monoclonal antibodies as probes. *Infect Immun* **59**: 407–14.

**63** CARROLL SF, COLLIER RJ (1988) Amino acid sequence homology between the enzymic domains of diphtheria toxin and *Pseudomonas aeruginosa* exotoxin A. *Mol Microbiol* **2**: 293–6.

**64** BRANDHUBER BJ, ALLURED VS, FALBEL TG, MCKAY DB (1988) Mapping the enzymatic active site of *Pseudomonas aeruginosa* exotoxin A. *Proteins* 1988; **3**: 146–54.

**65** CARROLL SF, COLLIER RJ (1987) Active site of *Pseudomonas aeruginosa* exotoxin A. Glutamic acid 553 is photolabeled by NAD and shows functional homology with glutamic acid 148 of diphtheria toxin. *J Biol Chem* **262**: 8707–11.

**66** WOZNIAK DJ, HSU LY, GALLOWAY DR (1988) His-426 of the *Pseudomonas aeruginosa* exotoxin A is required for ADP-ribosylation of elongation factor II. *Proc Natl Acad Sci USA* **85**: 8880–4.

**67** JINNO Y, CHAUDHARY VK, KONDO T, ADHYA S, FITZGERALD DJ, PASTAN I (1988) Mutational analysis of domain I of *Pseudomonas* exotoxin. Mutations in domain I of *Pseudomonas* exotoxin which reduce cell binding and animal toxicity. *J Biol Chem* **263**: 13203–7.

**68** KONDO T, FITZGERALD D, CHAUDHARY VK, ADHYA S, PASTAN I (1988) Activity of immunotoxins constructed with modified *Pseudomonas* exotoxin A lacking the cell recognition domain. *J Biol Chem* **263**: 9470–5.

**69** BATRA JK, JINNO Y, CHAUDHARY VK, *et al.* (1989) Antitumor activity in mice of an immunotoxin made with anti-transferrin receptor and a recombinant form of *Pseudomonas* exotoxin. *Proc Natl Acad Sci USA* **86**: 8545–9.

**70** CHAUDHARY VK, JINNO Y, FITZGERALD D, PASTAN I (1990) *Pseudomonas* exotoxin contains a specific sequence at the carboxyl terminus that is required for cytotoxicity. *Proc Natl Acad Sci USA* **87**: 308–12.

**71** SEETHARAM S, CHAUDHARY VK, FITZGERALD D, PASTAN I (1991) Increased cytotoxic activity of *Pseudomonas* exotoxin and two chimeric toxins ending in KDEL. *J Biol Chem* **266**: 17376–81.

**72** RAAG R, WHITLOW M (1995) Single-chain Fvs. *FASEB J* **9**: 73–80.

**73** WINTER G, MILSTEIN C (1991) Man-made antibodies. *Nature* **349**: 293–9.

**74** REITER Y, BRINKMANN U, LEE B, PASTAN I (1996) Engineering antibody Fv fragments for cancer detection and therapy: disulfide-stabilized Fv fragments. *Nat Biotechnol* **14**: 1239–45.

**75** CHOE M, WEBBER KO, PASTAN I (1994) B3(Fab)–PE38M: a recombinant immunotoxin in which a mutant form of *Pseudomonas* exotoxin is fused to the

Fab fragment of monoclonal antibody B3. *Cancer Res* **54**: 3460–7.

**76** HUSTON JS, LEVINSON D, MUDGETT-HUNTER M *et al.* (1988) Protein engineering of antibody binding sites: recovery of specific activity in an anti-digoxin single-chain Fv analogue produced in *Escherichia coli*. *Proc Natl Acad Sci USA* **85**: 5879–83.

**77** BIRD RE, HARDMAN KD, JACOBSON JW, *et al.* (1988) Single-chain antigen-binding proteins. *Science* **242**: 423–6.

**78** KREITMAN RJ, CHANG CN, HUDSON DV, QUEEN C, BAILON P, PASTAN I (1994) Anti-Tac(Fab)–PE40, a recombinant double-chain immunotoxin which kills interleukin-2-receptor-bearing cells and induces complete remission in an *in vivo* tumor model. *Int J Cancer* **57**: 856–64.

**79** DEBINSKI W, PASTAN I (1995) Recombinant F(ab′) C242–*Pseudomonas* exotoxin, but not the whole antibody-based immunotoxin, causes regression of a human colorectal tumor xenograft. *Clin Cancer Res* **1**. 1015 22.

**80** CHAUDHARY VK, QUEEN C, JUNGHANS RP, WALDMANN TA, FITZGERALD DJ, PASTAN I (1989) A recombinant immunotoxin consisting of two antibody variable domains fused to *Pseudomonas* exotoxin. *Nature* **339**: 394–7.

**81** BRINKMANN U, PAI LH, FITZGERALD DJ, WILLINGHAM M, PASTAN I (1991) B3(Fv)–PE38KDEL, a single-chain immunotoxin that causes complete regression of a human carcinoma in mice. *Proc Natl Acad Sci USA* **88**: 8616–20.

**82** BATRA JK, KASPRZYK PG, BIRD RE, PASTAN I, KING CR (1992) Recombinant anti-erbB2 immunotoxins containing *Pseudomonas* exotoxin. *Proc Natl Acad Sci USA* **89**: 5867–71.

**83** KUAN CT, PASTAN I (1996) Improved antitumor activity of a recombinant anti-Lewis(Y) immunotoxin not requiring proteolytic activation. *Proc Natl Acad Sci USA* **93**: 974–8.

**84** REITER Y, WRIGHT AF, TONGE DW, PASTAN I (1996) Recombinant single-chain and disulfide-stabilized Fv–immunotoxins that cause complete regression of a human colon cancer xenograft in nude mice. *Int J Cancer* **67**: 113–23.

**85** REITER Y, PASTAN I (1996) Antibody engineering of recombinant Fv–immunotoxins for improved targeting of cancer: disulfide-stabilized Fv–immunotoxins. *Clin Cancer Res* **2**: 245–52.

**86** BRINKMANN U, REITER Y, JUNG SH, LEE B, PASTAN I (1993) A recombinant immunotoxin containing a disulfide-stabilized Fv fragment. *Proc Natl Acad Sci USA* **90**: 7538–42.

**87** GLOCKSHUBER R, MALIA M, PFITZINGER I, PLUCKTHUN A (1990) A comparison of strategies to stabilize immunoglobulin Fv-fragments. *Biochemistry* **29**: 1362–7.

**88** REITER Y, PAI LH, BRINKMANN U, WANG QC, PASTAN I (1994) Antitumor activity and pharmacokinetics in mice of a recombinant immunotoxin containing a disulfide-stabilized Fv fragment. *Cancer Res* **54**: 2714–8.

**89** REITER Y, BRINKMANN U, JUNG SH, LEE B, KASPRZYK PG, KING CR, PASTAN I (1994) Improved binding and antitumor activity of a recombinant anti-erbB2 immunotoxin by disulfide stabilization of the Fv fragment. *J Biol Chem* **269**: 18327–31.

**90** MANSFIELD E, AMLOT P, PASTAN I, FITZGERALD DJ (1997) Recombinant RFB4 immunotoxins exhibit potent cytotoxic activity for CD22-bearing cells and tumors. *Blood* **90**: 2020–6.

**91** CHAUDHARY VK, FITZGERALD DJ, PASTAN I (1991) A proper amino terminus of diphtheria toxin is important for cytotoxicity. *Biochem Biophys Res Commun* **180**: 545–51.

**92** CHAUDHARY VK, GALLO MG, FITZGERALD DJ, PASTAN I (1990) A recombinant single-chain immunotoxin composed of anti-Tac variable regions and a truncated diphtheria toxin. *Proc Natl Acad Sci USA* **87**: 9491–4.

**93** STUDIER FW, MOFFATT BA (1986) Use of bacteriophage T7 polymerase to direct selective expression of cloned genes. *J Mol Biol* **189**: 113–30.

**94** KIYOKAWA T, SHIRONO K, HATTORI T, *et al.* (1989) Cytotoxicity of interleukin 2–toxin toward lymphocytes from patients with adult T-cell leukemia. *Cancer Res* **49**: 4042–6.

**95** KREITMAN RJ, CHAUDHARY VK, KOZAK RW, FITZGERALD DJP, WALDMANN TA, PASTAN I (1992) Recombinant toxins containing the variable domains of the anti-Tac monoclonal antibody to the interleukin-2 receptor kill malignant cells from patients with chronic lymphocytic leukemia. *Blood* **80**: 2344–52.

**96** KREITMAN RJ, CHAUDHARY VK, WALDMANN T, WILLINGHAM MC, FITZGERALD DJ, PASTAN I (1990) The recombinant immunotoxin anti-Tac(Fv)–*Pseudomonas* exotoxin 40 is cytotoxic toward peripheral blood malignant cells from patients with adult T-cell leukemia. *Proc Natl Acad Sci USA* **87**: 8291–5.

**97** ENGERT A, MARLIN G, AMLOT P, WIJDENES J, DIEHL V, THORPE P (1991) Immunotoxins constructed with anti-CD25 monoclonal antibodies and deglycosylated ricin A-chain have potent antitumor effects against human Hodgkin cells *in vitro* and solid Hodgkin tumors in mice. *Int J Cancer* **49**: 450–6.

**98** GHETIE M-A, RICHARDSON J, TUCKER T, JONES D, UHR JW, VITETTA ES (1991) Antitumor activity of Fab′ and IgG-anti-CD22 immunotoxins in disseminated human B lymphoma grown in mice with severe combined immunodeficiency disease: effect on tumor cells in extranodal sites. *Cancer Res* **51**: 5876–80.

**99** SKREPNIK N, ZIESKE AW, ROBERT E, BRAVO JC, MERA R, HUNT JD (1998) Aggressive administration of recombinant oncotoxin AR209 (anti-ErbB-2) in athymic nude mice implanted with orthotopic human non-small cell lung tumours. *Eur J Cancer* **34**: 1628–33.

**100** WAURZYNIAK B, SCHNEIDER EA, TUMER N, et al. (1997) *In vivo* toxicity, pharmacokinetics, and antileukemic activity of TXU (anti-CD7)–pokeweed antiviral protein immunotoxin. *Clin Cancer Res* **3**: 881–90.

**101** PURI RK, HOON DS, LELAND P, et al. (1996) Preclinical development of a recombinant toxin containing circularly permuted interleukin 4 and truncated *Pseudomonas* exotoxin for therapy of malignant astrocytoma. *Cancer Res* **56**: 5631–7.

**102** JAIN RK (1996) Delivery of molecular medicine to solid tumors. *Science* **271**: 1079–80.

**103** PAI LH, WITTES R, SETSER A, WILLINGHAM MC, PASTAN I (1996) Treatment of advanced solid tumors with immunotoxin LMB-1: an antibody linked to *Pseudomonas* exotoxin. *Nat Med* **2**: 350–3.

**104** PAI LH, PASTAN I (1998) Clinical trials with *Pseudomonas* exotoxin immunotoxins. *Curr Topics Microbiol Immunol* **234**: 83–96.

**105** PASTAN IH, PAI LH, BRINKMANN U, FITZGERALD DJ (1995) Recombinant toxins: new therapeutic agents for cancer. *Ann NY Acad Sci* **758**: 345–54.

**106** PASTAN IH, ARCHER GE, MCLENDON RE, et al. (1995) Intrathecal administration of single-chain immunotoxin, LMB-7 [B3(Fv)–PE38], produces cures of carcinomatous meningitis in a rat model. *Proc Natl Acad Sci USA* **92**: 2765–9.

**107** REITER Y, PAI LH, BRINKMANN U, WANG QC, PASTAN I (1994) Antitumor activity and pharmacokinetics in mice of a recombinant immunotoxin containing a disulfide-stabilized Fv fragment. *Cancer Res* **54**: 2714–8.

**108** BENHAR I, REITER Y, PAI LH, PASTAN I (1995) Administration of disulfide-stabilized Fv–immunotoxins B1(dsFv)–PE38 and B3(dsFv)–PE38 by continuous infusion increases their efficacy in curing large tumor xenografts in nude mice. *Int J Cancer* **62**: 351–5.

**109** SIEGALL CB, CHACE D, MIXAN B, et al. (1994) *In vitro* and *in vivo* characterization of BR96 sFv–PE40. A single-chain immunotoxin fusion protein that cures human breast carcinoma xenografts in athymic mice and rats. *J Immunol* **152**: 2377–84.

**110** WELS W, HARWERTH IM, MUELLER M, GRONER B, HYNES NE (1992) Selective inhibition of tumor cell growth by a recombinant single-chain antibody-toxin specific for the erbB-2 receptor. *Cancer Res* **52**: 6310–7.

**111** PAI-SCHERF LH, VILL J, PEARSON D, et al. (1999) Hepatotoxicity in cancer patients receiving erb-38, a recombinant immunotoxin that targets the erbB2 receptor. *Clin Cancer Res* **5**: 2311–5.

112 BENHAR I, PASTAN I (1995) Characterization of B1(Fv)PE38 and B1(dsFv)PE38: single-chain and disulfide-stabilized Fv–immunotoxins with increased activity that cause complete remissions of established human carcinoma xenografts in nude mice. *Clin Cancer Res* **1**: 1023–9.

113 LORIMER IA, KEPPLER-HAFKEMEYER A, BEERS RA, PEGRAM CN, BIGNER DD, PASTAN I (1996) Recombinant immunotoxins specific for a mutant epidermal growth factor receptor: targeting with a single chain antibody variable domain isolated by phage display. *Proc Natl Acad Sci USA* **93**: 14815–20.

114 CHOWDHURY PS, VINER JL, BEERS R, PASTAN I (1998) Isolation of a high-affinity stable single-chain Fv specific for mesothelin from DNA-immunized mice by phage display and construction of a recombinant immunotoxin with antitumor activity. *Proc Natl Acad Sci USA* **95**: 669–74.

115 LASKE DW, MURASZKO KM, OLDFIELD EH, *et al.* (1997) Intraventricular immunotoxin therapy for leptomeningeal neoplasia. *Neurosurgery* **41**: 1039–49.

116 GREENFIELD L, JOHNSON VG, YOULE RJ (1987) Mutations in diphtheria toxin separate binding from entry and amplify immunotoxin selectivity. *Science* **238**: 536–9.

117 LASKE DW, YOULE RJ, OLDFIELD EH (1997) Tumor regression with regional distribution of the targeted toxin TF-CRM1 07 in patients with malignant brain tumors. *Nat Med* **3**: 1362–8.

118 PURI RK, LELAND P, KREILMAN RJ, PASLAN I (1994) Human neurological cancer cells express interleukin-4 (IL-4) receptors which are targets for the toxic effects of IL-4–*Pseudomonas* exotoxin chimeric protein. *Int J Cancer* **58**. 574–81.

119 KREITMAN RJ, PURI RK, PASLAN I (1994) A circularly permuted recombinant interleukin 4 toxin with increased activity. *Proc Natl Acad Sci USA* **91**: 6889–93.

120 KREITMAN RJ, PASTAN I (1995) Targeting *Pseudomonas* exotoxin to hematologic malignancies. *Semin Cancer Biol* **6**: 297–306.

121 KREITMAN RJ, BAILON P, CHAUDHARY VK, FITZGERALD DJP, PASTAN I (1994) Recombinant immunotoxins containing anti-Tac(Fv) and derivatives of *Pseudomonas* exotoxin produce complete regression in mice of an interleukin-2 receptor-expressing human carcinoma. *Blood* **83**: 426–34.

122 KREITMAN RJ, WILSON WH, WHIE JD, *et al.* (2000) Phase I trial of recombinant immunotoxin anti-tac(Fv)–PE38 (LMB-2) in patients with hematological malignancies. *J Clin Oncol* **18**: 1622–36.

123 KREITMAN RJ, WILSON WH, ROBBINS D, *et al.* (1999) Responses in refractory hairy cell leukemia to a recombinant immunotoxin. *Blood* **94**: 3340–8.

124 MAVROUDIS OA, JIANG YZ, HENSEL N, *et al.* (1996) Specific depletion of alloreactivity against haplotype mismatched related individuals: a new approach to graft-versus-host disease prophylaxis in haploidentical bone marrow transplantation. *Bone Marrow Transplant* **17**: 793–9.

125 ENGERT A, OIEHL V, SCHNELL R, *et al.* (1997) A phase-1 study of an anti-CD25 ricin A-chain immunotoxin (RFT5–SMPT–dgA) in patients with refractory Hodgkin's lymphoma. *Blood* **89**: 403–410.

126 SCHNELL R, VITETTA E, SCHINDLER J, *et al.* (1998) Clinical trials with an anti-CD25 ricin A-chain experimental and immunotoxin (RFT5–SMPT–dgA) in Hodgkin's lymphoma. *Leuk Lymph* **30**: 525–37.

127 MONTAGNA O, YVON E, CALCATERRA V, *et al.* (1999) Depletion of alloreactive T cells by a specific anti-interleukin-2 receptor p55 chain immunotoxin does not impair *in vitro* antileukemia and antiviral activity. *Blood* **93**. 3550–7.

128 KREITMAN RJ, WYNDHAM H, BERGERON K, *et al.* (2001) Efficacy of the anti-CD22 recombinant immunotoxin BL22 in chemotherapy-resistant hairy cell leukemia. *N Engl J Med* **345**: 241–7.

129 AMLOT PL, STONE ML, CUNNINGHAM D, *et al.* (1993) A phase I study of an anti-CD22–deglycosylated ricin A chain immunotoxin in the treatment of B-cell

lymphomas resistant to conventional therapy. *Blood* **82**: 2624–33.

**130** SAUSVILLE EA, HEADLEE D, STETLER-STEVENSON M, *et al.* (1995) Continuous infusion of the anti-CD22 immunotoxin IgG–RFB4–SMPT–dgA in patients with B-cell lymphoma: a phase I study. *Blood* **85**: 3457–65.

**131** SENDEROWICZ AM, VITETTA E, HEADLEE D, *et al.* (1997) Complete sustained response of a refractory post-transplantation, large B-cell lymphoma to an anti-CD22 immunotoxin. *Ann Intern Med* **126**: 882–5.

**132** SCHEUERMANN RH, RACILA E (1995) CD19 antigen in leukemia and lymphoma diagnosis and immunotherapy. *Leuk Lymph* **18**: 385–97.

**133** STONE MJ, SAUSVILLE EA, FAY LW, *et al.* (1996) A phase I study of bolus versus continuous infusion of the anti-CD19 immunotoxin, IgG–HD37–dgA, in patients with B-cell lymphoma. *Blood* **88**: 1188–97.

**134** CONRY RM, KHAZAELI MB, SALEH MN, *et al.* (1995) Phase I trial of an anti-CD19 deglycosylated ricin A chain immunotoxin in non-Hodgkin's lymphoma: effect of an intensive schedule of administration. *J Immunother* **18**: 231–41.

**135** MULTANI PS, O'OAY S, NADLER LM, GROSSBARD ML (1998) Phase II clinical trial of bolus infusion anti-B4 blocked ricin immunoconjugate in patients with relapsed B-cell non-Hodgkin's lymphoma. *Clin Cancer Res* **4**: 2599–604.

**136** LEMAISTRE CF, SALEH MN, KUZEL TM, *et al.* (1998) Phase I trial of a ligand fusion-protein (DAB389IL-2) in lymphomas expressing the receptor for interleukin-2. *Blood* **91**: 399–405.

**137** RE GG, WATERS C, POISSON L, WILLINGHAM MC, SUGAMURA K, FRANKEL AE (1996) Interleukin 2 (lL-2) receptor expression and sensitivity to diphtheria fusion toxin DAB(389) lL-2 in cultured hematopoietic cells. *Cancer Res* **56**: 2590–5.

**138** WATERS CA, SCHIMKE PA, SNIDER CE, *et al.* (1990) Interleukin 2 receptor-targeted cytotoxicity. Receptor binding requirements for entry of a diphtheria toxin-related interleukin 2 fusion protein into cells. *Eur J Immunol* **20**: 785–91.

**139** OUVIC M, KUZEL T, OLSEN E, *et al.* (1998) Quality of life is significantly improved in CTCl patients who responded to DAB389ll-2 (ONTAK) fusion protein. *Blood* **92** (suppl 1): 2572.

**140** HUDSON PJ (1999) Recombinant antibody constructs in cancer therapy. *Curr Opin Immunol* **11**: 548–57.

**141** HUDSON PJ (2000) Recombinant antibodies: a novel approach to cancer diagnosis and therapy. *Exp Opin Invest Drugs* **9**: 1231–42.

**142** SMITH GP (1985) Filamentous fusion phage: novel expression vectors that display cloned antigens on the virion surface. *Science* **228**: 1315–7.

**143** ORLANDI R, GUSSOW DH, JONES PT, WINTER G (1989) Cloning immunoglobulin variable domains for expression by the polymerase chain reaction. *Proc Natl Acad Sci USA* **86**: 3833–7.

**144** CHIANG YL, SHENG-DONG R, BROW MA, LARRICK JW (1989) Direct cDNA cloning of the rearranged immunoglobulin variable region. *Biotechniques* **7**: 360–6.

**145** WARD ES, GUSSOW D, GRIFFITHS AD, JONES PT, WINTER G (1989) Binding activities of a repertoire of single immunoglobulin variable domains secreted from *Escherichia coli*. *Nature* **341**: 544–6.

**146** HUSE WD, SASTRY L, IVERSON SA, *et al.* (1989) Generation of a large combinatorial library of the immunoglobulin repertoire in phage lambda. *Science* **246**: 1275–81.

**147** BETTER M, CHANG CP, ROBINSON RR, HORWITZ AH (1988) *Escherichia coli* secretion of an active chimeric antibody fragment. *Science* **240**: 1041–3.

**148** SKERRA A, PLUCKTHUN A (1988) Assembly of a functional immunoglobulin Fv fragment in *Escherichia coli*. *Science* **240**: 1038–41.

**149** McCAFFERTY J, GRIFFITHS AD, WINTER G, CHISWELL DJ (1990) Phage antibodies: filamentous phage displaying antibody variable domains. *Nature* **348**: 552–4.

**150** HOOGENBOOM HR, GRIFFITHS AD, JOHNSON KS, CHISWELL DJ, HUDSON P, WINTER G (1991) Multi-subunit proteins on the surface of filamentous phage: methodologies for displaying antibody (Fab) heavy and light chains. *Nucleic Acids Res* **19**: 4133–7.

**151** GARRARD LJ, YANG M, O'CONNELL MP, KELLEY RF, HENNER DJ (1991) Fab assembly and enrichment in a monovalent phage display system. *Biotechnology* **9**: 1373–7.

**152** CHANG CN, LANDOLFI NF, QUEEN C (1991) Expression of antibody Fab domains on bacteriophage surfaces. Potential use for antibody selection. *J Immunol* **147**: 3610–4.

**153** MCGUINNESS BT, WALTER G, FITZGERALD K, *et al.* (1996) Phage diabody repertoires for selection of large numbers of bispecific antibody fragments. *Nat Biotechnol* **14**: 1149–54.

**154** CLACKSON T, HOOGENBOOM HR, GRIFFITHS AD, WINTER G (1991) Making antibody fragments using phage display libraries. *Nature* **352**: 624–8.

**155** PERSSON MA, CAOTHIEN RH, BURTON DR (1991) Generation of diverse high-affinity human monoclonal antibodies by repertoire cloning. *Proc Natl Acad Sci USA* **88**: 2432–6.

**156** BURTON DR, BARBAS CF III, PERSSON MA, KOENIG S, CHANOCK RM, LERNER RA (1991) A large array of human monoclonal antibodies to type 1 human immunodeficiency virus from combinatorial libraries of asymptomatic seropositive individuals. *Proc Natl Acad Sci USA* **88**: 10134–7.

**157** GRAUS YF, DE BAETS MH, PARREN PW, *et al.* (1997) Human anti-nicotinic acetylcholine receptor recombinant Fab fragments isolated from thymus-derived phage display libraries from myasthenia gravis patients reflect predominant specificities in serum and block the action of pathogenic serum antibodies. *J Immunol* **158**: 1919–29.

**158** CAI X, GAREN A (1995) Anti-melanoma antibodies from melanoma patients immunized with genetically modified autologous tumor cells: selection of specific antibodies from single-chain Fv fusion phage libraries. *Proc Natl Acad Sci USA* **92**: 6537–41.

**159** MARKS JD, HOOGENBOOM HR, BONNERT TP, MCCAFFERTY J, GRIFFITHS AD, WINTER G (1991) By-passing immunization. Human antibodies from V-gene libraries displayed on phage. *J Mol Biol* **222**: 581–97.

**160** BARBAS CF III, BAIN JD, HOEKSTRA DM, LERNER RA (1992) Semisynthetic combinatorial antibody libraries: a chemical solution to the diversity problem. *Proc Natl Acad Sci USA* **89**: 4457–61.

**161** WINTER G, GRIFFITHS AD, HAWKINS RE, HOOGENBOOM HR (1994) Making antibodies by phage display technology. *Annu Rev Immunol* **12**: 433–55.

**162** DALL'ACQUA A, CARTER P (1998) Antibody engineering. *Curr Opin Struct Biol.* **8**: 443–50.

**163** HOOGENBOOM HR, CHAMES P (2000) Natural and designer binding sites made by phage display technology. *Immunol Today* **21**: 371–8.

**164** HANES J, AND PLUCKTHUN A (1997) *In vitro* selection and evolution of functional proteins by using ribosome display. *Proc Natl Acad Sci USA* **94**: 4937–42.

**165** GEORGIOU G, STATHOPOULOS C, DAUGHERTY PS, NAYAK AR, IVERSON BL, CURTISS R III (1997) Display of heterologous proteins on the surface of microorganisms: from the screening of combinatorial libraries to live recombinant vaccines. *Nat Biotechnol* **15**: 29–34.

**166** BODER ET, WITTRUP KD (1997) Yeast surface display for screening combinatorial polypeptide libraries. *Nat Biotechnol* **15**: 553–7.

**167** HOOGENBOOM HR (1997) Designing and optimizing library selection strategies for generating high-affinity antibodies. *Trends Biotechnol* **15**: 62–70.

**168** JAKOBOVITS A (1998) Production and selection of antigen-specific fully human monoclonal antibodies from mice engineered with human Ig loci. *Adv Drug Del Rev* **31**: 33–42.

**169** YANG XD, JIA XC, CORVALAN JR, WANG P, DAVIS CG, JAKOBOVITS A (1999) Eradication of established tumors by a fully human monoclonal antibody to the epidermal growth factor receptor without concomitant chemotherapy. *Cancer Res* **59**: 1236–43.

**170** ANDERSEN PS, STRYHN A, HANSEN BE, FUGGER L, ENGBERG J, BUUS SA (1996) recombinant antibody with the antigen-specific, major histocompatibility complex-restricted specificity of T cells. *Proc Natl Acad Sci USA* **93**: 1820–4.

171 REITER Y, DI CARLO A, FUGGER L, ENGBERG J, PASTAN I (1997) Peptide-specific killing of antigen-presenting cells by a recombinant antibody–toxin fusion protein targeted to major histocompatibility complex/peptide class I complexes with T cell receptor-like specificity. *Proc Natl Acad Sci USA* **94**: 4631–6.

172 ENGBERG J, KROGSGAARD M, FUGGER L (1999) Recombinant antibodies with the antigen-specific, MHC restricted specificity of T cells: novel reagents for basic and clinical investigations and immunotherapy. *Immunotechnology* **4**: 273–8.

173 DE HAARD HJ, VAN NEER N, REURS A, *et al.* (1999) A large non-immunized human Fab fragment phage library that permits rapid isolation and kinetic analysis of high affinity antibodies. *J Biol Chem* **274**: 18218–30.

174 CHAMES P, HUFTON SE, COULIE PG, UCHANSKA-ZIEGLER B, HOOGENBOOM HR (2000) Direct selection of a human antibody fragment directed against the tumor T-cell epitope HLA-A1–MAGE-A1 from a nonimmunized phage-Fab library. *Proc Natl Acad Sci USA* **97**: 7969–74.

175 GRAM H, MARCONI LA, BARBAS CF III, COLLET TA, LERNER RA, KANG AS (1992) In vitro selection and affinity maturation of antibodies from a naive combinatorial immunoglobulin library. *Proc Natl Acad Sci USA* **89**: 3576–80.

176 CRAMERI A, CWIRLA S, STEMMER WP (1996) Construction and evolution of antibody-phage libraries by DNA shuffling. *Nat Med* **2**: 100–2.

177 CHOWDHURY PS, PASTAN I (1999) Improving antibody affinity by mimicking somatic hypermutation *in vitro*. *Nat Biotechnol* **17**: 568–72.

178 BEERS R, CHOWDHURY P, BIGNER D, PASTAN I (2000) Immunotoxins with increased activity against epidermal growth factor receptor vIII-expressing cells produced by antibody phage display. *Clin Cancer Res* **6**: 2835–43.

179 PAI LH, PASTAN I (1998) Clinical trials with *Pseudomonas* exotoxin immunotoxins. *Curr Topics Microbiol Immunol* **234**: 83–96.

180 SIEGALL CB, LIGGITT D, CHACE D, TEPPER MA, FELL HP (1994) Prevention of immunotoxin-mediated vascular leak syndrome in rats with retention of antitumor activity. *Proc Natl Acad Sci USA* **91**: 9514–8.

181 SIEGALL CB, LIGGIII D, CHACE D, MIXAN B, SUGAI J, DAVIDSON T, SIEINITZ M (1997) Characterization of vascular leak syndrome induced by the toxin component of *Pseudomonas* exotoxin-based immunotoxins and its potential inhibition with nonsteroidal anti-inflammatory drugs. *Clin Cancer Res* **3**: 339–45.

182 MCLAUGHLIN P, GRILLO-LOPEZ AJ, LINK BK, *et al.* (1998) Rituximab chimeric anti-CD20 monoclonal antibody therapy for relapsed indolent lymphoma: half of patients respond to a four-dose treatment program. *J Clin Oncol* **16**: 2825–33.

183 BALUNA R, VITETTA ES (1997) Vascular leak syndrome: a side effect of immunotherapy. *Immunopharmacology* **37**: 117–32.

184 KUAN C, PAI LH, PASTAN I (1995) Immunotoxins containing *Pseudomonas* exotoxin targeting Ley damage human endothelial cells in an antibody-specific mode: relevance to vascular leak syndrome. *Clin Cancer Res* **1**: 1589–94.

185 ROZEMULLER H, ROMBOUTS WJC, TOUW IP, *et al.* (1996) Treatment of acute myelocytic leukemia with interleukin-6 *Pseudomonas* exotoxin fusion protein in a rat leukemia model. *Leukemia* **10**: 1796–803.

186 LINDSTROM AL, ERLANDSEN SL, KERSEY JH, PENNELL CA (1997) An *in vitro* model for toxin-mediated vascular leak syndrome: ricin toxin A chain increases the permeability of human endothelial cell monolayers. *Blood* **90**: 2323–34.

187 BALUNA R, VITETTA ES (1999) An *in vivo* model to study immunotoxin-induced vascular leak in human tissue. *J Immunother* **22**: 41–47.

188 BALUNA R, RIZO J, GORDON BE, GHETIE V, VITETTA ES (1999) Evidence for a structural motif in toxins and interleukin-2 that may be responsible for

binding to endothelial cells and initiating vascular leak syndrome. *Proc Natl Acad Sci USA* **96**: 3957–62.

**189** ONDA M, KREITMAN RJ, VASMATZIS G, LEE B, PASTAN I (1999) Reduction of the nonspecific animal toxicity of anti-Tac(Fv)–PE38 by mutations in the framework regions of the Fv which lower the isoelectric point. *J Immunol* **163**: 6072–7.

**190** TSUTSUMI Y, ONDA M, NAGATA S, LEE B, KREITMAN RJ, PASTAN I (2000) Site-specific chemical modification with poly-ethylene glycol of recombinant immunotoxin anti-Tac(Fv)–PE38 (LMB-2) improves antitumor activity and reduces animal toxicity and immunogenicity. *Proc Natl Acad Sci USA* **97**: 8548–53.

**191** FRANKEL AE, LAVER JH, WILLINGHAM MC, BURNS LJ, KERSEY JH, VALLERA DA (1997) Therapy of patients with T-cell lymphomas and leukemias using an anti-CD7 monoclonal antibody–ricin A chain immunotoxin. *Leuk Lymph* **26**: 287–98.

# Glossary

### $\alpha_2$-Macroglobulin
A serum protease inhibitor with a broad range of specificities which blocks members of all four known classes of endopeptidases. It contains a unique thiol ester group which, when cleaved by the proteases, results in a covalent bond between protease and inhibitor. Concordantly, the protease becomes entrapped by a conformational change of the inhibitor. $\alpha_2$-Macroglobulin has been implicated to play a role in lipopolysaccharide sensitivity, neutralization of transforming growth factor-$\beta$ and in Alzheimer's disease. It binds to the cell surface receptor *CD91*.

### Adaptive immunity
Immunity to infectious or other antigens that improves in quality and intensity from the first to the second encounter with the *antigen*, in contrast to *innate immunity* which involves always the same immune reactions of the same intensity with every antigen challenge. Adaptive immunity is based on the selection and expansion of antigen-specific T and *B lymphocyte* clones. The B lymphocytes switch thereby from IgM to IgG production which have a higher affinity for the antigen.

### Adhesion molecule
Cell surface receptor for cell–cell and cell–matrix adhesiveness. They are implicated in stable cell–cell contacts in tissues as well as in the transient attachments of migrating cells, and play a role in transmigration of leukocytes through the endothelial cell layer of blood vessels and in the interaction of *T lymphocytes* with their stimulator or target cells. Several families of adhesion receptors with different functions have been described including cadherins, selectins, addressins, integrins, *Annexins* and members of the immunoglobulin superfamily, such as the intercellular adhesion molecules (ICAMs). Some adhesion molecules, e.g. some integrins, also transmit signals into the cell and/or out of the cell.

### Adjuvant
Material co-administered with specific *antigens* to improve the vaccination effects. Adjuvants are often derived from microorganisms but may also be cells like *dendritic cells*, subcellular components such as *heat shock proteins, cytokines, chemokines,* lipids of various origin, oligonucleotides or inorganic compounds such as aluminum hy-

droxide. Although the exact mechanism of the adjuvant effect of many of the compounds used is not well understood, they are thought to stimulate parts of the innate immune system (see *Innate immunity*) including the induction of inflammatory cytokines and chemokines, the recruitment and activation of *antigen-presenting cells*, and the expression of *co-stimulatory molecules*.

## Adoptive immunotherapy

Passive immunization involving the transplantation of immune *effector cells*, i.e. most often *T lymphocytes*, with the desired specificity into a patient. Lymphocytes may be autologous or, in animal models, syngeneic or allogeneic and be directly transferred from an immune individual into a non-immune individual or, as it is usually the case when applied for therapy, stimulated and expanded *in vitro*, and then injected into the patients.

## Angiogenesis

The process of forming new blood vessels in healthy as well as in malignant tissues. Angiogenesis is mediated by a variety of factors, most importantly vascular endothelial growth factor (VEGF) and basic fibroblast growth factor (bFGF). Often, the vascularization of tumors leads to atypical blood vessels some of which are dead-ended.

## Annexin

Widely expressed family of calcium dependent phospholipid-binding proteins involved in the aggregation, fusion and exocytosis of intracellular vesicles and granules, and in membrane recycling. Annexins are used as indicators for *apoptosis*. They bind to the phospholipids that appear at the cell surface early in *programmed cell death*. More than 10 Annexin family members have been identified to date. They are characterized by a common core domain of four or eight repeats of a 61-amino-acid domain. Annexin II, in its soluble form, inhibits *T lymphocyte* proliferation, and suppresses IgG and IgM secretion by *B lymphocytes*. High expression of Annexins has been correlated with higher-grade tumors.

## Antiangiogenesis

Therapeutic strategy that aims at inhibiting the formation of new blood vessels in tumors. Among the naturally occurring antiangiogenic proteins are angiostatin, endostatin, interferons (IFNs) and tissue inhibitors of metalloproteases. Some chemotherapeutic drugs used for cancer therapy such as thalidomide or IFNs have antiangiogenic activity.

## Antibody

Any protein (immunoglobulin) produced by *B lymphocytes* that binds *antigen*. Antibodies consist of an antigen-binding domain and a constant region. The gene segments for the variable domain, as it is the case for the *T cell receptor*, are formed by recombination of V, D and J segment to yield a clonotypic antigen receptor. The antibodies are homodimers of heterodimers of a heavy and a light chain. The light chain consists of two domains – one variable and one constant; the heavy chain, in addition to the variable domain, consists of three constant domains in the case of IgG, IgD and IgA or four in the case of IgE and IgM. In the case IgE and IgA these tetra-mers may form dimers. IgM is a pentamer of the basic dimeric unit. The B lympho-cytes that express specific antibodies can efficiently bind antigen and process it for presentation to *helper T cells*. They are thereby efficient *antigen-presenting cells* for their cognate antigen. Soluble-form antibodies bind and neutralize pathogens carrying the corresponding antigen, opsonize the antigen or antigen-bearing particle, and, thus, prepare it for specific phagocytosis and degradation by *macrophages* or serve as adaptor molecules that link antigen specificity to the antibody-dependent effector mechanisms of the immune system, such as complement and *antibody-dependent cellular cytotoxicity*. The type of immune effector function addressed is determined by the particular constant domains of the antibodies.

### Antibody-dependent cellular cytotoxicity (ADCC)

Destruction of target cells that are coated with a specific antibody by Fc receptor-expressing cytolytic cells. Fc receptors bind the constant region of the antibody. The *effector cells* in this context can be *cytotoxic T lymphocytes* and *natural killer cells*, but also macrophages or *neutrophils*. For cancer therapy, the application of *antibodies* with specificity for a molecule expressed at the surface of the tumor cells is meant to recruit Fc receptor-positive effector cells, leading to their activation and the destruction of the tumor cells. Examples for such therapeutic antibodies are anti-CD25 (interleukin-2 receptor) in cases of T cell lymphoma and anti-CD20 in cases of B lymphocyte lymphoma.

### Antigen

Any compound bound specifically by antigen receptors of the immune system, i.e. *antibodies* and *T cell receptors*. Whereas antibodies can be induced against molecules of virtually any chemical class, antigens recognized by *T lymphocytes* are almost exclusively proteins. Antibodies usually bind the entire molecule – in the case of proteins, the *epitopes* may be continuous stretches of the protein sequence (continuous epitopes) or combinations of elements contributed by different segments of the primary sequence of the protein (discontinuous epitopes). Epitopes for T lymphocytes are peptides generated inside the cells by limited proteolysis from the antigen, bound selectively by the *MHC* molecules and displayed as peptide/MHC complexes at the cell surfaces. The peptides for presentation by MHC class I molecules are mostly 8–9 amino acids; those for presentation by MHC class II molecules are mostly 11–15 amino acids long.

### Antigen presentation

Display of *MHC*-bound peptides at the surface of the cells for recognition by the *T cell receptor*. The MHC molecules select from a pool of peptides generated by limiting proteolysis inside the cells from antigen peptides that fulfill MHC allele-specific binding requirements. The MHC molecules come in two classes – MHC class I molecules present peptides for recognition by CD8$^+$ T lymphocytes and MHC class II molecules present peptides for recognition by CD4$^+$ T lymphocytes. Every cell that expresses MHC molecules presents antigens. However, *dendritic cells* do this particularly efficient and are therefore sometimes dubbed 'professional' *antigen-presenting cells*.

### Antigen-presenting cell (APC)

Term applied in particular to *dendritic cells* (DCs), but also a few other cell types such as *B lymphocytes*. APCs express *MHC* class I and II molecules, and thereby present antigens to CD4$^+$ and CD8$^+$ *T lymphocytes*. The high efficiency of *antigen presentation* by DCs correlates with a high efficiency of antigen uptake and processing, high expressions levels of the MHC molecules, co-expression of MHC class I and II molecules, expression of various *co-stimulatory molecules*, a particular morphology that allows for interactions of several T lymphocytes at the same time, an inducible mobility, and, upon activation, tropism for lymph nodes and the capacity to localize to particular areas of the secondary lymphatic organs to organize a cellular microenvironment that strongly promotes interactions between the DCs and *T lymphocytes* of the various types. DCs play a key role in the induction of immune responses.

### Antigen processing

All steps of antigen handling inside cells that lead to the presentation of T lymphocyte *epitopes* by *MHC* molecules. These steps include the limited proteolysis of the antigen by endopeptidases to generate peptides and the trimming of these peptides by exopeptidases to make them fit the MHC-binding requirements, the transport of the peptides to the site of the biosynthesis of the MHC molecule, loading of these molecules with the peptides, and the export of the MHC/peptide complexes for antigen presentation at the surfaces of the cells. The pathways of antigen processing are different for MHC class I- and II-restricted antigens. For presentation by MHC class I molecules, antigens are reduced to peptides by the cytosolic multicatalytic proteasomes, transported into the endoplasmic reticulum by TAP (transporter associated with antigen processing), trimmed by exopeptidases and, assisted by various chaperones, incorporated into nascent MHC class I molecules. Peptides for presentation by MHC class II molecules are generated in endolysosomes and bound to prepared MHC class II molecules. In both cases, there are indications that recycled MHC molecules can be reloaded with new peptides. Synthetic peptides can readily be loaded onto MHC molecules provided they fit the epitope-binding requirements. There is an on-going debate as to where synthetic peptides are incorporated into the MHC molecules. For some peptides, evidence has been presented for a peptide exchange at the surface of the cells.

### Apoptosis

Process of *programmed cell death* that ultimately leads to the disintegration of the cell. The apoptotic remainders are readily cleared by surrounding cells in the tissue. In contrast, in cases of necrosis the dead cells and tissues remain, and may induce inflammation and tissue destruction. Apoptosis is under the tight control of various regulator proteins inside the cells and at the cell surfaces. It can be induced by cell surface receptors such as Fas or by mechanisms inside the cell such as the tumor-suppressor gene products. Cytolysis by *cytotoxic T lymphocytes* or *natural killer* cells is also apoptosis. The typical changes associated with apoptosis involve flipping of phospholipids in the plasma membrane (*Annexin*), membrane blebbing and fragmentation of the DNA.

### B lymphocyte (B cell)

Antibody-expressing lymphocyte. They evolve from cells which are committed to the B cell linage but have not yet rearranged their immunoglobulin genes via different stages of pro-B development to pre-B cells with a partly rearranged immunoglobulin genome to immature B cells that express IgM, and mature B cells that secrete IgM and IgD. Upon contact with *antigen* and antigen-mediated interaction with *helper T cells* these mature B cells develop into clonally expanded, IgG-producing cells that either terminally differentiate into plasma cells or become memory cells and, thus, form the basis of secondary immune responses. Mature B cells express *MHC* class I and II molecules, and a number of adhesion and co-stimulating molcules that qualify them to serve as *antigen-presenting cells*. Their antigen receptor allows for a specific accumulation of their cognate antigen which is thus presented with high efficiency.

### Bone marrow transplantation (BMT)

Therapeutic transfer of bone marrow to reconstitute, replace or support the hematopoetic and immune system of the recipients. Generally, the recipient has received chemotherapy or radio-chemotherapy prior to BMT which has eliminated or substantially reduced the individual's own hematopoetic system. Two regimens are in use – the myeloablative approach (aimed at replacing the recipients bone marrow with autologous or allogeneic stem cells) and the non-myeloablative approach (resulting in a chimerism of host and donor stem cells). Because of incompatibility of minor or major histocompatibility gene products, continuous immunosuppression is necessary in most recipients.

### Carcinoembryonic antigen (CEA)

Glycoprotein expressed by many cell types in the developing fetus and by adenocarcinomas of endodermally derived intestinal epithelia, but also breast, lung, and some types of thyroid and ovarian cancers. CEA is used as a tumor marker and as a target *antigen* for cancer immune therapy. It has a molecular weight of 180 000 with about 60 % carbohydrate moieties. In healthy adults, CEA expression may be elevated due to smoking, inflammation, pancreatitis and liver cirrhosis.

### CD

Cluster of differentiation, nomenclature of differentiation antigens expressed by leukocytes. Regularly held international workshops allocate CD numbers to these antigens.

### CD91

Cell surface receptor for $\alpha_2$-macroglobulin and some *heat shock proteins* (gp96, HSP90, HSP70 and calreticulin). CD91 is expressed by *monocytes* and their derivatives including macrophages and *dendritic cells* and erythroblasts/reticulocytes. The molecule consists of two non-covalently associated chains – a 85-kDa transmembrane β subunit and a 515-kDa α subunit – derived by cleavage from a common precursor protein. Because of its similarity to the low-density lipoprotein receptor (LDL), CD91 was initially seen as the LDL receptor-related protein (LRP). $\alpha_2$-Macroglobulin was the first ligand identified for CD91.

## Central tolerance
Tolerance towards self-antigen established during the development of *T lymphocytes* in the thymus. T lymphocytes that bind with high affinity to *MHC*/peptide complexes by thymic *antigen-presenting cells* die by *apoptosis*.

## Chaperone
Stress protein; highly conserved proteins that non-covalently bind and thereby protect unfolded or nascent polypeptides to ensure correct folding. They also play a role as intermediate peptide carriers in *antigen processing*. There is indirect evidence for a shuttle function of some chaperones that transport peptides or T lymphocyte epitopes between cells. Some chaperones such as gp96 exhibit a non-specific immune stimulatory capacity. *Heat shock proteins* are a subset of the chaperones.

## Chemokine
Chemoattractive polypeptides. Chemokines play a major role in leukocyte trafficking, and direct lymphocytes, *monocytes* and other cells of the immune system to sites of inflammation and active immune responses.

## Chimeric receptor
Recombinant receptor molecule composed of domains of different proteins.

## Coley's toxin
Mixture of killed Gram-positive and Gram-negative bacteria, in some compositions including *Streptococcus* and *Proteus*, that was introduced in 1890 by William B. Coley to cancer therapy. Coley injected the toxin into sarcomas and observed tumor regression in many cases. It is not clear what the mechanisms of the clinical effects are. It has been suggested that lipopolysaccharide might play a role by stimulating polyclonal *B lymphocyte* responses or that *CpG motifs* of the bacterial DNA released from the toxin might serve as *adjuvant* to support the induction of antitumor immune responses by T lymphocytes.

## Co-stimulatory molecule
Molecule expressed at the surface of *antigen-presenting cells* or exchanged between interacting cells that induce signals in *T lymphocytes* to support the cellular response triggered by recognition of cognate *MHC*/peptide complexes. These signals can be essential supplements to the primary signals transduced via the *T cell receptor* to drive full activation or to direct the type of response, or to suppress activation-induced cell death of the T lymphocyte. Co-stimulatory signals are essential aspects of T lymphocyte activation and are dependent on the cooperation of the cells that ex-

press the proper receptor/counter-receptor pairs. These signals control the induction of T lymphocyte-mediated immune responses as well as the maturation of *B lymphocytes*. The 'two-signal hypothesis' was an earlier concept of the co-stimulation concept, initially seeing *interleukin-2* as the second and co-stimulating signal. Later, B7 with its receptor CD28 were recognized as a major co-stimulatory molecule combination.

## CpG motif
Immune-stimulating, unmethylated CG dinucleotides in various sequence contexts found in bacterial DNA. Vertebrate DNA contains 20 times fewer CG sequences that, usually, are methylated and in sequence contexts that are not immune stimulatory. The receptor for CpG is the *Toll-like receptor* 9 (TLR-9) which is expressed by *B lymphocytes* and plasmacytoid *dendritic cells*.

## Cross-priming
Induction of a T cellular immune response that is restricted by the *MHC* of the immunized individual rather than the MHC of the cells used for immunization. Cross-priming was originally reported for immunizations of $F_1$ mice against cells of one of the parental mouse strains. These immunizations resulted partly in the induction of $CD8^+$ *cytotoxic T lymphocyte* responses that were specific for minor histocompatibility antigens of one of the parent strains, but restricted by the MHC of the other parent. The term cross-priming is most often used to describe the ability of *antigen-presenting cells* to take up and present MHC class I-restricted antigens derived from other cells.

## Cytokine
Small soluble proteins and transfer signals from one cell to another. Cytokines include a number of different protein families such as *interferons, interleukins* or *chemokines* with various different functions in the immune system. They are important immune regulating molecules and serve as growth and differentiation factors or as suppressors of immune responses.

## Cytotoxic T lymphocyte (CTL)
Effector T lymphocyte that, upon specific, *MHC*-restricted *antigen recognition*, lyse other cells. Most of the CTLs express the CD8 accessory receptor and are MHC class I restricted. However, there are also $CD4^+$ MHC class II-restricted CTLs. Cytolysis may be achieved by (1) a mechanism depending on the pore-forming perforin and granzyme, and (2) a Fas/Fas ligand-dependent mechanism. The differential actions of these two mechanisms are not yet completely understood. In both cases, the attacked cell dies by *apoptosis*. Perforin by itself forms only pores and leads to necrosis. In conjunction with granzymes, the components of intracellular death pathways are accessible and induced. Of the eight described granzymes, only granzyme B was unequivocally linked to the induction of apoptosis. CTLs themselves are relatively resistant to their own cytolytic machineries – factors at the cell membrane that resemble the decay accelerating factor as well as cytosolic serine esterase inhibitors (Serpins) are involved in this protection.

## Dendritic cell (DC)

Migratory mononuclear cell found in nearly all tissues and characterized by typical filiform processes. DCs are highly efficient *antigen-presenting cells* and particularly important for the primary induction of immune responses. They are thought to harvest antigens in the tissues and, upon activation by inflammatory processes, for instance, migrate to the draining lymph nodes. These mature DCs express high levels of MHC class I and II molecules, and *co-stimulatory molecules*, and efficiently activate *T lymphocytes*. In man, two types of DCs have been described, the plasmocytoid DCs and the myeloid DCs. Myeloid DCs are derived from or related to *monocytes*. Plasmacytoid DCs, in addition to specific DC markers, express a set of cell surface molecules that are also found on cells of lymphatic lineage and synthesize type I *interferons*. Plasmacytoid and myeloid DCs express different sets of *Toll-like receptors*, and, thus, respond differently to pathogenic microorganisms.

## Donor lymphocyte infusion (DLI)

Therapeutic strategy of infusing into a patient subsequently to allogeneic *bone marrow transplantation* immune-competent *T lymphocytes* from the same donor. This therapy aims at induction of a graft-versus-leukemia (GvL) or graft-versus-tumor (GvT) effect of the donor lymphocytes.

## Effector cell

Cell with fully developed cytolytic capacity, usually activated $CD8^+$ *cytotoxic T lymphocytes* or *natural killer cells*.

## Epitope

Portion of an *antigen* that is actually bound by the immune receptors, antibodies or *T cell receptors* (TCR). For antibodies, epitopes may be continuous stretches of the primary sequence of a protein antigen (continuous epitopes) or composed of elements of different parts of the antigen (discontinuous epitopes). In addition to peptides, any small residue such as a hapten or a hapten in the context of a peptide can form an epitope for antibodies. Epitopes for *T lymphocytes* are always peptides derived from proteins by limited proteolysis that must be bound to *MHC* molecules for recognition by the TCR.

## Fas (APO-1, CD95)

Cell surface receptor of 43 kDa of the tumor necrosis factor (TNF) receptor superfamily which is one of the main triggers of receptor-mediated *apoptosis*. Fas is expressed in thymus, liver, heart and ovary, and by activated T lymphocytes and some tumors. It carries an intracellular death domain that, after engagement of Fas with its ligand (FasL), binds FADD, an intracellular adaptor molecule that initiates caspase-mediated pathways of apoptosis. FasL (CD95L), also a member of the TNF superfamily, is expressed predominantly by activated T lymphocytes. However, some tumors also express FasL and, thus, can induce apoptosis in *cytotoxic T lymphocytes* that attack the tumor. The actual role of receptor-mediated apoptosis in the control of tumors in patients has not yet been clarified.

**gp96**
See *Chaperone*.

**Graft-versus-host disease (GvHD)**
Immune reaction of donor *T lymphocytes* against the recipient's cells and tissue after allogeneic *bone marrow transplantation* (BMT) or hematopoietic stem cell transplantation. The grafted donor T lymphocytes recognize the host's body as foreign tissue and mount a T cellular immune reaction. The organs typically most affected are skin, liver, bowel and lung. *MHC* molecules can be the trigger and target for GvH reactions or, in cases where the transplantation was performed with matched MHC, minor histocompatibility antigens are the focus of the T lymphocyte reactions. GvHD usually does not affect recipients who have received hematopoietic stem cells of an identical twin. The GvHD patients usually require immunosuppressive treatments. While GvHD might cause substantial complications, it is generally accepted that an antileukemia or antitumor effect of BMT depends on the presence of immune-competent T lymphocytes in the graft. The issue in BMT, therefore, is often to achieve a therapeutic GvH reaction against the tumor cells and minimize the pathological effects on healthy tissues.

**Haploidentical cell transplantation**
Transplantation of donor stem cells that share half of the co-dominantly expressed *MHC* class I and II molecules with the recipient. Haploidentical transplantations are typically carried out by transferring bone marrow of a parent into a child (see *Bone marrow transplantation*).

**Heat shock protein (HSP)**
See *Chaperone*.

**Helper T cell**
CD4$^+$ *T lymphocytes* with a wide range of factors and processes that provide essential or supportive aid in the induction, activation and augmentation of effector immune responses mediated by *cytotoxic T lymphocytes* or *B lymphocytes*. T lymphocyte help for B lymphocyte differentiation is controlled by direct antigen-dependent interaction of T and B lymphocytes, which implies that the same antigen carries *epitopes* for both cells. This epitope linkage requirement is the basis for the hapten-carrier concepts for the induction of secondary humoral immune responses. In the case of T lymphocyte help for the induction of CD8$^+$ cytotoxic T lymphocytes, *antigen-presenting cells* (APCs) mediate the collaboration of the two T lymphocyte types. The APCs must present MHC class II- and I-restricted epitopes for the respective T lymphocyte types. The exact mechanisms of these cellular interactions and the identification of the factors involved are still under investigation.

**hTERT**
See *Telomerase*.

## Immune surveillance

Hypothesis proposing that the immune system provides the key instruments for the identification of and interference with malignant development. The immune surveillance hypothesis was originally proposed by F. M. Burnet who suggested that thymus-dependent immune cells, i.e. *T lymphocytes*, continuously scan the body for aberrant alterations which are then eliminated by destruction of the respective cells.

## Immunocytokine

Recombinant chimeric molecule that combine the specificity-determining fragment of an *antibody* with a *cytokine* in order to target the activity of the cytokine to a specific site and thereby alter the respective microenvironment in favor of protective immune responses.

## Immunoglobulin

See *Antibody*.

## Immunotoxin

Artificial molecule composed of specific antibodies or the specificity-determining domain thereof and a toxin. The toxin is thereby targeted to the site where it should exert its cytotoxic effect. Some immunotoxins are recombinant proteins of an antibody and a cytotoxic protein such as *Pseudomonas* exotoxin. In cancer therapy, immunotoxins for the treatment of B and T lymphocyte lymphomas are undergoing clinical trials. They target CD25 in cases of T lymphocyte lymphomas.

## Innate immunity

Protection provided by the non-acquired, non-adaptive elements and mechanisms of the immune system, including the skin as a physical barrier, antibiotic peptides, and cells that eliminate microbial and viral material by phagocytosis. The innate immune system phylogenetically predates *adaptive immunity*. It does not depend on lymphocytes, needs no priming and utilizes receptors such as the *Toll-like receptors* that are triggered by molecules present only in the microorganisms but not in the vertebrate host.

## Interferon (IFN)

*Cytokines* that are involved in inter-leukocyte communication and in the regulation of the differentiation of *T lymphocyte* and other cells of the immune system as well as in various cellular responses including the expression of *MHC molecules* and several components of the *antigen processing* machineries. The name refers to the capacity of the interferons to interfere with virus infection. They were originally identified in supernatants of virus-infected cells as factors that render other cells resistant to virus infection.

## Interleukin (IL)

A series of *cytokines* that exert various different functions in the regulation of immune reactions. They were originally described as soluble factors produced by leukocytes and addressing leukocytes. There are now, however, reports of ILs produced by other cells as well, such as IL-10 by keratinocytes, of ILs having a broad range of effects on non-leukocytes and of cell surface variants of some of the ILs, such as IL-1. Among the ILs which are particularly important in the context of tumor immunology and cancer immunotherapy are IL-2 as a growth and differentiation factor for *T lymphocytes*, IL-4 and IL-6 as factors regulating *B lymphocyte* differentiation, IL-10 as an immune-suppressive factor, and IL-12 which is thought to be particularly potent in supporting immune responses by $CD8^+$ effector T lymphocytes.

### Lymphokine-activated killer (LAK) cell

Lymphocytic cell generated in the absence of antigen by exposure to high doses of *cytokines* such as interleukin-2 exhibiting a high cytolytic capacity. LAK activity is perforin/granzyme dependent and not antigen specific. *Natural killer* cells are a major source for LAK cells.

### Major histocompatibility complex (MHC)

Gene complex that controls the rapid rejection of MHC-disparate transplants – hence its name. The MHC genes are highly polymorphic and map in humans [human leukocyte antigens (HLA)] to the short arm of chromosome 6 and in mice (H-2) to chromosome 17. Their gene products fall into two functionally and structurally distinct classes: MHC class I molecules (HLA-A, -B, and -C in humans or H-2K, -D and -C in mice) are heterodimers of the polymorphic transmembrane heavy chain and the non-covalently associated non-polymorphic $\beta_2$-microglobulin. They bind and present peptides that are usually 8–10 amino acids for recognition by $CD8^+$ *T lymphocytes*. MHC class II molecules (HLA-DP, -DQ and DR in humans, and H-2A and H-2E in mice) consist of two polymorphic non-covalently associated transmembrane polypeptides. They bind and present peptides of 11 or more amino acids for recognition by $CD4^+$ T lymphocytes. MHC class I molecules are expressed by most nucleated cells; MHC class II molecules, however, are expressed only by *antigen-presenting cells* and stimulated epithelial cells. In addition to MHC class I molecules, the MHC also encodes for the MHC class Ib molecules HLA-E, -F and -G, which resemble MHC class I molecules in their structure but exhibit a limited polymorphism and serve a range of different functions including the presentation of *N*-formylated peptides and lipids or, independent of any antigen presentation, as inhibitory receptors for *natural killer* cells.

### Monocyte

Mononuclear cell that circulate in the blood, emigrate into tissues and differentiate into phagocytic macrophages. Monocytes are a main source of *dendritic cells* of the myeloid type that are used in many protocols for cancer immune therapy.

### Natural killer (NK) cell

Large, lymphocyte-like cell with characteristic granula that play a role in natural resistance to tumors and in antibody-dependent cellular cytotoxicity. NK cells variably express killer cell immunoglobulin-like receptors (KIRs) and CD94/NKG2 that trans-duce variably inhibitory or activating signals after binding to *MHC* class I or Ib molecules. The absence of MHC expression may trigger NK cell activation.

## Neutrophil

A phagocytic polymorphonuclear leukocyte that can ingest and kill invading microorganisms. They play important parts in inflammatory reactions both in the removal of microorganisms and aged and damaged cells, and as a source for inflammatory agents such as *chemokines, cytokines,* leukotrienes and other lipid mediators of inflammation.

## Suicide gene

Inducible gene that codes for a protein which mediates cell death. One of the best-known examples is the herpes simplex virus thymidine kinase (HSV-*tk*) which converts the non-toxic prodrug gancyclovir into its cytotoxic phosphorylated form.

## Programmed cell death

see *Apoptosis.*

## T cell receptor (TCR)

Antigen receptor of *T lymphocytes.* The TCR consists of a disulfide-bonded $\alpha\beta$ or $\gamma\delta$ heterodimer expressed at the cell surface in association with the CD3 molecular complex as the signal-transducing unit of the receptor. The genes for the TCR are rearranged from the germline V, D, and J elements during the ontology of the T lymphocyte to form the clonotypic genes and gene products. The ligands of the TCR are *MHC*/peptide complexes.

## T lymphocyte (T cell)

Lymphocyte of the thymic linage which are subdivided into CD8-expressing *cytolytic T lymphocytes* (CTL) and CD4-expressing regulatory *helper T cells.* The precursors of T cells originate in the bone marrow and migrate as CD4/CD8 double-positive cells into the thymus where they differentiate into the mature T lymphocyte types. During thymic differentiation, the *T cell receptor* (TCR) genes are rearranged. T cells are selected to propagate whose TCR are *MHC*-restricted (positive selection) and are eliminated by apoptosis when they bind MHC/peptide complexes with high affinity; thus, they are potentially autoreactive (negative selection, see *Central tolerance*). T cells as regulator and effector T cells are key instruments of the adaptive immune system. Unlike *B lymphocytes,* T lymphocytes recognize their *epitopes* as complexes with MHC class I or I molecules.

## T body

*Cytotoxic T lymphocyte* genetically engineered to express a chimeric *antibody*/receptor surface molecule with specificity for an antigen on the surface of tumor cells. Usually the chimeric receptor consists of single-chain antibody fragments with the desired specificity fused to CD3$\zeta$ or Fc receptor $\gamma$ as signal transduction domains. T bodies have been developed with a number of different specificities. Anti-G250

T bodies are being tested for their antitumor activities in clinical trials with renal cell carcinoma patients.

**Telomerase, telomerase reverse transcriptase (hTERT)**
A ribonucleoprotein (larger than 100 kDa) with reverse transcriptase activity that, in concert with other molecules, adds multiple short telemetric DNA repeats to the 3′ end of chromosomes (telomeres) to preserve their structural integrity. Without telomerase activity cells progressively loose their terminal sequence with each cell cycle. Telomerase is expressed in self-replicating stem cells and in more than 85% of all tumors but rarely in normal cells. Telomerase expression is thought to be among the essential factors in tumorigenesis and therefore is considered as a potential universal *tumor-associated antigen*.

**T helper 1 ($T_h$1)/T helper 2 ($T_h$2) dichotomy**
Th1/Th2 dichotomy of the regulatory T lymphocyte responses where the immune reaction is polarized towards cellular or humoral immune responses. These different directions of the immune responses might, in some situations, be mutually suppressive. The polarity of the immune response is usually correlated to the *cytokine* profiles with interleukin (IL)-2, interferon (IFN)-$\gamma$ and tumor necrosis factor-$\alpha$ being indicative of a $T_h$1 response, and IL-4, -5 and -10 indicative of a $T_h$2 response. Selective activation of $T_h$1 cells is mediated by IFN-$\gamma$ and IL-12, and inhibited by IL-4 and -10, whereas IL-4 is essential for growth and differentiation of $T_h$2 cells.

**Toll-like receptor (TLR)**
Highly conserved cell surface receptors expressed preferentially on leukocytes but also on epithelial cells in lung, ovary or prostate. They are human homologs of the *Drosophila* Toll gene that is involved in dorsal/ventral differentiation. TLRs are important receptors in *innate immunity*. They bind microbial lipoproteins, DNA (see *GpG motif*) or lipopolysaccharide, and induce a range of cellular activities including proliferation and *cytokine* secretion. At least 10 TLRs have been identified to date that share a Toll/interleukin-1 receptor motif in the cytoplasmic domain and multiple copies of leucine-rich repeats in the extracellular domain. Activation of TLRs results in signaling via nuclear factor (NF)-$\kappa$B, MyD88 and IRAK TRAF6 molecules. Different types of *monocytes* express different spectra of the TLRs (pathogen-associated molecular pattern recognition profiles) which translate into differences in cytokine production depending on the nature of pathogens and, thus, in a polarization of the resulting adaptive immune response (see *Adaptive immunity*).

**Tumor antigen, tumor-associated antigen (TAA), tumor rejection antigen**
An *antigen* expressed exclusively or predominantly by tumor cells. Since the majority of the antigens described so far for various different tumors are not tumor-specific but expressed in non-malignant cells as well, the more cautious term TAA is usually preferred. TAA can be differentiation antigens shared with non-transformed cells of the tumor histotype, over-expressed proteins, embryonic antigens, antigens of the tumor-testis type, viral antigens in cases of tumor-associated viruses or mutations.

Only the latter group of antigens are tumor-specific. TAA are the focus of antitumor immune responses usually mediated by *cytotoxic T lymphocytes* and therefore potential vaccine antigens for cancer immune therapy.

### Tumor-infiltrating lymphocyte (TIL)

Lymphocyte of varying composition and numbers found in tumors. They largely comprise CD4$^+$ and CD8$^+$ T lymphocytes, and constitute an important component of the *tumor microenvironment*. Recent studies in melanoma have shown that a high portion of the CD8$^+$ TILs are specific for *tumor-associated antigens* expressed by the tumor. They are seen as an indication of an on-going struggle between the immune system and the tumor. The presence of TILs in many cancers is associated with a better prognosis for the patient. On the other hand, many studies have demonstrated functional impairment in TILs.

### Tumor microenvironment

Term describing the microenvironment in tumor lesions including the tumor cells, *tumor-infiltrating lymphocytes*, and other cells such as *monocytes* and *neurophils*, and various humoral factors such as *cytokines*, the extracellular matrix, stroma tissue and blood vessels. The tumor microenvironment is considered to be the primary battle ground for antitumor immune responses and the key to understanding cancer-related immune suppression.

### Tumor rejection antigen

See *Tumor antigen*.

# Index

*a*

acidic and basic fibroblast growth factor
  *see* fibroblast growth factor
activation-induced cell death (AICD)   110, 114, 234
–, effects of TGF-β   123
acute lymphocytic leukemia (ALL)   302
acute myelocytic leukemia (AML)   302, 305 f.
adaptive immunity, HSPs   253
ADCC   *see* antibody-dependent cellular cytotoxicity
add-back strategy, DLIs   306
adjuvants, definition   223
adoptive immunotherapy   301
adoptive T immunotherapy   5
adoptive transfer therapy   41
AICD   *see* activation-induced cell death
ALL   *see* acute lymphocytic leukemia
allogenic stem cell transplants   197
allogenic transplantation   361
allospecifities, MHC class I antigens   72
AML   *see* acute myelocytic leukemia
amplified-gene encoded antigens   22
angiogenesis
–, COX inhibitors   132
–, effects of IL-10   165
antiangiogenesis, immunocytokines   341 f.
anti-asialo-GM1 antiserum   274
antibodies
–, anti-IL-10   129
–, auto-   214
–, bacterial immunotherapy   274
–, cancer-specific   290
–, discovery   311
–, monoclonal   17 f., 277, 363–366
–, side effects of DC vaccinations   194
–, T-body approach   287
antibody 17-1A   313
antibody-cytokine fusion proteins   311 f.
antibody-dependent cellular cytotoxicity
  (ADCC)   277

antibody-dependent cytotoxicity   314
antibody fragments
–, immunotoxins   363–366
–, recombinant   354–357
antibody incidence, SEREX antigens   23
antibody responses, clinical significance   23
anti-CD20 antibody rituximab   17
antigen, definition   223
antigen identification   41–44
antigen loading, dendritic cells   186 f.
antigen loss
–, immunocytokines   331
–, MHC class I   66–69, 72–76
antigen presentation   30–39, 209 ff.
–, MHC pathway   59–62
antigen-presenting cells (APCs)   105, 210–214, 233
–, bacterial immunotherapy   276 f.
–, dendritic cells   196
–, effects of IL-10   158 f.
–, HCV   239 ff.
–, HSPs   258, 263
–, immunocytokines   318, 320
–, tumor cell killing   220
antigen processing   30–39
–, MHC pathway   59–62
antigen-processing machinery (APM)   60 ff.
–, MHC class I   70
–, MHC class II   79 ff.
antigen release, tumor cell killing   219 f.
antigenic complexity, of tumor cells   235
antigenic peptides, HSPs   254 f.
antigenicity
–, tumor   3–55, 155, 231 ff.
antigens
–, auto-   214
–, foreign   211, 224
–, near-self   224
–, self-   207, 209, 224
–, SEREX   19–27
–, shared   256

–, tumor   224
–, tumor-associated   231 ff.
antileukemia effect, HSV-tk engineered donor
   lymphocytes   305
antinuclear antibodies   194
antiserum, anti-asialo-GM1   274
anti-Tac(Fv)-PE38 (LMB-2), immunotoxins
   362, 368
antithyroid antibodies   194
antitumor immunity, models   205
antitumor response, MHC class II expression
   82 f.
antitumor vaccination   218–221
APCs   *see* antigen-presenting cells
APM   *see* antigen-processing machinery
apoptosis
–, DCs   105
–, effects of polyamines   133
–, immunotoxins   351
–, NK cells   101
–, T cell   123
–, T lymphocyte   111
–, tumor-induced   *see* tumor-induced
   apoptosis
apoptotic bodies, dendritic cells   187
arthritis, rheumatoid   215
autoantigens
–, cancer-related   22
–, non-cancer-related   23
autoimmune disease   209, 222
–, antigen presentation   211
–, genetic linkages   215 f.
autoimmune-like reactivity   221
autoimmune reactions   51, 194, 232, 235
autoimmunity   214–217
autologous HSPs   256 ff.


***b***

B cell leukemias   362
B cell lymphomas   17, 347
B cells
–, bacterial immunotherapy   272 ff.
–, HCV   238
–, lysis by hTERT specific CTL   10
–, tumor microenvironment   108
Bacillus Calmette-Guerin (BCG), cancer
   immunotherapy   268 f.
backbone, ODN classes   272 ff.
bacterial DNA, cancer immunotherapy
   268–286
bacterial extracts, cancer immunotherapy
   268 ff.
bacterial immunotherapy   268–286
bacterial toxins   352 ff.

BCG   *see* Bacillus Calmette-Guerin
BCG treatment   215
Bcr-Abl junction   211
bDNA   *see* bacterial DNA
β subunits of 20S proteasome   31–34, 69 ff.
$\beta_2$-m gene   67 ff.
biological activities, IL-10   157–161
Birbeck granules   180
bladder cancer, bacterial immunotherapy   268
blood DCs   180, 183–186
BMT   *see* bone marrow transplantation
bone marrow, immunocytokines   337 f.
bone marrow transplantation (BMT), immune
   therapy   299–310
breast cancer   361
–, clinical trials   190
–, immunotoxins   360


***c***

CAMEL, antigen   48
cancer
–, bladder   *see* bladder cancer
–, breast   *see* breast cancer
–, CEA expressing   *see* CEA expressing cancer
–, colon   *see* colon cancer
–, gastro-intestinal   *see* gastro-intestinal cancer
–, human   *see* human cancer
–, ovarian   *see* ovarian cancer
–, pancreas   *see* pancreas cancer
–, prostate   *see* prostate cancer
–, renal cell   *see* renal cell cancers
–, *see also* carcinoma
–, *see also* tumors
cancer genomics   10
cancer immunology, strategies   177–379
cancer immunome   24 f.
cancer immunosurveillance   204
cancer models, effects of IL-10   164
cancer patients, IL-10 expression   161–164
cancer-specific antibodies   290
cancer vaccination, dendritic cells   179–203
cancer vaccine, preventative   12
cancer vaccine development   25 f.
carbohydrate antigen Lewis Y (LeY)   347, 367
–, immunotoxin therapy   360
carbohydrates, complex   354
carcinoembryonic antigen (CEA)   135
–, immunocytokines   319–327
carcinoma
–, colon   *see* colon carcinoma
–, colorectal   *see* colorectal carcinoma
–, ovarian   *see* ovarian carcinoma
–, prostate   *see* prostate carcinoma
–, *see also* cancer

–, *see also* tumors
cationic lipids, bacterial immunotherapy 274
CD3 ζ chain 102, 288
CD4 helper T lymphocyte responses 195
CD4 T cell help, definition 223
CD4 T cells 49 ff., 79, 81 ff., 99 ff.
–, effects of IL-10 127, 159 f.
–, immunocytokines 320, 331 f., 335 f.
CD8 T cells 99 ff.
–, effects of IL-10 127
–, immunocytokines 330 ff., 335 f., 338 ff.
CD8+ cytotoxic T lymphocytes 232, 304, 315–318
–, *see also* cytotoxic T lymphocytes (CTL)
CD19 antigen 347
CD20 antigen 347
CD22 antigen 347, 361 f.
CD25 361 f.
CD28 T cells, T-body approach 289
CD40 322 ff., 332
CD54 *see* intercellular adhesion molecule
CD80 326
–, tumor microenvironment 110 ff.
CD95-CD95 (CD95L) ligand pathway *see also* FasL Pathway
CD123 DCɛ, lymphoid 180 f., 183
CDR *see* complementary-determining region
CEA *see* carcinoembryonic antigen
CEA expressing cancer, clinical trials 191
CEA/CD40 ligand trimer 322
cell damage, immunotoxins 367
cell death 211–214, 218–221
–, activation-induced 234
cell differentiation, polyamines 133
cell interaction, HCV 234
cell killing, tumor 218 f.
central tolerance
–, antigen presentation 211
–, definition 223
Cγ1 gene 312
ch14.18, immunocytokines *see* human/mouse antiganglioside GD₂ antibody
ch14.18-IL-2 fusion protein, immunocytokines 330–341
ch14.18-LT-α immunocytokine 333 f.
chaperons, HSPs 254 f.
chemical conjugate immunotoxins *see* first-generation immunotoxins
chemokines, effects of dendritic cells 181
chemotherapy 299
chimeric receptors (CRs) 288–295
chimeric toxins 350
chromium release assay, CTL monitoring 45
chronic myelogenous leukemia (CML) 301 ff.

chronic myeloid leukemia, clinical trials 189
CIITA *see* MHC class II transactivator
class II-associated Ii peptide (CLIP) *see* MHC class II-associated Ii peptide
clinical impact, HLA-G expression 88
clinical relevance, MHC class I alterations 76–79
clinical significance, antibody responses 23
clinical staging, GvHD 300
clinical trials
–, colateral carcinoma 293
–, DC preparations 188–194
–, HCV 238–241
–, HIV 293
–, HSPs 257 f.
–, HSV-tk-transduced donor lymphocytes 304 f.
–, hTERT 8–12
–, huKS1/4-IL2 immunocytokine 329
–, IL-10 therapy 167
–, leukemia 361 f.
–, ovarian carcinomas 294
–, polynucleotides 270
–, ricin-based immunoconjugates 361 f.
–, RNA vaccination 187
–, side effects of DC vaccinations 194
–, T bodies 293 f.
–, vaccination strategies 234 f.
CLIP *see* MHC class II-associated Ii peptide
CML *see* chronic myelogenous leukemia
CMV *see* cytomegalovirus
Coley's toxins 268, 278
colon cancer, immunotoxins 360
colon carcinoma, immunocytokines 322 ff.
colorectal carcinoma
–, immunocytokines 313–316
–, T-body approach 293
combinatorial peptide library approach 44
complementary-determining region (CDR)-grafted antibodies 363, 366
complex carbohydrates 354
co-stimulatory molecules 210, 212 ff.
–, definition 223
–, HCV 236 f.
–, T-body approach 289
counting, of DCs 183
COX inhibitors, prostaglandin (PG) E2 132
CpG-A and CpG-B classes of ODN 272–278
CpG DNA, usage of term 273
CpG motif receptors 271 f.
CpG motifs, from bacterial DNA 268–286
CRF2 *see* cytokine receptor family II
cross-presentation
–, of peptides to thymic T cells 263

–, tumor cell killing   220
cross-priming
–, CpG DNA   276
–, dendritic cells   181
–, HSPs   255
cross-reaction, with autoantigens   215
CRs   *see* chimeric receptors
CT antigens   21, 26 f.
CT26 colon carcinoma cells   314–318
CTL   *see* cytotoxic T lymphocytes
CTL epitopes   32, 34–37
–, identification   41–44
–, monitoring   44–49
–, tumor-immune system interaction
   66
CTL precursor (pCTL)   317
CTL responses
–, effects of IL-10   127
–, inhibition by MIF   130
–, low-affinity   194
–, MHC class I alterations   77 f.
–, mucins   135
–, tumor site   46–49
cyclophosphamide, suppression of IL-10
   129
cytochrom P450   11
cytokine gene therapy   327
cytokine-producing cells, flow cytometry
   detection   195
cytokine receptor family II (CRF2)   156
cytokines
–, bacterial immunotherapy   274
–, DCs   105
–, effects of dendritic cells   181
–, hybrid cell vaccination (HCV)   234
–, IL-2, IL-10   100
–, immunoinhibitory factors   109
–, in cancer immune therapy   311–346
–, interferon (IFN)-γ   31
–, macrophages   108
–, NK cells   102 ff.
cytolysis, hTERT specific   9 f.
cytomegalovirus (CMV), BMT   305 f.
cytotoxic epitopes, dendritic cells   187
cytotoxic T lymphocytes (CTL)
–, CD8⁺   3, 6, 8 ff., 41
–, GvHD   303
–, HCV   234
–, T-body approach   292
–, *see also* CTL responses

*d*
damage, cell   367
danger signal

–, definition   224
–, dendritic cells   181
–, immunocytokines   324 f.
–, tumor cell killing   218
–, tumor microenvironment   96 f.
databases, SEREX antigens   25
DC counts, in cancer patients   183
DC immunotherapy   195 ff.
DC mobilization, in cancer patients   183
DCs   *see* dendritic cells
delayed-type hypersensitivity (DTH)   188
ΔNGER   *see* low-affinity receptor for the nerve
   growth factor
dendritic cells (DCs)
–, and cancer   179–203
–, antigen presentation   210
–, effects of IL-10   128, 158 f.
–, effects of TGF-β   123 f.
–, gp96   262 f.
–, HCV   234–241
–, HSPs   254
–, immunocytokines   322 ff., 329
–, tumor cell killing   218
–, tumor microenvironment   105 ff.
dendritic-like cells, immunocytokines   320
deoxyspergualin   367
DFMO   *see* difluoromethyornithine
diabodies   364
differentiation antigens   21, 231
difluoromethyornithine (DFMO)   133
diphteria toxin (DT)   350–361
disease, autoimmune   209, 211, 215 f.
disialoganglioside (GD₂)
–, antibody   312 f., 341
–, immunocytokines   330 ff.
display technology, immunotoxins
   363–366
disulfide-stabilized Fvs (dsFvs)   355 ff.,
   360 f.
DLI   *see* donor lymphocyte infusion
DNA, bacterial   268–271
DNA backbone, ODN classes   272 ff.
DNA-based immunotoxins   351–357
DNA hot spots   366
DNA vaccine, CEA-based   321–327
donor lymphocyte infusions (DLIs)   275,
   301–307
dose-limiting toxicity, immunotoxins   367 f.
down regulation, MHC class I   69–76
drugs, suppression of IL-10   129
dsFvs   *see* disulfide-stabilized Fvs
DT   *see* diphteria toxin
DTH   *see* delayed-type hypersensitivity
dysfunction, immune cells in cancer   108 f.

**e**

EBV   *see* Epstein-Barr virus
EDR   *see* escalating doses regimen
EGF   *see* epidermal growth factor
ELISPOT   195
embryonic antigens   231
endosome, PRR receptors   271 f.
endotoxin, bacterial immunotherapy   269
eosinophils, tumor cell killing   218
Ep-CAM/KS antigen (KSA)   312–329, 341
epidermal growth factor (EGF) receptor   347,
   354, 365 f.
epitope deduction   6 ff.
epitope linkage   233
epitope spreading   214, 222
epitopes
–, CTL   32, 34–37, 41–44
–, definition   223
–, multiple peptide   187
–, near-self   209, 211
–, subdominant   211, 224
–, T cell   3–16
–, tumor antigen-associated   220
–, tumor-associated T cell   231 ff.
Epstein-Barr virus (EBV), IL-10 homologs   157
ER retention motif, gp96   262
erbB familiy, oncogenic receptors   290 ff.
erbB2 receptor   347, 354, 360 f., 368
escalating doses regimen (EDR)   303
Escherichia coli, immunotoxins   351 f.
evolutionary tuning, of the immunoresponse
   206–209
exosomes, dendritic cells   180
exotoxin, pseudomonas   *see* pseudomonas
   exotoxin
expression
–, hTERT   8
–, IL-10   155 f., 161–164
–, of HSPs   261 f.
–, *see also* gene expression

**f**

FACS   *see* fluorescence-activated cell sorting
FAP   *see* Fas-associated phosphatase
Fas-associated phosphatase (FAP)   111
Fas-FasL Pathway   110 ff.
–, *see also* CD95-CD95 (CD95L) ligand pathway
FasL   *see* Fas-FasL Pathway
FBP   *see* folate binding protein
Fc receptors (FcRs)   277
–, γ   102
–, T-body approach   288
FcRs   *see* Fc receptors
fever, modulation of HSPs   261

FGF   *see* fibroblast growth factor
fibroblast growth factor (FGF), immunotoxins
   350
first-generation immunotoxins   349 f.
flow cytometry detection of cytokine-producing
   cells   195
Flt-3L, dendritic cells   195
fluorescence-activated cell sorting (FACS)   64
folate binding protein(FBP)-specific CR   292 ff.
foreign antigens   211
–, definition   224
foscarnet   305
Freund's adjuvant, incomplete   234
fusion proteins
–, antibody-cytokine   311 f.
–, ch14.18-IL-2   330–341
–, HSP/peptide   260
–, lymphotoxin (LT)-α   313
fusion technology, HCV   236 f.
Fv   *see* variable region fragment

**g**

galactose-specific lectins, immunotoxins
   351
gancyclovir (GCV)   304 ff.
gangliosides
–, $GD_2$   312 f., 330 ff., 341
–, RCC-derived   100
–, tumor-associated   109
–, tumor-derived   105
gastro-intestinal cancer, clinical trials   191
GCV   *see* gancyclovir
$GD_2$   *see* disialoganglioside
gene expression   10, 18 f.
–, MHC antigens   63 f.
–, underexpressed genes   23
–, *see also* expression
genetic linkages to autoimmune diseases
   215 f.
genomics, cancer   10
glioma
–, clinical trials   191
–, HCV   239
Glucksberg grade, GvHD   300
glycoproteins, immunotoxins   351
GM-CSF   *see* granulocyte macrophage colony
   stimulating factor
gp70 envelope protein   316
gp96, HSPs   253 ff., 258–263
gp100 antigen   334 f.
graft-versus-host (GvH) reactions   299–307
graft-versus-host disease (GvHD)   299–307
–, leukemia   361 f.
graft-versus-leukemia (GvL) effect   301 ff.

graft-versus-tumor (GvT) effect   299, 301
granules, Birbeck   180
granulocyte macrophage colony stimulating
   factor (GM-CSF)
–, dendritic cells   184
–, effects of IL-10   165
granulocytes, FasL   112 f.
growth factor
–, fibroblast   *see* fibroblast growth factor
–, insulin-like   *see* insulin-like growth factor
–, nerve   *see* nerve growth factor
–, transforming   *see* transforming growth
   factor
–, vascular endothelial   *see* vascular endothelial
   growth factor
GvH   *see* graft-versus-host
GvHD   *see* graft-versus-host disease
GvL   *see* graft-versus-leukemia
GvT   *see* graft-versus-tumor

*h*

hairy cell leukemia (HCL)   362
haplo-cell transplantation   306
HCL   *see* hairy cell leukemia
HCT   *see* hematopoietic cell transplantation
HCV   *see* hybrid cell vaccination
heat shock proteins (HSP)   253–267
–, cancer immunotherapy   256–263
–, dendritic cells   181
–, HCV   240
–, tumor cell killing   218
helper epitopes, dendritic cells   187, 195
helper T cells   233, 324
–, HCV   236 f.
–, immunotoxins   367
hematopoietic cell transplantation (HCT)
   *see* bone marrow transplantation
hepatotoxicity   361
Heregulin   *see* Neuregulin differentiation
   factor
Herpes Simplex virus (HSV)   304 ff.
high-affinity bindings, immunotoxins
   363
high-affinity cytokine receptors   234
high-affinity responses   195
HIV, T-body approach   293
HLA   *see* human leucocyte antigen
HLA-C locus expression   78
HLA class II restricted tumor associated
   antigens   49 f.
HLA-G expression   85–89
HLA/peptide tetramer responses
–, dendritic cells   188, 195
Hodgkin lymphomas, effects of IL-10   163

HOM-MEL-40 antigen   21
HOM-TES-14 antigen   24
homologs, IL-10   157
hot spots, DNA   366
HSP   *see* heat shock proteins
HSP/peptide covalent complex   259 f.
HSP/peptide fusion proteins   260
HSP/peptide non-covalent complex   259
HSV   *see* Herpes Simplex virus
HSV-tk   *see* thymidine kinases of Herpes
   Simplex virus
hTERT   *see* human telomerase reverse
   transcriptase
huKS1/4-IL2 immunocytokine   316 f., 319,
   323–328, 340 f.
human cancer, dendritic cells   182 f.
human leucocyte antigen (HLA)   49 f., 60–76,
   215
–, immunotoxins   365
–, MHC class I expression   85–89
–, MHC class II expression   82
–, mutations   75
human telomerase reverse transcriptase
   (hTERT)   8–12
human/mouse antiganglioside GD$_2$ antibody
   (ch14.18)   312 ff., 337
hybrid cell vaccination (HCV)   230–252
–, dendritic cells   187
hybrid proteasomes   33
hybridoma technology   364
hyperthermia, modulation of HSPs   261

*i*

ICAM   *see* intercellular adhesion molecule
Id   *see* idiotype
idiotype (Id), antigen   276
IFA   *see* imcomplete Freund's adjuvant
IFN   *see* interferon
IGF   *see* insulin-like growth factor
IgG1 and IgG2 isotypes, bacterial immuno-
   therapy   276
IL-2   *see* interleukin-2
IL-10   *see* interleukin-10
–, immunosuppressive factors   120
IL-10 expression   155 f.
–, in cancer patients   161–164
IL-10 homologs   157
IL-10 presence, in cancer patients   163
IL-10 production, selectivity   162 f.
IL-10 receptor (IL-10R)   155 ff.
IL-12, immunosuppressive factors   122
ILT   *see* immunoglobulin-like transcript
imcomplete Freund's adjuvant (IFA)   234
immature DCs   220

immature Mo-DCs   184
immune cells
–, effects of IL-10   158, 160 f.
–, tumor microenvironment   95–118
immune effector mechanisms   65 f.
immune escape, IL-10 therapy   167
immune responses
–, evolution   77
–, recombinant immunotoxins   367 f.
–, *see also* immunoresponses
immune selection   96, 208
immune surveillance   230
immune system
–, and tumor progression   95 ff.
–, in cancer   204–229
immune tolerance   363
immuno-proteasomes   31–37, 60
immunobiological tolerance   206 f.
immunocytokines, overview   311–346
immunoediting   206
immunogenicity, of tumor cells   234
immunoglogulin-like transcript (ILT)
    molecules   180
immunological ignorance   12
immunological tolerance   12
immunology
–, cancer   177–379
–, reverse   *see* epitope deduction
immunome, cancer   24 f.
immunoresponses
–, inhibition   108 f.
–, MHC class I alterations   76–79
–, monitoring   194 f.
–, *see also* immune responses
immunosuppression
–, IL-10   155
–, tumor-induced   107
immunosuppressive factors   119–154
immunosurveillance   40, 65 f., 96
–, cancer   204
–, IL-10   155
–, interferon (IFN)-γ   83 ff.
immunotherapy, adoptive   301
immunotoxins   347–379
in vitro models, of tumors   218–221
in vivo models, of tumors   218–221
indiviualized immunotherapy   256
inflammation, immune responses   211
innate immunity, HSPs   253
insulin-like growth factor (IGF)-1   350
integrin $\alpha_v\beta_3$   341
intercellular adhesion molecule (ICAM)   320
interferon (IFN)-γ   31, 33 ff., 60
–, bacterial immunotherapy   273 f.

–, HLA-G expression   86 f.
–, hybrid cell vaccination (HCV)   234
–, immunocytokines   322 ff., 335 f., 339
–, immunosurveillance   83 ff.
–, MHC class I antigens   69–72, 78 ff.
–, MHC class II antigens   81 ff.
–, NK cells   102 ff.
–, T cells   100
interleukin-2 (IL-2)
–, hybrid cell vaccination (HCV)   234
–, immunocytokines   313 f., 327–341
–, immunotoxins   347, 354, 361 f.
–, T cells   100
–, T-body approach   293 ff.
–, *see also* cytokines
interleukin-10 (IL-10)
–, immunocytokines   339
–, immunosuppressive factors   125–129
–, in cancer immunity   155–175
–, T cells   100
–, *see also* cytokines
intracellular tyrosine activation motifs
    (ITAMs)   289
IRF transcription factor   83 f.
isotypes, IgG   276
ITAMs   *see* intracellular tyrosine activation
    motifs


**j**

JAK   *see* janus tyrosine kinase
janus tyrosine kinase (JAK)   83 ff.
–, IL-10   157
–, immunosuppressive factors   122 f.


**k**

Kaplan-Meier survival curves   107, 331
KARs   *see* killer activating receptors
KDEL, gp96   262
keyhole limpet hemocyanin (KLH)   191, 276
killer activating receptors (KARs)   102
killer inhibitory receptors (KIRs)   63, 88,
    102
KIRs   *see* killer inhibitory receptors
KLH   *see* keyhole limpet hemocyanin
KSA   *see* Ep-CAM/KS antigen


**l**

lactate dehydrogenase, antigen   20
Lagerhans cells (LCs)   179
LAK   *see* lymphokine-activated killer
LAP   *see* latency-associated peptide
latency-associated peptide (LAP)   119
latent TGF-β binding protein   119 ff.
LCs   *see* Lagerhans cells

leukemia
–, acute lymphocytic   302
–, acute myelocytic   302, 305 f.
–, B cell   362
–, chronic myelogenous   301 ff.
–, chronic myeloid   189
–, hairy cell   362
–, immunotoxins   361 f.
–, T cell   347, 362
LeY   *see* carbohydrate antigen Lewis Y
LFA-2   326
life cycle, of dendritic cells   185
lipids, cationic   274
lipopolysaccharides (LPSs), bacterial
   immunotherapy   269, 271 f., 273
liver metastases, immunocytokines   337 f.
LLC-CEA-KSA   324, 327
LMB2   *see* anti-Tac(Fv)-PE38
LMB7 and LMB9, immunotoxins   360
LMP2, LMP7   *see* β subunits of 20S
   proteasome
LOH   *see* loss of heterozygosity
loss
–, antigen   66–69, 72–76, 331
–, of heterozygosity (LOH), MHC class I   67,
   74 f.
low-affinity CTL responses   194
low-affinity receptor for the nerve growth factor
   (ΔNGER)   304 f.
low-avidity TCR   232
LPS   *see* lipopolysaccharides
LT-α   *see* lymphotoxin (LT)-α
lymphocyte migration, T bodies   295
lymphoid CD123 DCs   180 f.
lymphoid-derived DCs   105
lymphoid-like tissues, peripheral   333 f.
lymphokine-activated killer (LAK)
–, effects of prostaglandin (PG) E2   132
–, effects of TGF-β   123
lymphoma
–, B cell   347
–, Hodgkin lymphomas   163
–, immunotoxins   361 f.
–, non-Hodgkin lymphomas (NHL)   163,
   189
lymphotoxin (LT)-α, tumor targeting   333 f.
lymphotoxin (LT)-α fusion proteins   313
lymphotoxin (LT)-α immunocytokine   333 f.
lysis, hTERT specific   *see* cytolysis

***m***
mAb B3   360 f., 367
mAb e23   360 f.
mAbs   *see* monoclonal antibodies

macrophage migration inhibitory factor
   (MIF)   120, 130
macrophages
–, effects of IL-10   126, 158 f.
–, effects of polyamines   133 f.
–, effects of prostaglandin (PG) E2   131
–, effects of TGF-β   121
–, tumor cell killing   218
–, tumor microenvironment   107 f., 113
MAGE   *see* melanoma antigens
maintenance therapy, HCV   240 f.
major histocompatibility complex (MHC)   3,
   6 ff., 30, 44, 52, 59–94, 210
MAPKs   *see* mitogen-activated protein kinases
matrix metalloproteinases (MMPs)   110
–, effects of IL-10   165
maturation
–, dendritic cells   181, 185–187
MDA   *see* melanoma differentiation associated
   gene
melanoma
–, clinical trials   189, 193
–, HCV   239 f.
–, immunocytokines   330–336
melanoma antigens (MAGE)   19, 26
–, CTL monitoring   45–50
–, immunotoxins   365
melanoma differentiation associated gene
   (MDA)-7   157
melanoma metastases, treatment with
   immunocytokines   330 ff.
memory responses   195
memory T cells, immunocytokines   317
mesothelin   361
metalloproteinases
–, inhibitors   113
–, matrix   110
metastases
–, liver   337 f.
–, melanoma   330 ff.
methylation of cytosines, bacterial immunotherapy   269
MHC   *see* major histocompatibility complex
MHC antigens
–, expression determination   63 f.
–, HSPs   263
MHC class I alterations
–, impact on immuneresponses and clinical
   relevance   76–79
–, underlying molecular mechanisms
   66–76
MHC class I antigen
–, immunocytokines   316, 321, 326 f., 334 f.
–, immunotoxins   365

MHC class I antigen-processing machinery 60 f.
MHC class I antigen-processing pathway 30 ff.
MHC class I down regulation 69–76
MHC class I expression, effects of IL-10 166
MHC class I loss 66–69, 72–76
MHC class I molecules 43
MHC class I-restricted CD8+ T cells 234
MHC class II antigen-processing machinery 61 f., 79 ff.
MHC class II-associated Ii peptide (CLIP) 62
MHC class II expression
–, antitumor response 82 f.
–, modulation of immune response 81 f.
MHC class II-restricted T cell epitopes 232
MHC class II transactivator (CIITA) 81–84
MHC haplotypes 215, 222
MHC locus 59
microenvironment 47
–, tumor 311, 327
MIF *see* macrophage migration inhibitory factor
migration, dendritic cells 180 f.
MIIC, MHC class II compartment 62
mimicry, molecular 211, 222, 224
mimotopes 44
mitogen-activated protein kinases (MAPKs) 270 ff.
mixed lymphocyte tumor cell culture (MLTC) 41 f.
MLTC *see* mixed lymphocyte tumor cell culture
MMPs *see* matrix metalloproteinases
Mo-DCs 184–193
mobilization, DC 183
models
–, animal 230
–, of tumors 218–221
–, T-body approach 292 f.
modulation of the expression of HSPs 261 f.
modulation of the site of HSP expression 262 f.
molecular mimicry 211, 222
–, definition 224
monitoring
–, CTL responses 44–49
–, immunoresponses 194 f.
monoclonal antibodies (mAbs) 17 f.
–, bacterial immunotherapy 277
–, discovery 311
–, immunotoxin therapy 360 f.
–, immunotoxins 363–366
monocytes
–, effects of IL-10 126, 158 f.

–, effects of polyamines 133 f.
–, effects of prostaglandin (PG) E2 131
–, effects of TGF-β 121
–, plasmacytoid 179 f.
morphology, plasmacytoid 179
moxibustion, HSPs 261
mRNA, HCV 240
MUC1, HCV 238 f.
mucins, tumor-shed antigens 134 f.
multiple myeloma
–, clinical trials 189, 193
multiple peptide epitopes 187
mutated antigens 21 f., 231
mutations, oncogenic 206 ff.
myeloid APCs, effects of IL-10 158 f.
myeloid DCs 179
myeloid-derived DCs 105

**n**

natural killer (NK) cells 63, 65 f., 218
–, bacterial immunotherapy 273 ff.
–, effects of dendritic cells 181, 195
–, effects of IL-10 128, 160, 166
–, effects of polyamines 134
–, effects of prostaglandin (PG) E2 132
–, effects of TGF-β 123
–, HLA-G expression 88
–, immunocytokines 328 f., 338 f.
–, inhibition by MIF 130
–, tumor microenvironment 101–104
NDF *see* Neuregulin differentiation factor
near-self antigens, definition 224
near-self epitopes 209, 211
nerve growth factor, low-affinity receptor 304 f.
Neuregulin differentiation factor (NDF) 292
neuroblastoma, immunocytokines 337–342
neutrophils, FasL 112
NF-κB, T cells 100
NHL *see* non-Hodgkin lymphomas
nitric oxide (NO)
–, effects of IL-10 165
–, immune response inhibitor 81
NK *see* natural killer
NK inhibitory receptor *see* killer inhibitory receptors
NO *see* nitric oxide
non-Hodgkin lymphomas (NHL)
–, clinical trials 189
–, effects of IL-10 163
non-individualized tumor vaccine 332
NSX2 cells
–, neuroblastoma 337 f., 340
nuclease activity 272

nucleic acids, cancer immunotherapy   268 ff.
NY-ESO, antigen   48

**o**

ODC   *see* ornithine decarboxylase
ODN   *see* oligodeoxynucleotides
oligodeoxynucleotides (ODN), bacterial
   immunotherapy   269–277
oncogenic mutations   206 ff.
ornithine decarboxylase (ODC)   133
ovarian cancer
–, clinical trials   190
–, T-body approach   294
over-expressed cellular proteins   231

**p**

PA28, proteasome activator   31–36
palindromes, bacterial immunotherapy   269
pancreas cancer, clinical trials   191
PAP   *see* prostatic acid phosphatase
papillomavirus oncoproteins   209
pattern recognition receptors (PRR), CpG
   motif   271 f.
PBLs   *see* peripheral blood lymphocytes
PBMC, specific CTL monitoring   44 ff.
PCR   *see* polymerase chain reaction
pCTL   *see* CTL precursor
PE   *see* pseudomonas exotoxin
PE38   360 f., 367 f.
pediatric solid tumors, clinical trials   191
PEGylation   *see* polyethylene glycol
peptide library approach, combinatorial   44
peptide specificity, antigen-specific T cell
   responses   3
peptide vaccination   234
peptide/HLA tetramers   *see* HLA/peptide
   tetramer responses
peptides
–, antigenic   254 f.
–, complexes with HSP   257–260
–, HCV   240
–, latency-associated   119
–, MHC class II-associated Ii   62
–, multiple epitopes   187
pER-CEA
–, immunocytokines   320, 325 f.
peripheral blood lymphocytes (PBLs)   304
peripheral lymphoid-like tissues   333 f.
peripheral tolerance
–, contributions of HSPs   263
–, T cells   319
–, to self antigens   220
peritumoral lymphoid tissue   334
PG E2   *see* prostaglandin

phage antibody libraries   364
phenotype-genotype link   363 f.
phosphatidylinositol 3-kinase, IL-10   157
phosphodiester DNA backbone (PO), ODN
   classes   272 ff.
phosphorothioate (PS), DNA backbone   272 f.
plant toxins, immunotoxins   351 f.
plasmacytoid monocytes   179 f.
plasmacytoid morphology, dendritic cells   179
PO   *see* phosphodiester DNA backbone
pokeweed antiviral protein, immunotoxins
   352
polyamines
–, immunosuppressive factors   120, 132 ff.
polyethylene glycol (PEGylation), immunotoxins   368
polymerase chain reaction (PCR)   64
–, reverse-transcription   110
polynucleotides, bacterial immunotherapy
   268 ff.
polytopes, dendritic cells   187
PRAME, tumor associated antigen   36, 43
preclinical development, immunotoxins   358 f.
preclinical experimental models, T bodies
   292 f.
preclinical studies, HCV   237 f.
preventive cancer vaccines   12, 232
preventive immunotherapy   12
primary antibody libraries   364
prognostic value, IL-10   163 f.
prostaglandin (PG) E2
–, immunosuppressive factors   120, 131 f.
prostaglandins, macrophages   107
prostate cancer   327 ff.
–, clinical trials   190, 193
prostate-specific antigen (PSA)   293
–, dendritic cells   195
prostate-specific membrane antigen (PSMA)
   193, 293
prostatic acid phosphatase (PAP)   193
proteasomes
–, antigen processing   59 f.
–, immuno   31–37, 43
protein tyrosine kinases (PTKs)   288
proteins
–, antibody-cytokine fusion   311 f.
–, ch14.18-IL-2 fusion   330–341
–, folate binding   292 ff.
–, glyco-   351
–, gp70 envelope   316
–, heat shock   *see* heat shock proteins
–, HSP/peptide fusion   260
–, latent TGF-β binding   119 ff.
–, lymphotoxin (LT)-α fusion   313

–, onco-   209
–, over-expressed cellular   231
–, pokeweed antiviral protein   352
–, Smad   121
PRR   *see* pattern recognition receptors
PS   *see* phosphorothioate
PSA   *see* prostate-specific antigen
pseudomonas exotoxin (PE)   350–362, 367f.
PSMA   *see* prostate-specific membrane antigen
PTKs   *see* protein tyrosine kinases
pw-CEA, immunocytokines   320, 325f.

*r*

radioimmunoconjugates, CEA-specific   319
radiotherapy   299
RCC   *see* renal cell cancers
reactive oxygen metabolites (ROM)   107f., 113
receptors
–, CpG motif   271f.
–, epidermal growth factor   347
–, Fc   277
–, Fcγ   *see* Fcγ receptors
–, for the nerve growth factor   304f.
–, IL-10   155ff.
–, killer activating   *see* killer activating
   receptors
–, killer inhibitory   *see* killer inhibitory
   receptors
–, pattern recognition   271f.
–, serine-thronine kinase   121
–, T cell   210f.
–, toll-like   180
–, TRAIL-TRAIL   *see* TRAIL-TRAIL receptor
   pathway
–, transferrin   361
recombinant antibody-cytokine fusion
   proteins   311f.
recombinant antibody fragments, immunotoxins   354–357
recombinant immunotoxins   347–379
redox shuffling, immunotoxins   358
refolding reaction, immunotoxins   358
regression, of tumors   268
renal cell cancers (RCC)   24, 86f., 100
–, clinical trials   190
–, HCV   239f.
responses
–, antibody   *see* antibody responses
–, antitumor   *see* antitumor response
–, autoimmune   232
–, CTL   *see* CTL responses
–, immuno   *see* immunoresponses
–, T cell   *see* T cell responses
–, tumor antigen   209

restin, antigen   20
reverse immunology   43
–, *see also* epitope deduction
RFB4(dsFv)-PE38, immunotoxins   362
RFT5-SMPT-dgA, immunotoxins   362
rheumatoid arthritis   215
ricin, immunotoxins   351f., 361
Rituximab
–, immunotoxins   367
–, monoclonal antibody   277
RNA, bacterial   268ff.
RNA vaccination   187
ROM   *see* reactive oxygen metabolites

*s*

S100 staining, dendritic cells   182
SAGE   *see* serial analysis of gene expression
saporin, immunotoxins   352
scCRs   *see* single-chain CRs
scFcRs   *see* single-chain FcRs
scFvs   *see* single-chain Fvs
SCP-1 gene   24
screening, antigen   19
SCT   *see* stem-cell transplantation
second-generation immunotoxins   349f.
–, *see also* recombinant immunotoxins
selectivity, IL-10 production   162f.
self-antigens   204, 207, 209
–, definition   224
–, immunocytokines   319
self-tolerance   232
SEREX   *see* serological analysis of tumor
   antigens by recombinant cDNA expression
   cloning
serial analysis of gene expression (SAGE)
   10f.
serine-thronine kinase receptors   121
serological analysis of tumor antigens by
   recombinant cDNA expression cloning
   (SEREX)   18–25, 42, 232
serological determinants, tumor cells   17–29
shared antigens   256
shed tumor antigens, immunosuppressive
   factors   120
side effects, immunotoxins   361
signal transducers and activation of
   transcription (STAT)   83ff.
–, IL-10   157
–, immunosuppressive factors   122f.
significance
–, clinical   23
–, functional   24
single-chain CRs (scCRs)   288–291
single-chain FcRs (scFcRs)   288f.

single-chain Fvs (scFvs), immunotoxins 355 ff.
single-chain IL-12 340
Smad proteins 121
solid tumors
–, clinical trials 191
–, immunotoxin therapy 360 f.
somatic hypermutation 363
splice variants of genes, for encoding
    antigens 22
SSX gene 21
STAT *see* signal transducers and activation of
    transcription
stem-cell transplantation (SCT) 197, 306
stem cells, dendritic cells 183 f.
stressful death, tumor cell killing 218
subdominant epitopes 211
–, definition 224
suicide gene strategy, BMT 304
suppression
–, immuno 107, 119–154
–, of IL-10 129
surveillance, immune 40, 65 f., 230
survivin 11
synovial sarcomas, SSX gene 21
systemic effects, IL-10 163

*t*
T-B cell collaboration 233
T body approach, cancer immunotherapy
    287–298
T cell anergy, effects of IL-10 127
T cell apoptosis, effects of TGF-β 123
T cell epitopes, universal tumor associated
    3–16
T cell immunology
–, reverse 17, 24
T cell leukemias 347, 362
T cell receptor (TCR) 99 f., 210–214
–, immunocytokines 331
–, T-body approach 287, 290
T cells
–, γδ 129
–, antigen presentation 210 f.
–, antigen-specific responses 3
–, autoimmunity 215 ff.
–, bacterial immunotherapy 275
–, CD4 79, 81 ff.
–, effects of IL-10 159 f.
–, GvHD 303
–, hybrid cell vaccination (HCV) 231–241
–, immunocytokines 311–342
–, in tumor immunity 40–55
–, thymic 263
–, thymic selection 206 f.

–, tumor cell killing 218–221
–, tumor microenvironment 99 ff., 114
–, with surface CRs 287–298
–, *see also* T lymphocytes
T helper cells 233
–, HCV 236 f.
–, immunocytokines 324
–, immunotoxins 367
T helper lymphocytes 18
T immunotherapy, adoptive 5
T lymphocyte apoptosis 111
T lymphocytes 3
–, effects of IL-10 126 f.
–, effects of polyamines 134
–, effects of prostaglandin (PG) E2 131
–, effects of TGF-β 122 f.
–, *see also* T cells
T-T cell collaboration 233 f.
TAAs *see* tumor-associated antigens
TADC *see* tumor-associated DC
TAM *see* tumor-associated macrophages
TAP *see* transporter associated with antigen
    processing
TAP vaccines 77
tapasin 71
targeted cancer therapy 347 f.
targeting moiety, immunotoxins 348,
    354–357, 363–369
TATC *see* tumor associated T cells
TCR *see* T cell receptor
telomerase, COX inhibitors 132
tertiary lymphoid tissue 333
tetramers, CTL monitoring 45
TGF *see* transforming growth factor
TGF-β, FasL 112
therapeutic vaccination 5
therapy
–, adoptive transfer 41
–, chemo- 299
–, effects of IL-10 128 f., 167
–, implication of polyamine inhibition 134
–, implication of prostaglandin (PG) E2
    inhibition 132
–, implication of TGF-β inhibition 124 f.
–, MIF neutralization 130
–, radio- 299
–, thermo- 261
thermotherapy, and HSPs 261
three-cell interaction, HCV 234
thymic selection of T cells 206 f.
thymic T cells, cross-presentation of peptides
    263
thymidine kinases of Herpes Simplex virus
    (HSV-tk) 304 ff.

TICD   *see* tumor-induced cell death
TILNs   *see* tumor-infiltrated lymph nodes
TILs   *see* tumor-infiltrating lymphocytes
TIMP   *see* tumor inhibitor of metalloproteinase
TLR family, PRR receptors   271 f.
TNF   *see* tumor necrosis factor
TNF-α
–, dendritic cells   184 f.
–, MHC class I antigens   79
TNF-related activation induced cytokine
   receptor (TRANCE-R)   181
tolerance
–, central   211, 223
–, immunobiological   206 f.
–, peripheral   263
toll-like receptors, dendritic cells   180
total body radiation   299
toxin moiety, immunotoxins   351
toxins
–, bacterial   *see* bacterial toxins
–, chimeric   *see* chimeric toxins
–, Coley's   *see* Coley's toxins
–, diphteria   *see* diphteria toxin
–, endo-   *see* endotoxins
–, exo-   *see* pseudomonas exotoxin
–, immuno-   *see* immunotoxins
–, lympho-   *see* lymphotoxins
TRAIL-TRAIL receptor pathway, tumor microenvironment   112
TRANCE-R   *see* TNF-related activation induced
   cytokine receptor
transferrin receptor   361
transforming growth factor (TGF)   100
transforming growth factor (TGF)-β   119–125
–, effects of IL-10   165 f.
–, immunotoxins   350
transgenic mice   365
transplant-related mortality (TRM)   300
transplantation
–, allogenic   197, 361
–, bone marrow   *see* bone marrow transplantation
transporter associated with antigen processing
   (TAP)   31, 34, 60
–, MHC class I   69–73
tripartite CR   289, 293
TRM   *see* transplant-related mortality
TRP-2 antigen   334 f.
tumor antigen-associated epitopes   220
tumor antigen responses   209
tumor antigenicity   3–55, 155, 231 ff.
tumor antigens   17–29
–, definition   224
–, HSPs   254

tumor-associated antigens (TAAs)   5 f., 66, 209,
   220 f., 231 ff., 347
–, dendritic cells   194–197
–, HCV   236 f.
–, HLA class II restricted   49 f.
–, immunocytokines   311 f.
–, processing and presentation   30–39
–, relevance of MHC class I alterations   76 f.
–, tumor microenvironment   96
tumor-associated DC (TADC)   105 f.
tumor-associated macrophages (TAM)   107 f.
tumor-associated T cell epitopes   231 ff.
tumor-associated T cells (TATC)   99
tumor cell killing   218 f.
tumor-derived HSP/peptide complexes
   257 f.
tumor-derived molecules, immunosuppressive
   factors   120
tumor escape   99, 195
tumor growth, immunosurveillance   84 f.
tumor-immune system interaction   65 f.
tumor-induced apoptosis   105
–, T cells   110
tumor-induced cell death (TICD)   110, 114
tumor-induced immunosuppression   107
tumor-infiltrated lymph nodes (TILNs)
   46–49
tumor-infiltrating lymphocytes (TILs)
   41, 46–49, 333
–, microenvironment   97–101
tumor inhibition, effects of IL-10   165 f.
tumor inhibitor of metalloproteinase (TIMP)
   113
–, effects of IL-10   165
tumor lysates, HCV   240
tumor microenvironment   47, 95–118, 311,
   327, 340
tumor models   218–221
–, *see also* models
tumor necrosis factor (TNF)   101, 109, 112 f.
tumor penetration   355
tumor progression, and immune system
   95 ff.
tumor promotion, effects of IL-10   164 f.
tumor regression antigens   5, 42
tumor rejection antigens   5
tumor-shed antigens, immunosuppressive
   factors   120, 134
tumor-specific peptides   365
tumor-specific vaccines, HSPs   256 ff.
tumor-testis antigens   231
tumor vaccines, non-individualized   332
tumors
–, solid   360 f.

–, *see also* cancer
–, *see also* carcinoma
tuning, evolutionary   206–209

*u*
underexpressed genes   23
universal tumor antigens   3–16

*v*
vaccination
–, antitumor   218–221
–, cancer   179–203
–, CpG DNA as an adjuvant   276 f.
–, delivery and schedule   187 f.
–, hybrid-cell   187, 230–252
–, peptide   234
–, pw-CEA   320
–, RNA   187
–, therapeutic   5
–, virus   234
–, whole-cell   187, 221, 260 f.
vaccines
–, cancer   25 f.
–, DNA   321–327
–, non-individualized tumor   332
–, preventive cancer   232
–, TAP   77
–, tumor-specific   256 ff.
variable heavy chain (V$_H$)   355–358
variable light chain (V$_L$)   355–358
variable region fragment (Fv)
–, immunotoxins   355–362, 366–369

–, T-body approach   287 f.
vascular endothelial growth factor (VEGF)
   105
–, effects of IL-10   166
vascular leak syndrome (VLS)   367
V$_\beta$11 and V$_\beta$8 T cell receptor   340
VEGF   *see* vascular endothelial growth factor
vesicular stomatitis virus (VSV), HSPs   254
V$_H$   *see* variable heavy chain
V$_L$   *see* variable light chain
viral antigens   232
viral-gene encoded antigens   22
virus specific peptides, HSPs   255
virus vaccination   234
vitiligo   211, 220
–, HCV   240
VLS   *see* vascular leak syndrome
VSV   *see* vesicular stomatitis virus

*w*
whole-cell vaccination   221
–, dendritic cells   187
–, HSPs   260 f.

*x*
xenomice   *see* transgenic mice

*z*
ZAP-70 family, PTKs   289
ζ chain
–, CD3   102, 288
–, TCR-associated   106